WOMEN'S MENTAL HEALTH

Women's Mental Health

A Comprehensive Textbook

Edited by

SUSAN G. KORNSTEIN
ANITA H. CLAYTON

THE GUILFORD PRESS
New York   London

© 2002 The Guilford Press
A Division of Guilford Publications, Inc.
72 Spring Street, New York, NY 10012
www.guilford.com

Printed in the United States of America

This book is printed on acid-free paper.

Last digit is print number: 9 8 7 6 5 4 3 2

Library of Congress Cataloging-in-Publication Data
available from the Publisher

ISBN 1-57230-699-8

About the Editors

Susan G. Kornstein, MD, is Professor of Psychiatry and Obstetrics and Gynecology at the Medical College of Virginia campus of Virginia Commonwealth University (VCU), where she serves as Chair of the Division of Ambulatory Care Psychiatry. She is also the Executive Director of the VCU Mood Disorders Institute, Executive Director of the VCU Institute for Women's Health, and Director of Psychiatric Services for MCV Women's HealthCare, a multidisciplinary health center for women. Dr. Kornstein is a nationally recognized leader in mental health issues for women, and has written or cowritten more than 100 articles, chapters, and abstracts on topics related to depression and women's health. She serves on several editorial boards and national advisory boards, and has given many presentations at national and international meetings. She has been a principal investigator on over 30 research studies in the areas of depression, anxiety disorders, and premenstrual syndrome, and has received many awards for her research, service, and leadership. Dr. Kornstein is a Fellow of the American Psychiatric Association and a member of the American College of Psychiatrists.

Anita H. Clayton, MD, is Professor and Vice Chair of the Department of Psychiatric Medicine at the University of Virginia (UVA) Health System in Charlottesville, Virginia, and serves as the Medical Director of the UVA Center for Psychiatric Clinical Research. Articles and abstracts written by Dr. Clayton have appeared in numerous journals, including *Academic Psychiatry*, the *American Journal of Psychiatry*, *Biological Psychiatry*, the *Journal of Clinical Psychiatry*, and the *Journal of Sex and Marital Therapy*. She is a contributing author to the first book published by the National Depressive and Manic–Depressive Association, *Restoring Intimacy: The Patient's Guide to Maintaining Relationships during Depression*. Her clinical and research interests include mood and anxiety disorders associated with reproductive life events in women, and sexual dysfunction related to illness and medications. Dr. Clayton has served as principal investigator on many research grants, and has presented at numerous regional, national, and international meetings. She is a Fellow of the American Psychiatric Association, and has received many local and national awards for teaching, research, and clinical expertise.

Contributors

Cheryl S. Al-Mateen, MD, Department of Psychiatry, Medical College of Virginia campus, Virginia Commonwealth University, Richmond, Virginia

Margaret Altemus, MD, Department of Psychiatry, Cornell Medical College, New York, New York

Angela F. Arnold, MD, Department of Psychiatry and Behavioral Sciences, Emory University School of Medicine, Atlanta, Georgia

Lesley M. Arnold, MD, Women's Health Research Program, Department of Psychiatry, University of Cincinnati College of Medicine, Cincinnati, Ohio

Ineke Ayubi-Moak, MD, Department of Family Practice, Scottsdale Healthcare, Scottsdale, Arizona

Pamela Bachanas, PhD, Department of Psychiatry and Behavioral Sciences, Emory University School of Medicine, Atlanta, Georgia

Claudia Baugh, BA, Department of Psychiatry and Behavioral Sciences, Emory University School of Medicine, Atlanta, Georgia

Christine F. Blake, MD, Department of Obstetrics and Gynecology, University of Oklahoma Health Sciences Center–Tulsa, Tulsa, Oklahoma

Mary C. Blehar, PhD, Women's Mental Health Program, National Institute of Mental Health, Bethesda, Maryland

Leslie Born, MSc, Department of Psychiatry and Behavioural Neurosciences, McMaster University, Hamilton, Ontario, Canada; Women's Health Concerns Clinic and Father Sean O'Sullivan Research Centre, St. Joseph's Hospital, Hamilton, Ontario, Canada

Reid Brackin, BA, Department of Psychiatry and Human Behavior, Jefferson Medical College, Philadelphia, Pennsylvania

Bethany Brand, PhD, Psychology Department, Towson University, Towson, Maryland

Jennifer S. Brasch, MD, Emergency Psychiatric Service, St. Joseph's Healthcare, Hamilton, Ontario, Canada; Department of Psychiatry and Behavioural Neurosciences, McMaster University Medical Centre, Hamilton, Ontario, Canada

Olga Brawman-Mintzer, MD, Department of Psychiatry and Behavioral Sciences, Medical University of South Carolina, Charleston, South Carolina

Jessica Brown, BA, Department of Psychiatry and Behavioral Sciences, Emory University School of Medicine, Atlanta, Georgia

R. J. Canterbury, MD, Department of Psychiatric Medicine, University of Virginia Medical School, Charlottesville, Virginia

M. Beth Casey, PhD, Department of Counseling and Applied Developmental and Educational Psychology, Boston College, Chestnut Hill, Massachusetts

Emmie I. Chen, MS, Jefferson Medical College, Philadelphia, Pennsylvania

Frances M. Christian, PhD, LCSW, Department of Psychiatry, Medical College of Virginia campus, Virginia Commonwealth University, Richmond, Virginia

Cathryn M. Clary, MD, CNS Medical Group, Pfizer, Inc., New York, New York

Anita H. Clayton, MD, Department of Psychiatric Medicine, University of Virginia Health System, Charlottesville, Virginia

Michele Cofield, MD, Department of Obstetrics and Gynecology, Eastern Virginia Medical School, Norfolk, Virginia

Lee S. Cohen, MD, Perinatal and Reproductive Psychiatry Clinical Research Program, Clinical Psychopharmacology Unit, Department of Psychiatry, Massachusetts General Hospital, Boston, Massachusetts

Ian M. Colrain, PhD, Sleep Disorders Clinic and Research Center, Department of Psychiatry and Behavioral Sciences, Stanford University, Palo Alto, California

Catherine C. Crone, MD, Department of Psychiatry, Georgetown University School of Medicine, Washington, DC; Georgetown University Program, Inova Fairfax Hospital, Fairfax, Virginia

Diana L. Dell, MD, FACOG, Departments of Psychiatry and Behavioral Sciences and of Obstetrics and Gynecology, Duke University Medical Center, Durham, North Carolina

Howard L. Field, MD, Department of Psychiatry and Human Behavior, Jefferson Medical College, Philadelphia, Pennsylvania

Angela Fisher, BS, Department of Psychiatry and Behavioral Sciences, Emory University School of Medicine, Atlanta, Georgia

Marlene P. Freeman, MD, Women's Mental Health Program, Department of Psychiatry, University of Arizona Health Sciences Center, Tucson, Arizona

Jean S. Gearon, PhD, Department of Psychiatry, University of Maryland School of Medicine, Baltimore, Maryland

Preface

Interest in women's health has grown over the past two decades. The topic of "women's health" includes health issues and diseases that are unique to women, such as gynecological conditions; diseases that are more prevalent in women; and diseases that are expressed differently in women and men, meaning that women may present with different symptoms, have a more serious form or a different course of illness, or respond differently to interventions. Women's health also includes issues of access to care, quality of care, and prevention of disease. Many women experience barriers to good health care, including limited access, insensitive attitudes in the medical profession, and poorly coordinated referral systems. Whereas earlier views of women's health focused exclusively on reproductive health, there is now a broader multidisciplinary approach that encompasses all organ systems and includes not only biological but also psychological and sociocultural aspects of health and disease across the lifespan.

Until recently, women were excluded from clinical trials. What was learned from studies of men was presumed to carry over to women. Moreover, in the studies that did include women, the data usually were not analyzed separately by gender. It was simply assumed that there were no differences in the way men and women present with an illness or respond to various treatments. We are now learning that there are important gender differences to consider in both assessment and treatment. We are learning that some diseases do show different symptoms, a different course of illness, and/or different risk factors in men and women. We are learning that sex differences in pharmacokinetics exist, and that pharmacokinetics in women may vary across the menstrual cycle as well as with menopausal status or hormonal therapies. In addition, we are learning about gender differences in treatment response. If we study only men or do not analyze data by gender, we can never learn about these differences, which have important implications for treatment. Thus there are large gaps in our knowledge concerning the etiology, course, and treatment of diseases in women, and these very questions are what the women's health movement aims to address.

Women's health has now taken a seat at the forefront of our national health agenda, perhaps due to the increasing numbers of women in medicine. There is currently an Office of Research on Women's Health at the National Institutes of Health (NIH), as well as an Office of Women's Health in the U.S. Department of Health and Human Services.

Toni Tildon, MD, Department of Pediatrics, Albert Einstein College of Medicine, Bronx, New York

Adele C. Viguera, MD, Perinatal and Reproductive Psychiatry Clinical Research Program, Clinical Psychopharmacology Unit, Department of Psychiatry, Massachusetts General Hospital, Boston, Massachusetts

Julia K. Warnock, MD, PhD, Department of Psychiatry, University of Oklahoma Health Sciences Center–Tulsa, Tulsa, Oklahoma

Thomas N. Wise, MD, Department of Psychiatry, Georgetown University School of Medicine, Washington, DC; Department of Psychiatry, Inova Fairfax Hospital, Fairfax, Virginia

Barbara A. Wojcik, MD, Department of Psychiatry and Behavioral Sciences, Johns Hopkins School of Medicine, Baltimore, Maryland

William R. Yates, MD, Department of Psychiatry, University of Oklahoma–Tulsa, Tulsa, Oklahoma

Elizabeth A. Young, MD, Department of Psychiatry, University of Michigan Medical Center, Ann Arbor, Michigan

Daniel A. Monti, MD, Department of Psychiatry and Human Behavior, Jefferson Medical College, Philadelphia, Pennsylvania

Ruta Nonacs, MD, PhD, Perinatal and Reproductive Psychiatry Clinical Research Program, Clinical Psychopharmacology Unit, Department of Psychiatry, Massachusetts General Hospital, Boston, Massachusetts

Grayson Norquist, MD, MSPH, Division of Services and Intervention Research, National Institute of Mental Health, Bethesda, Maryland

H. George Nurnberg, MD, Department of Psychiatry, University of New Mexico, Albuquerque, New Mexico

Barbara L. Parry, MD, Department of Psychiatry, University of California at San Diego, La Jolla, California

Michael J. Pertschuk, MD, Departments of Psychiatry and Surgery, Division of Plastic Surgery, and Edwin and Fannie Gray Hall Center for Human Appearance, University of Pennsylvania School of Medicine, Philadelphia, Pennsylvania

Katharine A. Phillips, MD, Butler Hospital and Department of Psychiatry and Human Behavior, Brown University School of Medicine, Providence, Rhode Island

Teresa A. Pigott, MD, Clinical Trials Program, Department of Psychiatry, University of Florida College of Medicine, Gainesville, Florida

Pauline S. Powers, MD, Department of Psychiatry and Behavioral Medicine, College of Medicine, Health Sciences Center, University of South Florida, Tampa, Florida

Jill A. Rachbeisel, MD, Division of Community Psychiatry, University of Maryland School of Medicine, Baltimore, Maryland

David B. Sarwer, PhD, Departments of Psychiatry and Surgery, Division of Plastic Surgery, and the Edwin and Fannie Gray Hall Center for Human Appearance, University of Pennsylvania School of Medicine, Philadelphia, Pennsylvania

Diane K. Shrier, MD, Departments of Psychiatry and Pediatrics, George Washington University Medical College, Washington, DC

Christine Skotzko, MD, Baltimore Veterans Affairs Medical Center, Baltimore, Maryland; University of Maryland School of Medicine, Baltimore, Maryland

Catherine A. Staropoli, MD, Women's Health, Veterans Affairs Maryland Healthcare System, Baltimore Division, Baltimore, Maryland; Department of Medicine, University of Maryland School of Medicine, Baltimore, Maryland

Meir Steiner, MD, PhD, FRCPC, Departments of Psychiatry and Behavioural Neurosciences and of Obstetrics and Gynecology, McMaster University, Hamilton, Ontario, Canada; Women's Health Concerns Clinic and Father Sean O'Sullivan Research Centre, St. Joseph's Hospital, Hamilton, Ontario, Canada

Marie Stoner, MEd, Department of Psychiatry, Jefferson Medical College, Philadelphia, Pennsylvania

Zachary N. Stowe, MD, Departments of Psychiatry and Behavioral Sciences and of Gynecology and Obstetrics, Emory University School of Medicine, Atlanta, Georgia

Ondria C. Gleason, MD, Department of Psychiatry, University of Oklahoma–Tulsa, Tulsa, Oklahoma

Sherri Hansen, MD, Capitol Square Associates, Madison, Wisconsin

Wilma Harrison, MD, CNS Medical Group, Pfizer, Inc., New York, New York

Paula L. Hensley, MD, Department of Psychiatry, University of New Mexico, Albuquerque, New Mexico

Sarah E. Herbert, MD, MSW, Department of Psychiatry and Behavioral Sciences, Emory University School of Medicine, Atlanta, Georgia

Suzanne Holroyd, MD, Department of Psychiatric Medicine, University of Virginia Medical School, Charlottesville, Virginia

Russell Joffe, MD, Department of Psychiatry, UMDNJ–New Jersey Medical School, Newark, New Jersey

Rochelle L. Klinger, MD, Department of Psychiatry, Medical College of Virginia campus, Virginia Commonwealth University, Richmond, Virginia

Susan G. Kornstein, MD, Departments of Psychiatry and of Obstetrics and Gynecology, Institute for Women's Health, and Mood Disorders Institute, Medical College of Virginia campus, Virginia Commonwealth University, Richmond, Virginia

Ania Korszun, MD, Department of Psychiatry, University of Cardiff, Cardiff, Wales, United Kingdom

Elisabeth J. S. Kunkel, MD, Department of Psychiatry and Human Behavior, Jefferson Medical College, Philadelphia, Pennsylvania

Marcia Lasswell, MA, Departments of Psychology and of Marriage and Family, California State University–Pomona, Pomona, California

Kathryn A. Lee, PhD, RN, School of Nursing, Department of Family Health, University of California, San Francisco, California

Glenda MacQueen, MD, PhD, Mood Disorders Program, Department of Psychiatry and Behavioural Neurosciences, McMaster University Medical Centre, McMaster University, Hamilton, Ontario, Canada

Rachel Manber, PhD, Sleep Disorders Clinic and Research Center, Department of Psychiatry and Behavioral Sciences, School of Medicine, Stanford University, Palo Alto, California

Susan L. McElroy, MD, Biological Psychiatry Program, Department of Psychiatry, University of Cincinnati College of Medicine, Cincinnati, Ohio

Ruth B. Merkatz, PhD, Albert Einstein College of Medicine, Bronx, New York; Department of Women's Health, Pfizer, Inc., New York, New York

Asha Mishra, MD, Department of Psychiatry, Medical College of Virginia campus, Virginia Commonwealth University, Richmond, Virginia

There are U.S. Food and Drug Administration guidelines and NIH policies regarding the need for inclusion of women and for investigation of gender differences in research studies. There are nationwide women's health initiatives and efforts through the Association of American Medical Colleges to evaluate medical school curricula on women's health.

In no field is women's health more worthy of attention than in mental health. One of the most consistent findings in epidemiological research is that unipolar depression is about twice as common in women as in men. Women are also more likely to experience many anxiety disorders (including panic disorder, generalized anxiety disorder, and posttraumatic stress disorder), and over 90% of cases of eating disorders occur in women. Rates of bipolar disorder are similar in men and women; however, women are more likely to develop depressive episodes of bipolar illness and a rapid-cycling course. Although alcoholism is much more prevalent in men, mortality rates among individuals with alcoholism are considerably higher in women. Recent research also has shown gender differences in treatment response for some psychiatric disorders.

Reproductive cycle events are critical points with regard to women's mental health. Mental disorders in women are most common during the childbearing years, and often reproductive events may act as triggers for the onset or exacerbation of symptoms. This timing raises issues concerning the management of disorders and the safety of treatments during pregnancy and lactation. In addition, the menstrual cycle and menopausal status may influence both illness presentation and treatment response.

Psychosocial factors also play an important part in the mental health of women. Gender differences in socialization processes and rates of traumatic abuse, as well as the various social roles of women as wives, mothers, caretakers of elderly parents, and workers, all deserve consideration in understanding risk factors for mental illness and the effects of these disorders on women and their families. In addition, special issues arise in the mental health care of lesbian women, women of color, and aging women.

This book summarizes the current state of knowledge of women's mental health. It consists of five sections. Part I provides an overview of women's psychobiology and the reproductive life cycle. It includes chapters on sex differences in neurobiology and psychopharmacology, as well as on psychiatric aspects of the menstrual cycle, pregnancy, the postpartum period, hormonal contraception, and menopause.

Part II discusses the assessment and treatment of psychiatric disorders in women, with an emphasis on gender differences in epidemiology, risk factors, symptom presentation, course of illness, comorbidity, and treatment response. Specific disorders reviewed include depression, bipolar disorder, schizophrenia, anxiety disorders, alcohol and other substance use disorders, eating disorders, sexual dysfunction, body dysmorphic disorder, sleep disorders, somatoform disorders, and personality disorders. Part II concludes with a chapter on the use of complementary and alternative medicine for mental health problems in women.

Part III approaches women's mental health from the perspective of consultation–liaison psychiatry. The chapters in this section provide an overview of medical and psychiatric aspects of women's health topics in other specialties of medicine, including gynecology, oncology, rheumatological diseases, endocrinology, cardiovascular disease, gastrointestinal disorders, HIV/AIDS, neurology, and cosmetic surgery.

Part IV discusses sociocultural issues in women's mental health. Topics covered include developmental considerations, marriage and the family, career and the workplace, abuse and violence, and three special populations (lesbian women, women of color, and aging and elderly women).

Finally, Part V addresses research methodology and health policy issues in women's mental health.

This book is intended to serve as a comprehensive reference on women's mental health for clinicians, researchers, and students. It is our hope that it will enrich the knowledge of those who already have a strong interest in this area and will provide a new level of understanding for those who are just beginning to explore it.

SUSAN G. KORNSTEIN
ANITA H. CLAYTON

Contents

PART III. PSYCHIATRIC CONSULTATION IN WOMEN

PART IV. SOCIOCULTURAL ISSUES FOR WOMEN

PART V. RESEARCH AND HEALTH POLICY ISSUES

Part I

Women's Psychobiology and Reproductive Life Cycle

1

Sex Differences in Neuroendocrine and Neurotransmitter Systems

ELIZABETH A. YOUNG
ANIA KORSZUN
MARGARET ALTEMUS

THE RELATIONSHIP OF STRESS TO DEPRESSION AND ANXIETY

Depressive and anxiety disorders are widely regarded as stress-related conditions. Although genetic vulnerability is critical to the development of depression, the incidence of depressive disorders is very low in the absence of environmental stressors (Kendler et al., 1995). Conversely, in approximately 75% of cases of depression, there is a precipitating life event (Brown & Harris, 1978; Frank et al., 1994). Living organisms survive by maintaining a complex dynamic equilibrium or homeostasis that is constantly challenged by intrinsic or extrinsic stressors. These stressors set in motion responses aimed at preserving homeostasis, including activation of a wide variety of neurotransmitters and neuromodulators. Corticotropin-releasing hormone (CRH), vasopressin, and norepinephrine are the principal central effectors of the stress response (Chrousos & Gold, 1992). CRH triggers the release of adrenocorticotropic hormone (ACTH) from the anterior pituitary corticotrope, which in turn triggers the release of adrenal glucocorticoids. The stress response is turned off by glucocorticoid feedback at brain and pituitary sites.

Depression and anxiety have both been conceptualized as maladaptive, exaggerated responses to stress. Abnormalities of the hypothalamic–pituitary–adrenal (HPA) axis, as manifested by hypercortisolemia and disruption of the circadian rhythm of cortisol secretion, are well-established phenomena in depression (Carroll et al., 1976; Sachar et al., 1973). In addition, depressed patients are less likely than control subjects to suppress ACTH and cortisol secretion after receiving dexamethasone (Carroll et al., 1976), suggesting a decreased sensitivity to glucocorticoid feedback regulation. Numerous factors are activated in response to stress, but CRH, vasopressin, and norepinephrine are considered to be the principal central effectors of the stress response (Chrousos & Gold, 1992). The assumption that the pathophysiology of anxiety disorders and depression involves exaggerated responses to stress is supported by evidence that CRH, vasopressin, and noradrenergic systems are hyperactivated in patients with these disorders (Altemus et al., 1992; Charney et al., 1987; Bremner et al., 1997; Butler & Nemeroff, 1990; Southwick et al., 1993). These systems are also hyperactivated in animal models of anxiety disorders (Coplan et al., 1996; Heim et al., 1997). Consistent with this model linking the generation of anxiety and depression to chronic stress is the extremely high comorbidity of depression and anxiety disorders (Kendler, 1996).

SEX DIFFERENCES IN ANXIETY AND DEPRESSION

In addition to their association with stress, another striking feature of mood and anxiety disorders is the increased prevalence of these conditions in women. Several lines of evidence indicate that sex steroid hormones play a role in the increased vulnerability of women to anxiety disorders and depression. Women have an increased incidence of unipolar depression and panic disorder (Weissman & Olfson, 1995), which arises at puberty. The immediate postpartum period, in particular, is a time of greatly increased risk for new onset or recurrence of mood disorders (Altshuler et al., 1998; Dean et al., 1989). In some women, recurrent depressive and anxiety symptoms are limited to the premenstrual period; in others, chronic depression is often exacerbated premenstrually (Rubinow & Roy-Byrne, 1984). There is also some evidence that panic disorder symptoms are relieved during pregnancy (Klein et al., 1995), and that obsessive–compulsive disorder can be exacerbated during pregnancy (Altemus et al., in press; Altshuler et al., 1998). Recent reports indicate that estrogen may be an effective treatment for postpartum (Gregoire et al., 1996) and perimenopausal depression (Zweifel & O'Brien, 1997).

BASIC REGULATION OF STRESS SYSTEMS

HPA Axis Regulation

To provide a basis for understanding the sex differences in the neurobiology of stress-related psychiatric disorders, an outline of the basic mechanisms of stress regulation and current knowledge of gonadal steroid modulation is presented here. Glucocorticoids act via multiple mechanisms, at several sites, to inhibit their own release. At the pituitary level, glucocorticoids exert direct effects on transcription of the gene for the ACTH precursor prohormone, proopiomelanocorticotropin, and subsequent ACTH peptide stores in the anterior pituitary (Birnberg et al., 1979; Roberts et al., 1979; Schacter et al., 1982). Studies have demonstrated that glucocorticoids interact with the CRH receptors in the anterior pituitary, acutely inhibiting the binding of CRH to its receptor and chronically decreasing CRH receptor numbers (Childs et al., 1986; Schwartz et al., 1986). Such direct effects of glucocorticoids on CRH receptors may account for some of the inhibitory action of glucocorticoids on ACTH release *in vitro*.

In addition to pituitary sites of action, glucocorticoids act at brain sites to modulate HPA axis activity. Early work by McEwen et al. (1968) demonstrated a very high-affinity uptake of corticosterone in the hippocampus of adrenalectomized rats injected *in vivo* with radiolabeled steroids. These receptors were difficult to demonstrate in nonadrenalectomized rats, presumably because these sites were saturated under resting conditions (McEwen et al., 1970). The receptors were not labeled by [^{3}H]dexamethasone, suggesting multiple types of glucocorticoid receptors (deKloet et al., 1975). The observation of receptor heterogeneity has been expanded upon by deKloet and colleagues, who subsequently demonstrated two glucocorticoid receptor types: mineralocorticoid receptors, which have particularly high affinity for the glucocorticoid corticosterone; and glucocorticoid receptors, which preferentially bind dexamethasone (Reul & deKloet, 1985). The latter are widely distributed throughout the brain, while the former exist predominantly in the hippocampus. In addition to action at the pituitary and hypothalamus, there is strong evidence from animal experiments that the hippocampus is a major glucocorticoid feedback site in the brain.

The importance of hippocampal steroid receptors in feedback regulation of stress has been demonstrated in several studies (Sapolsky et al., 1986). Removal of the hippocampus leads to increases in anterior pituitary secretion of ß-endorphin in plasma, increased CRH messenger ribonucleic acid (mRNA) in the paraventricular nucleus (PVN) of the hypothalamus, and a limited induction of vasopressin mRNA in parvocellular neurons of the PVN (Herman et al., 1989). In a formulation that may be relevant to depressive disorders, Sapolsky et al. (1986) have proposed the glucocorticoid cascade hypothesis, a model that describes the effects of chronic stress on hippocampal neurons. According to this model, repeated stress or chronic glucocorticoid administration down-regulates hippocampal steroid receptors, but not hypothalamic or pituitary receptors (Sapolsky et al., 1986; Young & Vazquez, 1996). Animals with down-regulated hippocampal glucocorticoid receptors are slow to turn off the glucocorticoid response to stress, and demonstrate decreased sensitivity to glucocorticoid fast feedback (Young & Vazquez, 1996). This decrease in glucocorticoid receptors and insensitivity to negative feedback lead to prolonged hypercortisolism, which eventually can result in atrophy of hippocampal neurons and further glucocorticoid hypersecretion. Glucocorticoid hypersecretion and hippocampal neuronal atrophy are most pronounced in aged rats—a situation possibly analogous to human depression, in which there is a higher incidence of HPA axis feedback abnormalities in aged individuals (Akil et al., 1993; Halbreich et al., 1984; Lewis et al., 1984; Young et al., 1995).

There is evidence in both animals and humans that the stress response is sexually dimorphic, and that gonadal steroids play an important role in modulating the HPA axis, acting particularly on sensitivity to glucocorticoid negative feedback (Young et al., 1993). Gonadal steroids may influence the HPA axis feedback mechanisms through effects on glucocorticoid receptors, on brain CRH systems, or on pituitary responsiveness to CRH. Identification of the physiological processes underlying these sex differences and the effects of reproductive hormone fluxes on mood and anxiety disorders should provide a better understanding of the pathophysiology of depression and anxiety and form the basis of new treatment approaches. To enable an understanding of the influence of gonadal hormones on the HPA axis and other neurotransmitters, an overview of gonadal steroid mechanisms follows.

Mechanisms of Action of Reproductive Hormones

The increased vulnerability of women to mood and anxiety disorders is not an X-linked trait (Merikangas et al., 1985); rather, it appears to arise from interactions of sex-specific hormonal and environmental factors with non-sex-specific genes on other chromosomes.

Variations in reproductive hormone levels occur in both sexes *in utero* and at puberty, and in women during the menstrual cycle, pregnancy, lactation, and menopause. Although reproductive hormone levels in men are generally stable, a rise in androgens takes place at puberty, and a gradual reduction in androgen production occurs with age. Estrogen, progesterone, and androgens have been examined for their effects on stress- and anxiety-associated neural systems. Sex differences in mood and anxiety could arise either from the acute effects of changing reproductive hormones, or from sexual differentiation of brain structure and function during development (McEwen et al., 1997), or both. Gonadal steroids can affect brain systems known to mediate mood and anxiety through alterations in neural structure, neurotransmitter and neuropeptide signaling efficiency, neuronal excitability, and synaptic plasticity.

Classical intracellular gonadal steroid receptors have been identified in multiple brain areas previously implicated in the regulation of mood and autonomic reactivity, including the hypothalamus, amygdala, hippocampus, bed nucleus of the stria terminalis, and locus coeruleus (LC) (Simerly et al., 1990). Gonadal steroids easily pass through cellular membranes and bind to these intracellular receptors. Once the hormone is bound, the receptor is "activated" and moves into the nucleus to act as a transcription factor to regulate gene expression. The effects of circulating steroid hormones can be differentially regulated in brain areas by the presence or absence of steroid receptors, different receptor subtypes, receptor isoforms that have differing activities (Auricchio, 1989; Kuiper et al., 1997), and transcriptional cofactors that can modify the effects of the activated receptor on gene transcription (Katzenellenbogen et al., 1996). Another level of complexity has been added by the discovery that estrogen receptors, after estrogen is bound, can alter the activity of other steroid hormone transcription factors, including activated glucocorticoid, thyroid, and progesterone receptors (Meyer et al., 1989; Uht et al., 1997; Zhu et al., 1996). In addition, androgen-metabolizing enzyme activity in specific brain areas regulates the activity of androgen hormones on estrogen and androgen receptors. Testosterone can be metabolized in the brain (1) to dihydrotestosterone, a hormone with greater affinity for the androgen receptor; (2) to androstenedione, a hormone with less affinity for the androgen receptor; or (3) by aromatase to estradiol, causing activation of estrogen rather than androgen receptors. Male and female rodents have similar density of estrogen receptors in extrahypothalamic brain areas relevant to anxiety, including the hippocampus, the raphe nucleus, and the cortex.

In addition to affecting gene transcription through binding to the intracellular steroid receptors, gonadal steroids appear to act directly at the neuronal membranes. Direct membrane actions of gonadal steroids occur within seconds or minutes, more rapidly than the time required for gene transcription and protein synthesis through the classical mechanism. Direct membrane actions of gonadal steroids include uncoupling of intracellular G-protein-coupled second-messenger systems, regulation of ion channels, modification of neurotransmitter receptor structure, and ultrastructural membrane remodeling (Wong et al., 1996).

Several steroid hormone metabolites are classified as "neurosteroids" because they are synthesized by neurons and glial cells in the central nervous system (Robel & Baulieu, 1995). Many of the neurosteroid hormones are produced in the brain as well as in the periphery by the gonads and adrenal glands, which secrete them into the circulation. Thus the action of these neurosteroid hormones may vary with fluctuations in peripheral hormone and hormone precursor levels during pregnancy, across the menstrual cycle, and during stress. Neurosteroids modulate neurotransmission primarily by acting directly on the neuronal membrane, but also may have direct effects on gene transcription (Rupprecht et al., 1996). Neurosteroids have been shown to modulate the functioning of γ-aminobutyric acid$_A$ (GABA$_A$) receptors, glutamatergic N-methyl-D-aspartate (NMDA) receptors, and the nicotinic acetylcholine receptor. They can have excitatory or inhibitory effects on neuronal activity and behavior. The best-documented effects of neurosteroids are the facilitation of GABA action at GABA$_A$ receptors by pregnenalone sulfate and allopregnanolone, two progesterone metabolites. Both of these steroids have anesthetic, hypnotic, and anxiolytic effects. Potentiation of GABA transmission by these two neurosteroids is similar to the action of benzodiazepines, which act at an adjacent site within the GABA$_A$ receptor complex.

Links between HPA and Noradrenergic Function in Animal Studies: Relationship to Anxiety and Depression

Both epidemiological and symptom cluster data suggest that anxiety and depression are closely linked. Emerging studies on stress may provide a neurobiological mechanism to explain this symptom linkage. Basic science studies on the biology of stress have suggested a central role for CRH in the coordination and integration of the stress response throughout the brain (Dunn & Berridge, 1990; Butler & Nemeroff, 1990; Koob et al., 1993). Although the role of CRH from the PVN of the hypothalamus as the releasing factor for ACTH is well established (Plotsky et al., 1989), a wealth of information from studies in rodents suggests that CRH outside the PVN appears to mediate the general stress response, including the behaviors of decreased sleep, anorexia, inhibition of sexual receptivity, altered gastrointestinal motility, decreased locomotion, increased startle reflex, and decreased exploratory behavior in novel environments (Dunn & Berridge, 1990; Butler & Nemeroff, 1990; Koob et al., 1993). Moreover, a number of behavioral effects of stress have been demonstrated to be reversed by central administration of alpha-helical CRH (Butler & Nemeroff, 1990), a CRH antagonist (Koob et al., 1993). The other major central component of the generalized stress response, the LC, is a nucleus of noradrenergic neurons located in the midpons with terminal fields in the hypothalamus, hippocampus, and amygdala, and throughout the cerebral cortex (Moore & Bloom, 1979). The LC provides much of the brain's supply of norepinephrine, and numerous findings have demonstrated the importance of the LC in mediating arousal. Electrical stimulation of the LC in unanesthetized primates produces intense anxiety, hypervigilance, and inhibition of exploratory behavior, while spontaneous firing of the LC increases during threatening situations and diminishes during sleep, grooming, and feeding (Aston-Jones et al., 1994). In addition, acute stress in animals causes increased release of norepinephrine in several brain areas, including the hypothalamus and LC (Glavin, 1985), as well as increased production of tyrosine hydroxylase, the rate-limiting enzyme for norepinephrine synthesis, in the LC (Smith et al., 1991); chronic stress increases brain norepinephrine levels and the activity of tyrosine hydroxylase (Weiss et al., 1975). Although the LC is closely related anatomically to nuclei of the peripheral sympathetic nervous system and sympathomedullary system, both of which release catecholamines in the periphery during arousal, the degree of functional integration of the central and peripheral noradrenergic systems remains to be defined.

Following the initial isolation and sequencing of CRH by Vale et al. (1981), Brown et al. (1982) demonstrated that injection of CRH activates the sympathetic nervous system. Although it was long known that stress activated the LC, the studies by Valentino (1989) demonstrating direct effects of CRH on LC neurons were particularly critical for understanding the role of CRH in mediating arousal. Subsequent studies by Aston-Jones et al. (1991) have demonstrated that the main afferent fibers to the LC arise from the nucleus paragigantocellularis (PGi), and that these neurons contain CRH. Thus these anatomical data provide the mechanism for the LC production of arousal/anxiety behavior following CRH administration. Furthermore, studies by Plotsky (1987) found noradrenergic stimulation resulted in secretion of CRH into the hypophyseal portal blood. Consequently, it is possible that stimulation of LC noradrenergic outflow can result in activation of the HPA axis. Finally, studies examining the effects of the HPA axis on the LC have demonstrated that cortisol may inhibit LC activity; an increase in tyrosine hydroxylase mRNA levels in LC following adrenalectomy, and decreased sympathetic nervous system activation following increases in circulating plasma glucocorticoid levels, have been reported (McEwen, 1995). These studies on stress suggest an underlying mechanism by which activation of these two stress systems is both linked and dependent upon the actions of CRH. Consequently, one can conceptualize two different but related CRH systems: the PVN/HPA axis system and the PGi/LC system. In depression, there is clear evidence of HPA axis activation indicating CRH hypersecretion from the PVN and suggestive extra-PVN CRH hypersecretion (Butler & Nemeroff, 1990). However, animal studies suggest that central CRH administration is also an excellent model of anxiety (Butler & Nemeroff, 1990). In anxiety disorders, HPA axis activation is not prominent, but there is some evidence of extra-PVN CRH hypersecretion (Bremner et al., 1997; Altemus et al., 1992.

Chronic antidepressant treatment inhibits stress responsive systems at multiple sites, through reductions in CRH and tyrosine hydroxylase activity, enhanced glucocorticoid receptor activity (Brady et al., 1991; Barden et al., 1995), and down-regulation of arousal-producing ß-adrenergic receptors (Heninger & Charney, 1987). Chronic treatment with antidepressant agents also reduces both the behavioral and endocrine responses to stress (Murua & Molina, 1992; Reul et al., 1993; Barden et al., 1995). Benzodiazepines also restrain neuroendocrine stress responses, such as ACTH, corticosterone, and catecholamine responses (Breier et al., 1992). Furthermore, chronic stress and glucocorticoids exaggerate development of fear behaviors in animals (Conrad et al., 1999; Corodimas et al., 1994; Roozendaal & McGaugh, 1996).

EFFECTS OF GONADOSTEROIDS ON STRESS SYSTEM AND ANXIETY CIRCUITS

HPA Axis

Studies in rodents support the existence of sex differences in several of the elements of the HPA axis. Female rats appear to have a more robust HPA axis response to stress than do male rats, and there is evidence that estrogen is at least partly responsible for this sexual dimorphism. For example, compared with male rats, female rats have a faster onset of corticosterone secretion after stress and a faster rate of rise of corticosterone (Jones et al., 1972). The increased corticosterone response is accompanied by a greatly increased ACTH response to stress in female rodents (Young, 1996). Furthermore, corticosteroid-binding globulin (CBG) is positively regulated by estrogen and thus higher in female rats;

however, estrogen and progesterone have been demonstrated to affect the HPA axis independent of the effects of CBG (Young, 1996). In addition, chronic estrogen treatment of ovariectomized female rats enhances their corticosterone response to stress and slows their recovery from stress (Burgess & Handa, 1992). Studies by Viau and Meaney (1991) demonstrate a greater ACTH and corticosterone stress response in acute estradiol-treated rats compared with ovariectomized female rats or with estradiol-plus-progesterone-treated female rats after short-term (24 hours) but not long-term (48 hours) estradiol treatment. This greater ACTH response in females probably results from a greater central CRH response to stress. Interestingly, a partial estrogen response element is found on the CRH gene, which is able to confer estrogen enhancement of CRH expression in CV-1 transfected cells (Vamvakopoulos & Chrousos, 1993), providing a mechanism by which estradiol may enhance stress responsiveness in females.

Another mechanism by which estrogen might increase the HPA stress response is through inhibition of glucocorticoid feedback mechanisms. A steeper rate of rise of corticosterone is necessary to elicit glucocorticoid fast feedback in female rats than in male rats (Jones et al., 1972). Two sets of studies (Burgess & Handa, 1992; Viau & Meaney, 1991) demonstrate that estrogen treatment delays the ACTH and glucocorticoid shutoff following stress in estrogen-treated female rats compared with ovariectomized female rats. In addition, estradiol treatment blocks down-regulation of hippocampal glucocorticoid receptors following chronic administration of RU 28362, a glucocorticoid agonist in rats. Following long-term (21 days) estradiol treatment, the potent and selective glucocorticoid RU 28362 was ineffective in blocking ether-stress-induced ACTH secretion.

There is also evidence to indicate that progesterone, like estrogen, may dampen feedback mechanisms in the HPA axis. Work by Keller-Wood et al. (1988) in pregnant ewes and ewes given progesterone infusions demonstrates that progesterone can diminish the effectiveness of cortisol feedback on stress responsiveness *in vivo*. In addition, progesterone demonstrates antiglucocorticoid effects on feedback in intact rats *in vivo* and *in vitro* (Svec, 1988; Duncan & Duncan, 1979). Progesterone binds to the glucocorticoid receptor; although it does so with a faster binding time than glucocorticoid itself, progesterone binds to a different site on the receptor than glucocorticoid does (Svec, 1988). Progesterone can also increase the rate of dissociation of glucocorticoids from the glucocorticoid receptor (Rousseau et al., 1972). In addition, in cultured rat hepatoma cells dexamethasone and progesterone bind to the same receptor, and progesterone is a clear competitive antagonist of dexamethasone binding. Although the majority of these effects are exerted at the glucocorticoid receptor, binding studies with expressed human mineralocorticoid receptor have demonstrated an affinity of progesterone for the latter receptor in a range similar to that of dexamethasone (Arriza et al., 1987). Furthermore, there was an increase in mineralocorticoid receptor binding following progesterone treatment of female rats (Carey et al., 1995). Finally, female rats have a greater number of glucocorticoid receptors in the hippocampus than male rats do (Turner & Weaver, 1985), and progesterone modulates immunoreactive glucocorticoid receptor distribution in the hippocampus of adrenalectomized rats (Ahima et al., 1992). It should be noted that binding studies do not distinguish agonist effects from antagonist effects, so even increases in number could result from antagonist effects at glucocorticoid receptors.

Until recently, the lack of a reliable stress test limited studies on sex differences in stress response in humans. In the Trier Social Stress Test, subjects undergo a mock job interview in front of a panel of interviewers who are instructed not to provide any verbal or nonverbal feedback; it is a reliable and robust stressor in normal subjects (Kirschbaum et al., 1995). It has now been shown that oral contraceptives decrease the free cortisol response to a social stressor in women (Kirschbaum et al., 1995), and that the treatment of normal men with estradiol for 48 hours results in enhanced ACTH and cortisol response to a social stressor (Kirschbaum et al., 1996). These data regarding the effects of estrogen treatment in men are consistent with results of studies in rats (Burgess & Handa, 1992; Viau & Meaney, 1991). However, results from studies of oral contraceptives are harder to interpret because these are synthetic steroids given at constant doses for a prolonged period of time, and they may differ from endogenous steroids in their effects.

In addition to these studies on HPA responses to social stress, we and others have examined sex differences in the response of the HPA axis to pharmacological challenges. For example, we administered ovine CRH (oCRH) to men and women and found a 40% greater cortisol response in women, again consistent with animal studies (Young, 1995). Because oCRH acts at the level of the pituitary, these data suggest that ovarian steroids modulate both hypothalamic and pituitary systems separately. Data from several studies indicate that among depressed patients, women are more likely than men to have abnormalities in HPA axis regulation such as hypercortisolemia, and the generally reported hypercortisolemia of depression may be a result of the fact that samples of depressed patients usually include more women than men (Young et al., 1991).

With respect to the influence of changes in ovarian hormones across the menstrual cycle in women, recent studies by Altemus et al. (1997) have found increased resistance to dexamethasone suppression during the luteal phase of the menstrual cycle as compared to the follicular phase—a change that may again be related to either increased estradiol or progesterone during the luteal phase. In addition, ACTH, vasopressin, and cortisol responses to stress are enhanced in the luteal phase compared to the follicular phase of the menstrual cycle (Altemus et al., 1997; Galliven, 1997), suggesting that decreases in glucocorticoid receptors may explain the decreased response to dexamethasone. In a design that allows investigators to distinguish the effects of progesterone from those of estrogen, Roca et al. (1998a, 1998b) studied women who were first treated with leuprolide, a gonadotropin-releasing hormone agonist that causes suppression of both estrogen and progesterone secretion, and then given sequential replacement of the two hormones. They examined the response to exercise stress as well as to dexamethasone feedback, and found that the exercise stress response was increased and response to dexamethasone feedback was decreased during the progesterone "add-back" phase, but not during the estrogen "add-back" phase. Again, these data suggest that progesterone acts as a glucocorticoid antagonist. Thus the data from human studies so far suggest that ovarian steroids, and in particular progesterone, influence the HPA axis response to stress by modulating sensitivity to negative feedback. Furthermore, some data suggest that progesterone may have negative effects on mood particularly in women with premenstrual dysphoric disorder (PMDD), in whom depressive symptoms occur in the luteal phase of the menstrual cycle when progesterone levels are high. Although the exact role of sex hormones in this disorder has not been established (Hammaback et al., 1985), estrogen and progesterone suppression by leuprolide has been reported to produce significant symptom improvement in depression (Rosenbaum et al., 1996) and PMDD (Mortola et al., 1991).

The Sexually Dimorphic Impact of Stress on Behavior and Neural Structure

Although sex differences in HPA axis responsivity have been described above, sex differences in extrahypothalamic and behavioral responses to stress have only recently come to light. Surprisingly, there are sex differences in the impact of stress on performance of a number of learned behaviors, including classical conditioning, operant conditioning, and conditioned fear behaviors. In male rats, stress facilitates classical conditioning of behaviors such as eyeblinking when an air puff to the eye is paired with a tone signal; in female rats, stress impairs aquisition of eyeblink conditioning. This sex difference depends upon estrogen, since impairment of conditioning in females was abolished by ovariectomy or treatment with an estrogen receptor antagonist, and restored by estrogen replacement (Wood & Shors, 1998). Exposure to inescapable shock reduced subsequent movement into the open arm of an elevated plus maze and shuttlebox escape performance in male rats to a much greater degree than in females (Kirk & Blampied, 1985; Steenbergen et al., 1990). Female rats also showed a smaller magnitude of behavior changes after exposure to acute restraint stress, but a failure of behavioral adaptation to repeated restraint stress, indicating that behavioral reactivity to stress was more persistent in females (Kennet et al., 1986).

Another surprising finding is that effects of stress on neural structure are also sexually dimorphic. Chronic stress over 21 days produces atrophy of apical dendrites of CA3 hippocampal pyramidal neurons in male rats, but this effect is not seen in females (Galea et al., 1997). In a similar study, repeated swim stress over 30 days decreased CA3 and CA4 pyramidal cell number in male but not female rats (Mizoguchi et al., 1992). Similar results were found in male and female vervet monkeys following chronic stress (Uno et al., 1989). The reduced amounts of hippocampal atrophy found in females was unexpected, since females demonstrate greater corticosterone response to stress compared to males (Galea et al., 1997), and available evidence suggests that corticosterone mediates the CA3 dendritic atrophy (Jacobson & Sapolsky, 1991; Magarinos & McEwen, 1995). This suggests that premenopausal women may be relatively protected from the hippocampal atrophy associated with elevated cortisol levels in human disorders such as Cushing's syndrome (Starkman et al., 1992) and depression (Sheline et al., 1996), as well as the hippocampal atrophy associated with increased glucocorticoid receptor sensitivity in posttraumatic stress disorder (Bremner et al., 1995; Yehuda et al., 1995).

Sex differences in developmental responses to prenatal stress have also been found. Prenatal stress in rodents results in exaggerated behavioral and neuroendocrine stress responses in adulthood, including increased emotional reactivity, increased anxiety-associated behaviors, and reduced hippocampal glucocorticoid receptors. Prenatally stressed female rats have greater HPA axis responsivity and greater reductions in glucocorticoid receptor binding in the amygdala and septum (McCormick et al., 1995) as adults than prenatally stressed male rats do. Thus prenatal stress has a greater impact in females than in males on later HPA axis regulation. Perinatal manipulation of gonadal steroid hormones alters several components of brain stress response systems in adulthood, including glucocorticoid receptor binding, hypothalamic CRH and vasopressin gene expression, and HPA axis responsivity to estradiol (Patchev et al., 1995). Fear-associated behaviors were not examined in these studies of sex differences in the sequelae of prenatal and perinatal stress.

Sex Differences in Animal Anxiety Models

Although women are clearly more prone to develop panic disorder, posttraumatic stress disorder, and phobias, studies of sex differences in fear behaviors have produced mixed results. Female rats have been shown to exhibit reduced fear behavior in a contextual fear-conditioning task but not a cued fear-conditioning task in two studies (Maren et al., 1994; Markus & Zecevic, 1997). Similarly, in a conditioned avoidance paradigm in mice, males demonstrated stronger conditioned avoidance of a footshock than females (Farr et al., 1995). In addition, females demonstrate less learned helplessness than males after exposure to inescapable shock (Heinsbroek et al., 1991).

Increased activity levels in females compared to males, and sex differences in other behavioral parameters (such as information processing, pain sensitivity, and appetite), complicate interpretation of sex differences in animal models of anxiety. In addition, sex differences may be the result of varying hormone levels in females affecting retrieval (Markus & Zecevic, 1997); that is, females may be less likely to recall a fear association if it is learned while the rat is in one estrous cycle phase, but reexposure occurs in a different phase.

Estrous/Menstrual Cycle Influences on Anxiety Systems

Behavior changes noted across the estrous cycle reflect the actions of both estrogen and progesterone. In the estrous cycle, estrogen rises precede progesterone increases, which potentiate but later antagonize the effects of estrogen. In the rat, estrogen peaks in early proestrous, progesterone peaks in late proestrous, and both reach a nadir in metestrous. Because multiple hormones change with the estrous cycle, it is often difficult to gauge the influence of a particular gonadal steroid on a biological mechanism or behavior. However, it is inadequate to examine the behavioral effects of estrogen and progesterone only in isolation. Estrogen up-regulates progesterone receptors in multiple brain areas (Parsons et al., 1982). Consequently, many progesterone effects on behavior can only be observed following estrogen priming (Rodier, 1971). For example, acute injections of progesterone (5 hours prior to testing) in estrogen-primed rats have been shown to increase punished responding in females (Rodriguez-Sierra et al., 1984, 1986)—an effect not seen with either hormone administered individually.

Many behavioral effects of estrogen have been shown to peak at 24–48 hours after exogenous estrogen dosing (Diaz-Veliz et al., 1989). This 48-hour lag for behavioral effect suggests that estrogen is working through genomic rather than nongenomic mechanisms. In the natural estrous cycle, the anxiolytic effects of estrogen are shorter in duration, possibly due to progesterone antagonism of estrogen effects. In most behavioral paradigms, measures of fear behavior are reduced in proestrous and estrous only 24 hours after circulating estrogen rises, while progesterone antagonism of estrogen effects is apparent during metestrous and diestrous. Reduced anxiety during proestrous and estrous is shown by less defensive burying after a shock probe was introduced to the cage (Fernandez-Guasti & Picazo, 1990), increased activity in an open field (Anderson, 1940; Burke & Broadhurst, 1966; Gray & Levine, 1964), slower aquisition of avoidance responses to footshock (Farr et al., 1995), and increased entrance into the open arms of the plus maze (Bitran et al., 1991; Diaz-Veliz et al., 1997; Mora et al., 1996; Nomikos & Spiraki, 1988). Also, proestrous female rats are more sensitive to the anxiolytic effect of diazepam (Fernandez-Guasti & Picazo, 1990), suggesting that similar changes in benzodiazepine sensitivity may occur across the menstrual cycle in humans.

Female rats showed a reduction in conditioned freezing (a measure of anxiety) only on the afternoon of proestrous compared to the morning of proestrous and estrous (Markus & Zecevic, 1997), more tightly corresponding to elevated levels of circulating estrogen and progesterone. The relatively rapid shift in this measure of fear, compared to other animal models of anxiety, suggests a nongenomic mechanism of action of gonadal steroids on this behavior.

In contrast to the rat 4- to 5-day estrous cycle of the rat, the sequential rise in estrogen and progesterone occurs over a much longer time frame during the human menstrual cycle. Thus the behavioral effects of unopposed estrogen should be present through the late follicular and early luteal phase of the cycle, and progesterone antagonism of estrogen effects would occur in the midluteal phase, followed by a loss of estrogen and progesterone in the late luteal phase. Consequently, if estrogen has anxiolytic effects in humans, as seen in rats, these effects should be evident in the late follicular and early luteal phases of the cycle, and lost in the latter half of the luteal phase. Indirect support for this model comes from evidence that mood-elevating effects of estrogen in postmenopausal women are often reduced during periods of progesterone coadministration (Zweifel & O'Brien, 1997), and that women with PMDD generally experience increased anxiety in the late luteal phase of the cycle (Rubinow & Roy-Byrne, 1984).

Effects of Pregnancy on Stress and Anxiety Systems

In addition to varying with the estrous cycle, gonadal hormones change with other reproductive events as well. Pregnancy is accompanied by steep rises in both estrogen and progesterone, whereas the postpartum period is defined by a dramatic decrease in these steroids with the termination of gestation. Less is known of the behavioral and brain effects of androstenedione, dehydroepiandrosterone, and other adrenal androgens that also increase markedly during pregnancy and during the luteal phase of the menstrual cycle. Increases in plasma CBG and cortisol during pregnancy are well documented, and dexamethasone challenge studies indicate resistance to glucocorticoid negative feedback during pregnancy (Carr et al., 1981; Demey-Ponsart et al., 1982; Nolten & Rueckert, 1981). However, the degree to which postdexamethasone hypercortisolism is simply an artifact of increased CBG levels, leading to higher levels of plasma cortisol following dexamethasone administration, is not completely known. Although dexamethasone itself is not bound by CBG, pregnancy could alter the metabolism of dexamethasone, resulting in less dexamethasone bioavailability. At least one study (Nolten & Rueckert, 1981) demonstrated higher free cortisol during pregnancy, higher free cortisol production following an ACTH infusion, decreased suppression of free cortisol by dexamethasone, and a normal circadian rhythm of cortisol, pointing to a change in cortisol set point during pregnancy. Again, these data are compatible with those showing that both estrogen and progesterone can antagonize the effects of glucocorticoids on negative feedback.

In pregnant women, several reports suggest a reduction in panic disorder symptoms during pregnancy (Klein et al., 1995). In contrast, several case studies and a retrospective study of obsessive–compulsive disorder reported an increase in symptom severity during pregnancy (Altshuler et al., 1998; Nezeroglu et al., 1992). The differential course of these two disorders during pregnancy could be related to several factors, including increased cerebrospinal fluid GABA levels during pregnancy (Kendrick et al., 1988), and high progesterone levels (which facilitate transmission at $GABA_A$ receptors). GABA agonists are effective treatments for panic disorder, but are ineffective for obsessive–compulsive disorder. Furthermore, rising gonadal steroid levels during pregnancy may lower serotonergic activity, which may be more harmful to patients with obsessive–compulsive disorder than to patients with panic disorder.

Effects of Lactation on Stress and Anxiety Systems

Lactation is associated with the unique endocrine environment of episodic secretion of oxytocin and prolactin, and suppression of the hypothalamic–pituitary–gonadal axis (McNeilly et al., 1994). Studies of lactating rats demonstrate reductions in the endocrine responses to stress. These findings include reductions in plasma ACTH (Lightman, 1992; Walker et al., 1992), corticosterone (Lightman, 1992; Walker et al., 1992), catecholamine (Higuchi et al., 1989), and prolactin (Higuchi et al., 1989; Pohl et al., 1989) responses to stressors. The inhibition of the peripheral HPA axis response is likely to be centrally mediated, because lactating rats also show significant decreases in several central nervous system responses to stress, including hippocampal immediate early gene induction (Abbud et al., 1992), hypothalamic CRH mRNA production (Lightman & Young, 1989), and expression of fear behaviors (Fleming & Luebke, 1981; Hansen & Ferreira, 1986).

In women, lactation also suppresses endocrine responses to exercise stress (Altemus et al., 1995) and autonomic nervous system responses to distressed infant cries (Weisenfeld et al., 1985). In women with panic disorder, lactation seems to ameliorate symptoms, but panic symptoms recur with weaning. A retrospective study of women who had panic disorder with agoraphobia showed a dramatic decline of panic attack frequency, but not agorophobia, during pregnancy and lactation (Klein et al., 1995).

The physiological mechanisms mediating the reduction in stress responses in lactating women and animals are still unclear. GABA levels are increased in the cerebrospinal fluid of lactating rats (Qureshi et al., 1987). Oxytocin, a neuropeptide with anxiolytic properties (McCarthy & Altemus, 1997), is released centrally during lactation into the cerebrospinal fluid and at the hippocampus and lateral septum (Kendrick et al., 1986, 1988; Neumann & Landgraf, 1989) in both sheep and rats. The only study of central oxytocin administration in humans found an analgesic effect in subjects with back pain (Yang, 1994). Production of neuropeptide Y, an anxiolytic neuropeptide, is also greatly enhanced during lactation (Smith, 1993). In animals, prolactin has been demonstrated to blunt hormonal responses to stress (Endroczi & Nyakas, 1972; Schlein et al., 1974), but nonreproductive behavioral effects of prolactin have received little attention.

Lactation-induced suppression of endocrine, autonomic, and behavioral response to stress may have several adaptive functions for both a mother and her infant. For instance, conservation of energy needed for synthesis of milk would be promoted both by reduced tonic sympathetic outflow and by inhibition of HPA axis activation and the associated catabolic effects of glucocorticoid secretion. In addition, inhibition of CRH and catecholamine release could minimize psychological arousal or anxiety associated with the demands of infant care, thereby potentially facilitating maternal behaviors. Reduced psychological reactivity during lactation could also attenuate reductions in milk release known to occur with stress (Newton & Newton, 1948).

Stress Effects on Serotonin

Serotonergic systems play an important role in both stress responsivity and anxiety. A fundamental hypothesis of the etiology of anxiety and depressive disorders is that these disorders may be due to a relative deficiency of serotonin. This hypothesis is based primarily on animal studies, and also on the antidepressant and anxiolytic efficacy of serotonin reuptake blockers. Preclinical studies indicate that chronic administration of these drugs increases the efficiency of serotonergic neurotransmission in rats (el Mansari et al., 1995)). To date, 14 serotonin receptor subtypes have been identified, some of which may have separate and opposing actions with reference to anxiety. Activation of the 5-HT_3 postsynaptic receptor seems to produce anxiogenic effects, whereas activation of 5-HT_{1A} and possibly 5-HT_{2C} postsynaptic receptors appears to have a more anxiolytic effect.

Both stress and glucocorticoids modulate serotonin transmission. Acute stress levels of glucocorticoids increase serotonin turnover and increase the responsiveness of hippocampal neurons to 5-HT_{1A} receptor stimulation (Meijer & deKloet, 1998; McEwen, 1995). When elevated levels of glucocorticoids persist (such as following chronic social stress), down-regulation of hippocampal 5-HT_{1A} receptors occurs, while 5-HT_2 receptors in the cerebral cortex are up-regulated (McEwen, 1995). In addition, 5-HT_{2C} receptors are increased following corticosterone adrenectomy, and normalize following corticosterone replacement (Meijer & deKloet, 1998). Animal studies demonstrate that chronic treatment with high doses of glucocorticoids leads to decreased serotonin-receptor-mediated responses; this is similar to the picture observed in depressed patients, although the exact mechanism of this hypofunctional serotonin state is unclear (Meijer & deKloet, 1998). This hypofunctional serotonin state may have further consequences for glucocorticoid secretion, since serotonin appears to be an important regulator of glucocorticoid feedback. Antidepressants that increase serotonin cause increases in glucocorticoid receptor number and can reverse the increased glucocorticoid secretion seen in depressed humans and in transgenic mice, which have been genetically altered to demonstrate reduced glucocorticoid receptors and increased glucocorticoid secretion (partial glucocorticoid receptor knockout) (Barden et al., 1995). Lesions of the serotonergic input to the hippocampus, an important site in inhibiting glucocorticoid secretion, do produce decreased glucocorticoid receptor expression and increased glucocorticoid secretion (Seckl & Fink, 1992).

Sex Differences in Serotonin Systems

Gonadal steroids appear to modulate anxiety at least in part through effects on serotonergic systems. Overall, the literature suggests that estrogen enhances the efficiency of serotonergic neurotransmission. Basic science studies indicate that there are clear sex differences in brain serotonin systems, some of which may depend upon estrogen and others upon testosterone. The serotonin content and uptake in multiple areas of the forebrain, hypothalamus, and limbic system are higher in females than in males (Haleem et al., 1990; Borisova et al., 1996; Carlsson & Carlsson, 1988). 5-HT_{1C} and 5-HT_2 receptor binding in the dentate gyrus or CA4 regions of the hippocampus is similar in male and female rats; however, the 5-HT_{1A} receptor binding in the CA1 region of the hippocampus is higher in female rats, and ovariectomy had no effect on this sex difference (Mendelson

& McEwen, 1991). Stress has been shown to cause greater increases in serotonin in female rats in multiple brain areas (Heinsbroek et al., 1990). More recent studies have found that estradiol increases serotonin transporter binding in female rat brains (McQueen et al., 1997) and stimulates an increase in $5\text{-}HT_{2A}$ binding sites in limbic cortex (Fink et al., 1996). Limited evidence suggests that, like estrogen, progesterone may up-regulate $5\text{-}HT_2$ receptors (Biegon et al., 1983) and increase serotonin content (Pecins-Thompson et al., 1996). However, no consistent effects of progesterone administration on serotonin function have been identified. There also is evidence that testosterone has opposing effects to estrogen on serotonergic activity. Reductions in androgenic steroids have been associated with enhancement of central serotonergic activity (Bonson et al., 1994; Fischette et al., 1984; Matsuda et al., 1991). In addition, administration of testosterone has been associated with reductions in central serotonergic activity (Martinez-Conde et al., 1985; Mendelson & McEwen, 1990).

Studies of sex differences in serotonin systems in humans are more limited. Sex differences in the prolactin and cortisol responses to serotonin agonists have been reported, with women showing greater response to the serotonergic challenges (Monteleone et al., 1997; Ryan et al., 1992; Lerer et al., 1996; Gelfin et al., 1995). However, estrogen regulates prolactin synthesis as well as cortisol secretion, so greater responses to serotonergic challenges in women do not necessarily indicate serotonin receptor differences. One study examining $5\text{-}HT_2$ receptors on platelets in children found a suggestion of increased binding in teenage girls after the age of 14, but the study was clearly limited by a small sample size of postpubertal adolescents (Biegon & Greuner, 1992). Incubation of human platelets with sex steroids shows no direct effects on serotonin uptake (Ehrenkranz, 1976). Depressed women have a higher density of $5\text{-}HT_2$ receptors on platelets than depressed men do (Hrdina et al., 1995). No sex differences have been found in serotonin metabolites in cerebrospinal fluid of normal subjects (Leckman et al., 1994; Yoshino, 1982). One postmortem study examining serotonin binding in human brains found no sex differences (Marcusson et al., 1984), whereas another reported increased $5\text{-}HT_2$ binding in the frontal cortex in women (Arato et al., 1991). One positron emission tomography imaging study found no sex differences in $5\text{-}HT_{2A}$ in the brain (Baeken et al., 1998). It should be noted that many of the human studies were conducted before an understanding of multiple serotonin receptors existed, so many of the compounds used to detect serotonin receptors were nonspecific. It is likely that there are sex differences in serotonin systems in humans, and that the differences between depressed women and depressed men may be larger than the differences seen in normal subjects. Of note, the two disorders shown to have a specific response to serotonergic antidepressants—premenstrual syndrome (Eriksson et al., 1995) and obsessive–compulsive disorder (Greist et al., 1995)—appear to be particularly sensitive to changes in gonadal steroids.

Sex Differences in Glutamate Systems

Another factor influenced by ovarian hormones and involved in the stress response is glutamate. Glutamate is the primary excitatory transmitter in the brain. Activation of glutamate systems induces anxiety, long-term potentiation (an electrophysiological animal model of learning), and (in higher doses) seizures. Estrogen activation of the NMDA and non-NMDA types of glutamate receptors (Gazzaley et al., 1996; Smith, 1989; Weiland,

1992a; Wong & Moss, 1992) may contribute to estrogen and proestrous associated reductions in seizure threshold (Buterbaugh & Hudson, 1991; Terasawa & Timiras, 1967; Teyler et al., 1980), as well as to increases in long-term potentiation during estrogen plus progesterone treatment (Warren et al., 1995; Wong & Moss, 1992). These changes in seizure threshold and long-term potentiation are compatible with observations of increases in synaptic density and number of dendritic spines in the CA1 nucleus of the hippocampus during estrogen treatment and at proestrous (Woolley & McEwen, 1992). NMDA receptor activation has been shown to mediate estrogen-induced increases in synaptic density in the CA3 region of the hippocampus (Woolley & McEwen, 1994). The effects of estrogen on glutamatergic transmission appear to involve both genomic and nongenomic mechanisms.

Estrogen potentiation of glutamatergic receptors does not seem consistent with estrogen-associated reductions in anxiety, since glutamate agonists increase a variety of fear behaviors. However, although estrogen treatment reduces seizure threshold in the hippocampus and medial amygdala, it raises seizure threshold in the lateral nucleus of the amygdala (Terasawa & Timiras, 1967). The lateral nucleus plays an important role in generation of conditioned and unconditioned fear behaviors (LeDoux, 1996). These differential effects suggest a mechanism whereby estrogen may enhance memory, but also decrease anxiety. Another mechanism contributing to this inverse relationship between seizure threshold and fear behavior may be tonic inhibition of amygdala activity by the hippocampus (Gray, 1982). Rats with bilateral hippocampal lesions demonstrate enhanced fear-associated behaviors, including enhanced acquisition of conditioned avoidance (Pitman, 1982; Port et al., 1991) and delayed extinction of conditioned responses (Devenport, 1978; Schmaltz & Isaacson, 1967).

Sex Differences in GABA Systems

The amino acid GABA, synthesized from glutamate, is the primary inhibitory neurotransmitter in the brain. The $GABA_A$ subtype of GABA receptor, which is widely distributed in the central nervous system, primarily postsynaptically, inhibits neuronal firing by opening a Cl- channel. The $GABA_A$ receptor, the benzodiazapine binding site, and the Cl- ionophore are part of a single macromolecular complex. A number of progesterone metabolites and other neurosteroids potentiate GABA activity by binding to the $GABA_A$ receptor.

Estrogen also has multiple effects on GABA systems consistent with its anxiolytic effects. Estrogen increases GABA receptor binding in the hippocampus (Schumacher et al., 1989), and GABA activity is enhanced at proestrous in the lateral septum. Finally, production of mRNA for the enzyme glutamic acid decarboxylase, the rate-limiting step for GABA synthesis, is enhanced in the hippocampus (Weiland, 1992b) and midbrain central grey matter (McCarthy et al., 1995) during estrogen treatment. Progesterone administered alone had no effect on GABA receptor binding (Schumacher et al., 1989), but antagonized the estrogen-induced hippocampal glutamic acid decarboxylase mRNA increase when coadministered with estrogen (Weiland, 1992b). The observation that the response to diazepam is enhanced in estrogen-treated rats (McCarthy et al., 1995) is consistent with these neurobiological studies and suggests that estrogen may increase sensitivity to benzodiazepine treatment in humans.

CONCLUSIONS

The finding of an increased ACTH response to stress in females, compared with males, has important implications for our understanding of stress and stress responsiveness in women. Several stress-associated disorders are more common in women, such as depression and anxiety disorders, including posttraumatic stress disorder (Kessler et al., 1994). If indeed there is an exaggerated central CRH response to stress in women, this may explain some of their increased susceptibility to these disorders. In addition, resistance to the feedback effects of endogenous glucocorticoids, as described above, may contribute to the increased incidence of stress-related conditions in women. Indeed, Munck and Guyre (1986) hypothesize that the purpose of glucocorticoids is to terminate not just the HPA axis stress response, but the entire stress response. For example, studies suggest that glucocorticoids can inhibit the autonomic nervous system response (McEwen, 1995), supporting a role for glucocorticoids in terminating stress-induced activation of the autonomic stress system. Thus women's increased resistance to glucocorticoids, compared with men's, could exaggerate stress responsiveness in a number of physiological systems.

As described above, it is possible that estrogen and progesterone antagonism of glucocorticoid feedback mechanisms, and the increased stress responsiveness of females, contribute to the increased prevalence of anxiety disorders and autonomic hyperarousal in women compared with men. However, this is modulated by the fact that estrogen and progesterone also appear to be anxiolytic, independently of their effects on the HPA axis, so that it is not always possible to predict the final effects of ovarain steroids. Clinical data suggest that some reproductive hormones, particularly estrogen and androgens, may potentiate psychiatric symptoms in some individuals. Because the gonadal steroids have so many effects on multiple brain systems, effects of these hormones are likely to vary among individuals, based on underlying differences in target neurochemical systems. For example, women with low serotonin levels or low serotonergic tone may experience increases rather than decreases in anxiety and irritability in the premenstrual phase of the cycle, as progesterone antagonizes a proserotonergic effect of estrogen and then estrogen levels also drop. Future studies of inbred rat strains with stable neurobiological variations may identify strains with similar, paradoxical behavioral responses to estrogen and progesterone.

The fact that women have much greater and repetitive fluxes in reproductive hormones over the lifespan may enhance the potential for dysregulation of a wide variety of brain neurochemical systems. In addition, as noted above, organizational differences between male and female brains are caused by exposure to high levels of gonadal steroids in the pre- and perinatal periods. The interactions of these organizational effects in females with cyclical gonadal steroid hormone changes following puberty, followed then by menopause and the loss of these same steroids, suggest that stress responsiveness and susceptibility to stress-related disorders could vary substantially over the lifetime of women. There is certainly evidence that women's increased vulnerability to depression arises at puberty, when gonadal steroids could further enhance HPA axis responsiveness (Kessler et al., 1993). In addition, the evidence linking stress and glucocorticoids to hippocampal damage and subsequent memory problems (Issa et al., 1990), and the important role that gonadal steroids may play in protection from these effects in premenopausal women, imply that further research is needed into the interaction of stress, menopause, and memory impairment.

ACKNOWLEDGMENTS

We would like to acknowledge the support of National Institutes of Health Grant No. MH00427 to Elizabeth A. Young and Grant No. DE11972 to Ania Korszun.

REFERENCES

Abbud, R., Lee, W. S., Hoffman, G. E., et al. (1992). Lactation inhibits hippocampal and cortical activation of cFos expression by NMDA but not kainate receptor agonists. *Molecular Cell Neuroscience, 3*, 244–250.

Ahima, R. S., Lawson, A. N. L., Osei, S. Y. S., et al. (1992). Sexual dimorphism in regulation of type II corticosteroid receptor immunoreactivity in the rat hippocampus. *Endocrinology, 131*, 1409–1416.

Akil, H., Haskett, R., Young, E. A., et al. (1993). Multiple HPA profiles in endogenous depression: Effect of age and sex on cortisol and beta-endorphin. *Biological Psychiatry, 33*, 73–85.

Altemus, M., & Arleo, E. K. (1999). Modulation of anxiety by reproductive hormones. In E. L. Luft (Ed.), *Gender differences in mood and anxiety disorders* (pp. 53–89). Washington, DC: American Psychiatric Press.

Altemus, M., Deuster, P., Galliven, E., et al. (1995). Suppression of hypothalamic–pituitary adrenal axis responses to stress in lactating women. *Journal of Clinical Endocrinology and Metabolism, 80*, 2954–2959.

Altemus, M., Greenberg, B. D., Keuler, D., et al. (in press). Open trial of flutamide for treatment of obsessive–compulsive disorder. *Journal of Clinical Psychiatry.*

Altemus, M., Pigott, T., Kalogeras, K. T., et al. (1992). Abnormalities in the regulation of vasopressin and corticotropin releasing factor secretion in obsessive–compulsive disorder. *Archives of General Psychiatry, 49*, 9–20.

Altemus, M., Redwine, L., Yung-Mei, L., et al. (1997). Reduced sensitivity to glucocorticoid feedback and reduced glucocorticoid receptor mRNA expression in the luteal phase of the menstrual cycle. *Neuropsychopharmacology, 17*(2), 100–109.

Altshuler, L. L., Hendrick, V., & Cohen, I. S. (1998). Course of mood and anxiety disorders during pregnancy and the postpartum period. *Journal of Clinical Psychiatry, 59*(Suppl. 2), 29–33.

Anda, R., Williamson, D., Jones, C., et al. (1993). Depressed affect, hopelessness, and the risk of ischemic heart disease in a cohort of U. S. adults. *Epidemiology, 4*, 285–294.

Anderson, E. E. (1940). The sex hormones and emotional behavior: 1. The effect of sexual receptivity upon timidity in the female rat. *Journal of Genetic Psychology, 56*, 149–158.

Arato, M., Frecska, E., Tekes, K., et al. (1991). Serotonergic interhemispheric asymmetry: Gender difference in the orbital cortex. *Acta Psychiatrica Scandinavica, 84*(1), 110–111.

Arriza, J. L., Weinberger, C., Cerelli, G., et al. (1987). Cloning of human mineralocorticoid receptor complementary DNA: Structural and functional kinship with the glucocorticoid receptor. *Science, 237*, 268–275.

Aston-Jones, G., Shipley, M. T., Chouvet, G., et al. (1991). Afferent regulation of locus coeruleus neurons: Anatomy, physiology and pharmacology. *Progress in Brain Research, 88*, 47–75.

Aston-Jones, G., Rajkowski, J., Kubiak, P., & Alexinsky, T. (1994). Locus coeruleus neurons in monkey are selectively activated by attended cues in a vigilance task. *Journal of Neuroscience, 7*, 4467–4480.

Auricchio, F. (1989). Phosphorylation of steroid receptors. *Journal of Steroid Biochemistry, 32*, 613–622.

Baeken, C., D'haenen, H., Flamen, P., et al. (1998). 123I-5-I-R91150, a new single-photon emission tomography ligand for 5-HT2A receptors: Influence of age and gender in healthy subjects. *European Journal of Nuclear Medicine, 25*(12), 1617–1622.

Barden, N., Reul, J. M. H. M., & Holsboer, F. (1995). Do antidepressants stabilize mood through actions on the hypothalamic–pituitary–adrenocortical system? *Trends in Neuroscience, 18,* 6–10.

Biegon, A., Reches, A., Snyder, L., et al. (1983). Serotonergic and noradrenergic receptors in the rat brain: Modulation by chronic exposure to ovarian hormones. *Life Sciences, 32,* 2015–2021.

Biegon, A., & Greuner, N. (1992). Age-related changes in serotonin 5-HT2 receptors on human blood platelets. *Psychopharmacology, 108*(1–2), 210–212.

Birnberg, N. C., Civelli, O., Lissitzski, J. C., et al. (1979). Regulation of pro-opiomelanocortin gene expression in the pituitary and central nervous system. *Endocrinology, 110,* 134A.

Bitran, D., Hilvers, R. J., & Kellogg, C. K. (1991). Ovarian endocrine status modulates the anxiolytic potency of diazepam and the efficacy of gamma-aminobutyric acid–benzodiazepine receptor-mediated chloride ion transport. *Behavioral Neuroscience, 105,* 652–662.

Bonson, K. R., Johnson, R. G., Fiorella, D., et al. (1994). Serotonergic control of androgen-induced dominance. *Pharmacology Biochemistry and Behavior, 49,* 313–322.

Borisova, N. A., Proshlyakova, E. V., Sapronova, A. Y., et al. (1996). Androgen-dependent sex differences in the hypothalamic serotonergic system. *European Journal of Endocrinology, 134*(2), 232–235.

Brady, L., Whitfield, H. J., Fox, R. J., et al. (1991). Long-term antidepressant administration alters corticotropin releasing hormone, tyrosine hydroxylase and mineralocorticoid receptor gene expression in rat brain: Therapeutic implications. *Journal of Clinical Investigations, 87,* 831–837.

Breier, A., Davis, O., Buchanan, R., et al. (1992). Effects of alprazolam on pituitary–adrenal and catecholaminergic responses to metabolic stress in humans. *Biological Psychiatry, 15,* 880–890.

Bremner, J. D., Lincinio, J., Darnell, A., et al. (1997). Elevated CSF corticotropin-releasing factor concentrations in post-traumatic stress disorder. *American Journal of Psychiatry, 154,* 624–629.

Bremner, J. D., Randall, P., Scott, T. M., et al. (1995). MRI-based measurement of hippocampal volume in patients with combar-related posttraumatic stress disorder. *American Journal of Psychiatry, 152,* 973–981.

Brown, G. W., & Harris. T. (1978). *Social origins of depression: A study of psychiatric disorder in women.* New York: Free Press.

Brown, M. R., Fisher, L. A., Spiess, J., et al. (1982). Corticotropin releasing factor: Actions on sympathetic nervous system and metabolism. *Endocrinology, 111,* 928–931.

Burgess, L. H., & Handa, R. J. (1992). Chronic estrogen-induced alterations in adrenocorticotropin and corticosterone secretion, and glucocorticoid receptor-mediated functions in female rats. *Endocrinology, 131,* 1261–1269.

Burke, A. W., & Broadhurst, P. L. (1966). Behavioral correlates of the oestrous cycle in the rat. *Nature, 209,* 223–224.

Buterbaugh, G. G., & Hudson, G. M. (1991). Estradiol replacement to female rats facilitates dorsal hippocampal but not ventral hippocampal kindled seizure acquisition. *Experimental Neurology, 111,* 55–64.

Butler, P. D., & Nemeroff, C. B. (1990). Corticotropin releasing factor as a possible cause of comorbidity in anxiety and depressive disorders. In J. D. Maser & C. R. Cloninger (Eds.), *Comorbidity of mood and anxiety disorders* (pp. 413–435). Washington DC: American Psychiatric Press.

Carey, M. P., Deterd, C. H., de Koning, J., et al. (1995). The influence of ovarian steroids on hypothalamic–pituitary–adrenal regulation in the female rat. *Journal of Endocrinology, 144,* 311–332.

Carlsson, M., & Carlsson, A. (1988). A regional study in sex differences in rat brain serotonin. *Progress in Neuro-Psychopharmacology and Biological Psychiatry, 12*(1), 53–61.

Carr, B. R., Parker, C. R., Jr., Madden, J. D., et al. (1981). Maternal plasma adrenocorticotropin and cortisol relationships throughout human pregnancy. *American Journal of Obstetrics and Gynecology, 139,* 416–422.

Carroll, B. J., Curtis, G. C., & Mendels, J. (1976). Neuroendocrine regulation in depression: I. Limbic system–adrenocortical dysfunction. *Archives of General Psychiatry, 33,* 1039–1044.

Charney, D., Woods, S., Goodman, W., et al. (1987). Neurobiological mechanisms of panic anxiety: Biochemical and behavioral correlates of yohimbine-induced panic attacks. *American Journal of Psychiatry, 144,* 1030–1036.

Childs, G. V., Morell, J. L., Niendorf, A., et al. (1986). Cytochemical studies of corticotropin releasing factor receptors in anterior lobe corticotrophs: Binding, glucocorticoid regulation and endocytosis of [Biotinyl-Ser1] CRF. *Endocrinology, 119,* 2129.

Chrousos, G. P. (1998). A healthy body in a healthy mind—and vice versa—the damaging power of uncontrollable stress. *Journal of Clinical Endocrinology and Metabolism, 83,* 1842–1845.

Chrousos, G. P., & Gold, P. W. (1992). The concepts of stress and stress system disorders. Overview of physical and behavioral homeostasis. *Journal of the American Medical Association, 267,* 1244–1252.

Conrad, C. D., LeDoux, J. E., Magarinos, A. M., et al. (1999). Repeated restrain stress facilitates fear conditioning independently of causing hippocampal CA3 dendritic atrophy. *Behavioral Neurosciences, 5,* 902–913.

Coplan, J. D., Andrews, M. W., Rosenblum, L. A., et al. (1996). Persistent elevations of cerebrospinal fluid concentrations of corticotropin-releasing factor in adult nonhuman primates exposed to early-life stressors: Implications for the pathophysiology of mood and anxiety disorders. *Proceedings of the National Academy of Sciences USA, 93,* 1619–1623.

Corodimas, K. P., LeDoux, J. E., Gold, P. W., et al. (1994). Corticosterone potentiation of learned fear. *Annals of the New York Academy of Sciences, 746,* 392–393.

Dean, C., Williams, R. J., & Brockington, I. F. (1989). Is puerperal psychosis the same as bipolar manic-depressive disorder? A family study. *Psychological Medicine, 19,* 637–647.

deKloet, R., Wallach, G., & McEwen, B. S. (1975). Differences in corticosterone and dexamethasone binding to rat brain and pituitary. *Endocrinology, 96,* 598.

Demey-Ponsart, E., Foidart, J. M., Sulon, J., et al. (1982). Serum CBG, free and total cortisol and circadian patterns of adrenal function in normal pregnancy. *Journal of Steroid Biochemistry, 16,* 165–169.

Devenport, L. D. (1978). Schedule-induced polydipsia in rats: Adrenocortical and hippocampal modulation. *Journal of Comparative and Physiological Psychology, 92,* 651–660.

Diaz-Veliz, G., Alarcon, T., Espinoza, C., et al. (1997). Ketanserin and anxiety level: Influence of gender, estrus cycle, ovariectomy and ovarian hormones in female rats. *Pharmacology, Biochemistry and Behavior, 58,* 637–642.

Diaz-Veliz, G., Soto, V., Dussaubat, N., et al. (1989). Influence of the estrous cycle, ovariectomy and estradiol replacement upon the acquisition of conditioned avoidance responses in rats. *Physiology and Behavior, 46,* 397–401.

Duncan, M. R., & Duncan, G. R. (1979). An in vivo study of the action of antiglucocorticoids on thymus weight ratio, antibody titre and the adrenal–pituitary–hypothalamus axis. *Journal of Steroid Biochemistry, 10,* 245–259.

Dunn, A. J., & Berridge, C. W. (1990). Physiological and behavioral responses to corticotropin-releasing factor administration: Is CRF a mediator of anxiety or stress response? *Brain Research Reviews, 15,* 71–100.

Ehrenkranz, J. R. (1976). Effects of sex steroids on serotonin uptake in blood platelets. *Acta Endocrinologica, 83*(2), 420–428.

el Mansari, M., Bouchard, C., & Blier, P. (1995). Alteration of serotonin release in the guinea pig orbito-frontal cortex by selective serotonin reuptake inhibitors: Relevance to treatment of obsessive–compulsive disorder. *Neuropsychopharmacology, 13,* 117–127.

Endroczi, E., & Nyakas, C. S. (1972). Pituitary adrenal function during lactation and after LTH (prolactin) administration in the rat. *Acta Physiologica Academia Science Hungariea, 41,* 49–54.

Eriksson, E., Hedberg, M. A., Andersch, B., et al. (1995). The serotonin reuptake inhibitor paroxetine is superior to the noradrenaline reuptake inhibitor maprotiline in the treatment of premenstrual syndrome. *Neuropsychopharmacology, 12,* 167–176.

Farr, S. A., Flood, J. F., Scherrer, J. F., et al. (1995). Effect of ovarian steroids on footshock avoidance learning and retention in female mice. *Physiology and Behavior, 58,* 715–723.

Fernandez-Guasti, A., & Picazo, O. (1990). The actions of diazepam and serotonergic anxiolytics vary according to the gender and the estrous cycle phase. *Pharmacology, Biochemistry and Behavior, 37,* 77–81.

Fink, G., Sumner, B. E., Rosie, R., et al. (1996). Estrogen control of central neurotransmission: Effect on mood, mental state, and memory. *Cellular and Molecular Neurobiology, 16*(3), 325–344.

Fischette, C. T., Biegon, A., & McEwen, B. S. (1984). Sex steroid modulation of the serotonin behavioral syndrome. *Life Sciences, 35,* 1197–1206.

Fleming, A. S., & Luebke, C. (1981). Timidity prevents the virgin female rat from being a good mother: Emotionality differences between nulliparous and parturient females. *Physiology and Behavior, 27,* 863–868.

Frank, E., Anderson, B., Reynolds, C., et al. (1994). Life events and the Research Diagnostic Criteria endogenous subtype: A confirmation of the distinction using the Bedford College methods. *Archives of General Psychiatry, 51,* 519–524.

Galea, L. M., McEwen, B. S., Tanapat, P., et al. (1997). Sex differences in dendritic atrophy of CA3 pyramidal neurons in response to chronic restraint stress. *Neuroscience, 81,* 689–697.

Galliven, E. A., Singh, A., Michelson, D., Bina, S., Gold, P. W., & Deuster, P. A. (1997). Hormonal and metabolic responses to exercise across time of day and menstrual cycle phase. *Journal of Applied Physiology, 6,* 1822–1831.

Gazzaley, A. H., Weiland, N. G., McEwen, B. S., et al. (1996). Differential regulation of NMDAR1 mRNA and protein by estradiol in the rat hippocampus. *Journal of Neuroscience, 16,* 6830–6838.

Gelfin, Y., Lerer, B., Lesch, K. P., et al. (1995). Complex effects of age and gender on hypothermic, adrenocorticotrophic hormone and cortisol responses to ipsapirone challenge in normal subjects. *Psychopharmacology, 120*(3), 356–364.

Glavin, G. B. (1985). Methylphenidate effects on activity-stress gastric lesions and regional brain noradrenaline metabolism in rats. *Pharmacological Biochemical Behavior, 3,* 379–383.

Gray, A., & Levine, S. (1964). Effect of induced oestrus on emotional behaviour in selected strains of rats. *Nature, 201,* 1198–1200.

Gray, J. A. (1982). *The neuropsychology of anxiety: An enquiry into the functioning of the septohippocampal system.* New York: Oxford University Press.

Gregoire, A., Kumar, R., Everitt, B., et al. (1996). Transdermal oestrogen for treatment of severe postnatal depression. *Lancet, 347,* 930–933.

Greist, J. H., Jefferson, J. W., Kobak, K. A., et al. (1995). Efficacy and tolerability of serotonin transport inhibitors in obsessive–compulsive disorder. *Archives of General Psychiatry, 52,* 53–60.

Halbreich, U., Asnis, G. M., Zumoff, B., et al. (1984). The effect of age and sex on cortisol secretion in depressives and normals. *Psychiatry Research, 13,* 221–229.

Haleem, D. J., Kennett, G. A., & Curzon, G. (1990). Hippocampal 5–hydroxytryptamine synthesis is greater in female rats than in males and more decreased by the 5–HT1A agonist 8–OH-DPAT. *Journal of Neural Transmission, 79*(1–2), 93–101.

Hammaback, S., Backstrom, T., Holst, J., et al. (1985). Cyclical mood changes as in premenstrual tension syndrome during sequential estrogen–progestogen postmenopausal replacement therapy. *Acta Obstetricia Gynecologica Scandinavica, 64,* 393–397.

Hansen, S., & Ferreira, A. (1986). Food intake, aggression and fear behavior in the mother rat: Control by neural systems concerned with milk ejection and maternal behavior. *Behavioral Neuroscience*, *100*, 410–415.

Heim, C., Owens, M. J., Plotsky, P. M., et al. (1997). Persistent changes in corticotropin-releasing factor systems due to early life stress: Relationship to the pathophysiology of major depression and post-traumatic stress disorder. *Psychopharmacology Bulletin*, *33*, 185–192.

Heinsbroek, R. P., van Haaren, F., Feenstra, M. G., et al. (1990). Sex differences in the effects of inescapable footshock on central catecholaminergic and serotonergic activity. *Pharmacology, Biochemistry and Behavior*, *37*(3), 539–550.

Heinsbroek, R., van Haaren, F., Poll, N. V. D., et al. (1991). Sex differences in the behavioral consequences of inescapable footshocks depend on time since shock. *Physiology and Behavior*, *49*, 1257–1263.

Heninger, G. R., & Charney, D. S. (1987). Mechanism of action of antidepressant treatment: Implications for the etiology and treatment of depressive disorders. In H. Y. Meltzer (Ed.), *Psychopharmacology: The third generation of progress* (pp. 535–544). New York: Raven Press.

Herman, J. P., Schafer, M. K-H., Young, E. A., et al. (1989). Hippocampal regulation of the hypothalamo–pituitary–adrenocortical axis: In situ hybridization analysis of CRF and vasopressin messenger RNA expression in the hypothalamic paraventricular nucleus following hippocampectomy. *Journal of Neuroscience*, *9*, 3072–3082.

Higuchi, T., Negoro, H., & Arita, J. (1989). Reduced responses of prolactin and catecholamine to stress in the lactating rat. *Journal of Endocrinology*, *122*, 495–498.

Hrdina, P. D., Bakish, D., Chudzik, J., et al. (1995). Serotonergic markers in platelets of patients with major depression: Upregulation of 5–HT2 receptors. *Journal of Psychiatry and Neuroscience*, *20*(1), 11–19.

Issa, A. M., Rowe, W., & Meaney, M. J. (1990). Hypothalamic–pituitary–adrenal activity in aged, cognitively impaired and cognitively unimpaired rats. *Journal of Neuroscience*, *10*, 3247–3254.

Jacobson, L., & Sapolsky, R. (1991). The role of the hippocampus in feedback regulation of the hypothalamic–pituitary–adrenocortical axis. *Endocrine Review*, *12*, 118–134.

Jones, M. T., Brush, F. R., & Neame, R. L. B. (1972). Characteristics of fast feedback control of corticotrophin release by corticosteroids. *Journal of Endocrinology*, *55*, 489.

Katzenellenbogen, J., O'Malley, B., & Katzenellenbogen, B. (1996). Tripartite steroid hormone receptor pharmacology: Interaction with multiple effector sites as a basis for the cell- and promoter-specific action of these hormones. *Molecular Endocrinology*, *10*, 119–131.

Keller-Wood, M., Silbiger, J., & Wood, C. E. (1988). Progesterone attenuates the inhibition of adrenocorticotropin responses by cortisol in nonpregnant ewes. *Endocrinology*, *123*, 647–651.

Kendler, K. S. (1996). Major depression and generalized anxiety disorder. Same genes, (partly) different environments—revisited. *British Journal of Psychiatry*, *30*(Supp. l), 68–75.

Kendler, K. S., Kessler, R. C., Walters, E. E., et al. (1995). Stressful life events, genetic liability and onset of an episode of major depression in women. *American Journal of Psychiatry*, *152*, 833–842.

Kendrick, K. M., Keverne, E. B., Baldwin, B. A., et al. (1986). Cerebrospinal fluid levels of acetylcholinesterase, monoamines and oxytocin during labour, parturition, vaginocervical stimulation, lamb separation and suckling in sheep. *Neuroendocrinology*, *44*, 149–156.

Kendrick, K. M., Keverne, E. B., Chapman, C., et al. (1988). Intracranial dialysis measurement of oxytocin, monoamine and uric acid release from the olfactory bulb and substantia nigra of sheep during parturition, suckling, separation from lambs and eating. *Brain Research*, *439*, 1–10.

Kennet, G., Chaouloff, F., Marcou, M., et al. (1986). Female rats are more vulnerable than males in an animal model of depression: The possible role of serotonin. *Brain Research*, *382*, 416–421.

Kessler, R. C., McGonagle, K. A., Swartz, M., et al. (1993). Sex and depression in the National Comorbidity Survey: I. Lifetime prevalence, chronicity and recurrence. *Journal of Affective Disorders, 29*, 85–96.

Kessler, R. C., McGonagle, K. A., Zhao, S., et al. (1994). Lifetime and 12–month prevalence of DSM-III-R psychiatric disorders in the United States. *Archives of General Psychiatry, 51*, 8–19.

Kirk, R. C., & Blampied, N. M. (1985). Activity during inescapable shock and subsequent escape avoidance learning: Females and males compared. *New Zealand Journal of Psychology, 14*, 9–14.

Kirschbaum, C., Pirke, K.-M., & Hellhammer, D. H. (1995). Preliminary evidence for reduced cortisol responsivity to psychological stress in women using oral contraceptive medication. *Psychoneuroendocrinology, 20*, 509–514.

Kirschbaum, C., Schommer, N., Federenko, I., et al. (1996). Short-term estradiol treatment enhances pituitary–adrenal axis and sympathetic responses to psychosocial stress in healthy young men. *Journal of Clinical Endocrinology and Metabolism, 81*, 3639–3643.

Klein, D. F., Skrobala, A. M., & Garfinkel, R. S. (1995). Preliminary look at the effects of pregnancy on the course of panic disorder. *Anxiety, 1*, 227–232.

Koob, G. F., Heinrichs, S. C., Pich, E. M., et al. (1993). The role of corticotropin-releasing factor in behavioral responses to stress. *Ciba Foundation Symposium, 172*, 277–289.

Kuiper, G. G., Carlsson, B., Grandien, K., et al. (1997). Comparison of the ligand binding specificity and transcript tissue distribution of estrogen receptors ? and ß. *Endocrinology, 138*, 863–870.

Leckman, J. F., Goodwin, W. K., North, W. G., et al. (1994). The role of central oxytocin in obsessive–compulsive disorder and related normal behavior. *Psychoneuroendocrinology, 19*, 723–749.

LeDoux, J. (1996). *The emotional brain.* New York: Simon & Schuster.

Lerer, B., Gillon, D., Lichtenberg, P., et al. (1996). Interrelationship of age, depression, and central serotonergic function: Evidence from fenfluramine challenge studies. *International Psychogeriatrics, 8*(1), 83–102.

Lewis, D. A., Pfohl, B., Schlecte, J., et al. (1984). Influence of age on the cortisol response to dexamethasone. *Psychiatry Research, 13*, 213–220.

Lightman, S. L. (1992). Alterations in hypothalamic–pituitary responsiveness during lactation. *Annals of the New York Academy of Sciences, 652*, 340–346.

Lightman, S. L., & Young, W. S. (1989). Lactation inhibits stress-mediated secretion of corticosterone and oxytocin and hypothalamic accumulation of corticotropin-releasing factor and enkephalin messenger ribonucleic acids. *Endocrinology, 124*, 2358–2364.

Magarinos, A. M., & McEwen, B. S. (1995). Stress-induced atrophy of apical dendrites of hippocampal CA3c neurons: Involvement of glucocorticosteroid secretion and excitatory amino acid receptors. *Neuroscience, 69*, 89–98.

Marcusson, J., Oreland, L., & Winblad, B. (1984). Effect of age on human brain serotonin (S-1) binding sites. *Journal of Neurochemistry, 43*(6), 1699–1705.

Maren, S., DeOc, B., Fanselow, M. S. (1994). Sex differences in hippocampal long-term potentiation (LTP) and Pavlovian fear conditioning in rats: Positive correlation between LTP and contextual learning. *Brain Research, 661*, 25–34.

Markus, E. J., & Zecevic, M. (1997). Sex differences and estrous cycle changes in hippocampus-dependent fear conditioning. *Psychobiology, 25*, 246–252.

Martinez-Conde, E., Leret, M. L., & Diaz, S. (1985). The influence of testosterone in the brain of the male rat on levels of serotonin (5–HT) and 5–hydroxyindoleacetic acid (5–HIAA). *Comparative Biochemistry and Physiology, 80*, 411–414.

Matsuda, T., Nakano, Y., Kanda, T., et al. (1991). Gonadal hormones affect the hypothermia induced by serotonin1A (5-HT1A) receptor activation. *Life Sciences, 48*, 1627–1632.

McCarthy, M. M., & Altemus, M. (1997, June). Central nervous system actions of oxytocin and modulation of behavior in humans. *Molecular Medicine Today*, pp. 269–275.

McCarthy, M. M., Kaufman, L. C., Brooks, P. J., et al. (1995). Estrogen modulation of mRNA levels for the two forms of glutamic acid decarboxylase (GAD) in female rat brain. *Journal of Comparative Neurology, 360*, 685–697.

McCormick, C., Smythe, J., Sharma, S., et al. (1995). Sex-specific effects of prenatal stress on hypothalamic–pituitary–adrenal responses to stress and brain glucocorticoid receptor density in adult rats. *Brain Research: Developmental Brain Research, 84*, 55–61.

McEwen, S. B. (1995). Adrenal steroid actions on brain: Dissecting the fine line between protection and damage. In M. J. Friedman, D. S. Charney, & A. Y. Deutch (Eds.), *Neurobiological and clinical consequences of stress: From normal adaptation to PTSD* (pp. 135–147). Philadelphia: Lippincott–Raven.

McEwen, B. S., Alves, S. E., Bulloch, K., et al. (1997). Ovarian steroids and the brain: Implications for cognition and aging. *Neurology, 48*, S8–S15.

McEwen, B. S., Weiss, J. M., & Schwartz, L. S. (1968). Selective retention of corticosterone by limbic structures in the rat brain. *Nature, 220*, 911–913.

McEwen, B. S., Weiss, J. M., & Schwartz, L. S. (1970). Retention of corticosterone by cell nuclei from brain regions of adrenalectomized rats. *Brain Research, 17*, 471.

McNeilly, A. S., Tay, C. C. K., & Glasier, A. (1994). Physiological mechanisms underlying lactational amenorrhea. *Annals of the New York Academy of Sciences, 709*, 145–155.

McQueen, J. K., Wilson, H., & Fink, G. (1997). Estradiol-17 beta increases serotonin transporter (SERT) mRNA levels and the density of SERT-binding sites in female rat brain. *Brain Research: Molecular Brain Research, 45*(1), 13–23.

Meijer, O. C., & deKloet, R. (1998). Corticosterone and serotonergic neurotransmission in the hippocampus: Functional implications of central corticosteroid receptor diversity. *Critical Reviews in Neurobiology, 12*(1–2), 1–20.

Mendelson, S. D., & McEwen, B. S. (1990). Testosterone increases the concentration of (3H)8–hydroxy-2–(di-n-propylamino)tetralin binding at 5–HT1A receptors in the medial preoptic nucleus of the castrated male rat. *European Journal of Pharmacology, 181*, 329–331.

Mendelson, S. D., & McEwen, B. S. (1991). Autoradiographic analyses of the effects of restraint-induced stress on 5–HT1A, 5–HT1C and 5–HT2 receptors in the dorsal hippocampus of male and female rats. *Neuroendocrinology, 54*(5), 454–461.

Merikangas, K. R., Weissman, M. M., & Pauls, D. L. (1985). Genetic factors in the sex ratio of major depression. *Psychological Medicine, 15*, 63–69.

Meyer, M.-E., Gronemeyer, H., Turcutte, B., et al. (1989). Steroid hormone receptors compete for factors that mediate their enhancer function. *Cell, 57*, 433–442.

Mizoguchi, K., Kunishita, T., Chui, D. H., et al. (1992). Stress induces neuronal death in the hippocampus of castrated rats. *Neuroscience Letters, 138*, 157–160.

Monteleone, P., Catapano, F., Tortorella, A., et al. (1997). Cortisol response to d-fenfluramine in patients with obsessive–compulsive disorder and in healthy subjects: Evidence for a gender-related effect. *Neuropsychobiology, 36*(1), 8–12.

Moore, R. Y., & Bloom, F. E. (1979). Central catecholamine neuron systems: Anatomy and physiology of the norepinephrine and epinephrine systems. *Annual Review of Neuroscience, 2*, 113–168.

Mora, S., Dussaubat, N., & Diaz-Veliz, G. (1996). Effects of the estrous cycle and ovarian hormones on behavioral indices of anxiety in female rats. *Psychoneuroendocrinology, 21*, 609–620.

Mortola, J. F., Girton, L., & Fischer, U. (1991). Successful treatment of severe premenstrual syndrome by combined use of gonadotropin-releasing hormone agonist and estrogen/progestin. *Journal of Clinical Endocrinology and Metabolism, 72*, 252A–252F.

Munck, A., & Guyre, P. M. (1986). Glucocorticoid physiology, pharmacology and stress. *Advances in Experimental Medicine and Biology, 196*, 81–96.

Murua, V. S., & Molina, V. A. (1992). Effects of chronic variable stress and antidepressant drugs on behavioral inactivity during an uncontrollable stress: Interaction between both treatments. *Behavioral and Neural Biology, 57,* 87–89.

Neumann, I., & Landgraf, R. (1989). Septal and hippocampal release of oxytocin, but not vasopressin, in the conscious lactating rat during suckling. *Journal of Neuroendocrinology, 1,* 305–308.

Neumann, I. D., Johnstone, H. A., Hatzinger, M., et al. (1998). Attenuated neuroendocrine responses to emotional and physical stressors in pregnant rats involve adenohypophysial changes. *Journal of Physiology, 508,* 289–300.

Newton, M., & Newton, N. R. (1948). The let-down reflex in human lactation. *Journal of Pediatrics, 33,* 698–704.

Nezeroglu, F., Anemone, R., & Yaryura-Tobia, J. (1992). Onset of obsessive–compulsive disorder in pregnancy. *American Journal of Psychiatry, 149,* 947–950.

Nolten, W. E., & Rueckert, P. A. (1981). Elevated free cortisol index in pregnancy: Possible regulatory mechanisms. *American Journal of Obstetrics and Gynecology, 139,* 492–498.

Nomikos, G. G., & Spiraki, C. (1988). Influence of oestrogen in spontaneous and diazepam-induced exploration of rats in an elevated plus-maze. *Neuropharmacology, 27,* 691–696.

Parsons, B., Rainbow, T. C., MacLusky, N. J., et al. (1982). Progesterone receptor levels in rat hypothalamic and limbic nuclei. *Journal of Neuroscience, 2,* 1446–1452.

Patchev, V., Hayashi, S., Orikasa, C., et al. (1995). Implications of estrogen-dependent brain organization for gender difference in hypothalamic–pituitary–adrenal regulation. *FASEB Journal, 9,* 419–423.

Pecins-Thompson, M., Brown, N. A., Kohama, S. G., et al. (1996). Ovarian steroid regulation of tryptophan hydroxylase mRNA expression in rhesus macaques. *Journal of Neuroscience, 16,* 7021–7029.

Pitman, R. K. (1982). Neurological etiology of obsessive–compulsive disorders? *American Journal of Psychiatry, 139,* 139–140.

Plotsky, P. M. (1987). Facilitation of immunoreactive corticotropin-releasing factor secretion into the hypophyseal–portal circulation after activation of catechoaminergic pathways or central norepinephrine injection. *Endocrinology, 121,* 924–930.

Plotsky, P. M., Cunningham, E. T., & Widmaier, E. P. (1989). Catecholaminergic modulation of corticotropin-releasing factor and adrenocorticotropin secretion. *Endocrine Reviews, 10,* 437–458.

Pohl, C. R., Lee, L. R., & Smith, M. S. (1989). Qualitative changes in luteinizing hormone and prolactin responses to N-methyl-D-aspartic acid during lactation in the rat. *Endocrinology, 124,* 1905–1911.

Port, R. L., Sample, J. A., & Seybold, K. S. (1991). Partial hippocampal pyramidal cell loss alters behavior in rats: Implications for an animal model of schizophrenia. *Brain Research Bulletin, 26,* 993–996.

Qureshi, G. A., Hansen, S., & Sodersten, P. (1987). Offspring control of cerebrospinal fluid GABA concentrations in lactating rats. *Neuroscience Letters, 75,* 85–88.

Reul, J. M. H., & deKloet, E. R. (1985). Two receptor systems for corticosterone in rat brain: Microdistribution and differential occupation. *Endocrinology, 117,* 2505–2511.

Reul, J. M., Stec, I., Soder, M., et al. (1993). Chronic treatment of rats with the antidepressant amitriptyline attenuates the activity of the hypothalamic–pituitary adrenocortical system. *Endocrinology, 133,* 312–320.

Robel, P., & Baulieu, E. E. (1995). Neurosteroids: Biosynthesis and function. *Critical Reviews in Neurobiology, 9,* 383–394.

Roberts, J. L., Budarf, M. L., Baxter, J. D., & Herbert, E. (1979). Selective reduction of proadrenocorticotropin/endorphin proteins and messenger ribonucleic acid activity in mouse pituitary tumor cells by glucocorticoids. *Biochemistry, 22*, 4907–4915.

Roca, A. C., Altemus, M., Galliven, E., et al. (1998a). Effect of reproductive hormones on the hypothalamic–pituitary–adrenal axis response to stress. *Biological Psychiatry, 43*, 6S.

Roca, C. A., Schmidt, P. J., Altemus, M., et al. (1998b, June). *Effects of reproductive steroids on the hypothalamic–pituitary–adrenal axis response to low dose dexamethasone.* Abstract, Neuroendocrine Workshop on Stress, New Orleans, LA.

Rodier, W. I. (1971). Progesterone–estrogen interaction in the control of activity-wheel running in the female rat. *Journal of Comparative Physiology and Psychology, 74*, 365–373.

Rodriguez-Sierra, J. F., Hagkey, M. T., & Hendricks, S. E. (1986). Anxiolytic effects of progesterone are sexually dimorphic. *Life Sciences, 38*, 1841–1845.

Rodriguez-Sierra, J. F., Howard, J. L., Pollard, G. T., et al. (1984). Effects of ovarian hormones on conflict behavior. *Psychoneuroendocrinology, 9*, 293–300.

Roozendaal, B. J., & McGaugh, J. L. (1996). Amygdaloid lesions differentially affect glucocorticoid-induced memory enhancement in an inhibitory avoidance task. *Neurobiology of Learning and Memory, 65*, 1–8.

Rosenbaum, A. H., Ginsburg, K., Rosenberg, R., et al. (1996, August). *Treatment of major depression and manic–depressive illness with gonadotropin-releasing hormone-agonist therapy.* Abstract, International Society of Psychoneuroendocrinology XXVIIth Congress, Cascais, Portugal.

Rousseau, G. G., Baxter, J. D., & Tomkins, G. M. (1972). Glucocorticoid receptors: Relations between steroid binding and biological effects. *Molecular Biology, 67*, 99–115.

Rubin, R. T., Poland, R. E., Lesser, I. M., et al. (1987). Neuroendocrine aspects of primary endogenous depression I. Cortisol secretory dynamics in patients and matched controls. *Archives of General Psychiatry, 44*, 328–336.

Rubinow, D. R., Hoban, M., Grover, G. N., et al. (1998). Changes in plasma hormones across the menstrual cycle in patients with menstrually related mood disorder and in control subjects. *American Journal of Obstetrics and Gynecology, 158*, 5–11.

Rubinow, D. R., & Roy-Byrne, P. P. (1984). Premenstrual syndromes: Overviews from a methodologic perspective. *American Journal of Psychiatry, 141*, 163–172.

Rupprecht, R., Hauser, C. A., Trapp, T., et al. (1996). Neurosteroids: Molecular mechanisms of action and psychopharmacologic significance. *Journal of Steroid Biochemistry and Molecular Biology, 56*, 163–168.

Ryan, N., Birmaher, B., Perel, J. M., et al. (1992). Neuroendocrine response to L-5–hydroxytryptophan challenge in prepubertal major depression. *Archives of General Psychiatry, 49*(11), 843–851.

Sachar, E. J., Hellman, L., Roffwarg, H. P., et al. (1973). Disrupted 24 hour patterns of cortisol secretion in psychotic depressives. *Archives of General Psychiatry, 28*, 19–24.

Sapolsky, R. M., Krey, L. C., & McEwen, B. S. (1986). The neuroendocrinology of stress and aging: The glucocorticoid cascade hypothesis. *Endocrine Reviews, 7*, 284–301.

Schacter, B. S., Johnson, L. K., Baxter, J. D., et al. (1982). Differential regulation by glucocorticoids of proopiomelanocortin mRNA levels in the anterior and intermediate lobes of the rat pituitary. *Endocrinology, 110*, 1142.

Schlein, P. A., Zarrow, M. X., & Denenberg, V. H. (1974). The role of prolactin in the depressed or "buffered" adrenocorticosteroid response of the rat. *Journal of Endocrinology, 62*, 93–99.

Schmaltz, L. W., & Isaacson, R. L. (1967). Effect of bilateral hippocampal destruction on the acquisition and extinction of an operant response. *Physiology and Behavior, 2*, 291–298.

Schumacher, M., Coirini, H., & McEwen, B. (1989). Regulation of high-affinity GABAa receptors in the dorsal hippocampus by estradiol and progesterone. *Brain Research, 487*, 178–183.

Schwartz, J., Billestrup, N., Perrin, M., Rivier, J., & Vale, W. (1986). Identification of corticotropin releasing factor target cells and effects of dexamethasone on binding in anterior pituitary using a fluorescent analog of CRF. *Endocrinology, 119,* 2376.

Seckl, J. R., & Fink, G. (1991). Use of in situ hybridization to investigate the regulation of hippocampal corticosteroid receptors by monoamines. *Journal of Steroid Biochemistry and Molecular Biology, 40*(4–6), 685–688.

Sheline, Y. I., Wang, P. W., Gado, M. H., et al. (1996). Hippocampal atrophy in recurrent major depression. *Proceedings of the National Academy of Sciences USA, 93,* 3908–3913.

Simerly, R. B., Chang, C., Muramatsu, M., et al. (1990). Distribution of androgen and estrogen receptor mRNA-containing cells in the rat brain: An in situ hybridization study. *Journal of Comparative Neurology, 294,* 76–95.

Smith M. A., Brady, L. S., Glowa, J., Gold, P. W., & Herkenham, M. (1991). Effects of stress and adrenalectomy on tyrosine hydroxylase mRNA levels in the locus ceruleus by in situ hybridization. *Brain Research, 544,* 26–32.

Smith, M. S. (1993). Lactation alters neuropeptide-Y and proopiomelanocortin gene expression in the arcuate nucleus of the rat. *Endocrinology, 133,* 1258–1265.

Smith, S. S. (1989). Estrogen administration increases neuronal responses to excitatory amino acids as a long term effect. *Brain Research, 503,* 354–357.

Southwick, S., Krystal, J., & Morgan, C. (1993). Abnormal noradrenergic function in posttraumatic stress disorder. *Archives of General Psychiatry, 50,* 266–274.

Starkman, M. N., Gebarski, S., Berent, S., et al. (1992). Hippocampal formation volume, memory dysfunction, and cortisol levels in patients with Cushing's syndrome. *Biological Psychiatry, 32,* 756–765.

Steenbergen, H. L., Heinsbroek, R. P. W., VanHaaren, F., et al. (1990). Sex-dependent effects of inescapable shock administration on shuttlebox-escape performance and elevated plus-mase behavior. *Physiology and Behavior, 48,* 571–576.

Svec, F. (1988). Differences in the interaction of RU 486 and ketoconazole with the second binding site of the glucocorticoid receptor. *Endocrinology, 123,* 1902–1906.

Terasawa, E., & Timiras, P. S. (1967). Electrical activity during the estrous cycle of the rat: Cyclic changes in limbic structures. *Endocrinology, 83,* 207–216.

Teyler, T. J., Vardaris, R. M., Lewis, D., et al. (1980). Gonadal steroids: Effects on excitability of hippocampal pyramidal neurons. *Science, 209,* 1017–1019.

Turner, B. B., & Weaver, D. A. (1985). Sexual dimorphism of glucocorticoid binding in rat brain. *Brain Research, 343,* 16–23.

Uht, R., Anderson, C., Webb, P., et al. (1997). Transcriptional activities of estrogen and glucocorticoid receptors are functionally integrated at the AP-1 response element. *Endocrinology, 138,* 2900–2908.

Uno, H., Else, J. G., Suleman, M. A., et al. (1989). Hippocampal damage associated with prolonged and fatal stress in primates. *Journal of Neuroscience, 9,* 1705–1711.

Vale, W., Spiess, J., Rivier, J., et al. (1981). Characterization of a 41-residue ovine hypothalamic peptide that stimulates secretions of corticotropin and beta-endorphin. *Science, 213,* 1394–1397.

Valentino, R. J. (1989). Corticotropin-releasing factor: Putative neurotransmitter in the noradrenergic nucleus locus coeruleus. *Psychopharmacology Bulletin, 25,* 306–311.

Vamvakopoulos, N. C., & Chrousos, G. P. (1993). Evidence of direct estrogenic regulation of human corticotropin-releasing hormone gene expression. *Journal of Clinical Investigation, 92,* 1896–1902.

Viau, V., & Meaney, M. J. (1991). Variations in the hypothalamic–pituitary–adrenal response to stress during the estrous cycle in the rat. *Endocrinology, 129,* 2503–2511.

Walker, C. D., Lightman, S. L., Steele, M. K., et al. (1992). Suckling is a persistent stimulus to the adrenocortical system of the rat. *Endocrinology, 130,* 115–125.

Warren, S. G., Humphries, A. G., Juraska, J. M., et al. (1995). LTP varies across the estrous cycle: Enhanced synaptic plasticity in proestrus rats. *Brain Research, 703,* 26–30.

Watts, A. G., & Sanchez-Watts, G. (1995). Region specific regulation of neuropeptide mRNA levels in neurons of the limbic forebrain by adrenal steroids. *Journal of Physiology (London), 484,* 721–736.

Weiland, N. (1992a). Estradiol selectively regulates agonist binding sites on the N-methyl-D-aspartate receptor complex in the CA1 region of the hippocampus. *Endocrinology, 131,* 662–668.

Weiland, N. (1992b). Glutamic acid decarboxylase messenger ribonucleic acid is regulated by estradiol and progesterone in the hippocampus. *Endocrinology, 131,* 2697–2702.

Weisenfeld, A. R., Malatesta, C. Z., Whitman, P. B., et al. (1985). Psychophysiological response of breast- and bottle-feeding mothers to their infants' signals. *Psychophysiology, 22,* 79–86.

Weiss, J. M., Glazer, H. I., Pohorecky, L. A., Brick, J., & Miller, N. E. (1975). Effects of chronic exposure to stressors on avoidance-escape behavior and on brain norepinephrine. *Psychosomatic Medicine, 37,* 522–534.

Weissman, M. M., & Olfson, M. Depression in women: Implications for health care research. *Science, 269,* 799–801, 1995

Wong, M., & Moss, R. L. (1992). Long-term and short-term electrophysiological effects of estrogen on the synaptic properties of hippocampal CA1 neurons. *Journal of Neuroscience, 12,* 3217–3225.

Wong, M., Thompson, T. L., & Moss, R. L. (1996). Nongenomic actions of estrogen in the brain: Physiological significance and cellular mechanisms. *Critical Reviews in Neurobiology, 10,* 189–203.

Wood, G. E., & Shors, T. J. (1998). Stress facilitates classical conditioning in males, but impairs classical conditioning in female through activational effects of ovarian hormones. *Proceedings of the National Academy of Sciences USA, 95,* 4066–4071.

Woolley, C., & McEwen, B. S. (1992). Estradiol mediates fluctuation in hippocampal synapse density during the estrous cycle in the adult rat. *Journal of Neuroscience, 12,* 2549–2554.

Woolley, C. S., & McEwen, B. S. (1994). Estradiol regulates hippocampal dendritic spine density via an N-methyl-D-aspartate receptor-dependent mechanism. *Journal of Neuroscience, 14,* 7680–7687.

Yang, J. (1994). Intrathecal administration of oxytocin induces analgesia in low back pain involving the endogenous opiate peptide system. *Spine, 19,* 867–871.

Yehuda, R., Boisoneau, D., Lowy, M. T., et al. (1995). Dose–response changes in plasma cortisol and lymphocyte glucocorticoid receptors following dexamethasone administration in combat veterans with and without posttraumatic stress disorder. *Archives of General Psychiatry, 52,* 583–593.

Yoshino, K. (1982). [Concentrations of monoamines and monoamine metabolites in cerebrospinal fluid determined by high-performance liquid chromatography with electrochemical detection]. *Brain and Nerve, 34*(11), 1099–1106.

Young, E. A. (1996). Sex differences in response to exogenous corticosterone. *Molecular Psychiatry, 1,* 313–319.

Young, E. A., Haskett, R. F., Grunhaus, L., et al. (1994). Increased evening activation of the hypothalamic pituitary adrenal axis in depressed patients. *Archives of General Psychiatry, 51,* 701–707.

Young, E. A., Haskett, R. F., Watson, S. J., & Akil, H. (1991). Loss of glucocorticoid fast feedback in depression. *Archives of General Psychiatry, 48,* 693–699.

Young, E. A., Kotun, J., Haskett, R. F., et al. (1993). Dissociation between pituitary and adrenal suppression to dexamethasone in depression. *Archives of General Psychiatry, 50,* 395–403.

Young, E. A., Kwak, S. P., & Kottak, J. (1995). Negative feedback regulation following administration of chronic exogenous corticosterone. *Journal of Neuroendocrinology, 7,* 37–45.

Young, E. A., & Vazquez, D. (1996). Hypercortisolemia, hippocampal glucocorticoid receptors and fast feedback. *Molecular Psychiatry, 1,* 149–159.

Zhu, Y., Yen, P., Chin, W., et al. (1996). Estrogen and thyroid hormone interaction on regulation of gene expression. *Proceedings of the National Academy of Sciences USA, 93,* 12587–12592.

Zweifel, J. E., & O'Brien, W. H. (1997). A meta-analysis of the effect of hormone replacement therapy upon depressed mood. *Psychoneuroendocrinology, 22,* 189–212.

2

Sex Differences
in Psychopharmacology

OLGA BRAWMAN-MINTZER

For many years, researchers argued the lack of gender-related differences in drug metabolism in humans (Kato, 1974). Others stated that although gender differences may exist for a few agents, they are of minor clinical importance (Giudicelli & Tillement, 1977). Thus it is not surprising that research on potential gender differences in pharmacokinetics and pharmacodynamics in humans has received little attention, and that women have been significantly underrepresented in pharmacological clinical treatment trials. In contrast, gender differences in the pharmacokinetics and pharmacodynamics of many drugs have been well known in animals. For example, researchers reported as early as 1932 that female rats may require lower doses of some drugs (such as barbiturates) to obtain clinical effects similar to those seen in male rats (Skett, 1988). However, it was not until 1993 that the U.S. Food and Drug Administration (FDA) revised its old guidelines, which excluded women of childbearing potential from clinical trials, and the National Institutes of Health introduced similar changes for government-sponsored studies (FDA, 1993). To date, the available data on gender-related variation in the effects of psychotropic agents are still limited, but there is some evidence suggesting possible gender differences in the pharmacokinetics and pharmacodynamics of many drugs. It should be noted that the true extent and the clinical significance of these gender-related differences are still unclear and subject to debate. This chapter highlights the available data on the effects of gender on drug pharmacokinetics and pharmacodynamics, with a focus on psychotropic agents.

GENDER DIFFERENCES IN PHARMACOKINETICS

Pharmacokinetics

Pharmacokinetics is the study of the absorption, distribution, biotransformation, and elimination of drugs and their metabolites from the body. These processes play an important role in determining the pharmacological effects of drugs, and thus deserve special consideration. First, the route and rate of drug administration can be used to control the rate of drug availability and to determine the onset and duration of its pharmacological effects. For example, an intravenous injection ensures that the entire administered drug is available to the circulation. However, intramuscular administration, which is commonly thought to produce a rapid onset of effects, can also be slow and erratic (Greenblatt et al., 1974). Most psychotropic drugs are administered orally. Oral drug absorption is primarily a passive process occurring in the small intestine. The efficiency of oral absorption is influenced by the physiological state of the patient, drug properties, and the timing of administration. For example, the presence of food or antacid drugs in the stomach usually decreases the rate of drug absorption. The amount of drug that is absorbed from the gastrointestinal tract also depends on the acid base and lipophilic properties of the medication, as well as the physiology of the gastrointestinal tract. Many drugs undergo extensive metabolism as they move from the gastrointestinal tract to the systemic circulation. This process is called "first-pass effect" or "presystemic elimination." First-pass effect may lead to decreased amount of a drug's reaching the systemic circulation or to an increased amount of its metabolites; thus first-pass effect is a major source of pharmacokinetic variability. Drugs are metabolized in the gut by cytochrome P450 (CYP450 enzymes, which are present in the epithelium of the small intestine (Kolars et al., 1992). The 3A4 isoenzyme of CYP450 (or CYP3A4, for short) represents approximately 70% of the total CYP450 found in the human intestine, and therefore has a significant effect on presystemic metabolism.

Following absorption, drugs are distributed to various tissues. The rate of drug distribution plays an important role in the onset of its pharmacological effects. Several factors may affect the distribution of a drug in the body. Drug distribution depends on membrane permeability, differences in blood volume, cardiac output, and organ size (Gilman et al., 1990). Other variables include acid base, water and lipid solubility, and the affinity of the drug for plasma proteins and tissue components (Riester et al., 1980). The ratio of lean body mass to adipose tissue mass may also affect distribution. Only unbound drug is capable of being distributed between plasma and tissues. As drug concentration in plasma declines due to distribution out of the systemic circulation, drug concentration in the tissue increases. Equilibrium is eventually reached between the drug in plasma and in the tissue.

Finally, most drugs are eliminated from the body through renal excretion in an unchanged form, through biotransformation in the liver to polar metabolites, or both. Renal excretion is a major route of elimination for many drugs, especially their hydrophilic metabolites. The processes involved in renal excretion of a drug may be a combination of glomerular filtration, tubular secretion, and tubular reabsorption. The net drug excretion resulting from these processes can be further modulated by such factors as renal blood flow, protein binding, and urine pH and flow.

The biotransformation of drugs in the liver involves Phase I and Phase II reactions. Phase I reactions include the oxidation, hydroxylation, N-demethylation, reduction, and hydrolysis of different compounds. These reactions are mediated through the CYP450 system, which is involved in the oxidative metabolism of various endogenous compounds (such as steroids) and numerous drugs. Phase II reactions consist of glucoronidation, sulfation, methylation, and/or acetylation of parent molecules and Phase I reaction products.

With the appearance of the selective serotonin reuptake inhibitors (SSRIs) and the evidence of their ability to inhibit specific CYP450 isoenzymes, many psychopharmacologists began focusing on research of the biochemistry, genetics, and clinical pharmacology of the CYP450 system. Of the human CYP450 enzymes, three major isoenzyme families—the CYP1, CYP2, and CYP3 groups—appear to be involved in drug metabolism (Guengerich, 1992). CYP3A4 is considered clinically the most important CYP450 isoenzyme, constituting as much as 60% of the total CYP450 content of *in vitro* liver specimens (Guengerich, 1990). CYP3A4 is involved in the metabolism of a broad range of compounds, including alprazolam, midazolam, diazepam, terfenadine, astemizole, carbamazepine, tricyclic antidepressants (TCAs), nefazodone, calcium channel blockers, erythromycin, steroids, quinidine, lidocaine, and others (Pollock, 1994; Smith & Jones, 1992; Kerr et al., 1994; Murray, 1992; von Moltke et al., 1999). Importantly, there is *in vitro* evidence for varied inhibition of CYP3A3/4 by frequently prescribed antidepressants, such as nefazodone, fluvoxamine, and the fluoxetine metabolite norfluoxetine (von Moltke et al., 1995, 1999). Plasma concentrations of some drugs metabolized by this isoenzyme have been observed to increase during concomitant therapy with fluvoxamine, nefazodone, or fluoxetine, but only negligibly (or not at all) during therapy with sertraline, paroxetine, or venlafaxine (Anderson et al., 1991; Amchin et al., 1998; Greene et al., 1995). Although CYP3A4 participates in the metabolism of the largest number of drugs, CYP2D6 is probably the most extensively studied isoenzyme (Brosen, 1990). Approximately 5% to 10% of Caucasians lack this isoenzyme as a result of an autosomal recessive defect in gene expression. Such "poor metabolizers" may exhibit greater bioavailability, higher plasma concentrations, prolonged elimination half-lives, and possibly exaggerated pharmacological response from standard doses of drugs that are metabolized by CYP2D6. CYP2D6 metabolizes many different classes of drugs, including antidepressants, antipsychotics, ß-adrenergic blockers, Type 1C antiarrhythmics, dextromethorphan, and some chemotherapeutic agents. For example, codeine and venlafaxine are both O-demethylated by this enzyme (Otton et al., 1994; Brosen & Gram, 1989). Nortriptyline, desipramine, and imipramine are hydroxylated by CYP2D6. CYP2D6 is also involved in the clearance of paroxetine (Bloomer et al., 1992). A number of different drugs potentially inhibit CYP2D6, including quinidine, fluphenazine, haloperidol, thioridazine, amitriptyline, desipramine, and clomipramine. Of the SSRIs, fluoxetine and paroxetine are potent inhibitors of CYP2D6, whereas sertraline and fluvoxamine are nearly an order of magnitude lower. Citalopram, nefazodone, and venlafaxine are very weak CYP2D6 inhibitors (Brosen, 1990; Pollock, 1994; Crewe et al., 1992; Otton et al., 1993, 1996; von Moltke et al., 1999; Schmider et al., 1996).

CYP2C is a subfamily of enzymes that includes 2C9, 2C10, 2C19, and others. CYP2C enzymes demethylate diazepam, clomipramine, amitriptyline, and imipramine. In addition, warfarin (Rettie et al., 1992), phenytoin (Smith & Jones, 1992), tolbutamide (Knodell et al., 1987), and certain nonsteroidal anti-inflammatory agents (Newlands et al., 1992) are also believed to be metabolized by CYP2C enzymes. Based on the observed increases in plasma concentrations of concomitantly administered drugs that are metabolized by this family of enzymes, it is believed that the SSRIs fluvoxamine, fluoxetine, and sertraline may inhibit CYP2C isoenzymes (Jalil, 1992; Skjelbo & Brosen, 1992).

Finally, within the CYP1 isoenzyme family, CYP1A2 isoenzyme is involved in the metabolism of various commonly used compounds and drugs. CYP1A2 appears to be involved in the metabolism of theophylline, caffeine (Wrighton & Stevens, 1992), TCAs (Pollock, 1994; Brosen, 1993), clozapine (Jerling et al., 1994), and possibly thiothixene (Ereshefsky et al., 1991). CYP1A2 is induced by cigarette smoke, charcoal-broiled foods, and cabbage (Pollock, 1994; Brosen, 1993; Guengerich, 1992). Furthermore, CYP1A2 shows potent inhibition by fluvoxamine *in vitro* (Brosen et al., 1993). However, other SSRIs do not appear to inhibit this isoenzyme.

In summary, it is clear that the various pharmacokinetic processes described above may significantly affect the relationship between dosing and drugs' pharmacological effects. Therefore, the understanding of these processes is invaluable in the course of developing appropriate dosage regimens. There are also growing data indicating that drug absorption, bioavailability, distribution, and metabolism may be further affected by gender and gender-related variables, such as the use of exogenously administered female hormones. The following section reviews the potential gender-related differences in drug pharmacokinetics and their clinical significance.

Absorption and Bioavailability

It has been suggested that women secrete less gastric acid than men, which may lead to potential gender differences in absorption (Grossman et al., 1963). Subsequently, a decrease in gastric acid secretion may decrease enzymatic action and decrease the absorption of weak acids, but increase absorption of weak bases. There are also several studies that suggest gender differences in gastric emptying and gastrointestinal transit time (Sweeting, 1992; McBurney, 1991). For example, Wald et al. (1981) reported that gastrointestinal transit time was significantly prolonged in women during the luteal phase of the menstrual cycle. Other researchers (Datz et al., 1987) demonstrated similar results (i.e., that women empty solids from their stomachs more slowly than men do). The mechanism for these differences is unknown, but researchers hypothesize that it may be due to the effects of progesterone and estradiol on the gastrointestinal tract. It should also be noted that there some studies have failed to demonstrate significant effects of menstrual hormones on gastrointestinal transit time (e.g., Degen & Phillip, 1996).

Gender differences in the activity of various gastrointestinal enzymes may also affect drug metabolism. For example, CYP3A4 appears to be more active in women than in men (Kolars et al., 1991; Strobel et al., 1991). It is unknown, however, whether increased activity of CYP3A4 in the liver also affects the gastrointestinal enzyme analogue.

Despite the potential differences in gastric acid secretion, gastrointestinal transit time, and differences in enzyme activity, no consistent differences in the absorption and the bioavailability of various agents have been observed. For example, for some agents such as the antihistamine mizolastine, significant gender differences in the duration of absorption of the compound have been observed (3.09 hours for men vs. 0.67 hours for women) (Mesnil et al., 1998). In contrast, researchers found that following oral administration, aspirin (in the form of lysine salt) was absorbed more rapidly in women than in men, but the overall bioavailability did not differ between genders (Aarons et al., 1989). However, others have found higher bioavailability of aspirin (in its pure form) in women then men, resulting in higher plasma levels in females (Ho et al., 1985). The clinical significance of such differences has yet to be determined.

Distribution

Potential gender differences in drug distribution may be the result of different proportions of muscular and adipose tissue in men and women, lower weight in women, and higher percentage of their body mass as fat (Seeman, 1989). Physiological changes during the menstrual cycle, surges in hormones, and fluctuations in water and electrolyte balance may influence distribution as well. Although empirical data are lacking, it can be hypothesized that menstrual-phase-related increases in fluid retention may dilute the concentration of medications, resulting in lower plasma levels and vice versa. One study also found evidence of menstrual phase changes in transcapillary fluid dynamics, resulting in fluid shifts between intravascular and extravascular spaces (Pollan & Oian, 1986).

As mentioned, women have a lower ratio of lean body mass to adipose tissue; thus drugs with high affinity for adipose tissue, such as diazepam, would be expected to demonstrate a greater volume of distribution in females. Specifically, for these drugs the half-life may become prolonged and serum levels may be greater in patients with less lean body mass. Female patients with a higher percentage of fat at any given body weight may also require a higher initial dose, but maintenance over time of the same dose will cause drug accumulation, leading to potentially toxic effects.

Levels of plasma-binding proteins may also affect drug distribution. It has been shown that concentration of the binding protein α1-acid glycoprotein (AAG) is decreased by estrogen (Tuck et al., 1997). Thus plasma concentrations of AAG may be somewhat lower in females than in males. These differences may be considered when monitoring drug effects, because the free, unbound drug concentration determines its pharmacological activity.

Metabolism

O'Malley et al. (1971) first reported that the metabolism of phenazone (antipyrine) is influenced by gender. At that time, antipyrine metabolism was thought to reflect total CYP450 activity. However, in recent years many isoenzymes of CYP450 have been identified, and there are increasing data on potential gender differences in the activity of these various isoenzymes. Since the majority of antidepressants and antipsychotic drugs are either metabolized by one or more CYP450 isoenzymes, or inhibit these isoenzymes to varying degrees, the potential sex differences in the activity of these isoenzymes may be of particular relevance to the clinician.

CYP3A4 Activity

There are substantial data indicating that young women may have approximately 1.4 times the CYP3A4 activity of men. For example, erythromycin is metabolized 25% more rapidly by microsomes made from the human female liver than by microsomes made from the male liver (Hunt et al., 1992). Other drugs that show a similar sex difference in clearance include diazepam (Greenblatt et al., 1980a; Hulst et al., 1994), verapamil (Schwartz et al., 1994), and midazolam (Rugstad et al., 1986; Gilmore et al., 1992). It is possible that progesterone, which has been shown to activate CYP3A4 *in vitro* (Kerlan et al., 1992; Kerr et al., 1994), may be also responsible for the observed sex differences in enzyme activity *in vivo*. However, it should be noted that other researchers found no evidence for gender-related differences in CYP3A4-mediated drug metabolism. It is possible that these discrepancies may be due to interindividual variations in CYP3A4 activity (May et al., 1994; Lobo et al., 1986; Sitar et al., 1989; Yee et al., 1986; Shimada et al., 1994; Schmucker et al., 1990).

CYP2D6 Activity

Only a few studies have examined the influence of gender on CYP2D6-mediated metabolism. Gex-Fabry et al. (1990) have shown that the hydroxylation of clomipramine is higher in men than in women. Similarly, Abernethy et al. (1985) found that oral clearance of desipramine is greater in men than in women, although neither these authors nor Gex-Fabry et al. accounted for differences in body weight. Similar results were also shown for propranolol (Walle et al., 1985, 1989, 1994; Gilmore et al., 1992) and ondansetron (Pritchard et al., 1992). However, there are also data indicating that these two drugs may not be metabolized predominantly by the CYP2D6 system (Walle et al., 1989; Ashford et al., 1994). Overall, there is currently no convincing evidence suggesting that CYP2D6 activity is affected by gender.

CYP2C19 Activity

Research has shown that the activity of CYP2C19 may be higher in men than in women. Hooper and Qing (1990) have demonstrated that men clear methyl phenobarbital, a compound metabolized by CYP2C19, approximately 1.3 times faster than women. The metabolism of piroxicam exhibited a similar sex effect (Rugstad et al., 1986). However, others did not see these differences when adjustment for weight was performed (Richardson et al., 1985).

CYP1A2 Activity

Data regarding gender-related differences in the activity of CYP1A2 are scarce and conflicting. However, data from studies of caffeine and thiothixene metabolism suggest that CYP1A2 activity may be higher in men than in women (Ereshefsky et al., 1991; Relling et al., 1992). In contrast, Nafziger and Bertino (1989) reported that theophylline is cleared significantly faster in young women than in men. Interestingly, gender differences in theophylline metabolism do not appear to be present in elderly patients, suggesting that this difference could be hormone-dependent rather than due to genetic differences (Cuzzolin et al., 1990). Furthermore, clomipramine demethylation, which may be performed by CYP1A2, is not influenced by gender (Gex-Fabry et al., 1990). Thus, given the available data, no definite conclusions on the effects of gender on CYP1A2 activity can be drawn at this point.

Conjugation

Many drugs are excreted by the kidneys after conjugation with sulfate or glucuronic acid. Frequently, conjugation reactions are the second metabolic step after the drug has been metabolized, involving relatively slower cytochrome-mediated hydroxylation. Since cytochrome-mediated metabolism is often the rate-limiting step, it may not be possible to detect any gender-related differences in conjugation reactions for these drugs. However, several drugs are metabolized solely by conjugation, and these appear to display gender-related differences in their elimination. For example, the benzodiazepines temazepam and oxazepam, which are eliminated via conjugation, are cleared faster by men than by women (Greenblatt et al., 1980b; Divoll et al., 1981). Faster elimination in men was also observed for the clearance of digoxin (Yukawa et al., 1992), although the observed differences may be related to differences in renal function. The clearance of paracetamol was also greater (by 22%) in young men than in young women (Miners et al., 1983). Other compounds that are cleared by glucoronidation, such as ibuprofen, are not influenced by gender (Greenblatt et al., 1984).

In summary, although studies focusing on gender differences in the pharmcokinetics of various drugs are somewhat contradictory, gender differences exist and seem to be predominantly caused by differences in the activity of the metabolic enzyme systems.

GENDER DIFFERENCES IN PSYCHOTROPIC AGENTS

Although much is known about the determinants of pharmacokinetic variability, fewer data exist regarding the biochemical and physiological effects of drugs (i.e., pharmacodynamics). This relative paucity of data may be in part due to the fact that pharmacokinetic variables are often easier to determine and quantify than pharmacodynamic variables are. Subsequently, gender-related differences in drug effects are also more difficult to evaluate than the effect of gender on pharmacokinetics. There are, however, increasing data on potential gender differences in drug pharmacodynamics. Relevant to this chapter, this section reviews the available data on potential gender differences in psychotropic drugs, with a closer look at gender differences in drug pharmacodynamics.

Antipsychotic Agents

The literature analyzing pharmacokinetics, pharmacodynamics, and side effects of psychotropic agents by gender is the most substantial for antipsychotic drugs. The majority of studies found that women treated with antipsychotic medications experienced greater improvement than men. For example, Chouinard and Annable (1982) found that women had greater improvement than men following treatment with pimozide and chlorpromazine. Similarly, Szymanski et al. (1995) reported that female patients with schizophrenic had a better treatment response to antipsychotics than male patients did, whereas plasma drug levels did not differ significantly between men and women. However, there are also some reports indicating lack of gender differences in neuroleptic treatment response in male and female patients when subjects were matched for clinical, treatment, and demographic characteristics (Pinals et al., 1996).

Researchers hypothesized that the generally greater efficacy of neuroleptics in young women may be due to the presumed antidopaminergic effects of estrogen (Chouinard & Annable, 1982; Fields & Gordon, 1982; Villeneuve et al., 1978). Estrogen has been thought to play a protective (i.e., neuroleptic-like) role in the disease protection process of schizophrenia, leading to the delay of illness development (Seeman & Lang, 1990; Seeman, 1996) and a better response to neuroleptics in women. Interestingly, Kulkarni et al. (1996) found that women with schizophrenia who received estradiol in addition to neuroleptic treatment for 8 weeks improved more rapidly than did a group who received neuroleptics only. However, the difference was not sustained for the entire duration of the trial.

Researchers have also noted that women may require lower doses of neuroleptics than men, despite similarities in weight and age. It appears that women may achieve higher plasma levels of antipsychotics than men (Simpson et al., 1990; Chouinard et al., 1986). Simpson et al. (1990) found higher fluphenazine levels in women, despite comparable dosing, and similar age and weight characteristics. Chouinard et al. (1986) investigated fluspirilene, a long-acting injectable neuroleptic, and found that women required roughly half the dosage required by men, despite similar weight and age characteristics. In this trial, the prescribed doses were titrated to therapeutic efficacy, but serum levels were not available. Another study found that men had significantly higher oral clearance of thiothixene than women did, and that clearance did not necessarily correlate with body weight (Ereshefsky et al., 1991). The authors also found a reduction in clearance for subjects over the age of 50. Centorrino et al. (1994) reported that despite a 60% lower milligram per kilogram dose in women, the levels of clozapine were 40% higher in nonsmoking women than men and did not vary by diagnosis or age in the study sample. A recent study further confirmed that women possess higher plasma levels of clozapine and its metabolite norclozapine, but not the N-oxide metabolite (Lane et al., 1999). Similarly, plasma concentrations of the antipsychotic sertindole were higher in women compared to male subjects of similar age (Wong et al., 1997). Finally, recent studies indicate that women achieve higher plasma levels of other atypical antipsychotics, such as olanzapine (Kelly et al., 1999; Perry et al., 2001).

Gender-related differences were also observed in the expression of antipsychotic-induced side effects. Historically, it was assumed that women are more at risk of developing tardive dyskinesia (TD). For example, in earlier prevalence studies, the incidence of TD was reported as greater in women than in men (Chouinard et al., 1979; Smith & Dunn, 1979). Women have also been reported to suffer more severe TD symptoms. However, recent evidence suggests that this may only be the case in samples of older patients, whereas men are more at risk for developing TD in the younger age groups. Yassa and Jeste (1992) combined data from independent studies on prevalence, age, and sex differences in TD, and found that TD is more prevalent in older women. Chouinard et al. (1980) noted that young men reported a higher prevalence of severe TD than women did. The authors explained this discrepancy by suggesting that postmenopausal status and loss of estrogen-induced supersensitivity may favor the development of TD in postmenopausal women. However, in a recent study, van Os et al. (1999) examined a large sample of patients with chronic psychosis and found that female gender was associated with a lower risk of TD. The effect of gender was independent of other risk factors, such as older age, severity of negative symptoms, and past exposure to antipsychotic medication. It is possible that the authors could not demonstrate an interaction with age, due to the relatively young age of their patient sample (median age 36 years).

Data on the impact of gender on the development of parkinsonism are limited. Jeste (1995) reported that women who take lower doses of neuroleptic medications have similar or lower risks of parkinsonism compared to men.

In summary, the available literature indicates that there may be several clinically meaningful gender-related differences in the effects of neuroleptic medications.

Benzodiazepines

In contrast to the research on antipsychotic agents, relatively few studies have evaluated the therapeutic effects and side effects of benzodiazepines in women. The available studies have focused primarily on potential gender-related differences in the pharmacokinetics of benzodiazepines. For example, Greenblatt et al. (1980a) found that diazepam, which is oxidatively metabolized, has a higher clearance in younger women than in men. This difference disappeared in women 62–84 years old. MacLeod et al. (1979) found that women metabolized diazepam more slowly than men, regardless of age. Nitrazepam, a benzodiazepine metabolized by reduction, was not found to have gender-related differences in clearance (Jochemsen et al., 1982). The metabolism of alprazolam, a benzodiazepine that undergoes oxidation, was not influenced significantly by gender or menstrual cycle phase (Greenblatt & Wright, 1993; Kirkwood et al., 1991). However, temazepam and oxazepam, benzodiazepines that undergo conjugation, had slower clearance rates among female than among male patients in several studies (Smith et al., 1983; Greenblatt et al., 1980; Divoll et al., 1981). This difference was present regardless of age (Smith et al., 1983). The concomitant administration of oral contraceptives may also affect the pharmacokinetics of benzodiazepines. The clearance of triazolam, alprazolam (Stoehr et al, 1984), and nitrazepam (Jochemsen et al., 1982) was reduced when oral contraceptives were taken concomitantly. In contrast, temazepam showed higher clearance in the presence of oral contraceptives (Stoehr et al., 1984).

As mentioned, data regarding gender differences in the effects of benzodiazepines are limited. Ellinwood et al. (1984) found that cognitive and psychomotor tasks performed by women taking diazepam and oral contraceptives were more impaired during the week off hormones, because benzodiazepine levels peaked more quickly. They postulated that oral contraceptives decrease the rate of absorption of diazepam, and that during the week off hormones, the plasma levels quickly rose to intoxicating levels. Contrasting findings were reported by Kroboth et al. (1985) for other benzodiazepines, such as alprazolam, triazolam, and lorazepam. In the Kroboth et al. study, psychomotor changes were most marked in women who received oral contraceptives. However, in both cases, plasma levels did not correlate with the observed clinical effect. Interestingly, van Haaren et al. (1997) observed that high doses of chlordiazepoxide increased response efficiency in male rats, but decreased response efficiency in female rats in animal models. Finally, Pesce et al. (1994) found that the incidence of benzodiazepine withdrawal seizures produced by the administration of flumazenil was significantly lower in male than in female diazepam-treated mice.

In summary, it appears that despite the varied methodology in the available studies, current data suggest gender-related differences in the metabolism and potentially in the effects of the various benzodiazepines.

Antidepressants

Although mood disorders are more prevalent in women than in men (Kessler et al., 1996), little attention has been devoted to research on antidepressant effects in women. However, several gender-related differences in the pharmacokinetics and, to a lesser degree, the pharmacodynamics of antidepressants have been identified. For example, higher plasma levels of certain TCAs have been observed in women than in men. Moody et al. (1967) found that women had higher plasma levels of imipramine than men. Similarly, Preskorn and Mac (1985) reported that women and older subjects had higher plasma levels of amitriptyline than young male subjects did. Gex-Fabry et al. (1990) found that the hydroxylation clearance of clomipramine was lower in women than men, while Abernethy et al. (1985) reported that clearance of oral dose of desipramine was greater in men than in women. However, the authors of these two studies did not normalize for body weight. Dahl et al. (1996) found that depressed female patients had significantly higher plasma levels of nortriptyline than males. In contrast, in an earlier study, Ziegler and Biggs (1977) found no significant gender differences in plasma levels of amitriptyline and nortriptyline. Finally, Greenblatt et al. (1987) found that the volume of distribution of trazodone was greater in women and the elderly, but that clearance was significantly reduced only in older men. The activity of the monoamine oxidase inhibitors (MAOIs) may also show gender-related differences. There are data indicating that monoamine oxidase activity may be decreased by estrogens and increased by progesterone, suggesting menstrual variations in a critical metabolic pathway for most psychotropic drugs (Klaiber et al., 1979; Banwick, 1976). The clinical significance of these changes is unknown, however.

In recent years, data have also emerged on potential gender differences in the pharmacokinetics of the SSRIs and other new antidepressants. In fact, several researchers observed that plasma concentrations of sertraline were approximately 35% to 40% lower in young men than in women and elderly men (Ronfeld et al., 1997; Warrington, 1991). Similarly, plasma concentrations of fluvoxamine have been shown to be 40% to 50% lower in men than in women, with the magnitude of effect possibly greater at lower medication doses (Hartter et al., 1993). Of the other antidepressants, the levels of nefazodone were found to be higher in elderly women than in younger subjects and elderly men (Barbhaiya et al., 1996). In contrast, Klamerus et al. (1996) reported that gender did not substantially alter the disposition or the tolerance of venlafaxine.

As mentioned, data regarding gender-related differences in treatment response to antidepressants are limited. Several available studies indicate that women may respond less well to TCAs than men do, but may respond better to SSRIs and MAOIs. A study by Davidson and Pelton (1986) evaluated the efficacy of TCAs and MAOIs by gender in three types of atypical depression. The authors found that depressed women with panic attacks had a more favorable response to MAOIs than to TCAs, whereas men who were depressed and had panic attacks responded more favorably to TCAs. Similarly, Raskin (1974) found that women younger than 40 years responded less well to imipramine than older women and men did. Steiner et al. (1993) compared the effects of paroxetine, imipramine, and placebo in outpatients with major depression, and found that women responded better to paroxetine than to imipramine. Finally, Kornstein et al. (2000), found that women with chronic or double depression, were significantly more likely to respond to sertraline than to imipramine, while men responded better to imipramine than to sertraline. Postmenopausal women had similar response rates to both antidepressants.

Thus it appears that there may be some clinically meaningful gender-specific differences in the efficacy and tolerability of the antidepressant medications.

CONCLUSIONS

This chapter has reviewed current literature on potential gender-related differences in pharmacokinetics and pharmacodynamics of psychotropic medications. It is apparent that there are still many conflicting findings, as well as considerable gaps in the available data addressing these issues. Nevertheless, there is evidence suggesting certain, gender-related variations in the pharmacokinetics of various compounds. Furthermore, examination of the effects of specific psychotropic agents reveals that (1) the effects of benzodiazepines may be influenced by gender and the concurrent use of oral contraceptives; (2) antipsychotic agents may be more effective in women, although older women may be more likely to experience adverse drug reactions; and, finally, (3) women may respond better to different classes of antidepressant agents than men—specifically, the SSRIs and the MAOIs agents. These data also indicate the need for further well-controlled research in this field.

REFERENCES

Aarons, L., Hopkins, K., Rowland, M., et al. (1989). Route of administration and sex differences in the pharmacokinetics of aspirin administered as its lysine salt. *Pharmacological Research, 6,* 660–666.

Abernethy, D. R., Greenblatt, D. J., & Shader, R. I. (1985). Imipramine and desipramine disposition in the elderly. *Journal of Pharmacology and Experimental Therapeutics, 232,* 183–188.

Amchin, J., Zarycranaski, W., Taylor, K. P., et al. (1998). Effect of venlafaxine on the pharmacokinetics of alprazolam. *Psychopharmacology Bulletin, 34,* 211–219.

Anderson, B. B., Mikkelsen, M., Vesterager, A., et al. (1991). No influence of the antidepressant paroxetine on carbamazepine, valproate, and phenytoin. *Epilepsy Research, 10,* 201–204.

Ashford, E. I., Palmer, J. L., Bye, A., et al. (1994). The pharmacokinetics of ondansetron after intravenous injection in healthy volunteers phenotyped as poor or extensive metabolisers of debrisoquine. *British Journal of Clinical Pharmacology, 37,* 389–391.

Banwick, J. H. (1976). Psychological correlates of the menstrual cycle and oral contraceptive medications. In E. Sacher (Ed.), *Hormones, behavior and psychopathology.* New York: Raven Press.

Barbhaiya, R. H., Buch, A. B., & Greene, D. S. (1996). A study of the effect of age and gender on the pharmacokinetics of nefazodone after single and multiple doses. *Journal of Clinical Psychopharmacology, 16*(1), 19–25.

Bloomer, J. C., Woods, F. R., Haddock, R. E., et al. (1992). The role of cytochrome P4502D6 in the metabolism of paroxetine by human liver microsomes. *British Journal of Clinical Pharmacology, 33,* 521–523.

Brosen, K. (1990). Recent developments in hepatic drug oxidation: Implications for clinical pharmacokinetics. *Clinical Pharmacokinetics, 18,* 220–239.

Brosen, K. (1993). The pharmacogenetics of the selective serotonin reuptake inhibitors. *The Clinical Investigator, 71,* 1002–1009.

Brosen, K., & Gram, L. F. (1989). Clinical significance of the sparteine/debrisoquine oxidation polymorphism. *European Journal of Clinical Pharmacology, 36,* 537–547.

Brosen, K., Skjelbo, E., Rasmussen, B. B., et al. (1993). Fluvoxamine is a potent inhibitor of cytochrome P4501A2. *Biochemical Pharmacology, 45,* 1211–1214.

Centorrino, F., Baldessarini, R. J., Kando, J. C., et al. (1994). Clozapine and metabolites: Concentrations in serum and clinical findings during treatment of chronically psychotic patients. *Journal of Clinical Psychopharmacology, 14*(2), 119–125.

Chouinard, G., & Annable, L. (1982). Pimozide in the treatment of newly admitted schizophrenic patients. *Psychopharmacology (Berlin), 76,* 13–19.

Chouinard, G., Annable, L., Ross-Chouinard, A., et al. (1979). Factors related to tardive dyskinesia. *American Journal of Psychiatry, 136,* 79–83.

Chouinard, G., Annable, L., & Steinberg, S. (1986). A controlled clinical trial of fluspirilene, a long-acting injectable neuroleptic, in schizophrenia patients with acute exacerbation. *Journal of Clinical Psychopharmacology, 6,* 21–26.

Chouinard, G., Jones, B. D., Annable, L., et al. (1980). Sex differences and tardive dyskinesia [Letter to the editor]. *American Journal of Psychiatry, 137*, 507.

Crewe, H. K., Kennard, M. S., Tucker, G. T., et al. (1992). The effect of selective serotonin reuptake inhibitors on cytochrome P4502D6 (CYP2D6) activity in human liver microsomes. *British Journal of Clinical Pharmacology, 34*, 262–265.

Cuzzolin, L., Schinella, M., Tellini, U., et al. (1990). The effect of sex and cardiac failure on the pharmacokinetics of a slow-release theophylline formulation in the elderly. *Pharmacological Research, 22*, 137–138.

Dahl, M. L., Bertilsson, L., & Nordin, C. (1996). Steady-state plasma levels of nortriptyline and its 10–hydroxy metabolite: Relationship to the CYP2D6 genotype. *Psychopharmacology (Berlin), 123*, 315–319.

Datz, F. L., Christian, P. E., & Moore, J. (1987). Gender-related differences in gastric emptying. *Nuclear Medicine, 28*, 1204–1207.

Davidson, J., & Pelton, S. (1986). Forms of atypical depression and their response to antidepressant drugs. *Psychiatry Research, 17*, 87–95.

Degen, L. P., & Phillip, S. F. (1996). Variability of gastrointestinal transit in healthy women and men. *Gut, 39*(2), 299–305.

Divoll, M., Greenblatt, D. J., Harmatz, J. S., et al. (1981). Effects of age and gender on disposition of temazepam. *Journal of Pharmacological Science, 70*, 1104–1107.

Ellinwood, E. H., Easler, M. E., Linnoila, M., et al. (1984). Effects of oral contraceptives on diazepam-induced psychomotor impairment. *Clinical Pharmacology and Therapeutics, 35*, 360–366.

Ereshefsky, L., Saklad, S. R., Watanabe, M. D., et al. (1991). Thiothixene pharmacokinetic interactions: A study of hepatic enzyme inducers, clearance inhibitors, and demographic variables. *Journal of Clinical Psychopharmacology, 11*, 296–301.

Fields, J. Z., & Gordon, J. H. (1982). Estrogen inhibits the dopaminergic super-sensitivity induced by neuroleptics. *Life Sciences, 30*, 229–234.

Food and Drug Administration (FDA). (1993). Guideline for the study and evaluation of gender differences in the clinic evaluation of drugs. *Federal Register, 58*(139), 39406–39416.

Gex-Fabry, M., Balanta-Gorgia, A. E., Balant, L. P., et al. (1990). Clomipramine metabolism: Model-based analysis of variability factors from drug monitoring data. *Clinical Pharmacokinetics, 19*, 241–255.

Gilman, A. G., Rall, T. W., Nies, A. S., et al. (1990). *The pharmacological basis of therapeutics* (8th ed.). New York: Pergamon Press.

Gilmore, D. A., Gal, J., Gerber, J. G., et al. (1992.). Age and gender influence of the stereoselective pharmacokinetics of propranolol. *Journal of Pharmacology and Experimental Therapeutics, 261*, 1181–1186.

Giudicelli, J. F., & Tillement, J. P. (1977). Influence of sex on drug kinetics in man. *Clinical Pharmacokinetics, 2*, 157–166.

Greene, D. S., Salazar, D. E., Pittman, K., et al. (1995). Coadministration of nefazodone and benzodiazepines: III. A pahrmacokinetic interaction study with alprazolam. *Journal of Clinical Psychopharmacology, 15*, 399–408.

Greenblatt, D. J., Abernethy, D. A., Matlis, R., et al. (1984). Absorption and distribution of ibuprofen in the elderly. *Arthritis and Rheumatism, 27*, 1066–1069.

Greenblatt, D. J., Allen, M. D., Harmatz, J. S., et al. (1980). Diazepam disposition determinants. *Clinical Pharmacology and Therapeutics, 27*, 301–312.

Greenblatt, D. J., Divoll, M., Harmatz, J. S., et al. (1980). Oxazepam kinetics: Effects of age and sex. *Journal of Pharmacology and Experimental Therapeutics, 215*, 86–91.

Greenblatt, D. J., Freidman, H., Burstein, E. S., et al. (1987). Trazodone pharmacokinetics: Effect of age, gender and obesity. *Clinical Pharmacology and Therapeutics, 42*, 193–200.

Greenblatt, D. J., Shader, R. I., Koch-Wiser, J., et al. (1974). Slow absorption of intramuscular chlordiazepoxide. *New England Journal of Medicine, 291,* 1116–1118.

Greenblatt, D. J., & Wright, C. E. (1993). Clinical pharmacokinetics of alprazolam: Therapeutic implications. *Clinical Pharmacokinetics, 24*(6), 453–471.

Grossman, M. I., Kirsner, J. B., Gillespie, I. A. (1963). Basal and histalog stimulated gastric secretion in control subjects and in patients with peptic ulcer or gastric cancer. *Gastroenterology, 45,* 14–26.

Guengerich, F. P. (1990). Mechanism-based inactivation of human liver microsomal cytochrome P450 IIIA4 by gestodene. *Chemical Research in Toxicology, 3,* 363–371.

Guengerich, F. P. (1992). Human cytochrome P450 enzymes. *Life Sciences, 50,* 1471–1478.

Hartter, S., Wetzel, H., Hammes, E., et al. (1993). Inhibition of antidepressant demethylation and hydroxylation by fluvoxamine in depressed patients. *Psychopharmacology, 110,* 302–308.

Ho, P. C., Triggs, E. J., Bourn, D. W. A., et al. (1985). The effects of age and sex on the disposition of acetylsalicylic acid and its metabolites. *British Journal of Clinical Pharmacology, 19,* 675–684.

Hooper, W. D., & Qing, M.-S. (1990). The influence of age and gender on the stereoselective metabolism and pharmacokinetics of mephobarbital in humans. *Clinical Pharmacology and Therapeutics, 48,* 633–640.

Hulst, L. K., Fleishaker, J. C., Peters, G. R., et al. (1994). Effect of age and gender on tirilazad pharmacokinetics in humans. *Clinical Pharmacology and Therapeutics, 55,* 378–384.

Hunt, C. M., Westerkam, W. R., & Stave, G. M. (1992). Effect of age and gender on the activity of human hepatic CYP3A. *Biochemical Pharmacology, 44,* 275–283.

Jalil, P. (1992). Toxic reaction following the combined administration of fluoxetine and phenytoin: Two case reports [Letter to the editor]. *Journal of Neurology, Neurosurgery and Psychiatry, 55,* 412–413.

Jerling, M., Lindstrom, L., Bondesson, U., et al. (1994). Fluvoxamine inhibition and carbamazepine induction of the metabolism of clozapine: Evidence from a therapeutic drug monitoring service. *Therapeutic Drug Monitoring, 16,* 368–374.

Jeste, D. V. (1995). *Gender and ethnicity differences in pharmacology of neuroleptics.* Paper presented at the 148th Annual Convention of the American Psychiatric Association, Miami, FL.

Jochemsen, R., Van der Graaf, M., Boeijinga, J. K., et al. (1982). Influence of sex, menstrual cycle and oral contraception on the disposition of nitrazepam. *British Journal of Clinical Pharmacology, 13,* 319–324.

Kato, R. (1974). Sex-differences in drug metabolism. *Drug Metabolism Reviews, 3,* 1–31.

Kelly, D. L., Conley, R. R., & Tamminga, C. A. (1999). Diffential olanzapine plasma concentrations by sex in a fixed-dose study. *Schizophrenia Research, 40*(2), 101–104.

Kerlan, V., Dreano, Y., Bercovici, J. P., et al. (1992). Nature of cytochromes P450 involved in the 2–/4–hydroxylations of estradiol in human liver microsomes. *Biochemical Pharmacology, 44,* 1745–1756.

Kerr, B. M., Thummel, K. E., Wurden, C. J., et al. (1994). Human liver carbamazepine metabolism: Role of CYP3A4 and CYP2C8 in 10,11–epoxide formation. *Biochemical Pharmacology, 47,* 1969–1979.

Kessler, R. C., Nelson, C. B., McGonagle, K. A., et al. (1996). Comorbidity of DSM-III-R major depressive disorder in the general population: Results from the US National Comorbidity Survey. *British Journal of Psychiatry, 171*(Suppl. 30), 17–30.

Kirkwood, C., Moore, A., Hayes, P., et al. (1991). Influence of menstrual cycle and gender on alprazolam pharmacokinetics. *Clinical Pharmacology and Therapeutics, 50,* 404–409.

Klaiber, E. L., Broverman, D. M., Vogel, W., et al. (1979). Estrogen therapy for severe persistent depressions in women. *Archives of General Psychiatry, 36,* 550–554.

Klamerus, K. J., Parker, V. D., Rudolph, R. L., et al. (1996). Effects of age and gender on venlafaxine and O-desmethyl venlafaxine pharmacokinetics. *Pharmacotherapy, 16*(5), 915–923.

Knodell, R. G., Hall, S. D., Wilkinson, G. R., et al. (1987). Hepatic metabolism of tolbutamide: Characterization of the form of cytochrome P450 involved in methyl hydroxylation and relationship to in vivo disposition. *Journal of Pharmacology and Experimental Therapeutics, 241*, 1112–1119.

Kolars, J. C., Awni, W. M., Merion, R. M., et al. (1991). First-pass metabolism of cyclosporin by the gut. *Lancet, 338*, 1488–1490.

Kolars, J. C., Flockhart, D. A., Post, R. M., et al. (1992). The emerging role of cytochrome P450 3A in psychopharmacology. *Journal of Clinical Psychopharmacology, 15*, 387–398.

Kroboth, P. D., Smith, R. B., Stoehr, G. P., et al. (1985). Pharmacodynamic evaluation of the benzodiazepine–oral contraceptive interaction. *Clinical Pharmacology and Therapeutics, 38*, 525–532.

Kulkarni, J., de Castella, A., & Smith, D. (1996). A clinical trial of the effects of estrogen in acutely psychotic women. *Schizophrenia Research, 20*(3), 247–252.

Lane, H. Y., Chang, Y. C., Chang, W. H., et al. (1999). Effects of gender and age on plasma levels of clozapine and its metabolites: Analyzed by critical statistics. *Journal of Clinical Psychiatry, 60*(1), 36–40.

Lobo, J., Kack, D. B., & Kendall, M. J. (1986). The intra- and inter-subject variability of nifedipine pharmacokinetics in young volunteers. *European Journal of Clinical Pharmacology, 30*, 57–60.

MacLeod, S. M., Giles, H. G., Bengert, B., et al. (1979). Age and gender-related differences in diazepam pharmacokinetics. *Journal of Clinical Pharmacology, 19*, 15–19.

May, D. G., Porter, J., Wilkinson, G. R., et al. (1994). Frequency distribution of dapsone N-hydroxylase, a putative probe for P4503A4 activity in a white population. *Clinical Pharmacology and Therapeutics, 55*, 492–500.

McBurney, M. (1991). Starch malabsorption and stool excretion are influenced by the menstrual cycle in women consuming low fiber Western diets. *Scandinavian Journal of Gastroenterology, 28*, 880–886.

Mesnil, F., Mentre, F., Dubruc, C., et al. (1998). Population pharmacokinetic analysis of mizolastine and validation from sparse data on patients using the nonparametric maximum likelihood method. *Journal of Pharmacokinetics and Biopharmaceutics, 26*, 133–161.

Miners, J. O., Attwood, J., & Birkett, D. J. (1983). Influence of sex and oral contraceptive steroids on paracetamol metabolism. *British Journal of Clinical Pharmacology, 16*, 503–509.

Moody, J. P., Tait, A. C., & Todrick, A. (1967). Plasma levels of imipramine and desmethyl imipramine during therapy. *British Journal of Psychiatry, 113*, 183–193.

Murray, M. (1992). P450 enzymes: Inhibition mechanisms, genetic regulation and effects of liver disease. *Clinical Pharmacokinetics, 23*, 132–146.

Nafziger, A. N., & Bertino, J. S., Jr. (1989). Sex-related differences in theophylline pharmacokinetics. *European Journal of Clinical Pharmacology, 37*, 97–100.

Newlands, A. J., Smith, D. A., Jones, B. C., et al. (1992). Metabolism of nonsteroidal, anti-inflammatory drugs by cytochrome P450 2C [Abstract]. *British Journal of Clinical Pharmacology, 34*, 152P.

O'Malley, K., Crooks, J., Duke, E., et al. (1971). Effects of age and sex on human drug metabolism. *British Medical Journal, iii*, 607–609.

Otton, S. V., Ball, S. E., Cheung, S. W., et al. (1994). Comparative inhibition of the polymorphic enzyme CYP2D6 by venlafaxine (VF) and other 5HT uptake inhibitors (abstract PI-71). *Clinical Pharmacology and Therapeutics, 55*, 141.

Otton, S. V., Ball, S. E., Cheung, S. W., et al. (1996). Venlafaxine oxidation in vitro is catalyzed by CYP2D6. *British Journal of Clinical Pharmacology, 41*, 149–156.

Otton, S. V., Wu, D., Joffe, R. T., et al. (1993). Inhibition by fluoxetine of cytochrome P4502D6 activity. *Clinical Pharmacology and Therapeutics, 53*, 401–409.

Perry, P. J., Lund, B. C., Sanger, T., et al. (2001). Olanzapine plasma concentrations and clinical response: Acute phase results of the North American olanzapine trial. *Journal of Clinical Psychopharmacology, 21*(1), 14–20.

Pesce, M. E., Acevedo, X., Pinardi, G., et al. (1994). Gender differences in diazepam withdrawal syndrome in mice. *Pharmacology and Toxicology, 75*(6), 353–355.

Pinals, D. A., Malhotra, A. K., Missar, C. D., et al. (1996). Lack of gender differences in neuroleptic response in patients with schizophrenia. *Schizophrenia Research, 22*(3), 215–222.

Pollan, A., & Oian, P. (1986). Changes in transcapillary fluid dynamics—a possible explanation of the fluid retention in the premenstrual phase. In L. Dennerstein & I. Fraser (Eds.), *Hormones and behavior.* New York: Elsevier.

Pollock, B. G. (1994). Recent developments in drug metabolism of relevance to psychiatrists. *Harvard Review of Psychiatry, 2,* 204–213.

Preskorn, S. H., & Mac, D. S. (1985). Plasma level of amitriptyline: Effect of age and sex. *Journal of Clinical Psychiatry, 46,* 276–277.

Pritchard, J. F., Bryson, J. C., Kernodle, A. E., et al. (1992). Age and gender effects on ondansetron pharmacokinetics: Evaluation of healthy aged volunteers. *Clinical Pharmacology and Therapeutics, 51,* 51–55.

Raskin, A. (1974). Age–sex differences in response to antidepressant drugs. *Journal of Nervous and Mental Disease, 159,* 120–130.

Relling, M. V., Lin, J. S., Ayers, G. D., et al. (1992). Racial and gender differences in N-acetyltransferase, xanthine oxidase, and CYP1A2 activities. *Clinical Pharmacology and Therapeutics, 52,* 643–658.

Rettie, A. E., Korzekwa, K. R., Kunze, K. L., et al. (1992). Hydroxylation of warfarin by human cDNA-expressed cytochrome P450: A role for P4502C9 in the etiology of (S)-warfarin drug interactions. *Chemical Research in Toxicology, 5,* 54–59.

Richardson, C. J., Blocka, K. L. N., Ross, S. G., et al. (1985). Effects of age and sex on piroxicam disposition. *Clinical Pharmacology and Therapeutics, 37,* 13–18.

Riester, E. F., Pantuck, E. J., Pantuck, C. B., et al. (1980). Antipyrine metabolism during the menstrual cycle. *Clinical Pharmacology and Therapeutics, 28,* 384–391.

Ronfeld, R. A., Tremaine, L. M., & Wilner, K. D. (1997). Pharmacokinetics of sertraline and its N-dimethyl metabolite in elderly and young male and female volunteers. *Clinical Pharmacokinetics, 32*(Suppl. 1), 22–30.

Rugstad, H. E., Hundal, O., Holme, I., et al. (1986). Piroxicam and naproxen plasma concentrations in patients with osteoarthritis: Relation to age, sex, efficacy and adverse events. *Clinical Rheumatology, 5,* 389–398.

Schmider, J., Greenblatt, D. J., Harmatz, J. S., et al. (1996). Inhibition of cytochrome P450 by nefazodone in vitro: Studies of dextrometorphan O- and N-demethylation. *British Journal of Clinical Pharmacology, 41,* 339–343.

Schmucker, D. L., Woodhouse, K. W., Wang, R. K., et al. (1990). Effects of age and gender on in vitro properties of human liver microsomal monoxygenases. *Clinical Pharmacology and Therapeutics, 48,* 365–374.

Schwartz, J., Capili, H., & Daugherty, J. (1994). Aging of women alters S-verapamil pharmacokinetics and pharmacodynamics. *Clinical Pharmacology and Therapeutics, 55,* 509–517.

Seeman, M. V. (1989). Neuroleptic prescription for men and women. *Social Pharmacology, 3,* 219–236.

Seeman, M. V. (1996). The role of estrogen in schizophrenia. *Journal of Psychiatry and Neuroscience, 21*(2), 123–127.

Seeman, M. V., & Lang, M. (1990). The role of estrogens in schizophrenia gender differences. *Schizophrenia Bulletin, 16,* 185–194.

Shimada, T., Yamazaki, H., Mimura, M., et al. (1994). Interindividual variations in human liver cytochrome P-450 enzymes involved in the oxidation of drugs, carcinogens and toxic chemicals: Studies with liver microsomes of 30 Japanese and 30 Caucasians. *Journal of Pharmacology and Experimental Therapeutics, 270,* 414–423.

Simpson, G. M., Yadalam, K. G., Levinson, D. F., et al. (1990). Single dose pharmacokinetics of fluphenazine after fluphenazine decanoate administration. *Journal of Clinical Psychopharmacology, 10,* 417–421.

Sitar, D., Duke, P. C., Benthuysen, J. L., et al. (1989). Aging and alfentanil disposition in healthy volunteers and surgical patients. *Canadian Journal of Anaesthesiology, 36,* 149–154.

Skett, P. (1988). Biochemical basis of sex differences in drug metabolism. *Pharmacology and Therapeutics, 38,* 269–304.

Skjelbo, E., & Brosen, K. (1992). Inhibitors of imipramine metabolism by human liver microsomes. *British Journal of Clinical Pharmacology, 34,* 256–261.

Smith, D. A., & Jones, B. C. (1992). Speculations on the substrate structure–activity relationship (SSAR) of cytochrome P450 enzymes. *Biochemical Pharmacology, 44,* 2089–2098.

Smith, R. B., Divoll, M., Gillespie, W. R., et al. (1983). Effect of subject age and gender on the pharmacokinetics of oral triazolam and temazepam. *Journal of Clinical Psychopharmacology, 3,* 172–176.

Smith, J. M., & Dunn, D. D. (1979). Sex differences in the prevalence of severe tardive dyskinesia. *American Journal of Psychiatry, 136,* 1081–1082.

Steiner, M., Wheadon, D. E., Kreider, M. S., et al. (1993, May). *Antidepressant response to paroxetine by gender.* Paper presented at the 146th Annual Convention of the American Psychiatric Association, San Francisco.

Stoehr, G. P., Kroboth, P. D., Juhl, R. P., et al. (1984). Effect of oral contraceptives on triazolam, temazepam, alprazolam, and lorazepam kinetics. *Clinical Pharmacology and Therapeutics, 36*(5), 683–690.

Strobel, H. W., Hammond, D. K., White, T. B., et al. (1991). Identification and localization of cytochromes P450 in gut. *Methods in Enzymology, 206,* 648–655.

Sweeting, J. (1992). Does the time of the month affect the function of the gut? *Gastroenterology, 102,* 1084–1085.

Szymanski, S., Lieberman, J. A., Alvir, J. M., et al. (1995). Gender differences in onset of illness, treatment response, course, and biologic indexes in first-episode schizophrenic patients. *American Journal of Psychiatry, 152*(5), 698–703.

Tuck, C. H., Holleran, B., & Berglund, L. (1997). Hormonal regulation of lipoprotein(a) levels: Effects of estrogen replacement therapy on lipoprotein(a) and acute phase reactants in postmenopausal women. *Arteriosclerosis, Thrombosis, and Vascular Biology, 17*(9), 1822–1829.

van Haaren, F., Katon, E., & Anderson, K. G. (1997). The effects of chlordiazepoxide on low-rate behavior are gender dependent. *Pharmacology, Biochemistry and Behavior, 58*(4), 1037–1043.

van Os, J., Walsh, E., van Horn, E., et al. (1999). Tardive dyskinesia in psychosis: Are women really more at risk? *Acta Psychiatrica Scandinavica, 99,* 288–293.

Villeneuve, A., Langlier, P., & Bedard, P. (1978). Estrogens, dopamine and dyskinesias. *Canadian Psychiatric Association Journal, 23,* 68–70.

von Moltke, L. L., Greenblatt, D. J., Court, M. H., et al. (1995). Inhibition of alprazolam and desipramine hydroxylation in in vitro by paroxetine and fluvoxamine: Comparison with other selective serotonin reuptake inhibitor antidepressants. *Journal of Clinical Psychopharmacology, 15,* 125–131.

von Moltke, L. L., Greenblatt, D. J., Granda, B. W., et al. (1999). Nefazodone, meta-chlorophenyl piperazine, and their metabolites in vitro: Cytochromes mediating transformation, and P450–3A4 inhibitory actions. *Psychopharmacology (Berlin), 145,* 113–122.

Wald, A., Van Thiel, D. H., Hoechstetter, L., et al. (1981). Gastrointestinal transit: The effect of the menstrual cycle. *Gastroenterology, 80*(6), 1497–1500.

Walle, T., Byington, R. P., Furberg, C. D., et al. (1985). Biologic determinants of propranolol disposition: Results from 1308 patients in the beta-blocker heart attack trial. *Clinical Pharmacology and Therapeutics, 38,* 509–518.

Walle, T., Walle, U. K., Cowart, T. D., et al. (1989). Pathway-selective sex differences in the metabolic clearance of propranolol in human subjects. *Clinical Pharmacology and Therapeutics, 45,* 257–263.

Walle, T., Walle, U. K., Mathur, R. S., et al. (1994). Propranolol metabolism in normal subjects: Association with sex steroid hormones. *Clinical Pharmacology and Therapeutics, 56,* 127–132.

Warrington, S. J. (1991). Clinical implications of the pharmacology of sertraline. *International Clinical Psychopharmacology, 6,* 11–21.

Wong, S. L., Cao, G., Mack, R. J., et al. (1997). Pharmacokinetics of sertindole in healthy young and elderly male and female subjects. *Clinical Pharmacology and Therapeutics, 62,* 157–162.

Wrighton, S. A., & Stevens, J. C. (1992). The human hepatic cytochromes P450 involved in drug metabolism. *Critical Reviews in Toxicology, 22,* 1–21.

Yassar, J., & Jeste, D. V. (1992). Gender differences in tardive dyskinesia: A critical review of the literature. *Psychological Bulletin, 18*(4), 701–715.

Yee, G. C., Lennon, T. P., Gmur, D. J., et al. (1986). Age-dependent cyclosporine: Pharmacokinetics in marrow transplant recipients. *Clinical Pharmacology and Therapeutics, 40,* 438–443.

Yukawa, E., Mine, H., Higuchi, S., et al. (1992). Digoxin population pharmacokinetics from routine clinical data: Role of patient characteristics for estimating dosing regimes. *Journal of Pharmacy and Pharmacology, 44,* 761–765.

Ziegler, V. E., & Biggs, J. T. (1977). Tricyclic plasma levels: Effect of age, race, sex, and smoking. *Journal of the American Medical Association, 238,* 2167–2169.

3

Psychiatric Aspects of the Menstrual Cycle

MEIR STEINER
LESLIE BORN

Many women in their reproductive years, from menarche to menopause, report clinically significant menstrually-related emotional as well as physical symptoms (Steiner, 1999). The burden of illness associated with moderate to severe premenstrual symptoms can be profound, highly impacting women's occupational and social roles and especially their relationships with their partners and children (Hylan et al., 1999; Robinson & Swindle, 2000). A patient's report of such symptoms may be influenced by a number of factors, including subjective perception, cultural influences, retrospective versus prospective reporting, and a concurrent psychiatric condition. The need for accurate assessment and diagnosis of premenstrual complaints is therefore crucial. In general, the "premenstrual syndromes" include the more common premenstrual syndrome (PMS; World Health Organization [WHO], 1996), and the less prevalent premenstrual dysphoric disorder (PMDD; American Psychiatric Association [APA], 1994).

From antiquity to the present, menstruation and premenstrual symptomatology have been referred to as the "curse," contributing to a negative perception of a natural cyclical event. The importance of subjective perception in the experience of menstrual events has been underscored in a recent report on the significant reduction of negative symptoms in a sample of women with severe premenstrual symptomatology, following a psychosocially based intervention that emphasized positive reframing (positive connotation) (Morse, 1999). Social beliefs about menstruation, however, vary among different cultures and can influence expectations about the menstrual cycle as well as the reporting of symptoms (Sveindottir, 1998).

Age may also influence the reporting of premenstrual symptoms (Johnson, 1987) and the clinical presentation of PMS or PMDD. Onset of distressing symptoms occurs typically when women are in their late 20s to mid-30s (Freeman et al., 1995a), and there is some evidence of worsening premenstrual symptomatology following childbirth (Johnson, 1987), although this association has yet to be confirmed prospectively. In one prospective study, investigators found that older adolescents (16–18 years) had significantly more intense symptoms than younger teens (13–15 years) (Cleckner-Smith et al., 1998).

Thus far the bulk of research on premenstrual syndromes has occurred in the United States, although additional insights have been garnered from surveys of European, Mediterranean, Middle Eastern, Southeast Asian, and African populations. Affective symptoms (irritability, mood swings, tension) and weight gain appear to be more prevalent among U.S. women, compared with a higher frequency of somatic symptoms (swelling, breast pain, backache) in Italian and Bahraini groups (Dan & Monagle, 1994), as well as in Swiss, Indian, and Chinese samples (Merikangas et al., 1993; Chandra & Chaturvedi, 1989; Chang et al., 1995). One report has suggested that "menstrual socialization" may influence expectation and reporting of symptoms (Sveindottir, 1998).

Finally, associations between educational level and both severity and type of symptoms have been suggested (Dan & Monagle, 1994). Women with higher levels of education have been shown to report more severe symptoms (Marvan et al., 1998), as well as more psychological complaints of premenstrual symptoms (Dan & Monagle, 1994).

Thus it is important to consider that many factors—beliefs, age, cultural context, and level of education—may influence women's premenstrual experiences, and therefore the nature of what is relayed to clinicians.

The etiology of PMS and PMDD is still largely unknown. That PMS and PMDD are biological phenomena (as opposed to purely psychological or psychosocial events) is primarily underscored by recent convincing evidence of the heritability of premenstrual symptoms (Kendler et al., 1998) and the elimination of premenstrual complaints with suppression of ovarian activity (Schmidt et al., 1998) or surgical menopause (Casson et al., 1990; Casper & Hearn, 1990).

The current consensus is that normal ovarian function, rather than simple hormone imbalance (Roca, 1996), is the cyclical trigger for PMDD-related biochemical events within the central nervous system and other target tissues. (For a review of the normal hormonal events across the menstrual cycle, see Speroff, Glass, & Kase, 1994, Chapter 6). The serotogenic system is in close reciprocal relationship with the hypothalamic–pituitary–gonadal axis (Tuiten et al., 1995; Eriksson et al., 1994), and increasing evidence suggests that serotonin is pivotal in the pathogenesis of PMDD (Rojansky et al., 1991; Rapkin, 1992; Steiner, 1992; Yatham, 1993; Steiner et al., 1997c). Premenstrual irritability and dysphoria are probably linked to a difference in the sensitivity of the serotonin system in predisposed women, rendering them more vulnerable to cyclical hormonal fluctuations (Steiner et al., 1997c; Halbreich & Tworek, 1993; Leibenluft et al., 1994; Kouri & Halbreich, 1997). Indeed, the selective serotonin reuptake inhibitors (SSRIs) are emerging as the most effective treatment options for women with PMDD.

Therapeutic interventions for premenstrual syndromes range from conservative measures (lifestyle and stress management), to treatment with psychotropic medications or hormonal therapy, to surgical procedures for very severe and treatment-refractory cases. Although all of these treatments are successful in relieving symptoms for some women, none to date has proven to be effective for all. Most pharmacological therapies are now being tested in randomized controlled trials. In contrast, the efficacy of many non-pharmacological therapies has yet to be scientifically demonstrated, although there are numerous case reports of women who obtain relief with some of these approaches.

RISK FACTORS

Some factors that may increase the risk for premenstrual syndromes have been pin-pointed, although in most instances more explicit evidence is required.

1. *Age.* As noted above, some evidence suggests that women are most likely to present with PMDD during the late 20s to the mid-30s (Freeman et al., 1995a).

2. *Menstrual cycle characteristics.* There are mixed reports on the association of menstrual cycle characteristics with severity of premenstrual symptoms. One study found a higher prevalence of PMS in women whose menses lasted longer than 6 days (Deuster et al., 1999). Others have found an association between PMS symptoms and longer (Woods et al., 1982) or shorter (specifically in women with purely depressive symptoms; Hargrove & Abraham, 1982) menstrual cycle length.

3. *Past or current psychiatric illness.* A high proportion of women presenting with PMDD have a history of previous episodes of mood disorders, including major depression (Halbreich & Endicott, 1985; Yonkers, 1997a), minor depression (Pearlstein et al., 1990), postpartum depression (Pearlstein et al., 1990), seasonal affective disorder (Parry, 1995), and bipolar disorder (Pearlstein et al., 1990). Some women with PMDD have a history of suicide attempts (Harrison et al., 1989), anxiety disorders (panic disorder, generalized anxiety disorder, phobias) (Yonkers, 1997b), personality disorders (Pearlstein et al., 1990), or substance abuse (Pearlstein et al., 1990). For example, a life-time history of major depressive disorder among patients with PMDD has been reported in the range of 30–70% (Yonkers, 1997a). In addition, in prospective studies, 14–16% of women with PMDD have a lifetime history of anxiety disorder (Yonkers, 1997b). In a sample of 206 women diagnosed with PMDD, Bailey and Cohen (1999) found that approximately 39% of respondents met criteria for mood or anxiety disorders or both. Approximately one out of two women suffering from seasonal affective disorder may also meet criteria for PMDD (Praschak-Rieder et al., 2001). Women with an ongoing mood disorder report premenstrual magnification of symptoms and the emergence of new symptoms (Harrison et al., 1989; Fava et al., 1992; McLeod et al., 1993; Endicott, 1993; Bancroft et al., 1994; Kaspi et al., 1994; Graze et al., 1990).

4. *Family history.* Population-based twin studies of the familial risk factors for premenstrual symptoms have suggested that PMS is heritable (Condon, 1993; Kendler et al., 1998).

5. *Psychosocial stressors.* A substantial body of literature has focused on life stressors involving major life events, relationships with significant others, work, social support (Severino & Moline, 1989), or history of sexual abuse (Paddison et al., 1990). This research suggests that life stress is positively associated with PMS symptoms.

CLASSIFICATION

Premenstrual Syndrome

PMS can be defined as a pattern of emotional, behavioral, and physical symptoms that occur premenstrually and remit after menses. These symptoms typically include minor mood changes, breast tenderness, bloating, and headache (WHO, 1996). More than 100 physical and psychological symptoms have been attributed to the premenstruum (Budeiri et al., 1994).

Epidemiological surveys have estimated that as many as 75% of women with regular menstrual cycles experience some symptoms of PMS (Johnson, 1987). The majority of these women do not require medical or psychiatric intervention. Since the emergence of the term "premenstrual syndrome" in the 1950s (Greene & Dalton, 1953), PMS has become an increasingly discussed topic in popular media sources; thus the more effective self-management techniques are easily accessed by women through the mass media or through their peers. Women who feel they are unable to self-manage their PMS are most often seen in primary care settings or by gynecologists.

The *International Classification of Diseases*, 10th revision (ICD-10; WHO, 1996) criteria for PMS include mild psychological discomfort and symptoms of bloating and weight gain, breast tenderness and swelling, swelling of hands and feet, various aches and pains, poor concentration, sleep disturbance, and change in appetite. Only one of these symptoms is required for this diagnosis, although the symptoms must be restricted to the luteal phase of the menstrual cycle, reach a peak shortly before menstruation, and cease with the menstrual flow or soon after.

For women who have mild to moderate symptoms of PMS (and do not meet criteria for PMDD or for other physical or psychological disorders), conservative treatments are appropriate, and management *without* pharmacological interventions should be encouraged. Stressful life events should be queried and monitored. These women should also be taught to review their own monthly diaries and identify triggers of symptom exacerbation. Many will improve with individual or group psychotherapy in combination with diet and lifestyle changes.

Premenstrual Dysphoric Disorder

PMDD, usually consisting of extremely distressing emotional and behavioral symptoms (irritability, dysphoria, tension, and mood lability), first appeared in the appendix of the revised third edition of the *Diagnostic and Statistical Manual of Mental Disorders* (DSM-III-R; APA, 1987) as late luteal phase dysphoric disorder (LLPDD). It was later renamed PMDD and incorporated into the appendix of the fourth edition (DSM-IV; APA, 1994). PMDD affects 3–8% of women of reproductive age (Johnson et al., 1988; Rivera-Tovar & Frank, 1990; Andersch et al., 1986; Merikangas et al., 1993; Ramacharan et al., 1992; Angst, 2001). These women report premenstrual symptoms, primarily mood symptoms, that are severe enough to interfere seriously with their lifestyle and relationships (Freeman et al., 1985; O'Brien et al., 1995). Some women may show sustained improvement with nondrug treatment (Freeman & Rickels, 1999); however, in general, women with PMDD do not respond to conservative interventions.

Some investigators have defined subtypes of PMDD. Women who receive a diagnosis of "pure–pure" PMDD meet DSM-IV criteria for PMDD and have no other past and/or present psychiatric disorder. Women who receive a diagnosis of "pure" PMDD meet DSM-IV criteria for PMDD and have no other concurrent psychiatric disorder, but have a history of a past psychiatric disorder (Steiner & Wilkins, 1996).

The definition of PMDD in DSM-IV is much stricter than the definition of PMS in ICD-10. In order to apply the DSM-IV criteria, women must chart symptoms daily prospectively for at least two symptomatic cycles, and their chief complaints must include one of four core symptoms (irritability, tension, dysphoria, and lability of mood) and at least 5 of 11 total symptoms. The symptoms should have occurred with most menstrual cycles during the last year, and must have interfered with social or occupational roles as well as lifestyle (Apa, 1994). Some women may report significant seasonal variation in premenstrual symptoms (Maskall et al., 1997). In addition, the charting of troublesome symptoms should demonstrate both clear premenstrual onset and remission within a few days after the onset of menstruation ("on–offness"). A change in symptoms from the follicular to the luteal phase of at least 50% is suggested for a diagnosis of PMDD (Steiner et al., 1995).

Clinicians utilizing the DSM-IV criteria for PMDD are assumed to have a certain familiarity with the multiaxial system. Thus, for PMDD, any current Axis I (major mental disorders), Axis II (personality disorders), or Axis III (general medical conditions) illness or episode must be excluded.

PMDD appears in the body of the DSM-IV under the heading "depressive disorder not otherwise specified," and in Appendix B as one of the criteria sets provided for further study (APA, 1994). Questions regarding its status as a distinct clinical diagnostic entity (likely stemming from the high rates of comorbidity between PMDD and depressive and anxiety disorders) have repeatedly been raised. Researchers have attempted to resolve this question, for the most part, by either describing similarities in features between PMDD and other mood disorders (Yonkers, 1997a; Halbreich, 1997; Odber et al., 1998) and between PMDD and anxiety disorders (Yonkers, 1997b; Facchinetti et al., 1998), or concentrating on the measurement of PMDD—in particular, the methods (Steiner et al., 1999; Ekholm et al., 1998) and items (Gehlert et al., 1997, 1999) that easily delineate individuals with PMDD.

Recently, a group of experts reached a consensus that PMDD is a distinct clinical entity (Endicott et al., 1999). The group's findings are summarized as follows:

- PMDD has a distinct clinical picture with characteristic symptoms of irritability, anger, and internal tension.
- The onset and offset of its symptoms are closely linked to the luteal phase of the menstrual cycle.
- The genetic component of PMDD does not seem to be related to depressive disorders.
- In PMDD, there is no dysregulation of the hypothalamic–pituitary–adrenal axis, unlike in major depression.
- Eliminating the menstrual cycle will cure women with PMDD, but not those with other mood disorders (after pregnancy, symptoms return once cycles have been reestablished).

Moreover, PMDD differs from other mood disorders in its response to treatment with antidepressants (i.e., rapid onset of response, efficacy of intermittent dosing, maximal response at low doses, and rapid recurrence of symptoms with discontinuation of treatment) (Eriksson, 1999). Serotonergic antidepressants have greater effectiveness for the treatment of PMDD than nonserotonergic antidepressants such as maprotiline (Eriksson et al., 1995), desipramine (Freeman et al., 1996, 1999b), and bupropion (Pearlstein et al., 1997); however, the serotonergic and noradrenergic agents are equally effective in the treatment of depression (Eriksson & Humble, 1990).

Additional evidence regarding the distinctness of PMDD compared with major depression can also be found in biochemical markers (Rapkin et al., 1998) and circadian variables (Parry et al., 1999).

Premenstrual Exacerbation

The category of "premenstrual exacerbation (or magnification)" denotes the premenstrual worsening of a major psychiatric disorder or of a medical condition. Women with continuing psychiatric disorders (e.g., major depression, dysthymic disorder, bipolar disorder [especially the rapid-cycling type], anxiety disorders, schizophrenia, bulimia nervosa, and substance abuse) report premenstrual exacerbation of symptoms and sometimes an emergence of new symptoms (Hendrick et al., 1996; Yonkers, 1997a; Blehar et al., 1998). In a study of women with chronic depression, over 50% reported premenstrual worsening of symptoms, and over 25% showed a pattern of premenstrual exacerbation of depression using prospective charting (Kornstein et al., 1996; see Kornstein & Wojcik, Chapter 8). Comorbid anxiety diagnoses (commonly panic disorder, generalized anxiety disorder, and phobias) have been reported to be as high as 32% in women with PMDD (Yonkers, 1997b), and in one study, investigators found (via retrospective reporting) that women with obsessive–compulsive disorder showed a high rate of premenstrual worsening (Williams & Koran, 1997). In general, interpretation of the literature is limited by the lack of prospective assessment (Hendrick et al., 1996). Nonetheless, it is important to exclude the possibility that the presentation is of a different major psychiatric or medical problem with premenstrual exacerbation.

Women who manifest severe physical symptoms or a psychiatric disorder with premenstrual exacerbation should be treated for their primary condition. Premenstrual symptoms usually remit considerably with successful treatment of the primary condition (sometimes increasing an already prescribed dose premenstrually can be effective), and residual symptoms can be treated as indicated.

An increased rate of psychiatric emergencies and hospital admissions during the premenstruum has been noted (Targum et al., 1991). A significant association between some affective premenstrual symptoms (including depression, irritability, mood swings, and a sense of losing control) and suicidal ideation has been demonstrated (Chaturvedi et al., 1995). Yet, to date, a relationship between suicide attempts (Lester, 1990; Gisselmann et al., 1996; Baca-Garcia et al., 1998) or completed suicides (Vanezis, 1990) and the late luteal phase has not been clearly delineated.

Other Psychiatric Diagnoses Mistaken for PMS or PMDD

Occasionally, women do not have premenstrual symptoms that meet criteria for PMS or PMDD, but do have some symptoms that meet DSM-IV criteria for another psychiatric disorder. Women meeting criteria for dysthymic disorder, cyclothymic disorder, bipolar I and II disorders, anxiety disorders, bulimia nervosa, or substance abuse may fall into this category (Hendrick et al., 1996). It should be noted that the cyclical nature of their symptoms *may or may not* match the phases of their menstrual cycle.

Menstrual Psychosis

In some women, transient psychotic symptoms may appear in rhythm with the menstrual cycle. This proposed classification can incorporate a broad range of phenomena, which may be grouped according to onset within the menstrual cycle (premenstrual, catamenial, paramenstrual, or midcycle) or according to stage in the reproductive life cycle (prepubertal, postpartum, amenorrhoea, menopause) (Brockington, 1998). These relatively rare phenomena have been the focus of much debate, although the literature is for the most part confined to case reports.

Several features delineate menstrual psychosis (as cited in Brockington, 1998):

- Acute or sudden onset, against a background of normality.
- Brief duration, with full recovery.
- Psychotic features (i.e., confusion, delusions, hallucinations, stupor and mutism, or a manic syndrome).
- A circamenstrual (approximately monthly) periodicity, in regular relation with the menstrual cycle.

As Brockington (1998) has noted, in many cases the patients "have manifested non-menstrual bipolar disorder at another stage of life" in which the phasic psychosis metamorphosed into a chaotic, continuous illness. Confusion regarding diagnostic status of menstrually related psychotic symptoms (sometimes called "atypical psychosis", "periodic psychosis," or "cycloid psychosis"; Severino & Yonkers, 1993) has led many to question whether menstrual psychosis is indeed a discrete condition. Furthermore, a frequent association between puerperal psychoses and (subsequent) menstrual psychoses suggests a common etiological factor for these latter two phenomena—namely, the abrupt changes in concentrations of female reproductive hormones (Deuchar & Brockington, 1998).

The treatments for menstrual psychosis have included ovariectomy, hormonal supplementation, endocrine therapy, clomiphene, phenytoin, or acetazolamine. The reader is referred to the case literature for further detail (see Brockington, 1998). In some instances, patients have experienced complete remittance from symptoms with pregnancy or menopause.

SCREENING AND DIAGNOSIS

Table 3.1 summarizes the process of screening and diagnosis for psychiatric aspects of the menstrual cycle. As a result of the lack of objective diagnostic tests for PMS or PMDD (attempts to pinpoint hormonal measures have yielded little success; see Rubinow et al., 1998), screening must begin with a complete medical and psychiatric history. Women presenting with PMDD frequently have a history of previous episodes of mood disorders, and women with continuing mood disorders report premenstrual magnification of symptoms and an emergence of new symptoms (Halbreich & Endicott, 1985; Graze et al., 1990; Blehar et al., 1998). In addition to a retrospective history of the premenstrual symptoms, this interview also should include a complete review of physical systems and medical disorders (including gynecological and endocrinological problems, allergies, and the like), and a detailed review of family loading for mental illness. Because the symptoms of anemia and thyroid disease often mirror those of PMS or PMDD, the patient should undergo laboratory investigations if any hint of an underlying medical cause for the symptoms arises. A high prevalence rate of past sexual abuse (40%) has been found among women seeking treatment for premenstrual symptoms (Paddison et al., 1990); therefore, screening for past abuse as well as for current domestic violence is an essential aspect of the assessment. A similar prevalence of premenstrual mood and physical symptoms have been found in women who are or are not using oral contraceptives (Sveindóttir & Bäckström, 2000).

Prospective daily rating of symptoms is essential in making a diagnosis of PMS or

TABLE 3.1. Psychiatric Aspects of the Menstrual Cycle: Screening and Diagnosis

Interview
- Retrospective history of premenstrual symptoms
- Seasonal variation
- Complete medical and psychiatric history
- History of sexual (or other) abuse
- Family loading for mental illness, including substance use

Laboratory
- Laboratory testing, especially thyroid, anemia, and gonadal hormones

Daily chart
- Prospective daily self-rating of symptoms for two menstrual cycles (using, e.g., PRISM, COPE)

Within-cycle percent change:
- $\dfrac{\text{luteal score} - \text{follicular score}}{\text{luteal score}} \times 100$

Diagnosis of PMDD
- Meets DSM-IV criteria
- ≥ 30% change in symptoms from the follicular to the luteal phase
- Pharmacological treatment: ≥ 50% change in symptoms from the follicular to the luteal phase

PMDD. To date, there is no consensus among investigators as to the best instruments for confirming prospectively the diagnosis of PMDD; nor is there a consensus as to the instruments most appropriate to measure treatment effects in clinical trials. Women with PMS are most often seen in primary care or by their obstetrician/gynecologist. The results of a recent U.S. study on the experiences of women with PMS who sought medical attention suggested a high rate of missed diagnoses (Kraemer & Kraemer, 1998).

Two of the available daily recording instruments seem to be the most appropriate for use in a clinical setting and aid in the required prospective measurement of symptoms: the Prospective Record of the Impact and Severity of Menstruation (PRISM; Reid, 1985), and the Calendar of Premenstrual Experiences (COPE; Mortola et al., 1990). These instruments allow respondents to rate a variety of physical and psychological symptoms, indicate negative and positive life events, record concurrent medications, and track menstrual bleeding and cycle length. They contain the core symptoms and most of the additional symptoms considered for the DSM-IV diagnosis of PMDD. Ling (2000) has recently published a report containing both the COPE and the PRISM, along with two examples of documented symptoms showing a pattern typical of depression and one typical to PMS.

Scores on the PRISM or the COPE can be used to calculate the "within-cycle percent change" in symptoms. This is done by subtracting the follicular score from the luteal score, dividing by the luteal score, and multiplying by 100 (Steiner & Yonkers, 1998):

$$\% \text{ change} = \frac{\text{luteal score} - \text{follicular score} \times 100}{\text{luteal score}}$$

After completion of a two-cycle prospective diagnostic assessment phase, women may qualify for any of the above-described diagnostic categories. Figure 3.1 presents an algorithm for diagnosing and treating PMS/PMDD (Steiner, 2000).

In a detailed study of three prospective symptom rating scales (used to establish severity of premenstrual mood symptoms and measure efficacy during a multicenter controlled treatment trial for premenstrual dysphoria; Steiner et al., 1995), researchers found that single-item visual analogue scales (VASs) (for irritability, tension, depression, mood swings), as well as the Premenstrual Tension Syndrome Observer (PMTS-O) and Self-Rating (PMTS-SR) Scales (Steiner et al., 1980), were sensitive to premenstrual worsening of symptoms, to change over time, and to response to treatment. Furthermore, premenstrual mood symptoms as measured by VASs significantly correlated with PMTS-O and PMTS-SR scores, denoting an easy-to-administer, user-friendly, reliable, and valid method of data collection (Steiner et al., 1999).

Given the sometimes close resemblance between PMDD and rapid-cycling bipolar II disorder (e.g., Hendrick & Altshuler, 1998), Macmillan and Young (1999) have recommended the Bipolar Mood Diary (a daily mood record derived from the COPE) in conjunction with a PMS daily record to facilitate differentiation between these disorders, as well as to note the severity and impact of manic, hypomanic, and depressive symptoms.

THERAPEUTIC INTERVENTIONS

Nonpharmacological Approaches

Lifestyle/stress management principles are necessary adjuncts to any therapeutic intervention, and patients should be educated and encouraged to practice these principles. The nonpharmacological approaches should be tried as first-line therapy for milder symptoms.

Diet and Exercise

The elimination or reduction of caffeine (especially coffee), alcohol, chocolate, and tobacco, and adopting a diet composed of frequent high-protein and low-refined-sugar meals is strongly recommended. Patients should be encouraged to decrease sodium in the diet when edema or fluid retention occurs, and, if possible, to reduce weight to within 20% of their ideal. Regular exercise (including aerobic exercise) is important and particularly effective when combined with the regular practice of stress management techniques.

Nutritional Supplements

Vitamin B$_6$. There is limited evidence to suggest that daily doses of pyridoxine up to 100 mg/day are likely to be beneficial in treating overall premenstrual symptoms, and of some benefit in treating premenstrual depressive symptoms. No conclusive evidence has been found of neurological side effects at this dose range; however, women receiving vitamin B$_6$ should be monitored for muscle weakness, numbness, clumsiness, and paresthesia (Wyatt et al., 1999).

Calcium. A daily supplementation of calcium carbonate containing 1,200 mg of elemental calcium has been shown to reduce overall luteal phase symptoms effectively in a large sample of women with confirmed PMS (Thys-Jacobs et al., 1998), suggesting a link between calcium deficiency and PMS. Symptom reduction occurred by the third treatment cycle.

Magnesium. There is some evidence to suggest that a daily supplement of 200 mg of magnesium for a minimum of 2 months is of benefit in treating premenstrual symp-

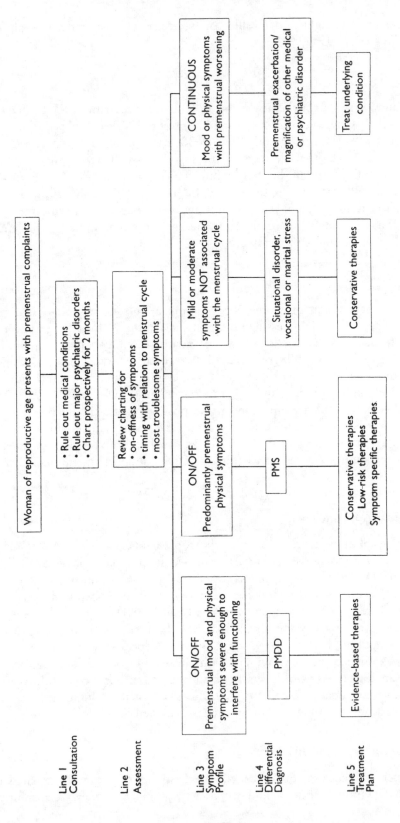

FIGURE 3.1. Algorithm for diagnosing and treating premenstrual syndrome and premenstrual dysphoric disorder.

Line 1
Consultation

Line 2
Assessment

Line 3
Symptom
Profile

Line 4
Differential
Diagnosis

Line 5
Treatment
Plan

toms of fluid retention (weight gain, swelling of extremities, breast tenderness, abdominal bloating) (Walker et al., 1998).

Light Therapy

Two studies found bright-light therapy to be an effective intervention for LLPDD as defined by DSM-III-R. One study utilized a minimum of 2,500-lux cool-white fluorescent light for 2 hours in the morning (6:30 A.M.–8:30 A.M.) or in the evening (7:00 P.M.–9:00 P.M.) during the symptomatic days in the luteal phase (Parry et al., 1993; Parry, 1998); the other utilized 10,000-lux cool-white fluorescent light for 30 minutes in the evening (7:00 P.M.–9:00 P.M.) during these days (Lam et al., 1999). Significant reductions in depression, irritability, and physical symptoms were observed. Furthermore, Parry (1998) found that the benefits of bright-light therapy were maintained in patients who completed at least 12 months of treatment.

Psychotherapy

Individual psychotherapy can aid women's psychological and social functioning, particularly those who have endured distressing premenstrual symptoms for a long time. There is some evidence from controlled studies that women with PMS may benefit from individual cognitive therapy (Blake et al., 1998) or coping skills training (Morse et al., 1991). There are conflicting reports, however, about the usefulness of cognitive-behavioral techniques such as restructuring, thought stopping, and anger management (Pearlstein, 1996).

There is also recent evidence of the benefits of positively reframing perceptions of the menstrual cycle (Morse, 1999) and structured group treatment using cognitive, behavioral, environmental, and dietary changes strategies (Taylor, 1999) among women with PMS. These latter studies affirm the usefulness of peer support in the management of PMS.

Pharmacological Approaches

The pharmacological approaches include psychotropic medications and hormonal interventions. The newer antidepressants in particular—including many of the SSRIs, as well as clomipramine (a tricyclic antidepressant with major serotonin-reuptake-inhibiting properties) and L-tryptophan (a serotonin precursor)—have demonstrated excellent efficacy and minimal side effects in women with PMS and PMDD who have not responded to conservative treatment. Two anxiolytics have also been successful in the reduction of psychological symptoms, but side effects and possible dependence may limit their use. There is likewise evidence of success with estradiol implants, gonadotropin-releasing hormone (GnRH) analogues, danazol (a synthetic androgen), and oral contraceptives; however, many women are unable to tolerate the side effects of these interventions. A summary of suggested pharmacological approaches is provided in Table 3.2.

Selective Serotonin Reuptake Inhibitors

There is consistent evidence for the efficacy and tolerability of many of the SSRIs in the treatment of PMDD (both emotional and somatic symptoms), and they are currently considered the first-line pharmacological treatments for premenstrual mood symptoms (Steiner et al., 1997a; Eriksson, 1999). More recently, several studies have indicated that intermittent (premenstrually only) treatment with SSRIs (Steiner et al., 1997b; Halbreich & Smoller, 1997; Sundblad et al., 1997; Young et al., 1998; Freeman et al., 1999a; Wikander et al., 1998; Jermain et al., 1999), clomipramine (Sundblad et al., 1992, 1993), and L-tryptophan (Steinberg et al., 1999) are equally effective in alleviating PMDD and may offer cheaper, easier-to-tolerate, and more attractive treatment options for a disorder that is itself intermittent. The SSRIs have also demonstrated benefit in the relief of physical symptoms that usually accompany PMS/PMDD, in particular breast tenderness and bloating (Eriksson et al., 1995; Wikander et al., 1998; Freeman et al., 1999b; Steiner et al., 2001). In a multicenter, placebo-controlled trial, women diagnosed with PMDD who were effectively treated with sertraline also showed significant improvement in quality of life and overall psychosocial functioning (Pearlstein et al., 2000).

PMS and PMDD respond to relatively low doses of SSRIs—for example, 10–20 mg/day of fluoxetine (Steiner et al., 1995; Diegoli et al., 1998; Romano et al., 1999) or 50–100 mg/day of sertraline (Jermain et al., 1999; Freeman et al., 1999a). As well, there is strong evidence that response to treatment with SSRIs or clomipramine will be relatively immediate (within the first month of treatment); therefore, if there is no change in symptomatology (even after several dosing increases), an alternative therapy should be considered within two to three menstrual cycles. A decreased clearance of sertraline and desmethylsertraline was reported in three of eight women treated for PMDD who were taking oral contraceptives (Brown et al., 2000), but there was no difference in the efficacy of sertraline or adverse events among any of these eight patients.

Anxiolytics

The efficacy of alprazolam (Smith et al., 1987; Harrison et al., 1990; Berger & Presser, 1994; Freeman et al., 1995b; Diegoli et al., 1998; Evans et al., 1998) and buspirone (Rickels et al., 1989) in the reduction of psychological symptoms has been demonstrated in randomized controlled trials; however, the effect is much smaller than that with the SSRIs. Intermittent dosing is also effective with both of these medications. The possibility of withdrawal symptoms with alprazolam portends a gradual taper during menses in some women. Dependence and tolerance are the major concerns, but weight gain is also a possible side effect of alprazolam (Evans et al., 1998).

Hormonal Interventions

The suppression of ovulation eliminates the symptomatology of PMS and PMDD, implying the involvement of ovarian hormones in the etiology of premenstrual syndromes in vulnerable women. The benefits and risks of this approach, however, should be carefully evaluated with the patient.

The gonadotropin-releasing hormone (GnRH) agonists leuprolide, buserelin, and goserelin have been shown to be effective in reducing physical and psychological symptoms in most (Bancroft et al., 1987; Hammarback & Backstrom, 1988; Brown et al., 1994; Mezrow et al., 1994; West & Hillier, 1994; Freeman et al., 1997; Schmidt et al., 1998; Leather et al., 1999; Sundström et al., 1999), but not in all studies and not for all symptoms (Brown et al., 1994; West & Hillier, 1994; Sundström et al., 1999).

TABLE 3.2. Pharmacological Therapies

Type	Recommended dose	References	Comments
Antidepressants			
Fluoxetine	20 mg/day	Steiner et al. (1995) Su et al. (1997) Pearlstein et al. (1997)	• SSRIs are the first-line treatments for premenstrual mood symptoms:
	20 mg/day 14 days before menses	Steiner et al. (1997b)[a]	• Highly efficacious and tolerable
	10 mg/day	Diegoli et al. (1998) (PMS)	• Intermittent use (luteal phase only) offers lower costs and side effect burdens
Sertraline	50–150 mg/day	Yonkers et al. (1997)	
	50–150 mg/day Luteal phase only	Halbreich & Smoller (1997) Young et al. (1998) Freeman et al. (1999a) (PMS) Jermaine et al. (1999)	
Paroxetine	10–30 mg/day	Eriksson et al. (1995)	
	5–30 mg Late luteal phase only	Sundblad et al. (1997)[a]	
Citalopram	20 ± 10 mg/day ovulation → Day 2	Wikander et al. (1998)	
Clomipramine	25–75 mg/day	Sundblad et al. (1992)	
	25–75 mg/day 14 days before menses	Sundblad et al. (1993)	
L-Tryptophan	6 g/day Ovulation → Day 3	Steinberg et al. (1999)	
Nefazodone	100–150 mg/day 14 days before menses	Kodesh et al. (2001)	
Venlafaxine	50–200 mg/day	Freeman et al. (2001)	
Anxiolytics			
Alprazolam	0.25–4 mg/day	Smith et al. (1987) Harrison et al. (1990) Diegoli et al. (1998)	• Dependence and tolerance can develop • Withdrawal symptoms can occur during menses
	0.25–2 mg/day 6–14 days before menses	Berger & Presser (1994) Freeman et al. (1995b)	• Mixed reports on improvement of psychological symptoms
Buspirone	25–60 mg/day 12 days before menses	Rickels et al. (1989)	
Ovulation suppression			
Danazol	200–400 mg/day During symptomatic days only	Sarno et al. (1987) Hahn et al. (1995) O'Brien & Abukhalil (1999)	• Efficacious treatment for premenstrual migraines and mastalgia • At lower dose (200 mg/day), ovulation is not suppressed (i.e., fewer side effects)
Leuprolide	3.75–7.5 mg i.m. injection monthly	Brown et al. (1994) Freeman et al. (1997)	• Potential risk for osteoporosis, cardiovascular disease with long-term use • Several months of use to reach full treatment effect

TABLE 3.2. (*continued*)

Type	Recommended dose	References	Comments
	7.5 mg i.m. injection monthly with "add-back" conjugated estrogen 0.625 mg/day (Monday to Saturday) and 10 mg medroxyprogesterone acetate orally for 10 days during every fourth cycle	Mezrow et al. (1994)	• "Add-back" estrogen plus progestin reduced physical and psychological symptoms. "Add-back" estrogen or progesterone alone was associated with recurrence of PMS
	3.75 mg/month with "add-back" transdermal estradiol 0.1 mg or progesterone vaginal suppository 200 mg twice daily	Schmidt et al. (1998)	• Lower dose relieved premenstrual depression and irritability, and some physical complaints
	3.75 mg i.m. injection monthly with "add-back" tibolone 2.5 mg/day orally at the onset of vasomotor symptoms	Di Carlo et al. (2001)	• "Add-back" tibolone significantly reduced hot flashes
Buserelin	100 µg/day Intranasal	Sundström et al. (1999)	• Low dose improved psychological symptoms, swelling and headache
	400–900 µg/day Intranasal	Bancroft et al. (1987)[a] Hammerback & Backstrom (1988)	• Not available in the United States
Goserelin	3.6 mg s.c. injection monthly	West & Hillier (1994)	• Significant physical but not psychological relief
	3.6 mg implant—four weekly	Leather et al. (1999	
Estradiol	100 g twice weekly patch with "add-back" dydrogesterone 10 mg or medroxyprogesterone 5 mg from days 17 to 26 of each cycle	Smith et al. (1995) Watson et al. (1989)	

Note. Double-blind, randomized, placebo-controlled studies, assessed prospectively for at least two complete cycles, in women with LLPDD/PMDD are cited, unless otherwise noted.

[a]Prospective case studies of PMDD.

The addition ("add-back") of estrogen *plus* progestin to depot leuprolide provided significant relief of premenstrual symptoms, and no significant changes in lipids, endometrium, or bone density were observed (Mezrow et al., 1994). Women who received "add-back" estrogen or progesterone *alone* with leuprolide acetate, on the other hand, had a significant recurrence of mood and physical symptoms (Schmidt et al., 1998). "Add-back" estrogen and progestin with goserelin, also did not significantly improve premenstrual symptomatology when compared with placebo (Leather et al., 1999). A preliminary report on "add-back" tibolone (a synthetic compound structurally related to noretinodrel) with depot leuprolide showed significant relief of mood and physical symptoms with less adverse effects (e.g., hot flashes, bone loss) in women with PMDD (Di Carlo et al., 2001).

Transdermal estradiol at a dose of 100µg with or without "add-back" progestogen for 10 days (mid to luteal phase) has been shown to be effective in the treatment of severe PMS (Watson et al., 1989; Smith et al., 1995). Danazol has demonstrated efficacy in the relief of premenstrual symptoms (Sarno et al., 1987), migraine (Hahn et al., 1995) and premenstrual mastalgia (O'Brien & Abukhalil, 1999). Some of the more troublesome adverse effects (nausea, acne, hirsutism) are significantly reduced with lower doses.

To date, only two controlled studies of oral contraceptives in the treatment of PMS have been published (Backstrom et al., 1992; Graham & Sherwin, 1992); the results indicate that a triphasic oral contraceptive effectively reduced physical symptoms (especially breast pain and bloating), but the reports on the relief of psychological symptoms with this intervention have been less firm.

Surgical Approach

A surgical approach should be the treatment of last resort for women with PMDD who have not found relief with pharmacological intervention, and a review with the patient of the implications of surgical menopause is recommended. Two studies have demonstrated the effectiveness of ovariectomy in the (complete) relief of severe premenstrual symptomatology (Casson et al., 1990; Casper & Hearn, 1990).

SUMMARY

The etiology of premenstrual syndromes has yet to be clarified in a comprehensive fashion. Notwithstanding, there is now a consensus that PMDD is a distinct clinical entity. We are now able to identify those women who present with severe psychological symptoms, to classify their symptoms, and to determine whether these symptoms are attributable only to the premenstruum or are a magnification of a physical or psychiatric disorder. Women who do not have a concurrent disorder and who meet criteria for PMS but not PMDD should be treated conservatively. Women who meet criteria for PMDD can be successfully treated with either low-dose SSRIs, clomipramine, or L-tryptophan on an intermittent (luteal phase only) or daily basis.

There is also some evidence for the efficacy of calcium, magnesium, and vitamin B_6, as well as bright artificial light, for premenstrual symptoms. Further replication studies with these interventions are still needed, however.

Using methods (pharmacological or surgical) to abolish the menstrual cycle, though very effective in eliminating symptoms of PMS and PMDD, poses an ethical dilemma: Such methods create a state of early menopause for young women, with all its potential ramifications.

REFERENCES

American Psychiatric Association (APA). (1987). *Diagnostic and statistical manual of mental disorders* (3rd ed., rev., pp. 367–369). Washington, DC: Author.

American Psychiatric Association (APA). (1994). *Diagnostic and statistical manual of mental disorders* (4th ed., pp. 717–718). Washington DC: Author.

Andersch, B., Wendestam, C., Hahn, L., et al. (1986). Premenstrual complaints: I. Prevalence of premenstrual symptoms in a Swedish urban population. *Journal of Psychosomatic Obstetrics and Gynaecology, 5,* 39–49.

Angst, J., Sellaro, R., Merikangas, K. R., & Endicott, J. (2001). The epidemiology of perimenstrual symptoms. *Acta Psychiatrica Scandinavica, 104,* 110–116.

Baca-Garcia, E., Sanchez-Gonzalez, A., Gonzalez Diaz-Corralero, P., et al. (1998). Menstrual cycle and profiles of suicidal behaviour. *Acta Psychiatrica Scandinavica, 97,* 32–35.

Backstrom, T., Hansson-Malmstrom, Y., Lindhe, B. A., et al. (1992). Oral contraceptives in premenstrual syndrome: A randomized comparison of triphasic and monophasic preparations. *Contraception, 46,* 253–268.

Bailey, J. W., & Cohen, L. S. (1999). Prevalence of mood and anxiety disorders in women who seek treatment for premenstrual syndrome. *Journal of Women's Health & Gender-Based Medicine, 8,* 1181–1184.

Bancroft, J., Rennie, D., & Warner, P. (1994). Vulnerability to perimenstrual mood change: The relevance of a past history of depressive disorder. *Psychosomatic Medicine, 56,* 225–231.

Berger, C. P., & Presser, B. (1994). Alprazolam in the treatment of two subsamples of patients with late luteal phase dysphoric disorder: A double-blind, placebo-controlled crossover study. *Obstetrics and Gynecology, 84,* 379–385.

Blake, F., Salkovskis, P., Gath, D., et al. (1998). Cognitive therapy for premenstrual syndrome: A controlled trial. *Journal of Pyschosomatic Research, 45,* 307–318.

Blehar, M. C., DePaulo, J. R., Jr., Gershon, E. S., et al. (1998). Women with bipolar disorder: Findings from the NIMH Genetics Initiative sample. *Psychopharmacology Bulletin, 34,* 239–243.

Brockington, I. (1998). Menstrual psychosis. *Archives of Women's Mental Health, 1,* 3–13.

Brown, C. S., Ling, F. W., Andersen, R. N., et al. (1994). Efficacy of depot leuprolide in premenstrual syndrome: Effect of symptom severity and type in a controlled trial. *Obstetrics and Gynecology, 84,* 779–786.

Brown, C. S., Parker, N., Ling, F., et al. (2000). Sertraline in contraceptive users with premenstrual dysphoric disorder. *Obstetrics and Gynecology, 95,* S29.

Budeiri, D. J., Li Wan Po, A., & Dornan, J. C. (1994). Clinical trials of treatment of premenstrual syndrome: Entry criteria and scales for measuring treatment outcomes. *British Journal of Obstetrics and Gynaecology, 101,* 689–695.

Casper, R. F., & Hearn, M. T. (1990). The effect of hysterectomy and bilateral oophorectomy in women with severe premenstrual syndrome. *American Journal of Obstetrics and Gynecology, 162,* 105–109.

Casson, P., Hahn, P. M., Van Vugt, D. A., et al. (1990). Lasting response to ovariectomy in severe intractable premenstrual syndrome. *American Journal of Obstetrics and Gynecology, 162,* 99–105.

Chandra, P. S., & Chaturvedi, S. K. (1989). Cultural variations in premenstrual experiences. *International Journal of Social Psychiatry, 35,* 343.

Chang, A. M., Holroyd, E., & Chau, J. P. (1995). Premenstrual syndrome in employed Chinese women in Hong Kong. *Health Care for Women International, 16,* 551–561.

Chaturvedi, S. K., Chandra, P. S., Gururaj, G., et al. (1995). Suicidal ideas during premenstrual phase. *Journal of Affective Disorders, 34,* 193–199.

Cleckner-Smith, C. S., Doughty, A. S., & Grossman, J. A. (1998). Premenstrual symptoms. Prevalence and severity in an adolescent sample. *Journal of Adolescent Health, 22,* 403–408.

Condon, J. T. (1993). The premenstrual syndrome: A twin study. *British Journal of Psychiatry, 162,* 481–486.

Dan, A. J., & Monagle, L. (1994). Sociocultural influences on women's experiences of perimenstrual symptoms. In J. H. Gold & S. K. Severino (Eds.), *Premenstrual dysphorias: Myths and realities* (pp. 201–211). Washington, DC: American Psychiatric Press.

Deuchar, N., & Brockington, I. (1998). Puerperal and menstrual psychoses: The proposal of a unitary etiological hypothesis. *Journal of Psychosomatic Obstetrics and Gynecology, 19,* 104–110.

Deuster, P. A., Adera, T., & South-Paul, J. (1999). Biological, social, and behavioral factors associated with premenstrual syndrome. *Archives of Family Medicine, 8,* 122–128.

DiCarlo, C., Palomba, S., Tommaselli, G. A., et al. (2001). Use of leuprolide acetate plus tibolone in the treatment of severe premenstrual syndrome. *Fertility and Sterility, 75,* 380–384.

Diegoli, M. S., da Fonseca, A. M., Diegoli, C. A., et al. (1998). A double-blind trial of four medications to treat severe premenstrual syndrome. *International Journal of Gynecology and Obstetrics, 62,* 63–67.

Ekholm, U. B., Ekholm, N. O., & Backstrom, T. (1998). Premenstrual syndrome: comparison between different methods to diagnose cyclicity using daily symptom ratings. *Acta Obstetricia et Gynecologica Scandinavica, 77,* 551–557.

Endicott, J. (1993). The menstrual cycle and mood disorders. *Journal of Affective Disorders, 29,* 193–200.

Endicott, J., Amsterdam, J., Eriksson, E., et al. (1999). Is premenstrual dysphoric disorder a distinct clinical entity? *Journal of Women's Health and Gender-Based Medicine, 8,* 663–679.

Eriksson, E. (1999). Serotonin reuptake inhibitors for the treatment of premenstrual dysphoria. *International Journal of Clinical Psychopharmacology, 14*(Suppl. 2), S27–S33.

Eriksson, E., Alling, C., Andersch, B., et al. (1994). Cerebrospinal fluid levels of monoamine metabolities: A preliminary study of their relation to menstrual cycle phase, sex steroids, and pituitary hormones in healthy women and in women with premenstrual syndrome. *Neuropsychopharmacology, 11,* 201–213.

Eriksson, E., Hedberg, M. A., Andersch, B., et al. (1995). The serotonin reuptake inhibitor paroxetine is superior to the noradrenaline reuptake inhibitor maprotiline in the treatment of premenstrual syndrome. *Neuropsychopharmacology, 12,* 167–176.

Eriksson, E., & Humble, M. (1990). Serotonin in psychiatric pathophysiology. A review of data from experimental and clinical research. In R. Pohl & S. Gershon (Eds.), *Progress in basic clinical pharmacology, 3rd edition. The biological basis of psychiatric treatment* (pp. 66–119). Basel: Karger.

Evans, S. M., Haney, M., Levin, F. R., et al. (1998). Mood and performance changes in women with premenstrual dysphoric disorder: Acute effects of alprazolam. *Neuropsychopharmacology, 19,* 499–516.

Facchinetti, F., Tarabusi, M., & Nappi, G. (1998). Premenstrual syndrome and anxiety disorders: A psychobiological link. *Psychotherapy and Psychosomatics, 67,* 57–60.

Fava, M., Pedrazzi, F., Guaraldi, G. P., et al. (1992). Comorbid anxiety and depression among patients with late luteal phase dysphoric disorder. *Journal of Anxiety Disorders, 6,* 325–335.

Freeman, E. W., Kunz, K., Rickels, K., et al. (2001). Efficacy and safety of venlafaxine for premenstrual dysphoric disorder. *Archives of Women's Mental Health, 3,* S37.

Freeman, E. W., & Rickels, K. (1999). Characteristics of placebo responses in medical treatment of premenstrual syndrome. *American Journal of Psychiatry, 156,* 1403–1408.

Freeman, E. W., Rickels, K., Arredondo, F., et al. (1999a). Full- or half-cycle treatment of severe premenstrual syndrome with a serotonergic antidepressant. *Journal of Clinical Psychopharmacology, 19,* 3–8.

Freeman, E. W., Rickels, K., Schweizer, E., et al. (1995a). Relationships between age and symptom severity among women seeking medical treatment for premenstrual symptoms. *Psychological Medicine, 25,* 309–315.

Freeman, E. W., Rickels, K., Sondheimer, S. J., et al. (1995b). A double-blind trial of oral progesterone, alprazolam, and placebo in the treatment of severe premenstrual syndrome. *Journal of the American Medical Association, 274,* 51–57.

Freeman, E. W., Rickels, K., Sondheimer, S. J., et al. (1999b). Differential response to antidepressants in women with premenstrual syndrome/premenstrual dysphoric disorder: A randomized controlled trial. *Archives of General Psychiatry, 56,* 932–939.

Freeman, E. W., Rickels, K., Sondheimer, S. J., et al. (1996). Sertraline versus desipramine in the treatment of premenstrual syndrome: An open-label trial. *Journal of Clinical Psychiatry, 57,* 7–11.

Freeman, E. W., Sondheimer, S. J., & Rickels, K. (1997). Gonadotropin-releasing hormone agonist in the treatment of premenstrual symptoms with and without ongoing dysphoria: A controlled study. *Psychopharmacology Bulletin, 33,* 303–309.

Freeman, E. W., Sondheimer, K., Weinbaum, P. H., et al. (1985). Evaluating premenstrual symptoms in medical practice. *Obstetrics and Gynecology, 65,* 500–505.

Gehlert, S., Chang, C. H., & Hartlage, S. (1997). Establishing the diagnostic validity of premenstrual dysphoric disorder using rasch analysis. *Journal of Outcome Measures, 1*, 2–18.

Gehlert, S., Chang, C. H., & Hartlage, S. (1999). Symptom patterns of premenstrual dysphoric disorder as defined in the *Diagnostic and Statistical Manual of Mental Disorders—IV. Journal of Women's Health, 8*, 75–85.

Gisselmann, A., Ait Ameur, A., Pinoit, J. M., et al. (1996). Attempted suicide and menstrual cycle: An epidemiologic study. *Annales Medico-Psychologiques (Paris), 154*, 136–139.

Graham, C. A., & Sherwin, B. B. (1992). A prospective treatment study of premenstrual symptoms using a triphasic oral contraceptive. *Journal of Psychosomatic Research, 36*, 257–266.

Graze, K. K., Nee, J., & Endicott, J. (1990). Premenstrual depression predicts future major depressive disorder. *Acta Psychiatrica Scandinavica, 81*, 201–205.

Greene, R., & Dalton, K. (1953). The premenstrual syndrome. *British Medical Journal, i*, 1007–1014.

Hahn, P. M., VanVugt, D. A., & Reid, R. L. (1995). A randomized, placebo-controlled crossover trial of danazol for the treatment of premenstrual syndrome. *Psychoneuroendocrinology, 20*, 193–209.

Halbreich, U. (1997). Premenstrual dysphoric disorders: A diversified cluster of vulnerability traits to depression. *Acta Psychiatrica Scandinavica, 95*, 169–176.

Halbreich, U., & Endicott, J. (1985). The relationship of dysphoric premenstrual changes to depressive disorder. *Acta Psychiatrica Scandinavica, 71*, 331–338.

Halbreich, U., & Smoller, J. W. (1997). Intermittent luteal phase sertraline treatment of dysphoric premenstrual syndrome. *Journal of Clinical Psychiatry, 58*, 399–402.

Halbreich, U., & & Tworek, H. (1993). Altered serotonergic activity in women with dysphoric premenstrual syndromes. *International Journal of Psychiatry in Medicine, 23*, 1–27.

Hammarback, S., & Backstrom, T. (1988). Induced anovulation as treatment of premenstrual tension syndrome. *Acta Obstetricia Gynecologica Scandinavica, 67*, 159–166.

Hargrove, J. T., & Abraham, G. E. (1982). The incidence of premenstrual tension in a gynecologic clinic. *Journal of Reproductive Medicine, 27*, 721–724.

Harrison, W. M., Endicott, J., & Nee, J. (1990). Treatment of premenstrual dysphoria with alprazolam: Controlled study. *Archives of General Psychiatry, 47*, 270–275.

Harrison, W. M., Endicott, J., Nee, J., et al. (1989). Characteristics of women seeking treatment for premenstrual syndrome. *Psychosomatics, 30*, 405–411.

Hendrick, V., & Altshuler, L. L. (1998). Recurrent mood shifts of premenstrual dysphoric disorder can be mistaken for rapid-cycling bipolar II disorder. *Journal of Clinical Psychiatry, 59*, 479–480.

Hendrick, V., Altshuler, L. L., & Burt, V. K. (1996). Course of psychiatric disorders across the menstrual cycle. *Harvard Review of Psychiatry, 4*, 200–207.

Hylan, T. R., Sundell, K., & Judge, R. (1999). The impact of premenstrual symptomatology on functioning and treatment-seeking behavior: Experience from the United States, United Kingdom, and France. *Journal of Women's Health and Gender-Based Medicine, 8*, 1043–1052.

Jermain, D. M., Preece, C. K., Sykes, R. L., et al. (1999). Luteal phase sertraline treatment for premenstrual dysphoric disorder: Results of a double-blind, placebo-controlled, crossover study. *Archives of Family Medicine, 8*, 328–332.

Johnson, S. R. (1987). The epidemiology and social impact of premenstrual symptoms. *Clinical Obstetrics and Gynecology, 30*, 367–376.

Johnson, S. R., McChesney, C., & Bean, J. A. (1988). Epidemiology of premenstrual symptoms in a nonclinical sample: I. Prevalence, natural history and help-seeking behavior. *Journal of Reproductive Medicine, 33*, 340–346.

Kaspi, S. P., Otto, M. W., Pollack, M. H. et al. (1994). Premenstrual exacerbation of symptoms in women with panic disorder. *Journal of Anxiety Disorders, 8*, 131–138.

Kendler, K. S., Karkowski, L. M., Corey, L. A., et al. (1998). Longitudinal population-based twin study of retrospectively reported premenstrual symptoms and lifetime major depression. *American Journal of Psychiatry, 155*, 1234–1240.

Kodesh, A., Katz, S., Lerner, A. G., et al. (2001). Intermittent, luteal phase nefazodone treatment of premenstrual dysphoric disorder. *Journal of Psychopharmacology, 15,* 58–60.

Kornstein, S. G., Yonkers, K. A., Schatzberg, A. F. et al. (May, 1996). *Premenstrual exacerbation of depression.* Paper presented at the 149th Annual Convention of the American Psychiatric Association, New York.

Kouri, E. M., & Halbreich, U. (1997). State and trait serotonergic abnormalities in women with dysphoric premenstrual syndromes. *Psychopharmacology Bulletin, 33,* 767–770.

Kraemer, G. R., & Kraemer, R. R. (1998). Premenstrual syndrome: Diagnosis and treatment experiences. *Journal of Women's Health, 7,* 893–907.

Lam, R. W., Carter, D., Misri, S., et al. (1999). A controlled study of light therapy in women with late luteal phase dysphoric disorder. *Psychiatry Research, 86,* 185–192.

Leather, A. T., Studd, J. W., Watson, N. R., et al. (1999). The treatment of severe premenstrual syndrome with goserelin with and without 'add-back' estrogen therapy: A placebo-controlled study. *Gynecological Endocrinology, 13,* 48–55.

Leibenluft, E., Fiero, P. L., & Rubinow, D. R. (1994). Effects of the menstrual cycle on dependent variables in mood disorder research. *Archives of General Psychiatry, 51,* 761–781.

Lester, D. (1990). Suicide and the menstrual cycle. *Medical Hypotheses, 31,* 197–199.

Ling, F. W. (2000). Recognizing and treating premenstrual dysphoric disorder in thr obstetric, gynecologic, and primary care practices. *Journal of Clinical Psychiatry, 61*(Suppl. 12), 9–16.

Macmillan, I., & Young, A. (1999). Bipolar II disorder vs. premenstrual dysphoric disorder. *Journal of Clinical Psychiatry, 60,* 409–410.

Marvan, M. L., Diaz-Erosa, M., & Montesinos, A. (1998). Premenstrual symptoms in Mexican women with different educational levels. *Journal of Psychology, 132,* 517–526.

Maskall, D. D., Lam, R. W., Misri, S., et al. (1997). Seasonality of symptoms in women with late luteal phase dysphoric disorder. *American Journal of Psychiatry, 154,* 1436–1441.

McLeod, D. R., Hoehn-Saric, R., Foster, G. V., et al. (1993). The influence of premenstrual syndrome on ratings of anxiety in women with generalized anxiety disorder. *Acta Psychiatrica Scandinavica, 88,* 248–251.

Merikangas, K. R., Foeldenyi, M., & Angst, J. (1993). The Zurich Study: XIX. Patterns of menstrual disturbances in the community: Results of the Zurich Cohort Study. *European Archives of Psychiatry and Clinical Neuroscience, 243,* 23–32.

Mezrow, G., Shoupe, D., Spicer, D., et al. (1994). Depot leuprolide acetate with estrogen and progestin add-back for long-term treatment of premenstrual syndrome. *Fertility and Sterility, 62,* 932–937.

Morse, C. A., Dennerstein, L., Farrell, E., et al. (1991). A comparison of hormone therapy, coping skills training, and relaxation for the relief of premenstrual syndrome. *Journal of Behavioral Medicine, 14,* 469–489.

Morse, G. (1999). Positively reframing perceptions of the menstrual cycle among women with premenstrual syndrome. *Journal of Obstetric, Gynaecologic and Neonatal Nursing, 28,* 165–174.

Mortola, J. F., Girton, L., Beck, L., et al. (1990). Diagnosis of premenstrual syndrome by a simple, prospective, and reliable instrument: The Calendar of Premenstrual Experiences. *Obstetrics and Gynecology, 76,* 302–307.

O'Brien, P. M., & Abukhalil, I. E. (1999). Randomized controlled trial of the management of premenstrual syndrome and premenstrual mastalgia using luteal phase-only danazol. *American Journal of Obstetrics and Gynecology, 180*(1, Pt. 1), 18–23.

O'Brien, P. M. S., Abukhalil, I. E. H., & Henshaw, C. (1995). Premenstrual syndrome. *Current Opinion in Obstetrics and Gynecology, 5,* 30–37.

Odber, J., Cawood, E. H., & Bancroft, J. (1998). Salivary cortisol in women with and without perimenstrual mood changes. *Journal of Psychosomatic Research, 45,* 557–568.

Paddison, P. L., Gise, L. H., Lebovits, A., et al. (1990). Sexual abuse and premenstrual syndrome: Comparison between a lower and higher socioeconomic group. *Psychosomatics, 31,* 265–272.

Parry, B. L. (1995). Mood disorders linked to reproductive cycle in women. In F. E. Bloom & D. J. Kupfer (Eds.), *Psychopharmacology: The fourth generation of progress* (pp. 1029–1042). New York: Raven Press.

Parry, B. L. (1998). Light therapy of premenstrual depression. In R. W. Lam (Ed.), *Seasonal affective disorder and beyond* (pp. 173–191). Washington, DC: American Psychiatric Press.

Parry, B. L., Mahan, A. M., Mostofi, N., et al. (1993). Light therapy of late luteal phase dysphoric disorder: An extended study. *American Journal of Psychiatry, 150*, 1417–1419.

Parry, B. L., Mostofi, N., LeVeau, B., et al. (1999). Sleep EEG studies during early and late partial sleep deprivation in premenstrual dysphoric disorder and normal control subjects. *Psychiatry Research, 85*, 127–143.

Pearlstein, T. B. (1996). Nonpharmacologic treatment of premenstrual syndrome. *Psychiatric Annals, 26*, 590–594.

Pearlstein, T. B., Frank, E., Rivera-Tovar, A., et al. (1990). Prevalence of Axis I and Axis II disorders in women with late luteal phase dysphoric disorder. *Journal of Affective Disorders, 20*, 129–134.

Pearlstein, T. B., Halbreich, U., Batzar, E. D., et al. (2000). Psychosocial functioning in women with premenstrual dysphoric disorder before and after treatment with sertraline or placebo. *Journal of Clinical Psychiatry, 61*, 101–109.

Pearlstein, T. B., Stone, A. B., Lund, S. A., et al. (1997). Comparison of fluoxetine, bupropion, and placebo in the treatment of premenstrual dysphoric disorder. *Journal of Clinical Psychopharmacology, 17*, 261–266.

Praschak-Rieder, N., Willeit, M., Neumeister, A., et al. (2001). Prevalence of premenstrual dysphoric disorder in female patients with seasonal affective disorder. *Journal of Affective Disorders, 63*, 239–242.

Ramacharan, S., Love, E. J., Fick, G. H., et al. (1992). The epidemiology of premenstrual symptoms in a population based sample of 2650 urban women: Attributable risk and risk factors. *Journal of Clinical Epidemiology, 45*, 377–392.

Rapkin, A. J. (1992). The role of serotonin in premenstrual syndrome. *Clinical Obstetrics and Gynecology, 35*, 629–636.

Rapkin, A. J., Cedars, M., & Morgan, M. (1998). Insulin-like growth factor-1 and insulin-like growth factor-binding protein-3 in women with premenstrual syndrome. *Fertility and Sterility, 70*, 1077–1080.

Reid, R. L. (1985). Premenstrual syndrome. *Current Problems in Obstetrics, Gynecology and Fertility, 8*, 1–57.

Rickels, K., Freeman, E., & Sondheimer, S. (1989). Buspirone in treatment of premenstrual syndrome [Letter to the editor]. *Lancet, i*, 777.

Rivera-Tovar, A. D., & Frank, E. (1990). Late luteal phase dysphoric disorder in young women. *American Journal of Psychiatry, 147*, 1634–1636.

Robinson, R. L., & Swindle, R. W. (2000). Premenstrual symptom severity: Impact on social functioning and treatment-seeking behaviors. *Journal of Women's Health and Gender-Based Medicine, 9*, 757–768.

Roca, C. A., Schmidt, P. J., Bloch, M., et al. (1996). Implications of endocrine studies of premenstrual syndrome. *Psychiatric Annals, 26*, 576–580.

Rojansky, N., Halbreich, U., Zander, K., et al. (1991). Imipramine receptor binding and serotonin uptake in platelets of women with premenstrual changes. *Gynecological and Obstetrical Investigations, 31*, 146–152.

Romano, S., Judge, R., Dillon, J., et al. (1999). The role of fluoxetine in the treatment of premenstrual dysphoric disorder. *Clinical Therapy, 21*, 615–633.

Rubinow, D. R., Schmidt, P. J., & Roca, C. A. (1998). Hormone measures in reproductive endocrine-related mood disorders: diagnostic issues. *Psychopharmacology Bulletin, 34*, 289–290.

Sarno, A. P., Miller, E. J., Jr., & Lundblad, E. G. (1987). Premenstrual syndrome: Beneficial effects of periodic low-dose danazol. *Obstetrics and Gynecology, 70*, 33–36.

Schmidt, P. J., Nieman, L. K., Danaceau, M. A., et al. (1998). Differential behavioral effects of go-nadal steroids in women with and in those without premenstrual syndrome. *New England Journal of Medicine, 338,* 209–216.

Severino, S. K., & Moline, M. L. (1989). *Premenstrual syndromes: A clinician's guide* (pp. 132–135). New York: The Guilford Press.

Severino, S. K., & Yonkers, K. A. (1993). A literature review of psychotic symptoms associated with the premenstruum. *Psychosomatics, 34,* 299–306.

Smith, R. N., Studd, J. W., Zamblera, D., & Holland, E. F. (1995). A randomised comparison over 8 months of 100 micrograms and 200 micrograms twice weekly doses of transdermal oestradiol in the treatment of severe premenstrual syndrome. *British Journal of Obstetrics and Gynaecology, 102,* 475–484.

Smith, S., Rinehart, J. S., Ruddock, V. E., & Schiff, I. (1987). Treatment of premenstrual syndrome with alprazolam: Results of a double-blind, placebo-controlled, randomized crossover clinical trial. *Obstetrics and Gynecology, 70,* 37–43.

Speroff, L., Glass, R. H., & Kase, N. G. (1999). *Clinical gynecologic endocrinology and infertility, 6th edition* (pp. 183–230). Baltimore: William & Wilkins.

Steinberg, S., Annable, L., Young, S. N., et al. (1999). A placebo-controlled clinical trial of L-tryptophan in premenstrual dysphoria. *Biological Psychiatry 45,* 313–320.

Steiner, M. (1992). Female-specific mood disorders. *Clinical Obstetrics and Gynecology, 35,* 599–611.

Steiner, M. (1999). Premenstrual syndromes. In M. P. Hopkins (Ed.), *Glass' office gynecology* (5th ed., rev., pp. 285–310). Baltimore: William & Wilkins.

Steiner, M. (2000). Premenstrual syndrome and premenstrual dysphoric disorder: Guidelines for management. *Journal of Psychiatry and Neuroscience, 25,* 459–468.

Steiner, M., Haskett, R. F., & Carroll, B. J. (1980). Premenstrual tension syndrome: The develop-ment of research diagnostic criteria and new rating scales. *Acta Psychiatrica Scandinavica, 62,* 177–190.

Steiner, M., Judge, R., & Kumar, R. (1997a). Serotonin re-uptake inhibitors in the treatment of premenstrual dysphoria: Current state of knowledge. *International Journal of Psychiatry in Clinical Practice, 1,* 241–247.

Steiner, M., Korzekwa, M., Lamont, J., et al. (1997b). Intermittent fluoxetine dosing in the treat-ment of women with premenstrual dysphoria. *Psychopharmacology Bulletin, 33,* 771–774.

Steiner, M., Lepage, P., & Dunn, E. J. (1997c). Serotonin and gender-specific psychiatric disorders. *International Journal of Psychiatry in Clinical Practice, 1,* 3–13.

Steiner, M., Romano, S. J., Babcock, S., et al. (2001). The efficacy of fluoxetine in improving physi-cal symptoms associated with premenstrual dysphoric disorder. *British Journal of Obstetrics and Gynecology, 108,* 462–468.

Steiner, M., Steinberg, S., Stewart, D., et al. (1995). Fluoxetine in the treatment of premenstrual dysphoria. *New England Journal of Medicine, 332,* 1529–1534.

Steiner, M., Streiner, D. L., Steinberg, S., et al. (1999). The measurement of premenstrual mood symptoms. *Journal of Affective Disorders, 53,* 269–273.

Steiner, M., & Wilkins, A. (1996). Diagnosis and assessment of premenstrual dysphoria. *Psychiat-ric Annals, 26,* 571–575.

Steiner, M., & Yonkers, K. (1998). Depression in women. In *Mood disorders associated with repro-ductive cyclicity* (p. 9). London: Martin Dunitz.

Su, T.-P., Schmidt, P. J., Danaceau, M. A., et al. (1997). Fluoxetine in the treatment of premenstrual dysphoria. *Neuropsychopharmacology, 16,* 346–356.

Sundblad, C., Hedberg, M. A., & Eriksson, E. (1993). Clomipramine administered during the luteal phase reduces the symptoms of premenstrual syndrome: A placebo-controlled trial. *Neuropsychopharmacology, 9,* 133–145.

Sundblad, C., Modigh, K., Andersch, B., et al. (1992). Clomipramine effectively reduces premenstrual irritability and dysphoria: A placebo controlled trial. *Acta Psychiatrica Scandinavica, 85,* 39–47.

Sundblad, C., Wikander, I., Andersch, B., et al. (1997). A naturalistic study of paroxetine in premenstrual syndrome: Efficacy and side-effects during ten cycles of treatment. *European Neuropsychopharmacology, 7,* 201–206.

Sundström, I., Nyberg, S., Bixo, M., et al. (1999). Treatment of premenstrual syndrome with gonadotropin-releasing hormone agonist in a low-dose regimen. *Acta Obstetricia et Gynecologica Scandinavica, 79,* 891–899.

Sveindottir, H. (1998). Prospective assessment of menstrual and premenstrual experiences of Icelandic women. *Health Care of Women International, 19,* 71–82.

Sveindottir, H., & Backstrom, T. (2000). Prevalence of menstrual cycle symptom cyclicity and premenstrual dysphoric disorder in a random sample of women using and not using oral contraceptives. *Acta Obstetricia et Gynecologica Scandinavica, 79,* 405–413.

Targum, S. D., Caputo, K. P., & Ball, S. K. (1991). Menstrual cycle phase and psychiatric admissions. *Journal of Affective Disorders, 22,* 49–53.

Taylor, D. (1999). Effectiveness of professional–peer group treatment: Symptom management for women with PMS. *Research in Nursing and Health, 22,* 496–511.

Thys-Jacobs, S., Starkey, P., Berstein, D., et al. (1998). Calcium carbonate and the premenstrual syndrome: Effects on premenstrual and menstrual symptoms. Premenstrual Syndrome Study Group. *American Journal of Obstetrics and Gynecology, 179,* 444–452.

Tuiten, A., Panhuysen, G., Koppeschaar, H., et al. (1995). Stress, serotonergic function, and mood in users of oral contraceptives. *Psychoneuroendocrinology, 20,* 323–334.

Vanezis, P. (1990). Deaths in women of reproductive age and relationship with menstrual cycle phase: An autopsy study of cases reported to the coroner. *Forensic Science International, 47,* 39–57.

Walker, A. F., DeSouza, M. C., Vickers, M. F., et al. (1998). Magnesium supplementation alleviates premenstrual symptoms of fluid retention. *Journal of Women's Health, 7,* 1157–1165.

Watson, N. R., Studd, J. W., Savvas, M., et al., (1989). Treatment of severe premenstrual syndrome with oestradiol patches and cyclical oral noresthisterone. *Lancet, 2,* 730–732.

West, C. P., & Hillier, H. (1994). Ovarian suppression with the gonadotrophin-releasing hormone agonist goserelin (Zoladex) in management of the premenstrual tension syndrome. *Human Reproduction, 9,* 1058–1063.

Wikander, I., Sundblad, C., Andersch, B., et al. (1998). Citalopram in premenstrual dysphoria: Is intermittent treatment during luteal phases more effective than continuous medication throughout the menstrual cycle? *Journal of Clinical Psychopharmacology, 18,* 390–398.

Williams, K. E., & Koran, L. M. (1997). Obsessive–compulsive disorder in pregnancy, the puerperium, and the premenstruum. *Journal of Clinical Psychiatry, 58,* 330–334.

Woods, N. F., Most, A., & Dery, G. K. (1982). Prevalence of perimenstrual symptoms. *American Journal of Public Health, 72,* 1257–1264.

World Health Organization (WHO). (1996). *International classification of diseases* (10th rev.). Geneva: Author.

Wyatt, K. M., Dimmock, P. W., Jones, P. W., et al. (1999). Efficacy of vitamin B-6 in the treatment of premenstrual syndrome: Systematic review. *British Medical Journal, 318,* 1375–1381.

Yatham, L. N. (1993). Is 5HT1A receptor subsensitivity a trait marker for late luteal phase dysphoric disorder? A pilot study. *Canadian Journal of Psychiatry, 38,* 662–664.

Yonkers, K. (1997a). The association between premenstrual dysphoric disorder and other mood disorders. *Journal of Clinical Psychiatry, 58,* 19–25.

Yonkers, K. (1997b). Anxiety symptoms and anxiety disorders: How are they related to premenstrual disorders? *Journal of Clinical Psychiatry, 58,* 62–67.

Yonkers, K., Halbreich, U., Freeman, E., et al. (1997). Sypmtomatic improvement of premenstrual dysphoric disorder with sertraline treatment: A randomized controlled trial Sertraline Premenstrual Dysphoric Collaborative Study Group. *Journal of the American Medical Association, 278,* 983–988.

Young, S. A., Hurt, P. H., Benedek, D. M., et al. (1998). Treatment of premenstrual dysphoric disorder with sertraline during the luteal phase: A randomized, double-blind, placebo-controlled crossover trial. *Journal of Clinical Psychiatry, 59,* 76–80.

4

Psychiatric Aspects of Pregnancy

RUTA NONACS
ADELE C. VIGUERA
LEE S. COHEN

Psychiatric illnesses, particularly mood and anxiety disorders, are common in women and typically emerge during the childbearing years (Kessler et al., 1993). With the advent of effective and well-tolerated pharmacological treatments for psychiatric disorders, a growing number of women are treated with psychotropic medications during their reproductive years. The clinician faces certain challenges when a woman with a psychiatric illness plans to conceive or inadvertently becomes pregnant. All psychotropic medications diffuse readily across the placenta, and no psychotropic drug has been approved by the U.S. Food and Drug Administration (FDA) for use during pregnancy. Although data accumulated over the last 30 years suggest that some medications may be used safely during pregnancy (Altshuler et al., 1996; Cohen & Altshuler, 1997), our knowledge regarding the risks of prenatal exposure to psychotropic medications is incomplete.

Given the potential for risk to the developing fetus, women have typically been encouraged to discontinue medications during pregnancy. Although pregnancy has typically been described as a time of emotional well-being for women, recent data reveal high rates of relapse during pregnancy in women with recurrent mood disorders who discontinue pharmacological treatment during pregnancy (Cohen et al., 1997; Viguera et al., 2000). While much attention has been focused on the risks of prenatal exposure to medications, the potential negative consequences of untreated psychiatric illness in the mother represent a significant, and often overlooked, risk (Orr & Miller, 1995; Steer et al., 1992).

The clinical challenge for the physician who cares for a woman with a psychiatric disorder during pregnancy is to minimize risk to the fetus while limiting morbidity from untreated psychiatric illness in the mother. Because no decision is absolutely free of risk, it is imperative that such clinical decisions be made collaboratively with patients and their partners. It is the physician's responsibility to provide accurate and up-to-date information on the reproductive safety of pharmacological treatment, and to help each patient to select the most appropriate treatment strategy. In this chapter we review the available information on psychotropic medication use during pregnancy, and provide guidelines for the treatment of psychiatric illness in pregnant women.

RISK–BENEFIT ASSESSMENT OF WOMEN OF CHILDBEARING POTENTIAL

Women with histories of psychiatric illness frequently present for consultation regarding the use of psychotropic medications during pregnancy, or they may seek treatment after recurrence of illness following conception. Not infrequently, women present with the first onset of psychiatric illness during pregnancy. All decisions regarding the continuation or initiation of treatment during pregnancy must reflect an assessment of the following risks: (1) risk of fetal exposure to medication, (2) risk of untreated psychiatric illness in the mother, and (3) risk of relapse associated with discontinuation of maintenance treatment. A discussion of each of these risks should be documented in the patient's medical record.

Potential Risks of Fetal Exposure to Pharmacotherapy

When considering the use of a psychiatric medication during pregnancy, the clinician must factor in three types of risk to the developing fetus: (1) risk of organ malformation or teratogenesis, (2) risk of neonatal toxicity or withdrawal syndromes during the acute neonatal period, and (3) risk of long-term neurobehavioral sequelae (Cohen & Altshuler, 1997).

To provide guidance to physicians seeking information on the reproductive safety of various prescription medications, the FDA has established a system that classifies medications into five risk categories (A, B, C, D, and X) based on data derived from human and animal studies. Category A medications are designated as safe for use during pregnancy, while Category X drugs are contraindicated and are known to have risks to the fetus that outweigh any benefit to the patient. Most psychotropic medications are classified as Category C, agents for which human studies are lacking and "risk cannot be ruled out." No psychotropic drugs are classified as safe for use during pregnancy (Category A). Unfortunately, this system of classification is frequently ambiguous and may sometimes be misleading. For example, tricyclic antidepressants (TCAs) are placed in category D and are linked with "positive evidence of risk," although the pooled available data do not support this assertion, and in fact suggest that TCAs are safe for use during pregnancy (Altshuler et al., 1996; Pastuszak et al., 1993). In contrast, bupropion, for which human studies are lacking, is classified in Category B. Therefore, the physician must rely on other sources of information when providing recommendations on the use of psychotropic medications during pregnancy. For obvious ethical reasons, it is not possible to conduct randomized, placebo-controlled studies on medication safety in pregnant populations. Therefore, many of the data on reproductive safety have been derived from retrospective studies and case reports, although more recent studies have utilized a prospective design (Chambers et al., 1996; Nulman et al., 1997; Pastuszak et al., 1993).

The baseline incidence of major congenital malformations in newborns born in the United States is estimated to be between 3% and 4% (Fabro, 1987). During the earliest stages of pregnancy, formation of major organ systems takes place; this is complete within the first 12 weeks after conception. A "teratogen" is defined as an agent that interferes with this process and produces some type of organ malformation or dysfunction. For each organ or organ system, there exists a critical period during which development takes place and may be susceptible to the effects of a teratogen (Moore & Persaud, 1998). For example, formation of the heart and great vessels takes place from 4 to 9 weeks after conception. Formation of lip and palate is typically complete by the 10th week. Neural tube folding and closure, which form the brain and spinal cord, occur within the first 4 weeks of gestation. Exposure to a toxic agent before 2 weeks of gestation is not associated with congenital malformations and is more likely to result in a nonviable, blighted ovum (Langman, 1985).

"Neonatal toxicity" or "perinatal syndromes" refer to a spectrum of physical and behavioral symptoms observed in the acute neonatal period that are attributed to drug exposure at or near the time of delivery. Although case reports over the last two decades describe a wide range of transient neonatal distress syndromes associated with exposure to (or withdrawal from) antidepressants, antipsychotics, benzodiazepines, and mood stabilizers, the incidence of these adverse events appears to be low. Anecdotal reports that attribute these syndromes to drug exposure must be cautiously interpreted, and larger samples must be studied in order to establish a causal link between exposure to a particular medication and a perinatal syndrome.

Because neuronal migration and differentiation occur throughout pregnancy and into the early years of life, the central nervous system (CNS) remains particularly vulnerable to toxic agents throughout pregnancy. However, insults that occur after neural tube closure produce changes in behavior and function, as opposed to gross structural abnormalities. "Behavioral teratogenesis" refers to the potential of a psychotropic drug administered prenatally to cause long-term neurobehavioral sequelae. For example, are children who have been exposed to an antidepressant *in utero* at risk for cognitive or behavioral problems at a later point during development? Animal studies demonstrate changes in behavior and neurotransmitter function after prenatal exposure to a variety of psychotropic agents (Ali et al., 1986; Vorhees et al., 1979; Vernadakis & Parker, 1980). The extent to which these findings are of consequence to humans has yet to be demonstrated. Studies of behavioral outcome following prenatal exposure to psychotropic medications, including TCAs, fluoxetine, benzodiazepines, and lithium, have been reported (Laegreid et al., 1992; Misri & Sivertz, 1991; Nulman et al., 1997; Schou, 1976); however, these studies vary significantly with respect to methodological rigor.

Impact of Untreated Psychiatric Illness in the Mother

Although clinicians have focused primarily on the impact of psychotropic medications on the developing fetus, untreated psychiatric illness in the mother also carries risk for the child during pregnancy. Current research suggests that maternal depression itself may adversely affect the developing fetus. Although it has been difficult to assess the impact of antenatal depression on fetal development and neonatal well-being, several studies have found an association between maternal depression and factors that predict poor neonatal outcome. Recent studies have found an association between maternal depressive symptoms and preterm birth, lower birthweight, smaller head circumference, and lower Apgar scores (Orr & Miller, 1995; Steer et al., 1992; Zuckerman et al., 1990). The physiological mechanisms by which symptoms of depression might affect neonatal outcome are not clear. However, increased serum cortisol and catecholamine levels, which are typically observed in patients with depression, may affect placental function by altering uterine blood flow and inducing uterine irritability (Glover, 1997; Teixeira et al., 1999). Dysregulation of the hypothalamic–pituitary–adrenal (HPA) axis, which is associated with depression, may also have a direct effect on fetal development. Animal studies suggest that stress during pregnancy is associated with neuronal death and abnormal development of neural structures in the fetal brain, as well as sustained dysfunction on the HPA axis in the offspring (Alves et al., 1997; Glover, 1997; Uno et al., 1990, 1994).

Psychiatric illness during pregnancy may also contribute to poor self-care and inattention to prenatal care. Women with depression often present with decreased appetite and consequently lower-than-expected weight gain in pregnancy—factors that have been associated with negative pregnancy outcomes (Zuckerman et al., 1989). In addition, pregnant women with depression are also more likely to smoke and to use either alcohol or illicit drugs (Zuckerman et al., 1989), which further increase risk to the fetus. Depression in the mother also places the rest of the family at risk. Depression is typically associated with interpersonal difficulties, and disruptions in mother–child interactions and attachment may have a profound impact on infant development. Research indicates that children of depressed mothers are more likely to have behavioral problems and to exhibit disruptions in motor, cognitive, and emotional development (Murray, 1992; Murray & Cooper, 1997; Weinberg & Tronick, 1998).

Risk of Medication Discontinuation

A growing body of literature on nongravid populations indicates that the discontinuation of maintenance pharmacological treatment is associated with high rates of relapse (Baldessarini & Tondo, 1998; Suppes et al., 1991; Viguera et al., 1997, 1998). For example, among patients with bipolar disorder, approximately 50% experience recurrence within 6 months of lithium discontinuation (Baldessarini et al., 1996; Baldessarini & Tondo, 1998; Suppes et al., 1991). This risk appears to be particularly high in the setting of abrupt, as opposed to more gradual, discontinuation of the mood stabilizer (Baldessarini et al., 1996; Faedda et al., 1993). In addition, studies have shown that the discontinuation of lithium in patients with bipolar disorder is followed by a dramatic increase in suicide risk (Tondo et al., 1998). Similar findings have been noted in patients with unipolar depression and in patients with anxiety disorders (Kupfer et al., 1992; Pollack & Smoller, 1995; Viguera et al., 1997, 1998).

When assessing the potential use of psychotropic medications during pregnancy, the clinician must also consider the potential risk for prolonged illness and treatment resistance in patients who experience relapse (Keller et al., 1983; Mueller et al., 1999; Post, 1992). Although the potential for teratogenesis is of serious concern, so too is the high risk of morbidity and mortality associated with discontinuation of maintenance medication. Given these findings, cessation of pharmacotherapy during pregnancy must be viewed as potentially dangerous. As such, the decision to discontinue maintenance treatment should be made only after careful consideration.

PHARMACOLOGICAL TREATMENT DURING PREGNANCY

Antidepressant Medications

Although early case reports suggested a possible association between first-trimester exposure to TCAs and limb malformation, 3 prospective studies and more than 10 retrospective studies have examined the risk of organ dysgenesis in over 400 cases of first-trimester exposure to TCAs (Altshuler et al., 1996; Cohen & Altshuler, 1997; Loebstein & Koren, 1997; McElhatton et al., 1996; Misri & Sivertz, 1991; Pastuszak et al., 1993). When evaluated on an individual basis and when pooled, these studies fail to indicate a significant association between fetal exposure to TCAs and risk for any major congenital anomaly.

Except for fluoxetine, information on the reproductive safety of the selective serotonin reuptake inhibitors (SSRIs) is limited. Four prospective studies have evaluated rates of congenital malformation in approximately 1,100 fluoxetine-exposed infants (Chambers et al., 1996; Goldstein et al., 1997; Nulman & Koren, 1996; Pastuszak et al., 1993). The postmarketing surveillance registry established by the manufacturer of fluoxetine, and one other retrospective study (McElhatton et al., 1996), complement these findings. These data collected from over 2,500 cases indicate no increase in risk of major congenital malformation in fluoxetine-exposed infants.

Although no study has observed an increase in risk for *major* congenital anomaly, Chambers et al. (1996) noted an increase in risk for multiple *minor* malformations in fluoxetine-exposed infants. In this study, "minor anomalies" were defined as structural defects that had no cosmetic or functional importance. In addition, this report suggested that late exposure to fluoxetine was associated with premature labor and poor neonatal adaptation. Interpretation of the findings in this study is limited by several methodological difficulties, however (Cohen & Rosenbaum, 1997; Robert, 1996). For example, the fluoxetine-exposed women and control groups differed significantly in terms of important variables such as age, presence of psychiatric illness, and exposure to other medications. In addition, raters who were aware of the groups' status were utilized, and only half of the fluoxetine-exposed infants were evaluated, which raises the question of selection bias. Although further data are needed to ensure clinical confidence, the data collected thus far on fluoxetine suggest that it is unlikely to be a significant human teratogen.

Information regarding the reproductive safety of sertraline, paroxetine, fluvoxamine, and citalopram use during pregnancy is gradually accumulating, but is limited in terms of sample size (Ericson et al., 1999; Inman et al., 1993; Kulin et al., 1998; McElhatton et al., 1996). One prospective study of 531 infants with first-trimester exposure to SSRIs (mostly citalopram; $n = 375$) did not demonstrate an increased risk of organ malformation (Ericson et al., 1999). In a retrospective study of 63 infants with first-trimester exposure to paroxetine, no increase in teratogenic risk was observed (Inman et al., 1993). In a prospective, controlled cohort study, Kulin et al. (1998) reported on outcomes in neonates exposed *in utero* to fluvoxamine ($n = 26$), paroxetine ($n = 97$), and sertraline ($n = 147$). Pregnancy outcomes did not differ between the exposed and nonexposed groups in terms of risk for congenital malformation or complications during pregnancy (e.g., miscarriage, stillbirth, or prematurity). Birthweights and gestational age were similar in both groups. Although this information on these SSRIs is reassuring, one of the major limitations of this study is that the analysis grouped the three antidepressants together, as opposed to analyzing *each* antidepressant separately for teratogenic risk. In addition, larger samples are required to establish the reproductive safety of these newer antidepressants. It is estimated that at least 500 to 600 exposures must be collected to demonstrate a twofold increase in risk for a particular malformation over what is observed in the general population (Shepard, 1989).

To date, prospective data on the use of mirtazapine, venlafaxine, nefazodone, trazodone, and bupropion are not available. Scant information is available regarding the reproductive safety of monoamine oxidase inhibitors (MAOIs). One study in humans described an increase in congenital malformations after prenatal exposure to tranylcypromine and phenelzine, although the sample size was extremely small (Heinonen et al., 1977). Moreover, during labor and delivery, MAOIs may produce a hypertensive crisis if tocolytic medications (such as terbutaline) are used to forestall delivery. Given this lack of data and the cumbersome restrictions associated with their use, MAOIs are typically avoided during pregnancy.

Various case reports have described perinatal syndromes in infants exposed to antidepressant medications near or at the time of delivery. These have included TCA withdrawal syndromes with characteristic symptoms of jitteriness, irritability and (less commonly) seizure (Cowe et al., 1982; Eggermont, 1973; Schimmel et al., 1991; Webster, 1973). Neonatal toxicity attributed to the anticholinergic effect of TCAs, such as functional bowel obstruction and urinary retention, have also been reported (Falterman & Richardson, 1980; Shearer et al., 1972). The extent to which prenatal exposure to fluoxetine or other SSRIs is associated with neonatal toxicity is still unclear. Case reports and one prospective study have described perinatal complications in fluoxetine-exposed infants, including poor neonatal adaptation, respiratory distress, feeding problems, and jitteriness (Chambers et al., 1996; Spencer, 1993). Other prospective studies have not observed perinatal distress in infants exposed to fluoxetine or other SSRIs (Cohen et al., 2000; Goldstein, 1995; Kulin et al., 1998).

With regard to long-term neurobehavioral sequelae in children exposed to either fluoxetine or TCAs, the data are limited but reassuring. In a landmark study, Nulman et al. (1997) followed a cohort of children up to preschool age who had been exposed to either TCAs (*n* = 80) or fluoxetine (*n* = 55) *in utero*, and compared these subjects to a cohort of nonexposed controls (*n* = 84). Results indicated no significant differences in IQ, temperament, behavior, reactivity, mood, distractibility, or activity level between exposed and nonexposed children. The authors concluded that their findings support the hypothesis that fluoxetine and TCAs are not behavioral teratogens. However, these data are preliminary; clearly, further investigation into the long-term neurobehavioral effects of prenatal exposure to antidepressants, as well as other psychotropic medications, is warranted.

Benzodiazepines

The consequences of prenatal exposure to benzodiazepines have been debated for over 25 years. Three prospective studies support the absence of increased risk of organ malformation following first-trimester exposure to benzodiazepines (Hartz et al., 1975; McElhatton, 1994; St. Clair & Schirmer, 1992). More controversial has been the issue of whether first-trimester exposure to benzodiazepines increases risk for specific malformations, such as cleft lip or cleft palate. Although several studies do not support this association (Rosenberg et al., 1983; Shiono & Mills, 1984), a meta-analysis (Altshuler et al., 1996) suggests an increased risk of oral cleft in infants with first trimester exposure to benzodiazepines. This risk is calculated to be 0.7%, approximately a 10-fold increase in risk for oral cleft over that observed in the general population (Altshuler et al., 1996). The limitations of risk estimates derived from this type of meta-analysis have previously been noted (Cohen & Altshuler, 1997; Dolovich et al., 1998). In general, methodological difficulties emerge when several studies are pooled that include exposure to different benzodiazepines at varying dosages and durations of treatment in populations ascertained in a noncontrolled fashion. Nonetheless, the likelihood that a woman exposed to benzodiazepines during the first trimester will give birth to a child with this congenital anomaly, although significantly increased, remains less than 1%.

A benzodiazepine withdrawal syndrome, characterized by symptoms of jitteriness, autonomic dysregulation and seizure, has been reported in infants exposed to benzodiazepines *in utero* (Athinarayanan et al., 1976; Mazzi, 1977; Rementaria & Bhatt, 1977; Rowlatt, 1978). In addition, case reports have described symptoms of neonatal toxicity in benzodiazepine-exposed infants, including impaired temperature regulation, apnea, depressed Apgar scores, muscular hypotonia and failure to feed (Gillberg, 1977; Speight, 1977; Fisher & Edgren, 1985; McElhatton, 1994). In one recent case series of 39 pregnant women with panic disorder treated with clonazepam alone (0.5 to 3.5 mg), Apgar scores were uniformly high, and no infants showed signs of neonatal withdrawal or toxicity (Weinstock et al., 2001).

Systematically derived data on the long-term neurobehavioral effects of benzodiazepine exposure are sparse. Several studies have reported motor and developmental delays (Laegreid et al., 1992; Milkovich & van den Berg, 1974; Viggedal et al., 1993), although these studies have been criticized for having significant ascertainment biases. Other studies have revealed no association between benzodiazepine exposure and developmental delay (Bergman et al., 1992; Hartz et al., 1975). Overall, the data do not support an identifiable impact on neurobehavioral function, although these data are too sparse to allow for any firm conclusions regarding the long-term impact of benzodiazepines on CNS development and function.

Currently, no systematic data are available on the reproductive safety of nonbenzodiazepine anxiolytic agents such as buspirone and zolpidem. Therefore, these medications are not recommended for use in pregnancy.

Antipsychotic Agents

Although an early case report describing limb malformations raised concerns regarding first-trimester exposure to haloperidol (Kopelman et al., 1975), other studies have not demonstrated teratogenic risk associated with high- or low-potency neuroleptic medications (Hanson & Oakley, 1975; Milkovich & van den Berg, 1976; Slone et al., 1977; van Waes & van de Velde, 1969; Waldman & Safferman, 1993). However, a meta-analysis of the studies available at that time noted a higher risk of congenital malformations after first-trimester exposure to low-potency neuroleptics (Altshuler et al., 1996). In clinical practice, higher-potency neuroleptic agents such as haloperidol and trifluoperazine are recommended over the lower-potency agents in managing pregnant women with psychiatric illness (Altshuler et al., 1996).

Information on the reproductive safety of atypical neuroleptic medications is sparse. There are no data on risperidone or quetiapine use in pregnancy. Recently the manufacturers of olanzapine have established a registry to collect information on prenatal exposure (Dickson & Dawson, 1998). To date, there are five published case reports of pregnant women maintained on clozapine during pregnancy, with no evidence of major congenital malformation (Barnas et al., 1994; Dickson & Hogg, 1998; Stoner et al., 1997; Waldman & Safferman, 1993). In addition, one manufacturer of clozapine has collected outcome information on babies exposed to clozapine (Novartis, personal communication, 1998). Of the 29 exposed neonates, 25 were noted to be healthy, and 4 babies showed a variety of abnormalities (neonatal convulsions, Turner's syndrome, collarbone fracture, facial deformity, congenital hip dislocation, and congenital blindness). However, a larger sample size is needed to support any causal relationship between neonatal outcome and drug exposure.

Case reports have documented transient extrapyramidal symptoms (e.g., motor restlessness, tremor, hypertonicity, dystonic movements, parkinsonism) in neonates exposed to neuroleptic drugs during pregnancy (Auerbach et al., 1992; Hill et al., 1966; Levy & Wisniewski, 1974). These problems have typically been of short duration, and infants exposed to neuroleptic medications *in utero* were noted to have normal motor development (Desmond et al., 1967). Limited data on the long-term neurobehavioral effects of prenatal exposure to antipsychotic agents are available. In one longitudinal study of IQ and behavior in children exposed to low-potency neuroleptics *in utero* and followed until 5 years of age, no significant abnormalities were noted (Slone et al., 1977).

Little information is available regarding the reproductive safety of medications used to treat the extrapyramidal side effects of neuroleptic medications. A possible association between exposure to benztropine and trihexyphenidyl and increased risk for congenital anomaly has been described (Heinonen et al., 1977). In contrast, studies evaluating the use of diphenhydramine during pregnancy have failed to reveal heightened risk of organ malformation (Aselton et al., 1985; Nelson & Forfar, 1971). Studies of ß-blockers, including propranolol and atenolol, during pregnancy have revealed no teratogenic risk (Rubin, 1981).

Mood Stabilizers

Lithium

From the early 1970s, there has been concern regarding the association between prenatal exposure to lithium and risk for major congenital anomalies. Reports from the International Register of Lithium Babies, a database derived from a voluntary physician reporting system, described increased rates of cardiovascular malformation (most notably Ebstein's anomaly) in lithium-exposed infants (Nora et al., 1974; Schou et al., 1973; Weinstein, 1976). The risk of this malformation in infants with first-trimester lithium exposure was initially determined to be 400 times higher than that observed in the general population. However, a significant methodological limitation of the register was an inherent bias toward the overreporting of adverse outcomes. More recent epidemiological studies suggest a more modest teratogenic risk associated with lithium exposure (Edmonds & Oakley, 1990; Jacobson et al., 1992; Kallen & Tandberg, 1983; Zalzstein et al., 1990). With a pooled analysis of the data, a revised risk for cardiovascular malformation after first-trimester exposure to lithium has been calculated (Cohen et al., 1994a) and is estimated to be between 1 in 2,000 (0.05%) and 1 in 1,000 (0.1%). Although this rate of cardiovascular malformation in lithium-exposed infants is 10 to 20 times higher than that observed in the general population (1 in 20,000), the absolute risk is small, and lithium remains the safest mood stabilizer for use during pregnancy.

Reports of neonatal toxicity in offspring exposed to lithium at the time of labor and delivery have included several cases of "floppy baby" syndrome, characterized by cyanosis and hypotonicity (Ananth, 1976; Schou & Amdisen, 1975; Woody et al., 1971). Isolated cases of neonatal hypothyroidism and nephrogenic diabetes insipidus have also been described (Ananth, 1976). A naturalistic survey of women treated with lithium found no direct evidence of neonatal toxicity in newborns whose mothers received lithium either during pregnancy or labor and delivery (Cohen et al., 1995). Limited data are available regarding behavioral outcomes of children exposed to lithium *in utero*. A 5-year follow-up investigation of children exposed to lithium during the second and third trimesters of pregnancy (*n* = 60) revealed no significant behavioral problems (Schou, 1976).

Anticonvulsants

Most data on the reproductive safety of the anticonvulsants have been collected in patients with a seizure disorder and not in women treated for psychiatric illness. The extent to which epilepsy may affect neonatal outcome is unknown. It remains controversial whether children of women with epilepsy have higher rates of congenital malformation, regardless of perinatal anticonvulsant exposure. However, it is well established that risk for congenital anomaly is increased in those exposed to anticonvulsants *in utero*, even after the effects of seizure activity during pregnancy are controlled for (Koch et al., 1992).

In comparison with lithium, anticonvulsants pose a more serious teratogenic risk. Fetal exposure to anticonvulsants is associated not only with multiple congenital anomalies, but also with relatively high rates of serious CNS lesions. Exposure to carbamazepine *in utero* is associated with a 0.5–1% risk for neural tube defect (Rosa, 1991). Infants exposed to carbamazepine prenatally are also at increased risk for craniofacial abnormalities, microcephaly, and growth retardation (Rosa, 1991; Holmes et al., 1990). Valproic acid may be a more severe teratogen, with rates of neural tube defect ranging from 1% to 6% (Omtzigt et al., 1992; Robert & Guibaud, 1982). Prenatal exposure to valproic acid has also been associated with characteristic craniofacial abnormalities, cardiovascular malformations, limb defects, and genital anomalies, as well as other CNS structural abnormalities, including hydrocephalus (Clayton-Smith & Donnai, 1995; Omtzigt et al., 1992; Lindhout & Omtzigt, 1994; Robert & Guibaud, 1982). Specific risk factors for teratogenesis include high maternal daily dosage or serum concentrations of anticonvulsant, low folate levels, and anticonvulsant polytherapy (Battino et al., 1992; Koch et al., 1992; Nakane et al., 1980; Omtzigt et al., 1992).

Data regarding the neurobehavioral sequelae of anticonvulsant exposure are limited. Although there is no evidence to support a risk for mental retardation, data suggest that antenatal exposure to anticonvulsants may produce subtle cognitive effects (Scolnik et al., 1994; Vanoverloop et al., 1992). Data also suggest that cognitive changes may occur even with "late" third-trimester exposure (Reinisch et al., 1995). In one study, prenatal exposure to carbamazepine did not appear to be associated with neurobehavioral dysfunction (Scolnik et al., 1994). In another study, however, clear cognitive deficits (i.e., depressed IQ scores, developmental delay) were noted in children exposed to carbamazepine compared to nonexposed children (Holmes et al., 1990; Jones et al., 1989). No systematic data on the reproductive safety of the newer anticonvulsants (e.g., gabapentin, lamotrigine) are available, save for a few case reports (Briggs et al., 1997). With few data supporting the reproductive safety of these newer anticonvulsants, it is difficult to justify their use during pregnancy at this time. However, a registry has recently been established for women taking anticonvulsants during pregnancy, in order to systematically collect information on the impact of anticonvulsants on fetal development (Anti-Epileptic Drug Registry; 888-233-2334).

GUIDELINES FOR THE TREATMENT
OF PSYCHIATRIC ILLNESS DURING PREGNANCY

Ideally, decisions regarding the use of psychotropic medications during pregnancy should be made prior to conception. A clinician must work collaboratively with a patient to arrive at the safest decision based on the available information. The patient's past psychiatric history, her current symptoms, and her attitude toward the use of psychiatric medications during pregnancy must be carefully assessed. Although the management of psychiatric illness during pregnancy remains largely empirical, with few definitive data and no controlled treatment studies during pregnancy, the most appropriate treatment algorithm depends on the severity of the disorder. In patients with milder forms of illness, it is appropriate to consider discontinuation of pharmacological therapy during pregnancy. For a woman with more severe or refractory illness, the patient and clinician may instead decide that the safest option is to continue pharmacological treatment during pregnancy. In any situation, close monitoring during pregnancy is essential, even if all medications are discontinued and there is no need for medication management. Psychiatrically ill women are at high risk for relapse during pregnancy, and early detection of recurrent illness may significantly reduce morbidity and facilitate treatment.

Nonpharmacological treatment strategies should always be explored and may be useful in either limiting or obviating the need for medication. These techniques may be used before conception to facilitate medication discontinuation, or during pregnancy either to treat or to prevent recurrent symptoms. In general, pharmacological treatment is pursued when it is felt that the risks associated with psychiatric illness outweigh the risks of fetal exposure to a particular medication.

In situations where pharmacological treatment is indicated, the clinician should attempt to select the safest medication regimen. Often this may necessitate switching from one psychotropic agent to another with a better reproductive safety profile—for example, switching from an MAOI to fluoxetine. In certain cases, one may decide to use a medication for which information regarding reproductive safety is sparse. For instance, a woman with refractory depressive illness who has responded only to one antidepressant for which data on reproductive safety are limited (e.g., sertraline, paroxetine) may choose to continue this medication during pregnancy, rather than to risk relapse if she were to discontinue this agent or switch to another antidepressant.

Many women, particularly those with refractory illness, require more than one medication to maintain euthymia. Every attempt should be made to simplify the medication regimen during pregnancy. This is especially true for a woman treated with multiple anticonvulsants; data suggest that combination anticonvulsant therapy confers more risk to the fetus than monotherapy does. Finally, one must use the appropriate dosage of medication. Unfortunately, many clinicians tend to undertreat psychiatric illness during pregnancy. Frequently the dosage of a medication will be reduced during pregnancy; however, this type of modification in treatment may instead place a woman at greater risk for recurrent illness. The woman is exposed, therefore, to all the risks of medication exposure without any of the benefits of pharmacological treatment.

Major Depression

Studies suggest that about 10% of women suffer from depression during pregnancy (O'Hara, 1986). Risk factors for antenatal depression include a personal history of mood disorder, a family history of depression, marital discord, poor psychosocial supports, recent adverse life events, and unwanted pregnancy (Gotlib et al., 1989; O'Hara, 1986). Women who have been maintained on an antidepressant medication prior to conception appear to be at high risk for relapse during pregnancy. Preliminary data suggest that among women with recurrent major depression who discontinue antidepressant medication proximate to conception, approximately 75% relapse during pregnancy, typically during the first trimester (Cohen et al., 1997).

Although more severe forms of depression illness may be readily detected, depression that emerges during pregnancy is frequently overlooked. Many of the neurovegetative signs and symptoms characteristic of major depression (e.g., sleep and appetite disturbance, diminished libido, low energy) are also observed in nondepressed women during pregnancy. In addition, certain medical disorders commonly seen during pregnancy, such as anemia, gestational diabetes, and thyroid dysfunction, may cause depressive symptoms and consequently may complicate the diagnosis of depression during pregnancy (Klein & Essex, 1995).

Women who develop mild depressive symptoms during pregnancy may benefit from nonpharmacological treatments such as interpersonal psychotherapy or cognitive-behavioral therapy (Beck et al., 1979; Klerman et al., 1984; Spinelli, 1997). Adjunctive interpersonal or cognitive-behavioral therapy may also be used prior to conception to facilitate the gradual tapering and discontinuation of an antidepressant medication in women planning to become pregnant.

Antidepressants during pregnancy are generally indicated for those patients who present with symptoms that interfere with maternal well-being and functioning, or for those who experience the symptoms of depression as intolerable. For women with histories of recurrent major depression, who have tried and failed to discontinue antidepressant therapy, remaining on maintenance antidepressant therapy during pregnancy may be the safest option. Among the TCAs, desipramine and nortriptyline are preferred, since they are least anticholinergic and least likely to exacerbate orthostatic hypotension (which occurs during pregnancy). Fluoxetine, with the most extensive literature supporting its reproductive safety, is a first-line choice. Data are not yet sufficient regarding the teratogenic risk of the newer SSRIs, including sertraline, paroxetine, and fluvoxamine. However, there is a growing literature on the reproductive safety of these newer SSRIs (Ericson et al., 1999; Kulin et al., 1998), and these agents may be useful in certain settings. In patients with severe depression who have not responded to either fluoxetine or a TCA, these newer agents may be considered, despite the limited information on their reproductive safety. Severely depressed patients with acute suicidality or psychosis require hospitalization, and electroconvulsive therapy (ECT) is frequently the treatment of choice. Two reviews of ECT use during pregnancy note the efficacy and safety of this procedure (Ferrill et al., 1992; Miller, 1994).

Based on a number of anecdotal reports of toxicity in infants born to mothers treated with antidepressants, some authors have recommended discontinuation of antidepressant medication several days or weeks prior to delivery, to minimize the risk of neonatal toxicity (Cowe et al., 1982; Eggermont, 1973; Schimmel et al., 1991; Webster,

1973). Given the low incidence of neonatal toxicity, this practice carries significant risk, since it withdraws treatment from patients precisely as they are about to enter the post-partum period—a time of heightened risk for mood disorders.

Bipolar Disorder

Although the postpartum period has been clearly defined as a period of risk for women with bipolar disorder (Kendell et al., 1987, Klompenhouwer & van Hulst, 1991; Reich & Winokur, 1970), the impact of pregnancy on the course of bipolar disorder has not been well characterized. Early reports suggested that pregnancy does not appear to increase risk for recurrence in women with bipolar illness, and that some patients are able to maintain euthymia during pregnancy despite medication discontinuation (Sharma & Persad, 1995; Targum et al., 1979). However, more recent studies suggest that recurrence of illness during pregnancy is not uncommon in women with bipolar disorder (Finnerty et al., 1996; Viguera et al., 2000). One recent study of pregnant women with bipolar disorder describes relapse rates of approximately 50% after lithium discontinuation (Viguera et al., 2000).

The decision to use lithium during pregnancy depends on illness severity. Patients with histories of a single past episode of mania with sustained affective well-being may be able to taper gradually (> 2 weeks) and discontinue lithium prior to conception. Women with more than one past episode of mania or depression offer a greater clinical challenge. Such a patient may choose to discontinue lithium gradually prior to conception. If the patient becomes symptomatic prior to conception, lithium may be reinitiated. Alternatively, lithium discontinuation may take place after early documentation of pregnancy. This strategy minimizes exposure and affords the longest period of antimanic prophylaxis while a woman attempts to conceive. However, this option involves a more abrupt discontinuation of lithium, which may actually provoke or hasten relapse, as has been previously reported in nonpregnant cohorts (Baldessarini et al., 1996; Faedda et al., 1993). As teratogenic risk for lithium is limited to the first trimester, some women choose to resume treatment during the second trimester of pregnancy. Preliminary data suggest that this strategy may limit risk for affective illness during the postpartum period (Nonacs et al., 1998).

For women with the most severe forms of bipolar disorder, maintenance of lithium treatment before and during pregnancy is advisable. Accepting the relatively small absolute increase in teratogenic risk associated with first-trimester exposure to lithium seems particularly justified, since these patients are at highest risk for clinical deterioration in the absence of treatment. A full-blown relapse of bipolar disorder during pregnancy is potentially dangerous to the mother and fetus and may require more aggressive treatment, including hospitalization and exposure to multiple psychotropic medications (e.g., neuroleptics, benzodiazepines). Therefore, patients with refractory bipolar disorder may opt to remain on lithium in order to maintain euthymia during pregnancy. All women who use lithium during the first trimester of pregnancy must be counseled about the increased risk of cardiovascular malformation. A Level II ultrasound at 16 to 18 weeks of gestation to detect cardiac anomalies is recommended (Cohen et al., 1994a).

For women with bipolar disorder who are maintained on valproic acid or carbamazepine and who wish to conceive, a switch to lithium is recommended. If a patient has a history of lithium nonresponse, then a trial of carbamazepine is recommended before using valproic acid. Patients who are only responsive to valproic acid may choose to remain on this medication during pregnancy and accept the teratogenic risks in order to maintain euthymia. Adjunctive treatment with a high-potency neuroleptic medication may also be helpful in situations where the response is partial. In general, avoiding exposure to anticonvulsants is recommended. However, if this is not possible, maintaining the lowest dose of anticonvulsant possible and folic acid supplementation (4 mg daily) may help reduce risk for spina bifida. Prenatal screening for neural tube defect, including Level II ultrasound and amniocentesis, is also recommended.

Finally, pregnant women with bipolar disorder should be clearly informed of the high risk for relapse during the postpartum period, and prophylaxis with a mood stabilizer (and/or a neuroleptic agent) should be recommended strongly. Lithium prophylaxis during the postpartum period significantly limits risk for relapse in women with bipolar disorder (Cohen et al., 1995; van Gent & Verhoeven, 1992).

Although typically lithium treatment is reinitiated after delivery, recent data suggest that earlier reintroduction of lithium may be more protective (Nonacs et al., 1998). The current practice of reducing lithium dosage prior to delivery due to concerns of neonatal lithium toxicity needs to be reevaluated. Rapid reductions in lithium serum concentration may precipitate relapse (Baldessarini et al., 1996; Rosenbaum et al., 1994), further increasing risk for affective instability during the postpartum period. In addition, reports linking lithium therapy during pregnancy to neonatal toxicity are extremely rare. Clinically, a more prudent option may be to follow serial serum lithium levels during labor and delivery, as well as during the first few postpartum days, and to adjust the dose accordingly.

Anxiety Disorders

Panic Disorder

The course of panic disorder in pregnancy is variable. Pregnancy may ameliorate symptoms of panic in some patients and may provide an opportunity to discontinue medication (Cowley & Roy-Byrne, 1989; George et al., 1987; Klein et al., 1994–1995; Villeponteaux et al., 1992). Other studies have noted the persistence or worsening of panic symptoms during pregnancy (Cohen et al., 1994b, 1996; Northcott & Stein, 1994).

For patients with panic disorder who wish to conceive, a slow taper of antipanic medications is recommended. Adjunctive cognitive-behavioral therapy may be of some benefit in helping patients discontinue antipanic agents and may increase the time to relapse (Robinson et al., 1992). Some patients may conceive inadvertently on antipanic medications and may present for emergent consultation. Abrupt discontinuation of antipanic maintenance medication is not recommended, given the risk for rebound panic symptoms or, at worst, a potentially serious withdrawal syndrome. However, gradual taper of benzodiazepine (i.e., >2 weeks) with adjunctive cognitive-behavioral therapy may be pursued in an effort to minimize fetal exposure to medication.

If a taper is unsuccessful or if symptoms recur during pregnancy, reinstitution of pharmacotherapy may be considered. For those patients with severe panic disorder, maintenance medication may be a clinical necessity. TCAs or fluoxetine are reasonable treatment options for the management of panic disorder during pregnancy (Altshuler et al., 1996). If patients do not respond to these antidepressants, the use of benzodiazepines may be considered (Weinstock et al., 2001). Although some may choose to avoid first-trimester exposure to benzodiazepines (given the data on risk for cleft lip and palate), benzodiazepines may be used without significant risk during the second and third trimesters, and may provide some advantage over antidepressant treatment because they may be used intermittently as needed.

Obsessive-Compulsive Disorder

For patients with premorbid obsessive–compulsive disorder (OCD), symptoms appear to worsen during pregnancy and the postpartum period (Buttolph & Holland, 1990; Sichel et al., 1993). In a prospective study of 14 patients who discontinued maintenance treatment during pregnancy, 43% required reinstitution of antiobsessional medications (Grush et al., 1996). Of those who remained medication-free during pregnancy, all had an exacerbation of their symptoms during the postpartum period. Several studies have also documented an association between pregnancy and new onset of OCD (Buttolph & Holland, 1990; Neziroglu et al., 1992). In one study, 52% of the women experienced the onset of OCD during their first pregnancy (Buttolph & Holland, 1990).

Behavioral techniques for the treatment of OCD symptoms should be considered as an alternative to medication during pregnancy, particularly for women with milder forms of this disorder. For those patients with moderate to severe symptoms, maintenance of pharmacological treatment throughout pregnancy may be indicated, given the potentially disabling sequelae of untreated OCD symptoms. Fluoxetine is an ideal first choice. The TCA clomipramine may also be used. Although not considered to be teratogenic, clomipramine may aggravate orthostatic hypotension. In addition, anecdotal data have linked clomipramine with neonatal seizures at the time of labor and delivery (Cowe et al., 1982). Clomipramine is not absolutely contraindicated for pregnant women who suffer from severe OCD; however, close monitoring during labor, delivery, and the acute postpartum period is required.

CONCLUSION

Although pregnancy is typically considered a time of emotional well-being for many women, pregnancy is not protective for women who suffer from psychiatric illness. Whereas nonpharmacological treatment strategies may be helpful for some women, others may require pharmacological treatment during pregnancy. Psychotropic medications may be used during pregnancy when the risk of untreated psychiatric illness in the mother outweighs the potential risks of fetal drug exposure. Although concerns regarding the teratogenic effects of psychotropic medications have kindled appropriate vigilance, discontinuation of these maintenance medications may result in significant morbidity for the patient. Of growing concern is the risk of untreated psychiatric illness on fetal development. When a patient presents with questions regarding the use of psychotropic medications during pregnancy, all of these risks must be weighed carefully, on a case-by-case basis, to arrive at the most appropriate treatment guideline.

In general, data support the relative reproductive safety of TCAs and fluoxetine as antidepressants. Emerging data on the other SSRIs are also reassuring. First-trimester exposure to lithium, benzodiazepines, and the anticonvulsants has been associated with increased risk of congenital malformation. However, these medications are not absolutely contraindicated during pregnancy. For some patients, the decision to accept an increase in teratogenic risk may be appropriate to ensure maternal stability during pregnancy.

The potential for long-term behavioral changes related to prenatal exposure to psychotropic agents requires more systematic study. Although animal studies suggest changes in neurotransmitter receptor number and function after prenatal exposure to various psychotropic medications, human studies are lacking. Large epidemiological follow-up studies of children exposed to psychotropic medications *in utero* are needed. Pending such studies, the clinician will continue to act in a state of relative uncertainty, weighing partially calculated risks in order to arrive at the most appropriate treatment strategy for a given patient.

The goal of the clinician who cares for women who either are planning to conceive or are pregnant should be to provide the best information regarding the spectrum of risks associated with either pursuing or deferring treatment with psychiatric medications during pregnancy. Coordinated care among a patient, her husband or partner, the obstetrician, and the psychiatrist is essential. Importantly, the goal is not to dictate treatment, but to provide accurate information that patients may utilize to make personal decisions regarding psychiatric treatment during pregnancy. Careful consideration of these issues allows for thoughtful treatment decisions that maximize both maternal and fetal well-being.

REFERENCES

Ali, S., Buelke, S. J., Newport, G. D., et al. (2986). Early neurobehavioral and neurochemical alterations in rats prenatally exposed to imipramine. *Neurotoxicology, 7,* 365–380.

Altshuler, L. L., Cohen, L. S., Szuba, M. P., et al. (1996). Pharmacologic management of psychiatric illness in pregnancy: Dilemmas and guidelines. *American Journal of Psychiatry, 153,* 592–606.

Alves, S. E., Akbari, H. M., Anderson, G. M., et al. (1997). Neonatal ACTH administration elicits long-term changes in forebrain monoamine innervation: Subsequent disruptions in hypothalamic–pituitary–adrenal and gonadal function. *Annals of the New York Academy of Sciences, 814,* 226–251.

Ananth, J. (1976). Side effects on fetus and infant of psychotropic drug use during pregnancy. *International Pharmacopsychiatry, 11,* 246–260.

Aselton, P., Jick, H., & Milunsky, A. (1985). First-trimester drug use and congenital disorders. *Obstetrics and Gynecology, 65,* 451–455.

Athinarayanan, P., Peirog, S. H., Nigam, S. K., et al. (1976). Chlordiazepoxide withdrawal in the neonate. *American Journal of Obstetrics and Gynecology, 124,* 212–213.

Auerbach, J. G., Hans, S. L., Marcus, J., et al. (1992). Maternal psychotropic medication and neonatal behavior. *Neurotoxicology and Teratology, 14(6),* 399–406.

Baldessarini, R., & Tondo, L. (1998). Effects of lithium treatment in bipolar disorders and post-treatment-discontinuation recurrence risk. *Clinical Drug Investigations, 15,* 337–351.

Baldessarini, R. J., Tondo, L., Faedda, G. L., et al. (1996). Effects of the rate of discontinuing lithium maintenance treatment in bipolar disorders. *Journal of Clinical Psychiatry, 57,* 441–448.

Barnas, C., Bergant, A., Hummer, M., et al: Clozapine concentrations in maternal and fetal plasma, amniotic fluid, and breast milk [Letter to the editor]. *American Journal of Psychiatry, 151,* 945.

Battino, D., Binelli, S., Caccamo, M. L., et al. (1992). Malformation in offspring of 305 epileptic women: A prospective study. *Acta Neurologica Scandinavica, 85,* 204–207.

Beck, A. T., Rush, A. J., Shaw, B. F., et al. (1979). *Cognitive therapy of depression*. New York: Guilford Press.

Bergman, U. F., Rosa, F. W., Baum, C., et al. (1992). Effects of exposure to benzodiazepine during fetal life. *Lancet, 340*, 694–696.

Briggs, G. G., Freeman, R. K., & Schofield, E. M. (1997). *Drugs in pregnancy and lactation: A reference guide to fetal and neonatal risk* (5th ed.). Baltimore, MD: William & Wilkins.

Buttolph, M. L., & Holland, A. (1990). Obsessive compulsive disorders in pregnancy and childbirth. In M. Jenike, L. Baer, & W. E. Minichiello (Eds.), *Obsessive compulsive disorders: Theory and management*. Chicago: Yearbook Medical.

Chambers, C. D., Johnson, K. A., Dick, L. M., et al. (1996). Birth outcomes in pregnant women taking fluoxetine. *New England Journal of Medicine, 335*(14), 1010–1015.

Clayton-Smith, J., & Donnai, D. (1995). Fetal valproate syndrome. *Journal of Medical Genetics, 32*(9), 724–727.

Cohen, L. S., & Altshuler, L. L. (1997). Pharmacologic management of psychiatric illness during pregnancy and the postpartum period. *Psychiatric Clinics of North America, 4*, 21–60.

Cohen, L. S., Friedman, J. M., Jefferson, J. W., et al. (1994). A reevaluation of risk of *in utero* exposure to lithium. *Journal of the American Medical Association, 271*(2), 146–150.

Cohen, L. S., Heller, V. L., Bailey, J., et al. (2000). Birth outcomes following prenatal exposure to fluoxetine. *Biological Psychiatry, 48*(10), 996–1000.

Cohen, L. S., Robertson, L., Grush, L., et al. (1997, May). *Impact of pregnancy on risk for relapse of MDD*. Paper presented at the 150th Annual Convention of the American Psychiatric Association, San Diego, CA.

Cohen, L. S., & Rosenbaum, J. R. (1997). Fluoxetine in pregnancy [Letter to the editor]. *New England Journal of Medicine, 336*, 872.

Cohen, L. S., Sichel, D. A., Dimmock, J. A., et al. (1994). Impact of pregnancy on panic disorder: A case series. *Journal of Clinical Psychiatry, 55*, 284–288.

Cohen, L. S., Sichel, D. A., Faraone, S. V., et al. (1996). Course of panic disorder during pregnancy and the puerperium: A preliminary study. *Biological Psychiatry, 39*, 950–954.

Cohen, L. S., Sichel, D. A., Robertson, L. M., et al. (1995). Postpartum prophylaxis for women with bipolar disorder. *American Journal of Psychiatry, 152*(11), 1641–1645.

Cowe, L., Lloyd, D. J., & Dawling, S. (1982). Neonatal convulsions caused by withdrawal from maternal clomipramine. *British Medical Journal, 284*, 1837–1838.

Cowley, D. S., & Roy-Byrne, P. P. (1989). Panic disorder during pregnancy. *Journal of Psychosomatic Obstetrics and Gynaecology, 10*, 193–210.

Desmond, M. M., Rudolph, A. J., & Hill, R. M. (1967). Behavioral alterations in infants born to mothers on psychoactive medication during pregnancy. In G. Farrell (Ed.), *Congenital mental retardation*. Austin: University of Texas Press.

Dickson, R. A., & Dawson, D. T. (1998). Olanzapine and pregnancy [Letter to the editor]. *Canadian Journal of Psychiatry—Revue Canadienne de Psychiatrie, 43*(2), 196–197.

Dickson, R. A., & Hogg, L. (1998). Pregnancy of a patient treated with clozapine. *Psychiatric Services, 49*, 1081–1083.

Dolovich, L. R., Addis, A., Vaillancourt, J. M., et al. (1998). Benzodiazepine use in pregnancy and major malformations or oral cleft: Meta-analysis of cohort and case–control studies. *British Medical Journal, 317*, 839–843.

Edmonds, L. D., & Oakley, G. P. (1990). Ebstein's anomaly and maternal lithium exposure during pregnancy. *Teratology, 41*, 551–552.

Eggermont, E. (1973). Withdrawal symptoms in neonates associated with maternal imipramine therapy. *Lancet, ii*, 680.

Ericson, A., Kallen, B., & Wiholm, B. (1999). Delivery outcome after the use of antidepressants in early pregnancy. *European Journal of Clinical Pharmacology, 55*(7), 503–508.

Fabro, S. E. (1987). *Clinical obstetrics*. New York: Wiley.

Faedda, G. L., Tondo, L., Baldessarini, R. J., et al. (1993). Outcome after rapid vs. gradual discontinuation of lithium treatment in bipolar disorders. *Archives of General Psychiatry, 50*(6), 448–455.

Falterman, C. G., & Richardson, C. J. (1980). Small left colon syndrome associated with maternal ingestion of psychotropic drugs. *Journal of Pediatrics, 97*, 308–310.

Ferrill, M. J., Kehoe, W. A., & Jacisin, J. J. (1992). ECT during pregnancy: Physiologic and pharmacologic considerations. *Convulsive Therapy, 8*(3), 186–200.

Finnerty, M., Levin, Z., & Miller, L. J. (1996). Acute manic episodes in pregnancy. *American Journal of Psychiatry, 153*, 261–263.

Fisher, J. B., Edgren, B. E., & Mammel, M. (1985). Neonatal apnea associated with maternal clonazepam therapy: A case report. *Obstetrics and Gynecology, 66*(Sept. Suppl.), 34–35.

George, D. T., Ladenheim, J. A., & Nutt, D. J. (1987). Effect of pregnancy on panic attacks. *American Journal of Psychiatry, 144*, 1078–1079.

Gillberg, C. (1977). 'Floppy infant syndrome' and maternal diazepam. *Lancet, ii*, 244.

Glover, V. (1997). Maternal stress or anxiety in pregnancy and emotional development of the child. *British Journal of Psychiatry, 171*, 105–106.

Goldstein, D. J. (1995). Effects of third trimester fluoxetine exposure on the newborn. *Journal of Clinical Psychopharmacology, 15*, 417–420.

Goldstein, D. J., Corbin, L. A., & Sundell, K. L. (1997). Effects of first-trimester fluoxetine exposure on the newborn. *Obstetrics and Gynecology, 89*, 713–718.

Gotlib, I. H., Whiffen, V. E., Mount, J. H., et al. (1989). Prevalence rates and demographic characteristics associated with depression in pregnancy and the postpartum. *Journal of Consulting and Clinical Psychology, 57*, 269–274.

Grush, L. R., Sichel, D. A., & Cohen, L. S. (1996, May). *Pharmacotherapy during pregnancy in women with OCD.* Paper presented at the 149th Annual Convention of the American Psychiatric Association, New York.

Hanson, J. W., & Oakley, G. P., Jr. (1975). Haloperidol and limb deformity [Letter to the editor]. *Journal of the American Medical Association, 231*, 26.

Hartz, S. C., Heinonen, O. P., Shapiro, S., et al. (1975). Antenatal exposure to meprobamate and chlordiazepoxide in relation to malformations, mental development, and childhood mortality. *New England Journal of Medicine, 292*, 726–728.

Heinonen, O., Sloan, D., & Shapiro, S. (1977). *Birth defects and drugs in pregnancy.* Littleton, MA: Publishing Services Group.

Hill, R. M., Desmond, M. M., & Kay, J. L. (1966). Extrapyramidal dysfunction in an infant of a schizophrenic mother. *Journal of Pediatrics, 69*, 589–595.

Holmes, L. B., Harvey, E. A., Coull, B. A., et al. (2001). The teratogenicity of anticonvulsant drugs. *New England Journal of Medicine, 344*(15), 1132–1138.

Inman, W., Kobotu, K., & Pearce, G. (1993). Prescription event monitoring of paroxetine. *PEM Reports PXL, 1206*, 1–44.

Jacobson, S. J., Jones, K., Johnson, K., et al. (1992). Prospective multicentre study of pregnancy outcome after lithium exposure during first trimester. *Lancet, 339*, 530–533.

Jones, K. L., Lacro, R. V., Johnson, K. A., et al. (1989). Pattern of malformation in the children of women treated with carbamazepine during pregnancy. *New England Journal of Medicine, 320*, 1661–1666.

Kallen, B., & Tandberg, A. (1983). Lithium and pregnancy. A cohort study on manic–depressive women. *Acta Psychiatrica Scandinavica, 68*(2), 134–139.

Keller, M. B., Lavori, P. W., Lewis, C., et al. (1983). Predictors of relapse in major depressive disorder. *Journal of the American Medical Association, 250*, 3299–3309.

Kendell, R. E., Chalmers, J. C., & Platz, C. (1987). Epidemiology of puerperal psychoses. *British Journal of Psychiatry, 150*, 662–673.

Kessler, R. C., McGonagle, K. A., Swartz, M., et al. (1993). Sex and depression in the National

Comorbidity Survey: I. Lifetime prevalence, chronicity and recurrence. *Journal of Affective Disorders, 29,* 85–96.

Klein, D. F., Skrobala, A. M., & Garfinkel, R. S. (1994–1995). Preliminary look at the effects of pregnancy on the course of panic disorder. *Anxiety, 1,* 227–232.

Klein, M. H., & Essex, M. J. (1995). Pregnant or depressed? The effects of overlap between symptoms of depression and somatic complaints of pregnancy on rates of major depression in the second trimester. *Depression, 2,* 308–314.

Klerman, G. L., Weissman, M. M., Rounsaville, B. J., et al. (1984). *Interpersonal psychotherapy of depression.* New York: Basic Books.

Klompenhouwer, J. L., & van Hulst, A. M. (1991). Classification of postpartum psychosis: A study of 250 mother and baby admissions in the Netherlands. *Acta Psychiatrica Scandinavica, 84,* 255–261.

Koch, S., Losche, G., Jager-Roman, E., et al. (1992). Major and minor birth malformations and antiepileptic drugs. *Neurology, 42*(Suppl. 5), 83–88.

Kopelman, A. E., McCullar, F. W., & Heggeness, L. (1975). Limb malformations following maternal use of haloperidol. *Journal of the American Medical Association, 231,* 62–64.

Kulin, N. A., Pastuszak, A., Sage, S. A., et al. (1998). Pregnancy outcome following maternal use of the new selective serotonin reuptake inhibitors: A prospective controlled multicenter study. *Journal of the American Medical Association, 279,* 609–610.

Kupfer, D., Frank, E., Prel, J., et al. (1992). Five-year outcome for maintenance therapies in recurrent depression. *Archives of General Psychiatry, 49,* 769–773.

Laegreid, L., Hagberg, G., & Lundberg, A. (1992). The effect of benzodiazepines on the fetus and the newborn. *Neuropediatrics, 23,* 18–23.

Langman, J. (1985). Human development—Normal and abnormal. In J. Langman (Ed.), *Medical embryology.* Baltimore: Williams & Wilkins.

Lindhout, D., & Omtzigt, J. G. (1994). Teratogenic effects of antiepileptic drugs: Implications for the management of epilepsy in women of childbearing age. *Epilepsia, 35*(Suppl. 4), S19–S28.

Levy, W., & Wisniewski, K. (1974). Chlorpromazine causing extrapyramidal dysfunction in newborn infant of psychotic mother. *New York State Journal of Medicine, 74,* 684–685.

Loebstein, R., & Koren, G. (1997). Pregnancy outcome and neurodevelopment of children exposed in utero to psychoactive drugs: The Motherisk experience. *Journal of Psychiatry and Neuroscience, 22,* 192–196.

Mazzi, E. (1977). Possible neonatal diazepam withdrawal: A case report. *American Journal of Obstetrics and Gynecology, 129,* 586–587.

McElhatton, P. R., Garbis, H. M., Elefant, E., et al. (1996). The outcome of pregnancy in 689 women exposed to theraputic doses of antidepressants: A collaborative study of the European Network of Teratology Information Services (ENTIS). *Reproductive Toxicology, 10,* 285–294.

McElhatton, P. R. (1994). The effects of benzodiazepine use during pregnancy and lactation. *Reproductive Toxicology, 8*(6), 461–475.

Milkovich, L., & van den Berg, B. J. (1974). Effects of prenatal meprobamate and chlordiazepoxide hydrochloride on human embryonic and fetal development. *New England Journal of Medicine, 291,* 1268–1271.

Miller, L. J. (1994). Use of electroconvulsive therapy during pregnancy. *Hospital and Community Psychiatry, 45*(5), 444–450.

Misri, S., & Sivertz, K. (1991). Tricyclic drugs in pregnancy and lactation: A preliminary report. *International Journal of Psychiatry in Medicine, 21*(2), 157–171.

Moore, K. L., & Persaud, T. V. N. (1998). *The developing human: Clinically oriented embryology.* Philadelphia: W. B. Saunders.

Mueller, T., Leon, A., Keller, M., et al. (1999). Recurrence after recovery from major depressive disorder during 15 years of observational follow-up. *American Journal of Psychiatry, 156,* 1000–1006.

Murray, L. (1992). The impact of postnatal depression on infant development. *Journal of Child Psychology and Psychiatry, 33*, 543–561.

Murray, L., & Cooper, P. (1997). Effects of postnatal depression on infant development. *Archives of Disease in Childhood, 77*, 99–101.

Nakane, Y., Okuma, T., Takahashi, R., et al. (1980). Multi-institutional study on the teratogenicity and fetal toxicity of antiepileptic drugs: A report of a collaborative study group in Japan. *Epilepsia, 21*, 663–680.

Nelson, M. M., & Forfar, J. O. (1971). Associations between drugs administered during pregnancy and congenital asbnormalities in the fetus. *British Medical Journal, i*, 523–527.

Neziroglu, F., Anemone, R., & Yaryura-Tobias, J. A. (1992). Onset of obsessive–compulsive disorder in pregnancy. *American Journal of Psychiatry, 149*(7), 947–950.

Nonacs, R., Viguera, A., Cohen, L., et al. (1998, May). *Risks of postpartum relapse in pregnant women with bipolar disorder.* Paper presented at the 151st Annual Convention of the American Psychiatric Association, Toronto.

Nora, J. J., Nora, A. H., & Toews, W. H. (1974). Lithium, Ebstein's anomaly and other congenital heart defects. *Lancet, ii*, 594–595.

Northcott, C. J., & Stein, M. B. (1994). Panic disorder in pregnancy. *Journal of Clinical Psychiatry, 55*(12), 539–542.

Nulman, I., & Koren, G. (1996). The safety of fluoxetine during pregnancy and lactation. *Teratology, 53*, 304–308.

Nulman, I., Rovet, J., Stewart, D. E., et al. (1997). Neurodevelopment of children exposed in utero to antidepressant drugs. *New England Journal of Medicine, 336*, 258–262.

O'Hara, M. W. (1986). Social support, life events, and depression during pregnancy and the puerperium. *Archives of General Psychiatry, 43*, 569–573.

Omtzigt, J. G., Los, F. J., Grobbee, D. E., et al. (1992a). The risk of spina bifida aperta after first-trimester exposure to valproate in a prenatal cohort. *Neurology, 42*(Suppl. 5), 119–125.

Orr, S. T., & Miller, C. A. (1995). Maternal depressive symptoms and the risk of poor pregnancy outcome: Review of the literature and preliminary findings. *Epidemiologic Reviews, 17*(1), 165–171.

Pastuszak, A., Schick-Boschetto, B., Zuber, C., et al. (1993). Pregnancy outcome following first-trimester exposure to fluoxetine (Prozac). *Journal of the American Medical Association, 269*(17), 2246–2248.

Pollack, M. H., & Smoller, J. W. (1995). The longitudinal course and outcome of panic disorder. *Psychiatric Clinics of North America, 18*, 785–801.

Post, R. M. (1992). Transduction of psychosocial stress into the neurobiology of recurrent affective disorder. *American Journal of Psychiatry, 149*, 999–1010.

Reich, T., & Winokur, G. (1970). Postpartum psychoses in patients with manic depressive disease. *Journal of Nervous and Mental Disease, 151*, 60–68.

Reinisch, J. M., Sanders, S. A., Mortensen, E. L., et al. (1995). In utero exposure to phenobarbital and intelligence deficits in adult men. *Journal of the American Medical Association, 724*, 1518–1525.

Rementeria, J. L., & Bhatt, K. (1977). Withdrawal symptoms in neonates from intrauterine exposure to diazepam. *Journal of Pediatriatrics, 90*, 123–126.

Robert, E. (1996). Treating depression in pregnancy. *New England Journal of Medicine, 335*, 1056–1058.

Robert, E., & Guibaud, P. (1982). Maternal valproic acid and congenital neural tube defects. *Lancet, ii*(8304), 937.

Robinson, L., Walker, J. R., & Anderson, D. (1992). Cognitive-behavioural treatment of panic disorder during pregnancy and lactation. *Canadian Journal of Psychiatry, 37*(9), 623–626.

Rosa, F. W. (1991). Spina bifida in infants of women treated with carbamazepine during pregnancy. *New England Journal of Medicine, 324*, 674–677.

Rosenbaum, J. F., Sachs, G. S., & Lafer, B. (1994). *High rates of relapse in bipolar patients abruptly changed from standard to low serum lithium levels in a double-blind trial.* Paper presented at the meeting of the American College of Neuropsychopharmacology, San Juan, Puerto Rico.

Rosenberg, L., Mitchell, A. A., Parsello, J. L., et al. (1983). Lack of relation of oral clefts to diazepam use during pregnancy. *New England Journal of Medicine, 309,* 1282–1285.

Rowlatt, R. J. (1978). Effect of maternal diazepam on the newborn. *British Medical Journal, 1, 985.*

Rubin, P. C. (1981). Current concepts: Beta-blockers in pregnancy. *New England Journal of Medicine, 305,* 1323–1326.

St. Clair, S. M., & Schirmer, R. G. (1992). First-trimester exposure to alprazolam. *Obstetrics and Gynecology, 80,* 843–846.

Schimmel, M. S., Katz, E. Z., Shaag, Y., et al. (1991). Toxic neonatal effects following maternal clomipramine therapy. *Journal of Toxicology: Clinical Toxicology, 29,* 479–484.

Schou, M. (1976). What happened later to the lithium babies? A follow-up study of children born without malformations. *Acta Psychiatrica Scandinavica, 54,* 193–197.

Schou, M., & Amdisen, A. (1975). Lithium and the placenta [Letter to the editor]. *American Journal of Obstetrics and Gynecology, 122,* 541.

Schou, M., Goldfield, M. D., Weinstein, M. R., et al. (1973). Lithium and pregnancy: I. Report from the Register of Lithium Babies. *British Medical Journal, ii,* 135–136.

Scolnik, D., Nulman, I., Rovet, J., et al. (1994). Neurodevelopment of children exposed in utero to phenytoin and carbamazepine monotherapy. *Journal of the American Medical Association, 271*(10), 767–770.

Sharma, V., & Persad, E. (1995). Effect of pregnancy on three patients with bipolar disorder. *Annals of Clinical Psychiatry, 7,* 39–42.

Shearer, W. T., Schreiner, R. L., & Marshall, R. E. (1972). Urinary retention in a neonate secondary to maternal ingestion of nortriptyline. *Journal of Pediatrics, 81,* 570–572.

Shepard, T. (1989). *Catalog of teratogenic agents.* Baltimore: Johns Hopkins University Press.

Shiono, P. H., & Mills, I. L. (1984). Oral clefts and diazepam use during pregnancy [Letter to the editor]. *New England Journal of Medicine, 311,* 919–920.

Sichel, D. A., Cohen, L. S., Dimmock, J. A., et al. (1993). Postpartum obsessive compulsive disorder: A case series. *Journal of Clinical Psychiatry, 54*(4), 156–159.

Slone, D., Siskind, V., Heinonen, O. P., et al. (1977). Antenatal exposure to the phenothiazines in relation to congenital malformations, perinatal mortality rate, birth weight, and intelligence quotient score. *American Journal of Obstetrics and Gynecology, 128,* 486–488.

Speight, A. (1977). Floppy infant syndrome and maternal diazepam and/or nitrazepam (Letter to the editor]. *Lancet, ii,* 878.

Spencer, M. J. (1993). Fluoxetine hydrochloride (Prozac) toxicity in the neonate. *Pediatrics, 92,* 721–722.

Spinelli, M .G. (1997). Interpersonal psychotherapy for depressed antepartum women: A pilot study. *American Journal of Psychiatry, 154,* 1028–1030.

Steer, R. A., Scholl, T. O., Hediger, M. L., et al. (1992). Self-reported depression and negative pregnancy outcomes. *Journal of Clinical Epidemiology, 45*(10), 1093–1099.

Stoner, S. C., Sommi, R. W., Jr., Marken, P. A., et al. (1997). Clozapine use in two full-term pregnancies [Letter to the editor]. *Journal of Clinical Psychiatry, 58,* 364–365.

Suppes, T., Baldessarini, R. J., Faedda, G. L., et al. (1991). Risk of recurrence following discontinuation of lithium treatment in bipolar disorder. *Archives of General Psychiatry, 48,* 1082–1088.

Targum, S. D., Davenport, Y. B., & Webster, M. J. (1979). Postpartum mania in bipolar manic–depressive patients withdrawn from lithium carbonate. *Journal of Nervous and Mental Disease, 167,* 572–574. •

Teixeira, J. M., Fisk, N. M., & Glover, V. (1999). Association between maternal anxiety in pregnancy and increased uterine artery resistance index: Cohort based study. *British Medical Journal, 318*(7177), 153–157.

Tondo, L., Baldessarini, R. J., Hennen, J., et al. (1998). Lithium treatment reduces risk of suicidal behavior in bipolar disorder patients. *Journal of Clinical Psychiatry, 59,* 405–414.

Uno, H., Eisele, S., Sakai, A,, et al. (1994). Neurotoxicity of glucocorticoids in the primate brain. *Hormones and Behavior, 28,* 336–348.

Uno, H., Lohmiller, L., Thieme, C., et al. (1990). Brain damage induced by prenatal exposure to dexamethasone in fetal rhesus macaques. *Developmental Brain Research, 53,* 157–167.

van Gent, E. M., & Verhoeven, W. M. (1992). Bipolar illness, lithium prophylaxis, and pregnancy. *Pharmacopsychiatry, 25,* 187–191.

Vanoverloop, D., Schnell, R. R., Harvey, E. A., et al. (1992). The effects of prenatal exposure to phenytoin and other anticonvulsants on intellectual function at 4 to 8 years of age. *Neurotoxicology and Teratology, 14,* 329–335.

van Waes, A., & van de Velde, E. (1969). Safety evaluation of haloperidol in the treatment of hyperemesis gravidum. *Journal of Clinical Psychopharmacology, 9,* 224–237.

Vernadakis, A., & Parker, K. (1980). Drugs and the developing central nervous system. *Pharmacology and Therapeutics, 11,* 593–647.

Viggedal, G., Hagberg, B. S., Laegreid, L., et al. (1993). Mental development in late infancy after prenatal exposure to benzodiazepines: A prospective study. *Journal of Child Psychology and Psychiatry, 34,* 295–305.

Viguera, A. C., Nonacs, R., Cohen, L. S., et al. (2000). Risk of recurrence of bipolar disorder in pregnant and nonpregnant women after discontinuing lithium maintenance. *American Journal of Psychiatry, 157*(2), 179–184.

Viguera, A. C., Baldessarini, R. J., & Friedberg, J. (1998). Discontinuing antidepressant treatment in major depression: Risks of interrupting continuation or maintenance treatment with antidepressants in major depressive disorders. *Harvard Review of Psychiatry, 5,* 293–306.

Viguera, A. C., Baldessarini, R. J., Hegarty, J. D., et al. (1997). Clinical risk following abrupt and gradual withdrawal of maintenance neuroleptic treatment. *Archives of General Psychiatry, 54,* 49–55.

Villeponteaux, V. A., Lydiard, R. B., Laraia, M. T., et al. (1992). The effects of pregnancy on preexisting panic disorder. *Journal of Clinical Psychiatry, 53,* 201–203.

Vorhees, C., Brunner, R., & Butcher, R. (1979). Psychotropic drugs as behavioral teratogens. *Science, 205,* 1220–1225.

Waldman, M. D., & Safferman, A. Z. (1993). Pregnancy and clozapine. *American Journal of Psychiatry, 150,* 168–169.

Webster, P. A. C. (1973). Withdrawal symptoms in neonates associated with maternal antidepressant therapy. *Lancet, ii,* 318–319.

Weinberg, M., & Tronick, E. (1998). The impact of maternal psychiatric illness on infant development. *Journal of Clinical Psychiatry, 59*(Suppl. 2), 53–61.

Weinstein, M. R. (1976). The international register of lithium babies. *Drug Information Journal, 50,* 81–86.

Weinstock, L., Cohen, L. S., Bailey, J. W., Blatman, R., & Rosenbaum, J. F. (2001). Obstetrical and neonatal outcome following clonazepam use during pregnancy: A case series. *Psychotherapy and Psychosomatics, 70*(3), 158–162.

Woody, J. N., London, W. L., & Wilbanks, G. D., Jr. (1971). Lithium toxicity in a newborn. *Pediatrics, 47,* 94–96.

Zalzstein, E., Koren, G., Einarson, T., et al. (1990). A case control study on the association between first-trimester exposure to lithium and Ebstein's anomaly. *American Journal of Cardiology, 65,* 817–818.

Zuckerman, B., Amaro, H., Bauchner, H., et al. (1989). Depressive symptoms during pregnancy: Relationship to poor health behaviors. *American Journal of Obstetrics and Gynecology, 160*(5, Pt. 1), 1107–1111.

Zuckerman, B., Bauchner, H., Parker, S., et al. (1990). Maternal depressive symptoms during pregnancy, and newborn irritability. *Journal of Developmental and Behavioral Pediatrics, 11*(4), 190–194.

5

Psychiatric Aspects of the Postpartum Period

ANGELA F. ARNOLD
CLAUDIA BAUGH
ANGELA FISHER
JESSICA BROWN
ZACHARY N. STOWE

Since its earliest documentation by Hippocrates in 400 B.C., the temporal relationship between childbirth and mental illness has been explored. Although many review articles, the lay press, and most patient support groups adhere to the theory that the onset of psychiatric illness during the postpartum period is biologically based, the current literature has failed to confirm this theory. Although the precise etiology remains unknown, the abundance of epidemiological data continues to pinpoint the childbearing years as a time of increased vulnerability for women to develop mood disorders in particular (Weissman & Olfson, 1995). The first postpartum year has been noted as the lifetime peak of psychiatric admissions for women, with up to 12.5% of all admissions in women occurring during this period (Duffy, 1983). Subsequently, Kendall et al. (1987) demonstrated a profound rise in psychiatric admissions during the first 3 months postpartum. The debate persists as to whether this increase in hospital admissions represents sufficient evidence for a classification as a distinct set of psychiatric disorders. Whether it is distinct in nature or not, there is considerable concern that maternal mental illness may have an impact on infant well-being. In light of the potential impact of postpartum mental disorders, effective identification and treatment are crucial. This chapter provides a review of the history and current research in the area of postpartum illness, focusing on the potential consequences for offspring, effective treatment planning, and treatment issues in breastfeeding women.

HISTORY OF THE POSTPARTUM DIAGNOSIS

Although the connection between the postpartum period and psychiatric disturbance was recognized over 2,000 years ago, it was not until the 19th century that clinicians began to ask the questions for which we still seek answers today. Esquirol (1845) described a variety of mood disturbances associated with the postpartum period and disputed their connection to lactation. Soon thereafter, Marcé, a French physician, published *Insanity in Pregnant, Puerperal, and Lactating Women* (1858). Marcé proposed that postpartum mental disorders encompass a variety of unique symptoms, which, when combined with the postpartum period, form a distinct syndrome that can be classified into two subgroups: symptoms with early onset (increased confusion or delirium), and those with late onset (more physical symptoms). As the century came to a close, the uniqueness of postpartum syndromes remained disputed. The distinct-diagnosis debate has consequently affected the diagnostic classification. Postpartum affective disorders were acknowledged briefly by the American Psychiatric Association (1968) in the second edition of the *Diagnostic and Statistical Manual of Mental Disorders* (DSM-II), in which "psychosis associated with childbirth" was listed as a psychosis caused by organic conditions. In the DSM-III and its revision, postpartum psychosis was noted only as an example of atypical psychosis (American Psychiatric Association, 1980). The American Psychiatric Association officially removed the term "postpartum" from the classification system, basing diagnosis on symptoms that were most apparent at the time of clinical presentation (Parry & Hamilton, 1999). The DSM-IV lists "postpartum onset" as an atypical-features modifier of mood disorders and brief reactive psychosis (American Psychiatric Association, 1994). Thus, if symptoms meeting criteria for any of the mood disorders or brief psychotic disorder appear within 4 weeks after the birth of a child, the specifier "with postpartum onset" may be applied to the diagnosis. Although diagnostic concerns do not constitute the entire controversy, these issues have provided an array of time periods for the diagnosis of postpartum disorders, rendering combinations of extant data difficult.

Theories of postpartum mental illness have pointed to intrapsychic conflict (Zilboorg, 1943), personality structure, and psychosocial adaptability (Jansson, 1963). Boyd was the first to propose a multifactorial etiology emphasizing individual vulnerability or predisposition to illness. He posed the question, "Is the patient's psychic reserve (hereditary constitution, training, personal psychologic organization) sufficient to resist the factors producing mental disorder (toxicity, endocrine imbalance, psychologic conflicts) engendered by pregnancy?" (quoted in Jansson, 1963). The purported temporal association with childbirth has contributed to the hypothesis that postpartum illnesses are biologically derived. However, the studies investigating potential biological aberrations have been remarkably negative or lack replication (Wisner & Stowe, 1997). Regardless of specific diagnostic recognition and etiological debate, most investigators have continued to group postpartum mental disturbances into three categories: postpartum blues (maternity blues), postpartum depression (PPD), and postpartum psychosis (PPP).

Postpartum Blues (Maternity Blues)

Postpartum blues is the most common and least severe postpartum illness, affecting between 50% and 80% of new mothers (Kennerley & Gath, 1989; O'Hara, 1991). The blues are not typically considered a "disorder" necessitating professional intervention. Postpartum blues are short-lived, with acute onset typically before 2 weeks postpartum and persisting from a few hours to a few days. A variety of symptoms have been described, including forgetfulness, irritability, headache, fatigue, confusion, anxiety, mild depression, and mood instability.

The etiology of postpartum blues is unknown; however, there has been much research focusing on the dramatic biological changes occurring during labor, delivery, and the immediate postpartum period. Of particular interest, several investigators have focused on the precipitous decline in progesterone (Dalton, 1985). Psychosocial and personality factors have also been studied (Condon & Watson, 1987; George & Wilson, 1981; Kennerley & Gath, 1989; O'Hara et al., 1991b). Risk factors that have been found to be associated with the blues include ambivalent feelings toward the pregnancy, fear of labor, poor social adjustment, a view of the pregnancy as emotionally difficult, and a history of severe premenstrual tension (Condon & Watson, 1987; Kennerley & Gath, 1989). O'Hara et al. (1991b) examined both biological and psychosocial factors, and found stressful life events and a personal or family history of depression to be associated with the blues.

Although the blues do not require intervention, it is important to note that this purportedly "normal" syndrome appears to be a risk factor for later depression. Up to 20% of women with the blues will experience major depression in the first postnatal year (Campbell et al., 1992; O'Hara, 1991).

Postpartum Depression

PPD constitutes a major depressive episode with clinical symptoms that may include irritability, anhedonia, sleep disturbance, fatigue, and anxiety. The majority of cases have an onset within 6 weeks postpartum (Stowe & Nemeroff, 1995) and demonstrate variability in symptom severity and duration (Wolkind et al., 1990). Rates of PPD have been reported to be between 6.8% and 16.5% in adult women (Gotlib et al., 1989; Pitt, 1968) and up to 26% in adolescent mothers (Troutman & Cutrona, 1990) during the first postpartum year. A review of 17 major studies examining the rates of PPD reported the prevalence to range from 5.2% to 22% (Richards, 1990). The wide variance in reports of prevalence is due in part to the lack of clearly defined diagnostic criteria, including conflicting definitions of the duration of the postpartum period. Distinguishing between depressive symptoms and the supposed "normal" sequelae of childbirth, such as changes in weight, sleep, and energy, is a challenge that complicates clinical diagnosis. Further confounding prevalence rates of PPD is the failure of previous studies to exclude possible physical causes (including anemia, diabetes, and thyroid dysfunction) that could possibly contribute to depressive symptoms (Pedersen et al., 1993).

A potential method of addressing the issues of diagnosis is the development of disorder-specific rating scales. The Edinburgh Postnatal Depression Scale (EPDS), a 10-item self-rated measure that does not include items on somatic symptoms, was developed to assess PPD in the community. This scale has been translated into over a dozen different languages and seems to be highly correlated with physician-rated depression measures (Cox et al., 1987). The Postpartum Depression Checklist, also developed as a screening tool for PPD, is intended for use by health professionals (Beck, 1995). Although these scales were developed for use in the postpartum period, identification of women at high risk for postpartum-onset illness prior to delivery is the emerging standard of care. Consequently, the EPDS has been validated for use in pregnancy as well as the puerperium (Glaze & Cox, 1991; Cox et al., 1996).

The risk factors contributing to PPD have undergone considerable scrutiny (Duffy, 1983; Gotlib et al., 1991; Marks et al., 1992; Stowe & Nemeroff, 1995). No association between demographic factors and onset of illness has been consistently found (Bagedahl Strindlund, 1986; Marks et al., 1992); however, evidence does exist that a personal or family history of mood disorder (Playfair & Gowers, 1981; Richards, 1990), depression or anxiety during pregnancy, and the maternity blues (Gotlib et al., 1991; O'Hara, 1986; O'Hara et al., 1991a) are all risk factors for the development of PPD. In addition, a previous episode of PPD has been found to put women at considerable risk for recurrent episodes following subsequent pregnancies (O'Hara, 1991). Psychosocial issues—including coping difficulties, marital/couple discord, infant medical problems, unwanted or unplanned pregnancies, lack of social support, and stressful life events during pregnancy (Righetti-Veltema et al., 1998; Gotlib et al., 1991; Graff et al., 1991; Marks et al., 1992; O'Hara et al., 1991b; Unterman et al., 1990)—also increase the risk of PPD. The chronic stressors of poverty have been found to constitute a further risk factor in women of low socioeconomic status (Seguin et al., 1999). This broad range of past history and psychosocial risk factors underscores the probable role of both genetic and stress-related variables in the development of PPD. Identification of these risk factors provides caregivers with the opportunity to observe high-risk individuals closely and identify illness early, making intervention and prevention possible.

Postpartum Psychosis

PPP is the most severe and least common postpartum mental disorder, reported to occur in only 1 or 2 of every 1,000 women (Kendell et al., 1987). This psychosis has an onset shortly after birth, usually within a few days and in most cases within the first 3 weeks (Brockington et al., 1981). The majority (>70%) of these psychoses represent either bipolar disorder or major depression with psychotic features. Brief reactive psychosis and schizophrenia also occur, but more infrequently (McGorry & Connell, 1990). Symptoms of PPP include delusions, hallucinations, an impaired concept of reality, rapid mood swings, insomnia, and abnormal or obsessive thoughts. It is estimated that up to 5% of women with PPP may commit suicide, and that 2–4% pose considerable direct risk to their infants (Knopps, 1993). PPP constitutes a psychiatric emergency, and a presumptive diagnosis of this psychosis always warrants hospitalization.

The prognostic investigations of recurrent psychotic symptoms following an index episode during the postpartum vary, though most studies agree that approximately 65% of these women will experience subsequent nonpuerperal psychotic episodes (Benvenuti et al., 1992; Schopf & Rust, 1994; Videbech & Gouliaev, 1995). It is noteworthy that up to two-thirds of these women will experience symptom relapse in subsequent pregnancies prior to delivery (Benvenuti et al., 1992; Schopf & Rust, 1994). However, compared to women who experience nonpostpartum psychosis, those who experience PPP are less likely to be readmitted to psychiatric hospitals, and spend less time there if readmitted (Platz & Kendell, 1988), suggesting a better prognosis.

OBSESSIVE–COMPULSIVE DISORDER AND PANIC
DISORDER IN PREGNANCY AND THE POSTPARTUM

The presence of anxiety and obsessions in postpartum-onset disorders has been noted in the DSM-IV, and epidemiological data suggest a high rate of comorbidity of depression and anxiety disorders in women (Kessler et al., 1994). Although mood disorders and psychosis have dominated the literature regarding the postpartum period, recent evidence suggests that both obsessive–compulsive disorder (OCD) and panic disorder may have their initial episodes during either pregnancy or the postpartum period. A retrospective study of 59 women with OCD found that 39% of them experienced symptom onset during pregnancy. Symptom onset was also reported during pregnancy in another 4 out of 5 women in this study who had an abortion or miscarriage (Neziroglu et al., 1992). Other studies have indicated that preexisting OCD is exacerbated during pregnancy (Brandt & Mackenzie, 1987; Williams & Koran, 1997), and symptoms of OCD have been reported to develop or worsen during the postpartum period as well (Williams & Koran, 1997). A recent report by Wisner et al. (1999) suggests a high prevalence of obsessive thoughts in women with PPD.

In contrast, earlier reports suggested that pregnancy might confer protection against panic attacks (George et al., 1987), followed by an increase in panic symptoms during the postpartum period (Klein et al., 1995; Metz et al., 1988). Subsequent studies have revealed a more complicated and variable course of panic disorder across gestation and the puerperium. In a retrospective study, 49 women with panic disorder reported similar rates of clinical improvement and symptom worsening during pregnancy (Cohen et al., 1994a). The same group found that out of a sample of 40 women, only a very small number (n = 3) reported symptom improvement in the postpartum period, while a larger number (n = 14) had their symptoms worsen, and the majority (n = 23) reported no change at all (Cohen et al., 1994b).

IMPACT OF MATERNAL MENTAL ILLNESS
AND MATERNAL SEPARATION ON OFFSPRING

The adverse impact of maternal mental illness and maternal separation on offspring has been documented in both the human and animal literature. It has been 50 years since the World Health Organization demonstrated the deleterious effects of prolonged maternal separation on human infants (Bowlby, 1951). The literature is teeming with studies specifically indicating the adverse impact of maternal mental illness on infants. These investigations have demonstrated detrimental effects on mother–infant attachment, infant cognitive competence, and child development and behavior (Avant, 1981; Brazelton, 1975; Campbell et al., 1995; Cogill et al., 1986; Cradon, 1979; Cutrona & Troutman, 1986; Murray & Cooper, 1996, 1997; Teti et al., 1995; Whiffen & Gotlib, 1989; Zahn-Waxler et al., 1984). A series of studies of depressed mothers demonstrated depressed infant behavior (Fields et al., 1988) and a decrease in mother–infant behavioral and electrocardiogram synchrony (Fields, 1990; Fields et al., 1989). Surprisingly, these effects were observed when the admission criterion for the depressed mothers was a Beck Depression Inventory (BDI) score over 12—a score representing only mild to moderate depression. Several other studies have shown that depression may affect not only a mother's interaction with her infant, but also the mother's perception of the infant. Depressed mothers have been shown to perceive their infants more negatively and as more difficult to care for than nondepressed controls view their infants (Murray et al., 1996; Whiffen & Gotlib, 1989). Murray (1992) concluded that "if normal maternal communication is experimentally disrupted for even brief periods, infants as young as 6 weeks old respond with distress and avoidance." Mandl et al. (1999) found that women whose infants had frequent problem-oriented primary care visits or emergency department visits were subsequently more likely to have depressive symptoms.

Similarly, early laboratory observations demonstrated adverse effects on socialization in maternally deprived offspring of primates (Harlow & Harlow, 1966). More contemporary animal models of maternal separation have demonstrated alterations in offspring that persist into adulthood. These changes are widespread and include (but are not limited to) alteration in neuroendocrine axes (Plotsky & Meaney, 1993), neurotransmitter systems (Matthew et al., 1996), behavior (Statham, 1998), central nervous system cytoarchitecture and receptors (McEwen et al., 1992; Sutanto et al., 1996), and neuronal firing patterns (Stowe et al., 1998b). The question remains as to whether laboratory investigations are applicable to clinical care, and whether such information affects treatment planning for women during the childbearing years.

EFFECTIVE TREATMENT PLANNING

Women of reproductive years may not be adequately represented in clinical trials, and the number of treatment studies specific to postpartum psychiatric illness is negligible by comparison. There are various treatment modalities for depression and anxiety that are not limited to the use of psychotropic medications; however, nonpharmacological options are even less well studied in pregnancy and lactation than are more standard medication approaches.

The treatment of psychiatric illness during pregnancy and lactation begins in the initial treatment planning for women of childbearing age. Considering that in North America 50% of pregnancies are not planned (Doering & Stewart, 1978), it is advantageous to assume that pregnancy is imminent for every patient of reproductive potential. Effective treatment planning for women with postpartum mental disorders or at high risk for such disorders should include the following: (1) professional and community education; (2) identification of women at risk, using antenatal and postnatal screening procedures; (3) treatment options, including a risk–benefit assessment for the use of psychotropic medication during breastfeeding; and (4) prevention strategies.

Education

With access to information expanding rapidly, it is important to utilize reputable sources of information about postpartum mental disorders, to avoid misleading and highly opinionated resources. There are several worthwhile sources, such as Depression After Delivery (800-944-4PPD), a national support group; volunteer contracts; and Web sites. There are also several informative books exploring postpartum mental illness; *This Isn't What I Expected* by Raskin and Kleinman (1994) provides a reasonable overview. More general information concerning mood disorders can be obtained from the National Depressive and

Manic Depressive Association (800-826-3632), one of the largest patient-operated support/information systems in the country. As the Internet expands, general medical Web sites such as WebMD and Vcure may also provide information. These valuable resources provide support for patients, their families, and the professionals involved in their care.

Identification of Women at Risk: Screening during Pregnancy and Postpartum

Despite data suggesting that many women who experience postpartum illness demonstrate symptom or illness onset during pregnancy, routine obstetrical documentation of mood or anxiety complaints during pregnancy seldom occur. When such symptoms are elicited, they are often attributed to the "normal" sequelae of pregnancy. Our group found that out of 181 women presenting with complaints of depression during the postpartum period, 17% reported symptom onset during pregnancy (Hostetter et al., 1999). As noted previously, over one-third of women with OCD also report onset of illness during pregnancy (Neziroglu et al., 1992). Although these retrospective studies are not conclusive, the data increasingly suggest that depression and/or anxiety during pregnancy may represent not a risk factor for PPD (O'Hara et al., 1991a), but rather the onset of illness.

The majority of risk factors that predispose women to the development of postpartum mental disorders are present prior to delivery. High-risk individuals identified during pregnancy may be screened more closely for additional risk factors. The use of a depression rating scale, such as the EPDS or the BDI, in early pregnancy establishes a baseline for comparison or subsequent assessment. Screening should include documentation of other risk factors, such as marital/couple discord and poor social support. Poor support from the husband or partner has been shown to be associated with a more chronic natural course for PPD, and thus short-term interventions are less cost-effective in the face of marital/couple dissatisfaction (Steinberg & Bellavance, 1999). Evaluation during the first 2 weeks following childbirth may identify cases of postpartum blues, further establishing risk for later depression. The lack of contact with clinicians focused on women's well-being after the 6-week postnatal check underscores the importance of identification prior to the postnatal appointment.

Treatment Options

In spite of the prevalence of postpartum mental disorders and their potential detrimental consequences, surprisingly few treatment studies have been conducted (see Table 5.1). In community-derived samples, a variety of psychotherapeutic treatment strategies (Rogerian therapy, cognitive-behavioral therapy [CBT], and psychodynamic approaches), as well as individual counseling (Wickberg & Hwang, 1996), have proven efficacious in treating women with PPD (O'Hara, 1994). The best-documented form of psychotherapy for women with PPD is interpersonal psychotherapy (IPT) (Stuart & O'Hara, 1995; O'Hara et al., 2000). The premise behind IPT is that women with PPD typically experience a disruption in interpersonal relationships, and thus that a therapy targeting these symptoms could be beneficial. A second community-based study ($n = 61$) demonstrated the effectiveness of CBT, fluoxetine monotherapy, and combination therapy for the treatment of PPD (Appleby et al., 1997). Additional studies with CBT have demonstrated

TABLE 5.1. Treatment and Prevention Studies in Postpartum Depression

Intervention	Design	Sample size[a]	Postpartum depression definition	Control group	Outcome measures	Results	Comments	Reference
Active treatment in women with postpartum depression								
Antidepressants								
Fluoxetine	Case series	4	DSM-III; onset unknown	None	HRSD, BDI	All patients made complete recovery (HRSD <7; CGI = 1) on fluoxetine 20 mg/day.	2 inpatients, 2 outpatients.	Roy, Cole, Goldman, et al. (1993).
Sertraline	Prospective, open-label	21	DSM-III, onset <24 weeks postpartum	None	SIGH-D, EPDS, BDI	In 20 women >50% reduction in SIGH-D scores; 14 women total recovery (SIGH-D <7, CGI = 1) by 8 weeks.	Highly efficacious and well-tolerated treatment for women with PPD; suggestion of earlier symptom onset associated with more rapid response.	Stowe, Casarella, Landry, et al. (1995).
Fluoxetine and/or CBT	Double-blind, placebo-controlled, randomized	61	RDC criteria for minor or major depression at 6–8 weeks postpartum	16 fluoxetine + 1s; 13 fluoxetine + 6s; 17 placebo + 1s; 15 placebo + 6s	HRSD, EPDS	CBT and fluoxetine superior to placebo single counseling session (1s); no significant advantage to combined fluoxetine and CBT (6 sessions [6s]).	Both fluoxetine and CBT are effective for PPD; no advantage in combining these therapies.	Appleby, Warner, Whitton, et al. (1997).
Venlafaxine	Prospective, open-label	15	DSM-IV; onset < 12 weeks postpartum	None	HRSD, Kellner Anxiety Scale	Statistically significant change in depression and anxiety by 4 weeks; 25% dropout rate.	Venlafaxine is effective in treatment of postpartum depression.	Cohen et al. (2001).
Antidepressants	Retrospective chart review	26	DSM-IV; onset < 4 weeks postpartum	25 with nonpostpartum MDE	Treatment course	Women with PPD are more anxious, recover more slowly, and require more medication than controls.	Trials are needed to assess anxiety and rapidity of response to medications.	Hendrick, Altshuler, Strouse, et al. (2000).
Psychotherapy								
Social support group	Prospective, controlled	152	CES, EPDS	44 support group 83 no intervention 15 information by mail	CES, EPDS	8 social support sessions did not improve mood more than no intervention or information by mail; multiple measures of adjustment also assessed—no differences.	Did not alleviate maternal depression; did increase mothers' attention to infants.	Fleming, Klein, & Corter (1992).
Counseling	Prospective, controlled	41	MADRS > 10; DSM-III-R criteria for MDE; onset unknown	20 counseling 21 control	MADRS, EPDS	31 women met DSM-III-R criteria, while 41 had MADRS > 10 and were included in analysis; after 6 visits with health nurse, 12 of 15 women with MDE recovered compared to 4 of 16 in control group.	Swedish health-care system: Counseling by health nurses is useful in treating PPD.	Wickberg & Hwang (1996).

Intervention	Design	N	Criteria	Control	Measure	Results	Comments	Reference
Counseling	Prospective, controlled	50	Goldberg's Standardized Psychiatric Interview; EPDS; symptom onset unknown	26 counseling 24 control	EPDS	Only 34 women met criteria for major depression at study entry.		Holden, Sagovsky, & Cox (1989).
IPT	Prospective, open trial	6	DSM-III-R criteria for MDE; onset unknown	None	HRSD, BDI, EPDS	Significant reduction in multiple depression measures after 12 weeks of IPT.	Good alternative to medicine; focus on changes in interpersonal relationship postpartum.	Stuart & O'Hara (1994).
IPT	Prospective, controlled	99	SCID, DSM-IV criteria for MDE	48 active 51 wait-list control	HRSD	Significant reduction in depressive symptoms in the IPT group compared to wait-list controls.	Approximately two-thirds of the participants had postpartum-onset major depression.	O'Hara, Stuart, Gorman, et al. (2000).
Other								
Bright light therapy	Case series	2	Clinical diagnosis; onset within 2 weeks postpartum	None	HRSD	75% reduction in HRSD score.		Corral, Kuan, & Kostaras (2000).
Transdermal estrogen	Double-blind placebo-controlled	61	RDC criteria for major depression; onset within 12 weeks postpartum	34 active 27 placebo	SADS change, EPDS	17-ß estrogen superior to placebo.	No evidence of endometrial hyperplasia; 47% of active group on antidepressants; dose duration of treatment guidelines needed.	Gregoire, Kumar, Everitt, et al. (1994).
Sublingual 17-ß estradiol	Case series	2	ICD-10 criteria for PPD	None	MADRS	Both patients' symptoms improved as serum estradiol levels increased; 8 weeks of treatment.	Subjects had low pretreatment estradiol levels, estradiol may be related to PPD.	Ahokas, Turtiainen, & Aito (1998)
Sublingual 17-ß estradiol	Prospective, open-label	23	ICD-10 criteria for PPD	None	MADRS	Serum estradiol levels increased and MADRS scores decreased by week 8.	Suggests link between low maternal serum estradiol and clinical response to 17-ß estradiol treatment.	Ahokas, Kaukoranta, Wahlbeck, et al. (2001).
Prevention studies in women with a history of PPD								
Antidepressants								
Nortriptyline (7), imipramine (2), fluoxetine (4), clomipramine (2)	Prospective, open-labeled, controlled	23	History of MDE by DSM-III-R during postpartum	15 active 8 observation	DSM-III-R criteria, IDD	6.7% on antidepressant prophylaxis suffered recurrence, compared to 62.5% without medication.	Antidepressant treatment effective prophylactic for PPD; some women on medication during pregnancy.	Wisner & Wheeler (1994).
Nortriptyline	Double-blind, placebo-controlled, randomized	51	History of PPD, SADS; onset within 12 weeks	26 active 25 placebo	RDC criteria for MDE, HRSD	Nortriptyline does not confer added prevention beyond that of placebo.	The rate of relapse in the placebo group was less than would be expected, suggesting benefit from participation and clinical contact.	Wisner, Perel, Peindl, et al. (2001).

(continued)

TABLE 5.1. (*continued*)

Intervention	Design	Sample size[a]	Postpartum depression definition	Control group	Outcome measures	Results	Comments	Reference
Other								
Progesterone	Prospective, controlled	315	History of PPD	94 active 221 control	Questionnaires to patients and clinicians	Women with history of PPD given progesterone prohylactically, only 9 (10%) had PPD recurrence compared to 68% in untreated group.	Progesterone only effective for prophylaxis; once symptoms have onset it is ineffective.	Daton (1985).
Estrogen	Prospective	11	History of MDE by DSM-III-R criteria onset within 2 weeks postpartum	None	Clinical interview	1 woman experienced relapse.	Seem to be effective treatment, although study conducted on small sample size.	Sichel, Cohen, Robertson, et al. (1995).
Prevention studies in community-based samples								
Psychosocial								
Antenatal education classes	Prospective, controlled	161	None	85 active 76 control	Clinician-rated 6-point scale	Only 15% of subjects who took classes had postpartum emotional upset, compared to 37% of controls.	Women who had their husbands attend class with them did better than those who did not.	Gordon & Gordon (1960).
Companionship at birth	Prospective, controlled	189	None	92 active 97 control	Pitt Depression Inventory	Support during labor and delivery reduced risk of anxiety and depression.		Wolman, Chalmers, Hofmeyer, et al. (1993).

Note. CBT, cognitive-behavioral therapy; IPT, interpersonal psychotherapy; ECT, electroconvulsive therapy; CGI, Clinical Global Impressions; MDE, major depressive episode; PPD, postpartum depression; PPP, postpartum psychosis; HRSD, Hamilton Rating Scale for Depression; SIGH-D, Structured Interview Guide for the HRSD; BDI, Beck Depression Inventory; EPDS, Edinburgh Postnatal Depression Scale; CES, Current Experiences Scale; IDD, Inventory to Diagnose Depression; RDC, Research Diagnostic Criteria; SADS, Schedule for Affective Disorders and Schizophrenia; SCID, Structured Clinical Interview for Diagnosis.
[a]Total sample size that completed treatment intervention.

comparable efficacy to alprazolam for the treatment of panic disorder during pregnancy and the postpartum (Klosko et al., 1990; Robinson et al., 1992), though with a more delayed response. Social support groups have not been found to be as effective as formal psychotherapy in alleviating symptoms of major depression (Fleming et al., 1992).

The use of gonadal hormones in the treatment of postpartum mental disorders has included progesterone treatment for PPP (Schmidt, 1943), and both sublingual and transdermal estrogen treatment for PPD (Ahokas et al., 1998; Gregoire et al., 1994, 1996; Murray, 1996). The largest hormone study (n = 34 active) demonstrated a positive response to 17ß-estradiol that was sustained at a 3-month follow-up, and no evidence of endometrial hyperplasia was found (Gregoire et al., 1996). It is noteworthy that depressive symptoms as measured by the EPDS were only modestly decreased, and that over one-third of these women were also on antidepressants during the study. The first open pharmacological trial (n = 21) conducted at a tertiary referral center demonstrated a dramatic response in 20 women after 8 weeks of treatment with sertraline monotherapy (Stowe et al., 1995). An initial report commented on successful treatment of women with PPD with the tricyclic antidepressant (TCA) nortriptyline (Wisner & Perel, 1991). Our group found a dramatic treatment response (>90% by 8 weeks) to sertraline monotherapy combined with education, supportive psychotherapy, and behavioral modification (Strader et al., 1997).

The total number of women actively treated in these case reports and studies was 186. It is difficult to compare the efficacy of the various treatment modalities employed, as diagnostic criteria, depression rating scales, and sample recruitment were not consistent across studies. Clearly, further study is needed to compare the efficacy of various treatments. In brief, the variety of risk factors, degree of neuroendocrine alterations, and probable multifactorial etiology of PPD may require a multidisciplinary treatment model.

Prevention Strategies

It is essential for health care practitioners involved in the care of pregnant and postpartum women (obstetricians, midwives, nurses, family practitioners, and pediatricians) to identify those at high risk for onset or relapse of mental disorders during pregnancy and the postpartum. The risks and benefits of prophylaxis should be weighed in women at high risk for recurrence of symptoms that have historically produced significant functional impairment or suicidal potential. Our experience suggests that many women with a history of postpartum illness develop symptoms during the latter part of pregnancy, making prevention more difficult if treatment is implemented after delivery (Hostetter et al., 1999).

The postpartum period carries the potential for the exacerbation of psychiatric symptoms in women with preexisting mental illness. In women with histories of psychiatric illness who may be on active treatment or in remission, the postpartum period represents an increased risk for relapse or worsening of the current illness. It is optimal to develop a treatment plan for this scenario prior to delivery. This plan should include common complications that may exacerbate psychiatric illness (e.g., complicated delivery, extended hospital stay, lack of social support, patient expectations), criteria for intervention, and identification of symptoms indicative of relapse. No clear guidelines or consensus have been forthcoming for postpartum prevention, but one of three approaches may be required, depending on history and severity:

1. *Active treatment/prevention*—initiation of treatment prior to delivery, so that the patient is euthymic and stable prior to entering the postpartum period.
2. *Postpartum prevention*—initiation of treatment upon delivery.
3. *Close observation*—discussion of criteria for intervention (e.g., symptoms for >3 days) prior to delivery. A follow-up visit between 10 and 14 days postpartum is preferable, as any symptom presentation would limit confusion with the maternity blues.

Few prophylactic treatment studies have been conducted, and they have demonstrated mixed success. Wisner and Wheeler (1994) investigated prophylactic treatment, beginning at delivery, in women with a history of PPD. Two groups of women were compared: those who chose postpartum monitoring and prophylactic treatment with an antidepressant ($n = 15$), and those who chose postpartum monitoring alone ($n = 7$). Four patients in the monitoring-only group experienced relapse, compared to only one in the medication-plus-monitoring group. These findings should be interpreted with caution, however, due to the fact that 10 of the participants in the study experienced depressive symptoms and were on medication at some point during their pregnancy. More recently, prophylactic treatment with nortriptyline, initiated at delivery in women with a history of PPD, was not successful in preventing recurrent episodes (Wisner, 1999). Psychosocial intervention, such as support during labor and delivery and psychoeducation of parents and children, has also been found to provide some benefit for women in preventing recurrent PPD (Beardslee et al., 1997; Wolman et al., 1993). Although progesterone therapy has shown success in preventing PPD, it does not treat symptoms once they have begun (Dalton, 1985). These results with progesterone therapy have not been duplicated. One group using intravenous estrogen in a select group of women ($n = 11$) with severe mood disorder demonstrated effectiveness in preventing recurrence (Sichel et al., 1995). For women with histories of bipolar disorder or PPD, prophylactic lithium administration was superior to haloperidol in decreasing the recurrence and severity of the illness (Cohen et al., 1995; Stewart et al., 1991).

The data on active treatment and prevention of postpartum mental illness, though limited in number, show promise. However, somatic intervention is complicated by a woman's decision to breastfeed.

ANTIDEPRESSANTS AND BREASTFEEDING

In the past 20 years, the number of women planning to breastfeed has increased, with an estimated 60% of pregnant women now planning to nurse (Briggs et al., 1998). Most professional groups support breast milk as the ideal source of nutrition for infants (American Academy of Pediatrics, Committee on Nutrition, 1993). The use of psychotropic medication, and specifically antidepressants, by nursing mothers has been reviewed by numerous groups (Baum & Misri, 1996; Buist et al., 1990; Llewellyn & Stowe, 1998; Misri & Sivertz, 1991; Mortola, 1989; Robinson et al., 1986; Stowe et al., 1998a; Wisner & Perel, 1988; Wisner et al., 1996). All psychotropic medications that have been investigated are excreted into breast milk; therefore, a nursing infant is always exposed to such medications. The literature includes reports on 49 women treated with TCAs, with the largest data set on nortriptyline ($n = 17$) (Birnbaum et al., 1999; Wisner & Perel,

1988; Wisner et al., 1996). The information on selective serotonin reuptake inhibitors (SSRIs) in lactation now exceeds the available data on any other class of medications (see Table 5.2). Reports on infant serum monitoring for the SSRIs with the largest data sets include reports on fluoxetine and sertraline. Direct comparison of the breastfeeding studies is difficult because of variations in methodology and assay sensitivity. Our group has completed detailed studies of sertraline, paroxetine, and fluoxetine, demonstrating a complex pattern of excretion, but indicating that an infant's maximum oral dose over 12 months (milligrams per year) of nursing is less than 3 times the maternal daily dose (i.e., maternal daily dose x 3 > infant dose for 12 months). As a class, the antidepressants have a considerable amount of data relative to other classes of medications.

It is important to conduct a thorough risk–benefit assessment in which all treatment options, as well as the risks of untreated maternal mental illness, are discussed with the patient and all significant others (see Table 5.3). A recent study showed that the majority of women who developed PPD in the first 2 postpartum months insisted on continuing to nurse despite the severity of their illness (Misri et al., 1997). If the choice to use an antidepressant is made, the treatment should first be based on the patient's history (i.e., "use what has worked previously"). A different medication may have more data available on its use during breastfeeding, but may be ineffective at controlling the patient's illness; therefore, the infant could be exposed to multiple medications as well as illness. In the absence of personal and familial history, available data on use of the medication during breastfeeding and side effect profiles are the primary determinants of antidepressant choice.

In all postpartum treatment scenarios, the goal is to minimize simultaneous exposure of the infant to maternal illness and medication. Once a decision to treat is made, it is imperative to treat effectively and adjust the treatment dose as needed. The optimal duration of treatment for postpartum illness remains unclear; the most conservative approach would be to approach these illnesses as nonunique. Therefore, treatment for at least 12 months would be reasonable. If a shorter duration is preferable, treatment should extend beyond other hormonal changes (e.g., return of menstrual cycle).

CONCLUSIONS AND FUTURE DIRECTIONS

Despite the prevalence of postpartum mental disorders, women continue to suffer in silence and with minimal assistance. Whether or not these disorders represent a distinct and separate set of diagnoses is a debate best left to research and is of limited clinical utility. The postnatal environment is a unique clinical, neuroendocrine, and psychosocial situation that may represent the crucible in which women with subclinical symptoms and/or a genetic predisposition may decompensate. Research has begun to focus on the treatment of postpartum disorders, with data now supporting the efficacy of both psychological and pharmacological interventions in the treatment and prevention of these disorders. Nevertheless, such data are of little use if we fail to identify those at risk for onset or relapse of illness. Awareness of the prevalence, risk factors, and potential adverse impact of these disorders, as well as emerging data on the use of medications in breastfeeding, will provide the foundation for early identification and treatment planning. Certainly, further study will shed light on the etiological debate; until then, however, it is advantageous to view postpartum mental disorders as a heterogeneous group of disorders with a multifactorial etiology that, once identified, can be effectively treated.

TABLE 5.2. Published Studies of Newer Antidepressants in Lactation

Medication	Mother–infant pairs[a] (n)	Mothers providing serum samples (n)	Mother providing breast milk samples (n)	Infant serum samples obtained (n)	Adverse events reported	Reference
Bupropion	1	1	1	1	None	Briggs, Samson, Ambrose, et al. (1993)
Citalopram	1	1	1	1	None	Jensen, Oleson, Bertelson, et al. (1997)
	2	3	3	0	None	Spigset, Carleborg, Korstrum, et al. (1996)
	1	1	1	1	1—Uneasy sleep	Schmidt, Olsesen, & Jensen (2000)
	7	7	7	7	None	Rampono, Kristensen, Hackett, et al. (2000)
Fluoxetine	1	1	1	0	None	Isenberg (1990).
	1	1	1	0	None	Burch & Wells (1992)
	1	0	1	1	1—Crying, emesis, diarrhea,poor sleep, high infant serum concentration[c]	Lester, Cucca, Andreozzi, et al. (1993)
	11	3	11	1[b]	None	Taddio, Ito, & Koren (1996)
	4	4	4	2	None	Yoshida, Smith, Craggs, et al. (1998)
	13	0	0	13	None	Birnbaum, Cohen, Bailey, et al. (1999)
	14	14	13	9	1—Colic, 1—hyperactive, 2—possible withdrawal	Kristensen, Ilett, Dusci, et al. (1998)
	46	39	25	42	None	Cohen et al. (2001)
Fluvoxamine	1	1	1	0	None	Wright, Dawling, & Ashford (1991)
	1	1	1	0	None	Yoshida, Smith, Craggs, et al. (1998)
	2	2	0	2	None	Piontek, Wisner, Perel, et al. (2001)
	4	2	0	4	None	Hendrick, Altshuler, Strouse, et al. (2000)
Nefazodone	2	0	2	0	None	Dodd (2001)

Drug				Adverse effects	Reference
Paroxetine	1	1	0	None	Spigset, Carleborg, Norstrom, et al. (1996)
	2	0	2	None	Birnbaum, Cohen, Bailey, et al. (1999)
	7	7	0	None	Ohman, Hagg, Carleborg, et al. (1999)
	16	14	16	None	Stowe, Cohen, Hostetter, et al. (2000)
	24	24	24	None	Misri, Kim, et al. (2000)
	16	16	16	None	Hendrick, Altshuler, Strouse, et al. (2000)
Sertraline	1	1	1	None	Altshuler, Cohen, et al. (1996)
	4	4	0	None	Epperson, Anderson, et al. (1997)
	8	0	8	None	Kristensen, Ilett, Dusci, et al. (1998)
	3	3	0	None	Mammen, Perel, Rudolph, et al. (1997)
	12	11	12	None	Stowe, Owens, Landry, et al. (1997)
	9	9	9	None; 1—high infant serum concentration[c]	Wisner, Perel, & Blumer (1998)
	3	0	3	None	Birnbaum, Cohen, Bailey, et al. (1999)
	10	10	10	None	Dodd (2001); Dodd, Stocky, Buist, et al. (2001)
	26	22	22	None, 1—high infant serum concentration[c]	Stowe, Hostetter, Owens, et al. (2001)
	30	29	30	None	Hendrick, Altshuler, Strouse, et al. (2000)
	14	13	11	None	Epperson, Czarkowski, Ward-O'Brien, et al. (2001)
Venlafaxine	3	3	3	None	Illett (1998)

[a] Total number of mother–infant nursing pairs that involved infant exposure to medication.

[b] Urine samples collected from 5 infants.

[c] High infant serum concentration defined as > 25% of maternal serum concentration.

TABLE 5.3. Risk–Benefit Assessment of Medication Use during Lactation

The postpartum period

- Over 60% of women plan to breastfeed during the puerperium.
- From 5% to 17% of all nursing women take a prescription medication during breastfeeding.
- From 12% to 20% of nursing women smoke cigarettes.
- Benefits of breastfeeding to infant: Support by all professional organizations as ideal form of nutrition for infants.
- The postnatal period is a high-risk time for onset/relapse of psychiatric illness.

Impact of illness

- Untreated maternal mental illness has an adverse impact on mother–infant attachment and later infant development.
- Laboratory and clinical data indicate that maternal separation has an adverse impact on offspring.

Impact of treatment

- All psychotropic medications studied to date are excreted in breast milk; therefore, the infant is always exposed to such medications.
- Adverse infant reports are limited to single-case reports (citalopram, fluoxetine, doxepin).
- Long-term effects of exposure to psychotropic medications through breastfeeding are unknown.

REFERENCES

Ahokas, A. J., Kaukoranta, J., Wahlbeck, K., et al. (2001). Estrogen deficiency in severe postpartum depression: Successful treatment with sublingual physiologic 17beta-estradiol: A preliminary study. *Journal of Clinical Psychiatry, 62*, 332–336.

Ahokas, A. J., Turtiainen, S., & Aito, M. (1998). Sublingual oestrogen treatment of postnatal depression. *Lancet, 351*, 109.

American Academy of Pediatrics, Committee on Nutrition. (1993). *Pediatric nutrition handbook* (3rd ed.). Elk Grove Village, IL: American Academy of Pediatrics.

American Psychiatric Association. (1968). *Diagnostic and statistical manual of mental disorders* (2nd ed.). Washington, DC: Author.

American Psychiatric Association. (1980). *Diagnostic and statistical manual of mental disorders* (3rd ed.). Washington, DC: Author.

American Psychiatric Association. (1994). *Diagnostic and statistical manual of mental disorders* (4th ed.). Washington, DC: Author.

Appleby, L., Warner, R., Whitton, A., et al. (1997). A controlled study of fluoxetine and cognitive-behavioural counselling in the treatment of postnatal depression. *British Medical Journal, 314*, 932–936.

Altshuler, L. L., Cohen, L., et al. (1996). Pharmacologic management of psychiatric illness in pregnancy: Dilemmas and guidelines. *American Journal of Psychiatry, 153*(5), 592–606.

Avant K. (1981). Anxiety as a potential factor affecting maternal attachment. *Journal of Obstetric, Gynecologic, and Neonatal Nursing, 10*, 416–419.

Bagedahl Strindlund, M. (1986). Peripartum mental illness: Timing of illness onset and its relation to symptoms and sociodemographic characteristics. *Acta Psychiatrica Scandinavica, 74*, 490–496.

Baum, A. L., & Misri, S. (1996). Selective serotonin-reuptake inhibitors in pregnancy and lactation. *Harvard Review of Psychiatry, 4*, 117–125.

Beardslee, W. R., Salt, P., Versage, E. M., et al. (1997). Sustained change in parents receiving preventive interventions for families with depression. *American Journal of Psychiatry, 154*, 510–555.

Beck, C. T. (1995). Screening methods for postpartum depression. *Journal of Obstetric, Gynecologic, and Neonatal Nursing, 24*, 308–312.

Begg, E. J., Duffull, S. B., Saunders, D. A., et al. (1999). Paroxetine in human milk. *British Journal of Clinical Pharmacology, 48,* 142–147.

Benvenuti, P., Cabras, P. L., Servi, P., et al. (1992). Puerperal psychoses: A clinical case study with follow-up. *Journal of Affective Disorders, 26,* 25–30.

Birnbaum, C. S., Cohen, L. S., Bailey, J. W., et al. (1999). Serum concentrations of antidepressants and benzodiazepines in nursing infants: A case series. *Pediatrics, 104,* 11.

Birnbaum, C. S., Cohen, L. S., Grush, L. R., et al. (1999). Serum concentrations of antidepressants and benzodiazepines in nursing infants: Implications for treatment. *Pediatrics, 140*(1), 1–6.

Bowlby, J. (1951). *Maternal care and mental health* (WHO Monograph Series No. 2). Geneva: World Health Organization.

Brandt, K. R., & Mackenzie, T. B. (1987). Obsessive–compulsive disorder exacerbated during pregnancy: A case report. *International Journal of Psychiatry in Medicine, 17,* 361–367.

Brazelton, T. B. (1975). Mother–infant reciprocity. In M. H. Klaus, T. Leger, & M. A. Trause (Eds.), *Maternal attachment and mothering disorders: A roundtable* (pp. 49–54). North Brunswick, NJ: Johnson & Johnson.

Brent, N., & Wisner, K. (1998). Fluoxetine and carbamazepine concentrations in a nursing mother–infant pair. *Clinical Pediatrics, 37,* 41–44.

Briggs, G. G., Freeman, R. K., & Yaffe, S. J. (1998). *Drugs in pregnancy and lactation* (5th ed.). Baltimore, MD: Williams & Wilkins.

Briggs, G. G., Samson, J. H., Ambrose, P. J., et al. (1993). Excretion of buproprion in breast milk. *Annual Pharmacotherapy, 27,* 431–433.

Brockington, I. F., Cernik, K. F., Schofield, E. M., et al. (1981). Puerperal psychosis: Phenomena and diagnosis. *Archives of General Psychiatry, 38,* 829–833.

Buist, A., Norman, T. R., & Dennerstein, L. (1990). Breastfeeding and the use of psychotropic medication: A review. *Journal of Affective Disorders, 19,* 197–206.

Burch, K. J., & Wells, B. G. (1992). Fluoxetine/norfluoxetine concentrations in human breast milk. *Pediatrics, 89,* 676–677.

Campbell, S. B., Cohn, J. F., Flanagan, C., et al. (1992). Course and correlates of postpartum depression during the transition to parenthood. *Development and Psychopathology, 4,* 29–47.

Campbell, S. B., Cohn, J. F., & Meyers, T. (1995). Depression in first-time mothers: Mother–infant interaction and depression chronicity. *Development and Psychopathology, 31,* 349–357.

Chambers, C. D., Anderson, P. O., Thomas, R. G., et al. (1999). Weight gain in infants breastfed by mothers who take fluoxetine. *Pediatrics, 104,* 5.

Cogill, S. R., Caplan, H. L., Alexandra, H., et al. (1986). Impact of maternal postnatal depression on cognitive development of young children. *British Medical Journal, 292,* 1165–1167.

Cohen, L. S., Sichel, D. A., Dimmock, J. A., et al. (1994a). Impact of pregnancy on panic disorder: A case series. *Journal of Clinical Psychiatry, 55*(7), 284–288.

Cohen, L. S., Sichel, D. A., Dimmock, J. A., et al. (1994b). Postpartum course in women with pre-existing panic disorder. *Journal of Clinical Psychiatry, 55*(7), 289–292.

Cohen, L. S., Sichel, D. A., Robertson, L. M., et al. (1995). Postpartum prophylaxis for women with bipolar disorder. *American Journal of Psychiatry, 152,* 1641–1645.

Cohen, L. S., Viguera, A. C., Collins, M. H., et al. (in press). Venlafaxine in the treatment of postpartum depression. *Biological Psychiatry.*

Condon, J. T., & Watson, T. L. (1987). The maternity blues: Exploration of a psychological hypothesis. *Acta Psychiatrica Scandinavica, 76,* 164–171.

Corral, M., Kuan, A., & Kostaras, D. (2000). Bright light therapy's effect on postpartum depression [Letter to the editor]. *American Journal of Psychiatry, 157,* 2.

Cox, J. L., Chapman, G., Murray, D., et al. (1996). Validation of the Edinburgh Postnatal Depression Scale (EPDS) in non-postnatal women. *Journal of Affective Disorders, 39,* 185–189.

Cox, J. L., Holden, J. M., & Sagovsky, R. (1987). Detection of postnatal depression. *British Journal of Psychiatry, 150,* 782–786.

Cradon, A. J. (1979). Maternal anxiety and neonatal wellbeing. *Journal of Psychosomatic Research, 23*, 113–115.

Cutrona, C. E., & Troutman, B. R. (1986). Social support, infant temperament, and parenting self-efficacy: A mediational model of postpartum depression. *Child Development, 57*, 1507–1518.

Dalton, K. (1985). Progesterone prophylaxis used successfully in postnatal depression. *Practitioner, 229*, 507–508.

Dodd, S. (2001). Sertraline in paired blood plasma and breast-milk samples from nursing mothers. *Human Pharmacology, 15*, 261–264.

Dodd, S., Maguire, K. P., Burrows, G. D., et al. (2000). Nefazadone in the breastmilk of nursing mothers: A report of two patients. *Journal of Clinical Psychopharmacology, 20*(6), 717–718.

Dodd, S., Stocky, A., Buist, A., et al. (2001). Sertraline analysis in the plasma of breast-fed infants. *Australian New Zealand Journal of Psychiatry, 35*(4), 545–546.

Doering, J., & Stewart, R. (1978). The extent and character of drug composition during pregnancy. *Journal of the American Medical Association, 239*, 843–846.

Duffy, C. L. (1983). Postpartum depression: Identifying women at risk. *Genesis, 11*, 21.

Epperson, C. N., Anderson, G. M., et al. (1997). Sertraline and breast-feeding (letter to the editor). *New England Journal of Medicine, 336*(16), 1189–1190.

Epperson, N., Czarkowski, K. A., Ward-O'Brien, D., et al. (2001). Maternal sertraline treatment and serotonin transport in breast-feeding mother–infant pairs. *American Journal of Psychiatry, 158*, 1631–1637.

Esquirol, E. (1845). *Des maladies mentales, considerées sous les rapports medical, hygienique et médico-legal*. Philadelphia: Lea & Blanchard.

Fields, T. (1990). Behavior-state matching and synchrony in mother–infant interactions of nondepressed versus depressed dyads. *Developmental Psychology, 26*, 7–14.

Fields, T., Healy, B., Goldstein, S., et al. (1988). Infants of depressed mothers show "depressed" behavior even with nondepressed adults. *Child Development, 59*, 1569–1579.

Fields, T., Healy, B., & LeBlanc, W. G. (1989). Sharing and synchrony of behavior states and heart rate in nondepressed versus depressed mother–infant interactions. *Infant Behavior and Development, 12*, 357–376.

Fleming, A. S., Klein, E., & Corter, C. (1992). The effects of a social support group on depression, maternal attitudes and behavior in new mothers. *Journal of Child Psychology and Psychiatry, 33*, 685–698.

George, A. J., & Wilson, K. C. (1981). Monoamine oxidase activity and the puerperal blues syndrome. *Journal of Psychosomatic Research, 25*, 409–413.

George, D. T., Ladenheim, J. A., & Nutt, D. J. (1987). Effect of pregnancy on panic attacks. *American Journal of Psychiatry, 144*, 1078–1079.

Glaze, R., & Cox, J. L. (1991). Validation of a computerised version of the 10-item (self-rating) Edinburgh Postnatal Depression Scale. *Journal of Affective Disorders, 22*(1–2), 73–77.

Gordon, R. E., & Gordon, K. K. (1960). Social factors in the prevention of postpartum emotion problems. *Obstetrics and Gynecology, 15*, 433–438.

Gotlib, I. H., Whiffen, V. E., Mount, J. H., et al. (1989). Prevalence rates and demographic characteristics associated with depression in pregnancy and postpartum. *Journal of Consulting and Clinical Psychology, 57*, 269–274.

Gotlib, I. H., Whiffen, V. E., Wallace, P. M., et al. (1991). Prospective investigation of postpartum depression: Factors involved in onset and recovery. *Journal of Abnormal Psychology, 100*, 122–132.

Graff, L. A., Syck, D. G., & Schallow, J. R. (1991). Predicting postpartum depressive symptoms: A structural modeling analysis. *Perceptual and Motor Skills, 73*, 1137–1138.

Gregoire, A. J. P., Henderson, A., Kumar, R., et al. (1994). A controlled trial of oestradiol therapy for postnatal depression. *Neuropsychopharmacology, 10*, 901S.

Gregoire, A. J. P., Kumar, R., Everitt, B., et al. (1996). Transdermal oestrogen for treatment of severe postnatal depression. *Lancet, 347,* 930–933.

Harlow, H. F., & Harlow, M. K. (1966). Social deprivation of monkeys. *Scientific American, 207,* 136–146.

Hendrick, V., Altshuler, L., Strouse, T., et al. (2000). Postpartum and nonpostpartum depression: Differences in presentation and response to pharmacologic treatment. *Depression and Anxiety, 11,* 66–72.

Holden, J. M., Sagovsky, R., & Cox, J. L. (1989). Counselling in a general practice setting: Controlled study of health visitor intervention in treatment of postnatal depression. *British Medical Journal, 298,* 223–226.

Hostetter, A. L., Baugh, C. L., & Stowe, Z. N. (1999). *Postpartum depression—Distinct entity or coincidence?* American Psychiatric Association Annual Meeting, Poster Abstract.

Illet, K., et al. (1998). Distribution and excretion of venlafaxine and O-desmethylvenlafaxine in human milk. *British Journal of Clinical Pharmacology, 45,* 459–462.

Isenberg, K. E. (1990). Excretion of fluoxetine in human breastmilk. *Journal of Clinical Psychiatry, 51*(4), 169.

Jansson, B. (1963). *Psychic insufficiencies associated with childbirth* (Suppl. 172, Vol. 39). Göteborg, Sweden: University Psychiatric Clinic.

Jensen, P., Oleson, O., Bertelson, A., et al. (1997). Citalopram and desmethylcitalopram concentrations in breast milk and in serum of mother and infant. *Therapy Drug Monitoring, 19,* 236–239.

Kendell, R. E., Chalmers, J. C., & Platz, C. (1987). Epidemiology of puerperal psychosis. *British Journal of Psychiatry, 150,* 662–673.

Kennerley, H., & Gath, D. (1989). Maternity blues: Associations with obstetric, psychological, and psychiatric factors. *British Journal of Psychiatry, 155,* 367–373.

Kessler, R. C., McGonagle, K. A., Zhao, S., et al. (1994). Lifetime and 12 month prevalence of DSM-III-R psychiatric disorders in the United States. *Archives of General Psychiatry, 51,* 8–19.

Klein, D. F., Skrobala, A. M., & Garfinkel, R. S. (1995). Preliminary look at the effects of pregnancy on the course of panic disorder. *Anxiety, 1,* 227–232.

Klosko, J. S., Barlow, D. H., Tassinari, R. B., et al. (1990). A comparison of alprazolam and cognitive behavior therapy in the treatment of panic disorder. *Journal of Consulting and Clinical Psychology, 58,* 77–84.

Knopps, G. G. (1993). Postpartum mood disorders: A startling contrast to the joy of birth. *Postgraduate Medicine, 93,* 103–116.

Kristensen, J. H., Ilett, K. F., Dusci, L. J., et al. (1998). Distribution and excretion of sertraline and N-desmethylsertraline in human milk. *British Journal of Clinical Pharmacology, 45,* 453–457.

Lester, B. M., Cucca, J., Andreozzi, L., et al. (1993). Possible association between fluoxetine hydrochloride and colic in an infant. *Journal of the American Academy of Child and Adolescent Psychiatry, 32*(6), 1253–1255.

Llewellyn, A., & Stowe, Z. N. (1998). Invited review: Psychotropic medications during lactation. *Journal of Clinical Psychiatry, 59*(Suppl. 2), 41–52.

Mammen, O. K., Perel, J. M., Rudolph, G., et al. (1997). Sertraline and norsertraline levels in three breastfed infants. *Journal of Clinical Psychiatry, 58*(3), 100–103.

Mandl, K., Tronick, E. Z., Brennan, T. A., et al. (1999). Infant health care use and maternal depression. *Archives of Pediatriatrics and Adolescent Medicine, 153,* 808–813.

Marcé, L. V. (1958). *Traite de la folie des femmes enceintes, des nouvelles accouchées et des norrices, et considerations médico-legales qui se rattachent a ce sujet.* Paris: Baillière.

Marks, M. N., Wieck, A., Checkley, S. A., et al. (1992). Contribution of psychological and social factors to psychotic and non-psychotic relapse after childbirth in women with previous histories of affective disorder. *Journal of Affective Disorders, 29,* 253–263.

Matthew, K., Scott, H. F., Wilkinson, L. S., et al. (1996). Retarded acquisition and reduced expression of conditional locomotor activity in adult rats following repeated early maternal separation: Effects of prefeeding, D-amphetamine, dopamine antagonists, and clonidine. *Psychopharmacology, 26,* 75–84.

McEwen, B. S., Gould, E. A., & Sakai, R. R. (1992). The vulnerability of the hippocampus to protective and destructive effects of glucocorticoids in relation to stress. *British Journal of Psychiatry, 15,* 18–23.

McGorry, P., & Connell, S. (1990). The nosology and prognosis of puerperal psychosis: A review. *Comprehensive Psychiatry, 31,* 519–534.

Metz, A., Sichel, D. A., & Goff, D. C. (1988). Postpartum panic disorder. *Journal of Clinical Psychiatry, 49,* 278–279.

Misri, S., Kim, J., et al. (2000). Paroxetine levels in postpartum depressed women, breastmilk and infant serum. *Journal of Clinical Psychiatry, 61*(11), 828–832.

Misri, S., Sinclair, D. A., & Kuan, A. J. (1997). Breast-feeding and postpartum depression: Is there a relationship? *Canadian Journal of Psychiatry, 42,* 1061–1065.

Misri, S., & Sivertz, K. (1991). Tricyclic drugs in pregnancy and lactation: A preliminary report. *International Journal of Psychiatry Medicine, 21,* 157–171.

Mortola, J. F. (1989). The use of psychotropic agents in pregnancy and lactation. *Psychiatric Clinics of North America, 12,* 69–87.

Murray, D. (1996). Oestrogen and postnatal depression. *Lancet, 347,* 918–919.

Murray, L. (1992). The impact of postnatal depression on infant development. *Journal of Child Psychology and Psychiatry, 33,* 543–561.

Murray, L., & Cooper, P. J. (1996). The impact of postpartum depression on child development. *International Review of Psychiatry, 8,* 55–63.

Murray, L., & Cooper, P. J. (1997). Postpartum depression and child development. *Psychological Medicine, 27,* 253–260.

Murray, L., Fiori-Cowley, A., & Hooper, R. (1996). The impact of postnatal depression and associated adversity on early mother–infant interactions and later infant outcome. *Child Development, 67,* 2512–2526.

Neziroglu, F., Anemone, R., & Yaryura-Tobias, J. A. (1992). Onset of obsessive–compulsive disorders in pregnancy. *American Journal of Psychiatry, 149,* 947–950.

O'Hara, M. W. (1986). Social support, life events and depression during pregnancy and the puerperium. *Archives of General Psychiatry, 43,* 569–573.

O'Hara, M. W. (1991). Postpartum mental disorders. In N. Droegemueller & J. Sciarra (Eds.), *Gynecology and obstetrics* (Vol. 6, pp. 1–13). Philadelphia: Lippincott.

O'Hara, M. W. (1994). *Psychosocial therapies in the postpartum period.* Paper presented at Workshop on Mental Disorders during Pregnancy and Postpartum, National Institute of Mental Health, Bethesda, MD.

O'Hara, M. W., Schlechte, J. A., Lewis, D. A., et al. (1991a). Controlled prospective study of postpartum mood disorders: Psychological, environmental, and hormonal variables. *Journal of Abnormal Psychology, 100,* 63–73.

O'Hara, M. W., Schlechte, J. A., Lewis, D. A., et al. (1991b). Prospective study of postpartum blues: Biologic and psychosocial factors. *Archives of General Psychiatry, 48,* 801–806.

O'Hara, M. W., Stuart, S., Gorman, L. L., et al. (2000). Efficacy of interpersonal psychotherapy for postpartum depression. *Archives of General Psychiatry, 57,* 1039–1045.

Ohman, R., Hagg, S., Carleborg, L., et al. (1999). Excretion of paroxetine into breastmilk. *Journal of Clinical Psychiatry, 60*(8), 519–523.

Parry, B. L., & Hamilton, J. A. (1999). Postpartum psychiatric syndromes. In S. C. Risch & D. S. Janowsky (Eds.), *The art of psychopharmacology.* New York: Guilford Press.

Pedersen, C. A., Stern, R. A., Pate, J., et al. (1993). Thyroid and adrenal measures during late pregnancy and the puerperium in women who have been major depressed or who become dysphoric postpartum. *Journal of Affective Disorders, 29,* 201–211.

Piontek, C. M., Wisner, K. L., Perel, J. M., et al. (2001). Serum fluvoxamine levels in breastfed infants. *Journal of Clinical Psychiatry, 62,* 111–113.

Pitt, B. (1968). "Atypical" depression following childbirth. *British Journal of Psychiatry, 114,* 1325–1335.

Platz, C., & Kendell, R. E. (1988). A matched-control follow-up and family study of 'puerperal' psychoses. *British Journal of Psychiatry, 153,* 90–94.

Playfair, H. R., & Gowers, J. I. (1981). Depression following childbirth—A search for predictive signs. *Journal of the Royal College of General Practitioners, 31,* 201–208.

Plotsky, P. M., & Meaney, M. J. (1993). Early, postnatal experience alters hypothalamic corticotropin-releasing factor (CRF) mRNA, median eminence CRF content and stress-induced release in adult rats. *Brain Research: Molecular Brain Research, 18,* 195–200.

Rampono, J., Kristensen, J. H., Hackett, L. P., et al. (2000). Citalopram and demethylcitalopram in human milk; distribution, excretion, and effects in breast fed infants. *British Journal of Clinical Pharmacology, 50*(3), 263–268.

Raskin, V. D., & Kleinman, K. R. (1994). *This isn't what I expected: Overcoming postpartum depression.* New York: Bantam Doubleday Dell Publishing Group, Inc.

Richards, J. P. (1990). Postnatal depression: A review of recent literature. *British Journal of General Practice, 40,* 472–476.

Righetti-Veltema, M., Conne-Perreard, E., Bousquet, A., et al. (1998). Risk factors and predictive signs of postpartum depression. *Journal of Affective Disorders, 49,* 167–180.

Robinson, G. E., Stewart, D. E., & Flak, E. (1986). The rational use of psychotropic drugs in pregnancy and postpartum. *Canadian Journal of Psychiatry, 31,* 183–190.

Robinson, L., Walker, J. R., & Anderson, D. (1992). Cognitive-behavioral treatment of panic disorder during pregnancy and lactation. *Canadian Journal of Psychiatry, 37,* 623–626.

Roy, A., Cole, K., Goldman, Z., et al. (1993). Fluoxetine treatment of postpartum depression. *American Journal of Psychiatry, 150,* 8.

Schmidt, H. J. (1943). The use of progesterone in the treatment of postpartum psychosis. *Journal of the American Medical Association, 121,* 190–193.

Schmidt, K., Olesen, O. V., & Jensen, P. N. (2000). Citalopram and breast feeding: Serum concentration and side effects in the infant. *Biological Psychiatry, 47,* 164–165.

Schopf, J., & Rust, B. (1994). Follow-up and family study of postpartum psychoses. *European Archives of Psychiatry and Clinical Neuroscience, 244,* 101–111.

Seguin, L., Potvin, L., St-Denis, M., et al. (1999). Depressive symptoms in the late postpartum among low socioeconomic status women. *Birth, 26*(3), 157–163.

Sichel, D. A., Cohen, L. S., Robertson, L. M., et al. (1995). Prophylactic estrogen in recurrent postpartum affective disorder. *Biological Psychiatry, 38,* 814–818.

Spigset, O., Carleborg, B., & Korstrom, A., et al. (1996). Paroxetine level in breastmilk. *Journal of Clinical Psychiatry, 57*(1), 39.

Statham, A. (1998). Current evidence from animal investigations of a role for early mother–infant relationships in the aetiology of major depressive illness. *Neurosciences in Psychiatry, 1,* 40–44.

Steinberg, S. I., & Bellavance, F. (1999). Characteristics and treatment of women with antenatal and postpartum depression. *International Journal of Psychiatry in Medicine, 29*(2), 209–233.

Stewart, D. E., Klompenhouwer, J. L., Kendall, R. E., et al. (1991). Prophylactic lithium in postpartum affective psychosis: The experience of three centers. *British Journal of Psychiatry, 158,* 393–397.

Stowe, Z. N., Casarella, J., Landry, J., et al. (1995). Sertraline in the treatment of women with postpartum major depression. *Depression, 3,* 49–55.

Stowe, Z. N., Cohen, L. S., Hostetter, A., et al. (2000). Paroxetine in human breast milk and nursing infants. *American Journal of Psychiatry, 157*(2), 185–190.

Stowe, Z. N., Hostetter, A., Owens, M. J., et al. (2001). *The pharmacokinetics of sertraline excretion in human breast milk: Determinants of infant serum concentrations.* Manuscript submitted for publication.

Stowe, Z. N., & Nemeroff, C. B. (1995). Women at risk for postpartum-onset major depression. *American Journal of Obstetrics and Gynecology, 173,* 639–645.

Stowe, Z. N., Owens, M. J., Landry, J. C., et al. (1997). Sertraline desmethylsertraline in human breast milk and nursing infants. *American Journal of Psychiatry, 154*(9), 1255–1260.

Stowe, Z. N., Strader, J. R., & Nemeroff, C. B. (1998). Psychopharmacology during pregnancy and lactation. In A. F. Schatzberg & C. B. Nemeroff (Eds.), *APA textbook of psychopharmacology* (pp. 979–996). Washington, DC: American Psychiatric Press.

Stowe, Z. N., Tang, Z., & Plotsky, P. M. (1998b). *Impact of neonatal stress on neuronal activity.* American Psychiatric Association Annual Meeting, Poster Abstract.

Strader, R., Llewellyn, A., Stowe, Z. N., et al. (1997). *Predictors of treatment response in postpartum depression.* American Psychiatric Association Annual Meeting, Young Investigator Slide Presentation—Abstract.

Stuart, S., & O'Hara, M. W. (1994). Interpersonal psychotherapy for postpartum depression: A treatment program. *Journal of Psychotherapy Practice Research, 4,* 18–29.

Sutanto, W., Rosenfeld, P., de Kloet, E. R., et al. (1996). Long-term effects of neonatal maternal deprivation and ACTH on hippocampal mineralocorticoid and glucocorticoid receptors. *Developmental Brain Research, 92,* 156–163.

Taddio, A., Ito, S., & Koren, G. (1996). Excretion of fluoxetine and its metabolite, norfluoxetine, in human breastmilk. *Journal of Clinical Pharmacology, 36,* 42–47.

Teti, D. M., Messinger, D. S., Gelfand, D. M., et al. (1995). Maternal depression and the quality of early attachment: An examination of infants, preschoolers, and their mothers. *Developmental Psychology, 31,* 364–376.

Troutman, B., & Cutrona, C. (1990). Nonpsychotic postpartum depression among adolescent mothers. *Journal of Abnormal Psychology, 99,* 69.

Unterman, R. R., Posner, N. A., & Williams, K. N. (1990). Postpartum depressive disorders: Changing trends. *Birth, 17*(3), 131–137.

Videbech, P., & Gouliaev, G. (1995). First admission with puerperal psychosis: 7–14 years of follow up. *Acta Psychiatrica Scandinavica, 91,* 167–173.

Weissman, M. M., & Olfson, M. (1995). Depression in women: Implications for health care research. *Science, 269,* 799–801.

Whiffen, V. E., & Gotlib, I. H. (1989). Infants of postpartum depressed mothers: Temperament and cognitive status. *Journal of Abnormal Psychology, 98,* 274–279.

Wickberg, B., & Hwang, C. P. (1996). Counseling of postnatal depression: A controlled study on a population based Swedish sample. *Journal of Affective Disorders, 39,* 209–216.

Williams, K. E., & Koran, L. M. (1997). Obsessive–compulsive disorder in pregnancy, the puerperium, and the premenstrum. *Journal of Clinical Psychiatry, 58,* 330–334.

Wisner, K. L. (1999). *Prevention and treatment of postpartum mood disorders.* Paper presented at the American Psychiatric Association Annual Meeting.

Wisner, K. L., Peindl, K. S., et al. (1999). Obsessions and compulsions in women with postpartum depression. *Journal of Clinical Psychiatry, 60*(3), 176–180.

Wisner, K. L., & Perel, J. M. (1988). Psychopharmacologic agents and electroconvulsive therapy during pregnancy and the puerperium. In R. L. Coehn (Ed.), *Psychiatric consultation in childbirth settings: Parent- and child-oriented approaches.* New York: Plenum Press.

Wisner, K. L., & Perel, J. M. (1991). Serum nortriptyline levels in nursing mothers and their infants. *American Journal of Psychiatry, 149,* 1234–1236.

Wisner, K. L., Perel, J. M., & Blumer, J. (1998). Serum sertraline and N-desmethylsertraline levels in breast-feeding mother–infant pairs. *American Journal of Psychiatry, 155*, 690–692.

Wisner, K. L., Perel, J. M., & Findling, R. L. (1996). Antidepressant treatment during breastfeeding. *American Journal of Psychiatry, 153*, 1132–1137.

Wisner, K. L., Perel, J. M., Peindl, K. S., et al. (2001). Prevention of recurrent postpartum depression: A randomized clinical trial. *Journal of Clinical Psychiatry, 62*, 82–86.

Wisner, K. L., & Stowe, Z. N. (1997). Psychobiology of postpartum mood disorders. *Seminars in Reproductive Endocrinology, 15*, 77–89.

Wisner, K. L., & Wheeler, S. B. (1994). Prevention of recurrent postpartum major depression. *Hospital and Community Psychiatry, 45*, 1191–1196.

Wolkind, S., Zajicek, E., & Ghodsian, J. (1990). Continuities in maternal depression. *International Journal of Family Psychiatry, 99*, 69.

Wolman, W., Chalmers, B., Hofmeyr, G. J., et al. (1993). Postpartum depression and companionship in the clinical birth environment: A randomized, controlled study. *American Journal of Obstetrics and Gynecology, 168*, 1388–1393.

Wright, S., Dawling, S., & Ashford, J. J. (1991). Excretion of fluvoxamine in breast milk. *British Journal of Clinical Pharmacology, 31*, 209.

Yoshida, K., Smith, Craggs, M., et al. (1998). Fluoxetine in breastmilk and developmental outcome of breastfed infants. *British Journal of Psychiatry, 172*, 175–179.

Zahn-Waxler, C., Cummings, E. M., Lonoff, R. J., et al. (1984). Young offspring of depressed patients: A population of risk for affective problems and childhood depression. In D. Cicchetti & Schneider-Rosen (Eds.), *Childhood depression* (pp. 81–105). San Francisco: Jossey-Bass.

Zilboorg, G. (1943). *Mind, medicine, and man.* New York: Harcourt, Brace.

6

Psychiatric Aspects
of Hormonal Contraception

JULIA K. WARNOCK
CHRISTINE F. BLAKE

Modern contraception is a 20th century development that has contributed enormously to women's quality of life by relieving them of the burden of consecutive pregnancies (Huezo, 1998). Roughly one-fourth of sexually active, fertile women in the United States use oral contraceptives because they provide the most effective reversible pregnancy prevention available. Most of the oral contraceptive formulations are combinations of an estrogen and a progestin, although progestin-only products are available. In this chapter, the term "oral contraceptive pill" (OCP) is used to refer to the combination oral contraceptive preparations containing ethinyl estradiol (EE) as the estrogen component, and one of the 19-nortestosterones as the progestin component.

Over the past 40 years, the formulations of OCPs have changed significantly. Burkman and Schulman (1998) note that prior to 1992, OCPs in the United States contained either EE or mestranol (3-methylether of EE). Since then, low-dose OCPs, formulations containing less than 50 µg of EE, have become standard. The low-androgenic progestins, norgestimate and desogestrel, were also introduced in 1992. The OCPs with these progestin formulations have significantly less adverse androgenic effects. The mechanism of action of OCPs is primarily inhibition of ovulation via negative feedback on the hypothalamic–pituitary axis. The progestin component of the OCP is what contributes to the suppression of pituitary gonadotropin secretion and causes changes in the cervical mucus and in the endometrium that inhibit implantation. The estrogen portion of the OCP maintains the endometrium, prevents breakthrough bleeding, and acts synergistically with the progestin to inhibit the pituitary (Burkman & Schulman, 1998).

COMBINATION HORMONAL CONTRACEPTIVES

The process of choosing the right contraceptive method for any woman involves finding the right balance among the multiple issues of efficacy, safety, availability, cost, reversibility, compliance issues, and personal and partner acceptability. Before a woman can decide on a hormonal method of contraception, she must be informed of the common side effects of each of the methods. In the United States, hormonal contraceptive methods include pills (combination estrogen–progesterone and progesterone only), injectables (Depo Provera), and implantables (Norplant). Other forms of injectables, patches, and vaginal rings for contraception are currently under development and investigation.

Efficacy of OCPs

Failure rates for contraceptive methods are usually expressed as number of pregnancies with use of a method for 1 year among 100 women ("woman-years"). In general, for women using no method of contraception who are sexually active for 1 year, approximately 85 of 100 will conceive. Estimates of the efficacy of OCPs may be expressed as either method (perfect use) rates or actual use rates. Because of this, failure rates range from less than 1/100 woman-years in very compliant women up to 15/100 woman-years in adolescents. Most authorities estimate average combination OCP failure rates to be 3–8/100 woman-years.

Side Effects of OCPs

Up to half of women who initiate OCPs for contraception discontinue use within the first year, secondary to side effects such as breakthrough bleeding, headache, nausea, weight gain, and amenorrhea (Thorneycroft, 1999). The single most common reason for discontinuation is breakthrough bleeding. In general, breakthrough, or intermenstrual, bleeding occurs in approximately 25% of women during the first 3 months of OCP usage and becomes progressively less common thereafter (American College of Obstetricians and Gynecologists [ACOG], 1994). OCP formulations containing phasic (or the lower, 20-μg) doses of EE are associated with somewhat higher rates of breakthrough bleeding than monophasic (30- to 35-μg formulations. The problem of breakthrough bleeding may be addressed by either adding estrogen supplementation for several days or changing to a higher-estrogen-dose OCP.

Androgenicity of Progestins

Much has been published in recent years on the new third-generation progestins (desogestrel, gestodene, and norgestimate), which are derived from levonorgestrel, and the diminished androgenic potential of these formulations as compared to previous progestins. Careful review of the available data shows that the progestins in the current OCPs in the United States have no clinically significant virilizing effects. In addition, the androgenic effects are not consistent from person to person (Thorneycroft, 1999). Although only one pill formulation currently has a U.S. Food and Drug Administration (FDA) indication for the treatment of acne, for the most part all combination OCPs are antiandrogenic, in that they suppress endogenous production of ovarian androgens and decrease free testosterone by increasing sex-hormone-binding globulin (Van der Vange et al., 1990). Thus most patients will have improvement in acne on OCPs. However, about 3–5% of women on OCPs will experience worsening or new-onset acne.

Cardiovascular Risk

The risk of venous thromboembolism (VTE) is decreased with pills containing 35 µg of EE as compared to the 50-µg pills. Among nonsmokers without other significant risk factors for cardiovascular disease, use of 30- to 35-µg pills is not associated with an excess risk of myocardial infarction or stroke. Although in theory the use of 20-µg pills might be associated with an additional reduction in risk, there is thus far no direct scientific evidence to support this conclusion (Kaunitz, 1998).

Breast Cancer Risk

The Collaborative Group on Hormonal Factors in Breast Cancer (1996) has published a reanalysis of the available data addressing the possible association between OCP use and an increased risk of breast cancer. In this review of 54 studies, the overall risk of breast cancer was not increased by OCP use occurring 10–20 years previously. A slightly increased risk was noted in women who were current users, with a relative risk of 1.24 (95% confidence interval = 1.15–1.33), and in women who had used OCPs within the last 1–4 years, with a relative risk of 1.16 (95% confidence interval = 1.08–1.23). The evidence analyzed implied that while there was a small increase in risk of diagnosis, there was also a trend toward earlier detection in users of OCPs. Thus the authors speculated that the excess risk may be in part due to an early detection bias.

Noncontraceptive Benefits of OCPs

Although the risks of OCPs are generally widely known, women are not as well informed of the health benefits associated with their use (Peipert & Gutmann, 1993). There is strong evidence that the health benefits of OCPs clearly outweigh the risks, especially with current pill formulations. In particular, for women who are healthy and do not smoke, an extensive list of health benefits continues to emerge (Grimes & Wallach, 1997).

Bone Density

It has long been established that estrogen replacement therapy in postmenopausal women is an important factor in the prevention of osteoporosis. A review by DeCherney (1996) evaluates the data regarding OCPs in premenopausal women as a protective factor against bone loss. Eight of 12 published research papers indicate that women using OCPs have greater bone mass than nonusers. Evidence also demonstrates an increasing protective effect of OCPs with longer duration of use. In particular, women who reported greater than 10 years of OCP use were afforded the greatest bone mineral density protection (Kleerekoper et al., 1991).

Ovarian Cancer

Approximately 26,000 women in the United States are diagnosed with ovarian cancer each year. The disease is often fatal because it typically remains asymptomatic until Stage III or IV. It is well established that OCPs protect against ovarian cancer. After 4 years of OCP use, the risk is reduced by about 40%, and the risk may be reduced by as much as 60–80% after 10–12 years of use (Hankinson et al., 1992; Cancer and Steroid Hormone Study of the Centers for Disease Control, etc., 1987).

Endometrial Cancer

Endometrial cancer is the most common gynecological cancer, with about 34,000 U.S. women receiving new diagnoses each year (American Cancer Society, 1996). Fortunately, the cumulative evidence strongly suggests that OCPs provide duration-dependent protection against endometrial cancer (Schlesselman, 1984). It appears that the decline in risk persists for at least 15 years after OCP discontinuation (Cancer and Steroid Hormone Study, 1987), which is important in light of the fact that most endometrial cancers occur in women after 50 years of age. It is speculated that the mechanism of the effect of OCPs on the endometrium is mediated by the progestin. Thus protection may vary by OCP formulation, with larger amounts of progestin offering the greatest protective benefit (Grimes & Wallach, 1997).

Ectopic Pregnancy and Salpingitis

OCPs offer a woman protection against ectopic pregnancy and the associated mortality and morbidity. In addition, woman taking OCPs are afforded less risk for salpingitis— possibly because of OCP related changes in cervical mucus, which becomes viscous and thick, and thus less penetrable to infectious organisms (Grimes & Wallach, 1997). Over 250,000 women per year develop serious sequelae of these disorders, including tubal damage, chronic pelvic pain, and infertility. One study indicates that women using OCPs with no history of salpingitis have a 50% lower risk of being hospitalized with the disease than nonusers (Peterson & Lee, 1989).

Other Benefits

Other important health benefits of OCP use include a reduction in the incidence of fibroadenomous and fibrocystic disease, as well as a decrease in menstrual blood loss, acne, and dysmenorrhea. Other possible benefits of OCP usage include less risk of colorectal cancer, uterine fibroids, toxic shock syndrome, and rheumatoid arthritis (Grimes & Wallach, 1997).

Contraindications

In general, contraceptive doses of estrogen are contraindicated in the following groups of women: women over age 35 who smoke, women with uncontrolled hypertension, women with coronary artery disease, women at increased risk of VTE, women with diabetes and macrovascular disease, women with active liver disease, women with history of classic migraine with neurological symptoms, and women with a personal history of estrogen-dependent cancer.

PROGESTIN-ONLY HORMONAL CONTRACEPTIVES

Depot Medroxyprogesterone Acetate

Depot medroxyprogesterone acetate (Depo Provera; abbreviated DMPA) is the only injectable form of hormonal contraception currently available in the United States. Despite the fact that it was not approved by the FDA until October 1992, substantial data on the safety and efficacy of this drug exist, as it has been used widely elsewhere in the world for over 25 years. DMPA is an aqueous suspension of microcrystals resulting in pharmacologically active systemic levels for 3–4 months after injection of the 150-mg dose. Ovulation will not occur for 14 weeks, and as the recommendation is for injections every 12 weeks, there is a 2-week grace period for repeat injections. Ideally, DMPA should be given within 5 days of the onset of menses, to ensure prevention of ovulation the first month. In addition, the clinician should determine that the patient is not pregnant when an injection is given.

Similar to birth control pills, the high level of progesterone suppresses gonadotropin secretion, inhibits ovulation, and also creates a viscous cervical mucus that hinders passage of sperm. The major advantage of this method of contraception is the decreased compliance responsibilities compared to OCPs or to coitus-related forms of contraception. The lack of an estrogen component also makes this method a good choice for women with contraindications to estrogen, such as those patients with a history of VTE.

Efficacy of DMPA

Because there is essentially no user influence on efficacy, failure rates are quite low, ranging from 0 to 0.7/100 woman-years. The typical failure rate is about 0.3/100 woman-years.

Side Effects of DMPA

Common side effects of DMPA include breakthrough bleeding, headaches, bloating, and mood changes. The most common side effect is unpredictable bleeding or spotting, which may last 7 or more days per month with initial injections. With additional injections, the frequency of irregular bleeding decreases. By 1 year, one-half of women on DMPA will be amenorrheic. For some women, amenorrhea is a welcome side effect; for others, it causes ongoing anxiety about the possibility of contraceptive failure and pregnancy. As with OCPs, troublesome irregular bleeding can be treated with oral estrogen supplementation, but the symptom will often recur when supplementation is discontinued. DMPA may also significantly decrease estradiol levels, which in some studies have resulted in decreased bone density levels in chronic users, though no increased risk of fractures or osteoporosis has been demonstrated (Cundy et al., 1991).

Cosmetic side effects associated with DMPA may include worsening of acne in some women, as well as bloating and weight gain. Patients can be reassured that in general, weight gain is only 3–6 pounds, if it occurs. In addition, some women will experience increased hair loss consistent with the telogen effluvium seen after pregnancy. One potentially significant side effect is that ovulation may be inhibited for 1 year or more after a single injection of DMPA. For this reason, DMPA is not considered a readily reversible form of contraception.

Benefits of DMPA

Use of DMPA may decrease the risk of pelvic inflammatory disease, reduce menstrual blood loss, and cause improvement in anemia. This potential for decreased menstrual blood loss may be an advantage in women with chronic illnesses such as sickle cell anemia or end-stage renal disease. The World Health Organization examined the effects of DMPA use in multiple large case–control studies and found an even greater reduction of risk for endometrial cancer than that of OCPs, as well as a lack of evidence to demonstrate any increase in breast, ovarian, or cervical cancers (ACOG, 1994).

Contraindications

In general, the majority of contraindications to combination OCPs are due to the estrogen component and thus do not apply to DMPA. There is limited data to suggest that DMPA is safe in women at risk for VTE and in women with active liver disease. Since the medication is administered intramuscularly, its use in women on full anticoagulation is controversial.

Norplant

Norplant is a long-acting subdermal implant system that releases a continuous dose of levonorgestrel, a synthetic progestin that inhibits ovulation and protects from pregnancy through the formation of hostile cervical mucus and impaired oocyte maturation for up to 5 years. As with DMPA, failure rates are quite low, at 0.8/100 users over 5 years. The failure rates do rise slightly over time to 2/100 woman-years by the 6th year (ACOG, 1994).

The health benefits for Norplant are not well established at this time. The common side effects of Norplant use include headache and breakthrough bleeding. Norplant may result in irregular bleeding in many women using it, with approximately one-third experiencing regular cycles. There are case reports of idiopathic intracranial hypertension; therefore, while a woman is on Norplant, any change in pattern of or new onset of headache should be evaluated. Though occurring less commonly than with DMPA, cosmetic problems with acne or hair loss may occur. Unlike those of DMPA, the contraceptive effects of Norplant are readily reversible with removal of the implants, and the medication is usually cleared from the system within several days of removal.

Progestin-Only Pills

Whereas combination OCPs are used by up to 26% of women in the United States, progestin-only pills (POPs) are used by only 1% (Kaunitz, 1997). There are currently two formulations approved for use in the United States, one containing 0.35 mg norethindrome (Micronor) and one containing 0.075 mg norgestrel (Ovrette). POPs are taken continuously and have active hormone in all 28 pills in a cycle pack. Mechanisms of action include blunting of the midcycle luteinizing hormone surge and creation of viscous cervical mucus. Because of the relatively short half-life of these pills, it is critical to take them at exactly the same time each day. If a user is more than 3 hours late, or forgets a pill altogether, normal use should be resumed and backup contraception used for at least 48 hours. Estimates of efficacy are primarily from data in women less likely to ovulate (lactating and older women); they suggest that failure rates are about 1/100 women per year, but may be as high as 10 per 100 woman-years.

Side effects are similar to those of Norplant, with approximately half of users experiencing irregular bleeding episodes. Other effects are rare. The rate of ectopic pregnancy among POP failures is as high as 10%, but the overall risk is still less than with no contraception.

POPs may be helpful in providing contraception for women who are breastfeeding, smokers older than age 35, women with vascular disease, complicated migraine patients, or patients at increased risk of thromboembolic disease (Kaunitz, 1997). POPs should not be used by women taking hepatic-enzyme-inducing drugs, as efficacy of the contraceptive will be reduced.

Thus far, there is not sufficient evidence to document reduction in ovarian or breast cancer with the use of POPs. However, the limited available data imply no increased risk, as well as a decreased risk of endometrial cancer.

EMERGENCY CONTRACEPTION

"Emergency contraception" refers to contraceptive methods that may be utilized after intercourse to prevent pregnancy. Two of three methods available include "morning-after pills" and the insertion of a copper IUD. The "morning-after pill" or Yuzpe method consists of the ingestion of a total of 200 μg of EE and 1.0 mg of levonorgestrel in a 12-hour time period within 72 hours of unprotected intercourse. This regimen is easily achieved with the use of four Ovral tablets, or eight Lo-Ovral, Tri-Levlen, Nordette, or Triphasil tablets. Half the dose is taken within 72 hours of unprotected intercourse, and the second half 12 hours later. One product specifically designed for this use has been marketed. The product, Preven, includes the four 50-μg EE/0.25-mg levonorgestrel tablets, as well as a pregnancy test to exclude previously existing pregnancy prior to usage. Commonly reported side effects are nausea and vomiting, which occur in 15–30% of women and may last up to 48 hours. This method can reduce the risk of unwanted pregnancy by up to 75% after unprotected intercourse (Dull & Blythe, 1998). The same contraindications as those for OCPs should be considered in emergency contraception. The FDA has recently approved the first POP for prevention of pregnancy after a contraceptive accident or unprotected sex. The product, called Plan B, consists of two 0.75-mg tablets of levonorgestrel. Again, women take the first pill within 72 hours after sex and take the second pill 12 hours after the first pill. There are reports of less nausea and vomiting. Adverse effects of Plan B include abdominal pain, fatigue, and headaches.

SPECIAL POPULATIONS

Adolescents

An estimated 1 million teen pregnancies occur in the United States each year, and approximately 82% of these are unintended (Dull & Blythe, 1998). Because of the significant emotional social and medical costs associated with teen pregnancy, prevention or reduction could provide significant societal benefit.

Contraceptive counseling techniques for adolescents must not only provide the appropriate patient education concerning various contraceptive methods, but also actively seek to dispel misinformation and myths surrounding their use. In addition, intensive counseling regarding protection from sexually transmitted diseases is of paramount importance in this population. Accessibility and cost are common barriers to the acquisition and continuation of use of contraception among adolescents. Thus a respectful, open discussion, which includes the financial options and assistance available in the local community, is necessary to increase adolescent compliance.

Compliance with coitus-related contraceptive methods will typically be lower among adolescents than with older women. Pregnancy rates in 15- to 19-year-old adolescents using only barrier methods were 13–27% after 1 year (Dull & Blythe, 1998). For an adolescent population, use of a reliable hormonal method for contraception and a barrier method such as condoms with or without spermicide is optimal for pregnancy prevention and protection from sexually transmitted diseases.

OCPs are the most popular contraceptive method among adolescents in the United States. Careful counseling regarding potential side effects and instructions regarding missed pills are critical to optimizing compliance and minimizing discontinuation (Stevens-Simon, 1998). Adolescents have higher method failure rates than adults do. The OCP usage failure rates in adolescents may be as high as 6–13/100 woman-years (Dull & Blythe, 1998).

The cosmetic consequences of OCP usage are of interest to adolescents. Although many OCP formulations reduce acne in a majority of patients, currently the only formulation with an FDA indication for acne treatment is Ortho Tri-Cyclen. In addition, the issue of the potential for weight gain must be directly addressed to provide accurate information and dispel fears and concerns that may create barriers to utilization.

For some adolescents, DMPA and/or Norplant may be viable contraceptive options. As with any patients, but particularly with adolescents, sensitive counseling regarding the benefits and the side effects of DMPA and Norplant are crucial to maximizing compliance. Finally, the adolescent population should be targeted for education about emergency contraceptive options and the ideal time frame for implementation. Given the high rates of noncompliance and method failure in this population, it is critically important that if a teen perceives an acute event placing her at increased risk of conception, she is aware of all her options to try to prevent an unwanted pregnancy.

Perimenopausal Women

Although OCP use declines significantly in women over the age of 35, the pill is a safe and effective birth control method for healthy, nonsmoking women up through menopause (Burkman & Shulman, 1998). During the perimenopausal years (ages 45 to 55), OCPs have the benefit of not only preventing unintended pregnancies, but also maintaining regular bleeding cycles and providing a consistent hormonal pattern right up to menopause. Estrogen supplementation in the form of low-dose OCPs can help manage hot flushes, which frequently begin during the perimenopausal period. A hot flush is experienced as a recurrent, transient period of flushing, sweating, or a sensation of heat. The flush may be accompanied by palpitations, a feeling of anxiety, and or occasionally chills (Kronenberg, 1990). Although the pathophysiology of the downward resetting of the hypothalamic thermoregulatory mechanism precipitating a hot flush is not fully understood, there appears to be a relationship between estrogen and the thermoregulatory mechanism. In particular, the severity of hot flushes may be related to the steepness of decline in estrogen levels (Bäckström, 1995).

The other preventive health benefits of OCPs, such as protection against bone loss and cancer prevention, may be of more interest to perimenopausal women as compared to younger women. For a perimenopausal woman desirous of maintaining or restoring cycle control, the use of OCPs containing 30–35 μg of EE appears to be superior to lower-dose formulations (Burkman & Shulman, 1998).

Of concern to some clinicians is that the perimenopause is a time in which women in community-based samples report an increase in dysphoric mood symptoms (Pearlstein, 1995). Brace and McCauley (1997), in reviewing the literature of the last two decades regarding the association between estrogen levels and psychological well-being, note that a subgroup of women appears to be at risk of mood and psychological disturbance during periods of hormonal change such as the perimenopause. There is increasing evidence that estrogen may alleviate minor mood symptoms in perimenopausal women (Rubinow et al., 1998). Thus, for a perimenopausal woman who has dysphoric mood symptoms and who also desires contraception, the clinician should consider monophasic OCPs. In addition, for a patient reporting dysphoric mood symptoms during the 7 days of placebo pills in the OCP packet, the clinician may consider Mircette, a relatively new formulation of OCP that offers a tapering dose of EE instead of abrupt discontinuation during the last 7 days of the OCP cycle. Alternatively, the patient may be placed on continuous monophasic OCPs, in which a 21-day pack is utilized or placebo pills omitted, thereby eliminating the hormone-free interval. If continuous pill usage is chosen, generally a pill-free or placebo week should be inserted every 3 months. However, if the patient's depressive symptoms are severe enough to meet criteria for major depression, then an antidepressant should be considered.

Women with Eating Disorders

Anorexia nervosa is an eating disorder that commonly results in anovulation and a hypoestrogenic state. This disorder places an underweight patient at higher risk of osteoporosis than her peers. With this population, the combination OCPs not only provide estrogen for bone mineral density maintenance, but also provide the additional benefit of reliable contraception, as gonadotropin-releasing hormone pulsatility and ovulatory function are recovered with increasing body mass index (Jimerson et al., 1996).

NEUROPSYCHIATRIC ASPECTS OF HORMONAL CONTRACEPTIVES

Since the introduction of OCPs in the 1960s, the potential psychiatric complications of their use have been the subject of considerable debate and discussion. Over the past four decades, the formulations have changed considerably, with the daily doses of EE in the combination OCPs reduced from 150 or 100 µg to 30 or 35 µg. Today, OCP formulations with as little as 20 µg of EE are available. The dose and type of progestogen in combination OCPs have also changed over the years, which may affect potential neuropsychiatric symptoms. Prior to 1992, the OCPs in the United States contained one of four progestins: norethindrone; norgestrel and its active isomer, levonorgestrel; norethindrone acetate; or ethynodiol diacetate. Although these progestins are readily available, two low-androgenic progestins, norgestimate and desogestrel, were introduced in OCPs in 1992 (Burkman & Shulman, 1998).

Mood and Anxiety Symptoms

The debate regarding neuropsychiatric symptoms associated with the older, higher-dose OCPs used in the 1960s and 1970s was well summarized in a review article by Slap (1981). Her review was prompted by a concern that dysphoric mood changes may contribute to the decision by some women to discontinue OCPs. Although 9 of 12 clinical trial studies reported significant depressive symptoms in 16–56% of women using OCPs, there were major flaws in most of the trials reviewed, including selection bias, lack of control groups, poor assessment of baseline rates of depressive symptoms, and an unclear definition or measurement of depression. More recently, Yonkers and Bradshaw (1999) have argued that the widely held belief that OCPs induce negative mood changes is not uniformly supported by the literature. They have noted that there are only a total of four placebo-controlled studies addressing the effects of OCPs on mood in the past 30 years. Their summary of the four studies suggests that there is limited support for OCP-induced mood deterioration. Patten and Love (1994) note that given the paucity of evidence that OCPs can cause depression, it is not surprising that there are few published guidelines as to its management.

Bancroft and Sartorius (1990) have noted that although most women currently taking OCPs do not experience significant mood disturbance, a minority of women may experience a disturbance of mood and are likely to discontinue use because of their symptoms. Evidence has been accumulating that fluctuating levels of steroid hormones may be associated with an increase in psychiatric symptoms in vulnerable women (Bancroft, 1993; Pearlstein, 1995; Schmidt et al., 1998). Thus, if a particular woman complains of dysphoric mood symptoms on OCPs, it is recommended that the clinician select a formulation in which neither the estrogen nor the progestin components fluctuate. Van Lunsen and Laan (1997) speculate that mood changes in OCP users could be related to the changes in levels of steroid hormones in the blood that occur during the pill-free interval, and also possibly to changes in dosage in some formulations. A monophasic OCP may have advantages in women psychiatrically vulnerable to changes in steroid hormones.

As described earlier, Norplant releases a continuous subdermal dose of levonorgestrel, a synthetic progestin, which is also a component of some formulations of OCPs. Wagner and Berenson (1994) and Wagner (1996) report on a total of seven cases of young women of reproductive age with no prior psychiatric history who developed major depression and/or anxiety symptoms while on subdermal levonorgestrel. In all of the case reports, the symptoms remitted following removal of the implants in about 2 months. The complaints of both depression and loss of libido, while not common, were noted in a study evaluating the efficacy and side effects of immediate postcoital administration of levonorgestrel 0.75 mg used repeatedly for contraception. Because of the numerous side effects, high dose levonorgestrel pills are unsuitable for regular postcoital contraception. Panic disorder with agoraphobia has been associated with the progesterone component of an OCP in two anecdotal reports (Deci et al., 1992; Ushiroyama et al., 1992). Deci and colleagues noted that the symptoms resolved once the patient discontinued the triphasic OCP. In a triphasic OCP, the progesterone dose increases over a 21-day period. They speculated that the progesterone component may have precipitated the panic disorder by its effect of respiratory stimulation and reduction of CO_2 at sensitive CO_2 receptors. One possible mechanism of progesterone-induced dysphoria is its effect of increasing mono-amine oxidase activity in the brain, which in turn lowers the level of various neuro-transmitters, such as serotonin. Bethea et al. (1998) suggest that the molecular action of synthetic progestins (e.g., medroxyprogesterone, levonorgestrel) differs significantly from the action of natural progesterone in serotonin neurons. It is speculated that the adminis-tration of synthetic progestins in some women may attenuate the beneficial effects of es-trogen on mood. However, well-controlled prospective studies are required to fully exam-ine the possible depressive or anxiety symptoms induced by various types and dosages of progestins. Clinicians should be aware of the possibility of progestin-induced psychiatric symptoms.

Sexual Functioning

Graham and Sherwin (1993) noted that little attention has been paid to possible adverse effects of OCPs on sexual functioning. Graham et al. (1995) have suggested that adverse effects on well-being and sexual functioning may explain the relatively high discontinua-tion rates of OCPs. Decreased libido or sexual desire has been reported in 5–13% of OCP users (Slap, 1981). The impairment of sexual desire and interest is a potential side effect that may affect one's quality of life (Dei et al., 1997). Although the mechanism of action of the OCPs on female sexual functioning remains unclear, one possibility is the reduction in free testosterone, which affects sexual interest in women (Bancroft et al., 1991). All of the androgen parameters investigated in a study by Coenen et al. (1996) decreased while female patients were taking any of the four recent formulations of OCPs containing a component of the third-generation progestins. With the use of these formulations, as the androgen-binding proteins increase, the free testosterone, androstenedione and dehydro-epiandrosterone sulfate decline. Ovarian synthesis of these androgens is also decreased. The net effect of these changes in binding proteins and hormone synthesis is that a sub-stantial decrease in biologically active testosterone occurs. Thus the authors note that during the use of any of the four newer OCPs, the endogenous androgen environment changed in the direction of hypoandrogenism. Thus lower androgen levels resulting from OCPs may negatively interfere with sexual desire.

Another possible explanation of OCPs' negative impact on sexual functioning may be provided by a woman's sexual functioning prior to the initiation of OCPs. Graham et al. (1995) noted a negative effect on sexual interest (and, to a lesser extent, the frequency of sexual activity) in 50% of oral contraceptive users in Edinburgh, but not in Manila. The difference in the two populations may be attributed to the difference in the sexual re-lationship existing prior to the use of the OCPs. The Edinburgh group of women de-scribed more enjoyable sexual relationships, associated with relatively high levels of sex-ual interest and preparedness to initiate lovemaking with their partners prior to the start of the OCPs, as compared to the Manila group. Thus it may be that women involved in a satisfying sexual relationship prior to the initiation of OCPs may be better able to articulate the adverse sexual side effects of these medications.

In terms of managing women with complaints of decreased sexual desire on OCPs, Darney (1997) offers insightful suggestions. Progestins in OCPs can be divided into various (high, medium, and low) levels of androgenic activity. Clinically, OCPs need to be titrated according to hypo- or hyperandrogenic symptoms. For example, women with pre-existing acne may benefit from monophasic OCPs with a low-androgenic progestin such as desogestrel. In contrast, a woman with complaints of decreased sexual desire on OCPs may benefit from a formulation with a progestin with higher androgenic activity such as norgestrel, which may compensate for the decrease in free testosterone.

METABOLIC EFFECTS AND PHARMACOKINETICS

Metabolic Changes

Estrogen affects the metabolism of both endogenous and exogenous substances. The adverse effects on metabolism attributed to EE are caused primarily by its effects on the liver. EE causes dose-dependent alterations in the synthesis of numerous endogenous proteins, such as various coagulation and fibrinolysis factors, angiotensin, and both high- and low-density lipoproteins (Hoffmann et al., 1998). These multiple metabolic effects interact to produce the increased risk of VTE and hypertension associated with OCP use.

Information regarding the neuroendocrine effects of estrogen on mood disorders is unfolding. There are good data suggesting that estrogen and progesterone affect the synthesis and the metabolism of neurotransmitters associated with mood, specifically serotonin and norepinephrine (Szewczyk & Chennault, 1997). Estrogen may affect the synthesis and availability of serotonin in multiple ways. One proposed mechanism focuses on estrogen's induction of tryptophan oxygenase, which may lead to a functional pyridoxine deficiency, resulting in depletion of serotonin and catecholamines (Gangat et al., 1986). Estrogen may also increase serotonin availability by several mechanisms. Estrogen increases the rate of degradation of monoamine oxidase, the enzyme responsible for the catabolism of serotonin, thus increasing the level of serotonin. In addition, estrogen displaces tryptophan from albumin, resulting in higher free levels available for serotonin synthesis (Panay & Studd, 1998).

Drug Interactions with Oral Contraceptives

Any time a woman on OCPs is prescribed a concurrent medication, the possibility of drug interactions becomes a concern. As more information has become available about the clinical pharmacology of contraceptive steroids, there has evolved an increased awareness of the individual variation in both the pharmacokinetic and the pharmacodynamic response to OCPs. The potential for problems in this area has actually increased because of the trend toward prescribing very low-dose formulations whenever possible. As a result, Shenfield and Griffin (1991) note that there have been increasing reports of "pill failure" because of the influence of interacting drugs. Fortunately, a clinically important decrease in the efficiency of OCPs because of interactions with other drugs appears to occur in a very small minority of women (<5%) (Fotherby, 1990).

The hepatic cytochrome P450 (CYP450) isoenzyme system is involved in the majority of serious drug interactions. CYP450 is a term used to identify a group of heme-containing isoenzymes located on the membrane of the smooth endoplasmic reticulum, located primarily in the liver, but also in the intestinal tract, kidneys, and brain. The CYP450 isoenzyme system mediates the Phase I reactions, which involve oxidative, reductive, and hydrolytic reactions. The reactions either unmask or introduce a functional group such as a hydroxyl moiety to the parent compound. These types of reactions often result in an increase of the drug's polarity (Ozdemi et al., 1999).

The potential for drug interactions with OCPs is present because the CYP450 system is important in the metabolism of steroid hormones as well as many other drugs. The drug interactions between OCPs and other drugs can be divided into two general categories: (1) other drugs' interference with OCP efficacy, and (2) OCPs' interference with the metabolism of other drugs (Back & Orme, 1990).

Other Drugs' Interference with OCP Efficacy

An unintended pregnancy can be an emotional hardship. Approximately half of the 2.7 million unintended pregnancies in the United States are the results of contraceptive failure ("FDA Reduces Warning on Preven Emergency Contraceptive Kit," 1999). Although the most common reason for pregnancy while the patient is taking OCPs is the failure to take the medication as prescribed, drug interactions can also affect the efficacy of OCPs. Over the past 30 years, case reports and clinical studies have documented various medications that cause an induction of CYP3A4 substrate, a P450 isoenzyme that may lead to a lowering of plasma levels of synthetic estrogens and progestogens. The decreased plasma level of the steroid hormones can result in the failure of the OCPs.

Various anticonvulsant drugs have been identified as causing failure of contraception or breakthrough bleeding in women taking OCPs. Phenytoin, phenobarbital, methyphenobarbital, topiramate (Rosenfeld et al., 1997), primidone, carbamazepine, and ethosuximide have all been implicated (Back & Orme, 1990) (see Table 6.1). In contrast, valproate (Crawford et al., 1986), lamotrigine (Holdich et al., 1991), and gabapentin do not cause hepatic enzyme induction and appear to have less potential for an interaction with OCPs (Eldon et al., 1998).

Clinicians should be mindful of the antiepileptics or mood stabilizers that do not interact with oral contraceptives when treating women of childbearing potential who are using OCPs for birth control. However, if a woman requires carbamazepine (for example) as a mood stabilizer, in order to minimize the possible consequences of an interaction with an OCP, the patient should be prescribed a contraceptive preparation with a higher estrogen content (e.g., 50 µg of EE). Note that this does not completely eliminate the risk, and an additional method of contraception may be advisable (Spina, Pisani, & Perucca, 1996).

Several broad spectrum antibiotics have been implicated in causing contraception failure in women on OCPs. Rifampin, an agent used in treating tuberculosis, is an inducer of CYP3A4, which causes a fourfold increase in the metabolism of the OCP (Barditch-Crovo et al., 1999). Although rifampin is the only antibiotic that is scientifically documented to interfere with the effectiveness of OCPs (Hersh, 1999), cases involving more commonly prescribed antibiotics have been reported over the past 25 years. These antibiotics have a weak association with OCP failure: amoxicillin, ampicillin, fluconazole, metronidazole, and tetracycline (Munckhof, 1998). Patients taking any antibiotic (other

TABLE 6.1. Drugs That May Interfere with Efficacy of OCPs

Decrease efficacy of OCPs	Increase efficacy of OCPs
Anticonvulsants/mood stabilizers	Vitamins
Phenytoin	Ascorbic acid
Phenobarbital	Antidepressants
Primidone	Nefazodone
Carbamazepine	Fluvoxamine
Ethosuximide	Fluoxetine
Topiramate	Sertraline
Antibiotics	Paroxetine
Rifampin (strong association)	Venlafaxine
Amoxycillin (weak association)	
Ampicillin (weak association)	
Tetracycline (weak association)	
Fluxonazol (weak association)	
Metronidazole (weak association)	

Note. The data are from Shenfield and Griffin (1991) and Tanaka (1998).

than rifampin) should be instructed that the risk of pregnancy while taking the OCP is about 1–3% per year, and that it is uncertain whether taking an antibiotic alters the baseline risk of pill failure (Munckhof, 1998). If a patient is taking an antibiotic for a short period of time, a barrier method may be suggested in addition to the OCP. If a woman if required to take an antibiotic for several months, a preparation containing 50 µg of EE should be considered.

Ascorbic acid is one example of a drug that may actually increase the therapeutic effect of oral contraceptive steroids. The bioavailability of EE has been reported to be increased over 60% shortly after 1 g of ascorbic acid was administered (Back & Orme, 1990) (see Table 6.2). Several antidepressants are CYP3A inhibitors, which may theoretically increase the steroid hormone in OCPs. The order of CYP3A inhibitory potency for these frequently used antidepressants appears to be nefazodone > fluvoxamine > sertraline > paroxetine > venlafaxine (Ketter et al., 1995). A clinically significant drug–drug interaction is unlikely to occur unless a particular patient is vulnerable to adverse effects of increased estrogens or progestins.

OCPs' Interference with Efficacy of Other Drugs

There are some reports suggesting that OCPs may have a negative effect (albeit normally a small one) on the efficacy of several concurrently administered drugs. Shenfield and Griffin (1991) review evidence suggesting that plasma levels of the tricyclic antidepressants amitriptyline, nortriptyline, and imipramine may increase in women taking OCPs (see Table 6.2). Some of the benzodiazepines, including diazepam, chlordiazepoxide, and alprazolam, are metabolized by hepatic microsomal oxidation. The OCPs inhibit enzyme activity and reduce clearance, thus possibly increasing sedative effects. On the other hand, other benzodiazepines (such as temazepam, which is metabolized by glucuronic acid conjugation) have a decrease in plasma concentration in some women taking OCPs (Back & Orme, 1990). In addition, the clearance of both theophylline and caffeine may be reduced in OCP users.

TABLE 6.2. OCPs' Interference with Efficacy of Other Drugs

Drugs with increased plasma concentration due to OCPs	Drugs with decreased plasma concentration due to OCPs
Antidepressants	Benzodiazepines
Amitriptyline	Lorazepam
Nortriptyline	Oxazepam
Imipramine	Temazepam
Benzodiazepines	Other
Diazepam	Acetaminophen
Chlordiazepoxide	Apomorphine
Triazolam	Morphine
Alprazolam	
Other	
Theophylline	
Caffeine	
Corticosteroids	
Cyclosporin	

Note. The data are from Fazio (1991), Shenfield and Griffin (1991), Back and Orme (1991), and Johnson et al. (1999).

CONCLUSIONS/FUTURE DIRECTIONS

Pharmaceutical companies continue to research and develop new forms of hormonal contraceptives. Efforts will probably be made to reduce the amount of estrogen to the lowest contraceptively effective dose and combine it with a type of progestational agent that provides predictable cyclic control while minimizing side effects. In the future, more attention and research need to be focused on decreasing the potential for neuropsychiatric effects of hormonal contraceptives in vulnerable women. Clinicians need to evaluate the various types of hormonal contraceptives and their effects, in particular, on women's mood, anxiety, and sexual functioning.

REFERENCES

American Cancer Society. (1996). *Cancer facts and figures—1996*. Atlanta, GA: Author.

American College of Obstetricians and Gynecologists (ACOG). (1994). *Hormonal contraception* (Technical Bulletin No. 198). Washington, DC: Author.

Back, D. J., & Orme, M. L. (1990). Pharmacokinetic drug interactions with oral contraceptives. *Clinical Pharmacokinetics, 18*(6), 472–484.

Bäckström, T. (1995). Symptoms related to the menopause and sex steroid treatments. *Ciba Foundation Symposium, 191,* 171–186.

Bancroft, J. (1993). The premenstrual syndrome: A reappraisal of the concept and the evidence. *Psychological Medicine, 24*(Suppl.), 1–47.

Bancroft, J., & Sartorius, N. (1990). The effects of oral contraceptives on well-being and sexuality. *Oxford Reviews of Reproductive Biology, 12,* 57–92.

Bancroft, J., Sherwin, B. B., Alexander, G. M., et al. (1991). Oral contraceptives, androgens, and the sexuality of young women: II. The role of androgens. *Archives of Sexual Behavior, 20,* 121–135.

Barditch-Crovo, P., Trapnell, C. B., Ette, E., et al. (1999). The effects of rifampin and rifabutin on the pharmacokinetics and pharmacodynamics of a combination oral contraceptive. *Clinical Pharmacology and Therapeutics, 65,* 428–438.

Bethea, C. L., Pecins-Thompson, M., Schutzer, W. E., et al. (1998). Ovarian steroids and serotonin neural function. *Molecular Neurobiology, 18*(2), 87–123.

Brace, M., & McCauley, E. (1997). Oestrogens and psychological well-being. *Annals of Medicine, 29*(4), 283–290.

Burkman, R. T., & Shulman, L. P. (1998). Oral contraceptive practice guidelines. *Contraception, 58*(3, Suppl.), 35S–43S.

Cancer and Steroid Hormone Study of the Centers for Disease Control and the National Institute of Child Health and Human Development. (1987). The reduction in risk of ovarian cancer associated with oral-contraceptive use. *New England Journal of Medicine, 316,* 650–655.

Coenen, C. M., Thomas, C. M., Borm, G. F., et al. (1996). Changes in androgens during treatment with four low-dose contraceptives. *Contraception, 53,* 171–176.

Collaborative Group on Hormonal Factors in Breast Cancer. (1996). Breast cancer and hormonal contraceptives: Collaborative reanalysis of individual data on 53,297 women with breast cancer and 100,239 women without breast cancer from 54 epidemiological studies. *Lancet, 347,* 1713–1727.

Crawford, P., Chadwick, D., Cleland, P., et al. (1986). The lack of effect of sodium valproate on the pharmacokinetics of oral contraceptive steroids. *Contraception, 33,* 23–29.

Cundy, T., Evans, M., Roberts, H., et al. (1991). Bone density in women receiving depot medroxyprogesterone acetate for contraception. *British Medical Journal, 303,* 13–16.

Darney, P. D. (1997). OC practice guidelines: Minimizing side effects. *International Journal of Fertility, 42*(Suppl. 1), 158–169.

DeCherney, A. (1996). Bone-sparing properties of oral contraceptives. *American Journal of Obstetrics and Gynecology, 174*(1, Pt. 1), 15–20.

Deci, P. A., Lydiard, R. B., Santos, A. B., et al. (1992). Oral contraceptives and panic disorder. *Journal of Clinical Psychiatry, 53,* 163–165.

Dei, M., Verni, A., Bigozzi, L., et al. (1997). Sex steroids and libido. *European Journal of Contraception and Reproductive Health Care, 2*(4), 253–258.

Dull, P., & Blythe, M. J. (1998). Preventing teenage pregnancy. *Primary Care, 25,* 111–122.

Eldon, M. A., Underwood, B. A., Randinitis, E. J., et al. (1998). Gabapentin does not interact with a contraceptive regimen of norethindrone acetate and ethinyl estradiol. *Neurology, 50,* 1146–1148.

Fazio, A. (1991). Oral contraceptive drug interactions: Important considerations. *Southern Medical Journal, 84,* 997–1002.

FDA reduces warning on Preven emergency contraceptive kit. (1999). In [Online]. Available: http://www.pslgroup.com/dg/iocfea.htm [1999, June 28].

Fotherby, K. (1990). Interactions with oral contraceptives. *American Journal of Obstetrics and Gynecology, 163*(6, Pt. 2), 2153–2159.

Gangat, A. E., Simpson, M. A., & Naidoo, L. R. (1986). Medication as a potential cause of depression. *South African Medical Journal, 70,* 224–226.

Graham, C. A., Ramos, R., Bancroft, J., et al. (1995). The effects of steroidal contraceptives on the well-being and sexuality of women: A double-blind, placebo-controlled, two-centre study of combined and progestogen-only methods. *Contraception, 52,* 363–369.

Graham, C. A., & Sherwin, B. B. (1993). The relationship between mood and sexuality in women using oral contraceptive as a treatment for premenstrual symptoms. *Psychoneuroendocrinology, 18*(4), 273–281.

Grimes, D. A., & Wallach, M. (Eds.). (1997). *Modern contraception: Updates from the contraception report.* Totowa, NJ: Emron.

Hankinson, S. E., Colditz, G. A., Hunter, D. J., et al. (1992). A quantitative assessment of oral contraceptive use and risk of ovarian cancer. *Obstetrics and Gynecology, 8,* 708–714.

Hersh, E. V. (1999). Adverse drug interactions in dental practice: Interactions involving antibiotics. *Journal of the American Dental Association, 130*, 236–251.

Hoffmann, H., Moore, C., Zimmermann, H., et al. (1998). Approaches to the replacement of ethinylestradiol by natural 17beta-estradiol in combined oral contraceptives. *Experimental and Toxicologic Pathology, 50*, 458–464.

Holdich, T., Whiteman, P., Orme, M., et al. (1991). Effect of lamotrigine on the pharmacology of the combined oral contraceptive pill [Abstract]. *Epilepsia, 32*(Suppl. 1), 96.

Huezo, C. M. (1998). Current reversible contraceptive methods: A global perspective. *International Journal of Gynaecology and Obstetrics, 62*(Suppl. 1), S3–S15.

Jimerson, D. C., Wolfe, B. E., Brotman, A. W., et al. (1996). Medications in the treatment of eating disorders. *Psychiatric Clinics of North America, 19*, 739–754.

Johnson, M. D., Newkirk, G., & White, J. R., Jr. (1999). Clinically significant drug interactions. *Postgraduate Medicine, 105*(2), 193–206.

Kaunitz, A. M. (1997). Revisiting progestin-only OCs. In *Contemporary OB/GYN archive* [On-line]. Available: http://www.pdr.net/cog/psrecord.htm [1997, December].

Kaunitz, A. M. (1998). Oral contraceptive estrogen dose considerations. *Contraception, 58*(3, Suppl.), 15S–21S.

Ketter, T. A., Flockhart, D. A., Post, R. M., et al. (1995). The emerging role of cytochrome P450 3A in psychopharmacology. *Journal of Clinical Psychopharmacology, 15*, 387–398.

Kleerekoper, M., Brienza, R. S., Schultz, L. R., et al. (1991). Oral contraceptive use may protect against low bone mass: Henry Ford Hospital Osteoporosis Cooperative Research Group. *Archives of Internal Medicine, 151*, 1971–1976.

Kronenberg, F. (1990). Hot flashes: Epidemiology and physiology. *Annals of the New York Academy of Sciences, 592*, 52–86.

Munckhof, W. J. (1998). Concurrent prescribing: Beware of drug interactions. *Australian Family Physician, 27*(10), 895–901.

Ozdemi, V., Masellis, M., Basile, V. S., et al. (1999). Variability in response to clozapine: Potential role of cytochrome P450 1A2 and the dopamine D4 receptor gene. *CNS Spectrums, 4*(6), 30–56.

Panay, N., & Studd, J. W. (1998). The psychotherapeutic effects of estrogens. *Gynecological Endocrinology, 12*, 353–365.

Patten, S. B., & Love, E. J. (1994). Drug-induced depression: Incidence, avoidance and management. *Drug Safety, 10*(3), 203–219.

Pearlstein, T. B. (1995). Hormones and depression: What are the facts about premenstrual syndrome, menopause, and hormone replacement therapy? *American Journal of Obstetrics and Gynecology, 173*(2), 646–653.

Peipert, J. F., & Gutmann, J. (1993). Oral contraceptive risk assessment: A survey of 247 educated women. *Obstetrics and Gynecology, 82*, 112–117.

Peterson, H. B., & Lee, N. C. (1989). The health effects of oral contraceptives: Misperceptions, controversies, and continuing good news. *Clinical Obstetrics and Gynecology, 32*, 339–355.

Rosenfeld, W. E., Doose, D. R., Walker, S. A, et al. (1997). Effect of topiramate on the pharmacokinetics of an oral contraceptive containing norethindrone and ethinyl estradiol in patients with epilepsy. *Epilepsia, 38*(3), 317–323.

Rubinow, D. R., Schmidt, P. J., & Roca, C. A. (1998). Estrogen–serotonin interactions: Implications for affective regulation. *Biological Psychiatry, 44*(9), 839–850.

Schlesselman, J. J. (1984). Cancer of the breast and reproductive tract in relation to the use of oral contraceptives. *Contraception, 40*, 1–38.

Schmidt, P. J., Nieman, L. K., Danaceau, M. A., et al. (1998). Differential behavioral effects of gonadal steroids in women with and in those without premenstrual syndrome. *New England Journal of Medicine, 338*(4), 209–216.

Shenfield, G. M., & Griffin, J. M. (1991). Clinical pharmacokinetics of contraceptive steroids: An update. *Clinical Pharmacokinetics, 20*(1), 15–37.

Slap, G. B. (1981). Oral contraceptives and depression: Impact, prevalence and cause. *Journal of Adolescent Health Care, 2*(1), 53–64.

Spina, E., Pisani, F., & Perucca, E. (1996). Clinically significant pharmacokinetic drug interactions with carbamazepine: An update. *Clinical Pharmacokinetics, 31*(3), 198–214.

Stevens-Simon, C. (1998). Providing effective reproductive health care and prescribing contraceptives for adolescents. *Pediatrics in Review, 19*, 409–417.

Szewczyk, M., & Chennault, S. A. (1997). Women's health: Depression and related disorders. *Primary Care, 24*, 83–101.

Tanaka, E. (1998). Clinically important pharmacokinetic drug–drug interactions: Role of cytochrome P450 enzymes. *Journal of Clinical Pharmacy and Therapeutics, 23*(6), 403–416.

Thorneycroft, I. H. (1999). Cycle control with oral contraceptives: A review of the literature. *American Journal of Obstetrics and Gynecology, 180*(2, Pt. 2), 280–287.

Ushiroyama, T., Okamoto, Y., Toyoda, K., et al. (1992). A case of panic disorder induced by oral contraceptive. *Acta Obstetricia et Gynecologica Scandinavica, 71*(1), 78–80.

Van der Vange, N., Blankenstein, M. A., Kloosterboer, H. J., et al. (1990). Effects of seven low-dose combined oral contraceptives on sex hormone binding globulin, corticosteroid binding globulin, total and free testosterone. *Contraception, 41*(4), 345–352.

Van Lunsen, R. H., & Laan, E. (1997). Sex, hormones and the brain. *European Journal of Contraception and Reproductive Health Care, 2*(4), 247–251.

Wagner, K. D. (1996). Major depression and anxiety disorders associated with Norplant. *Journal of Clinical Psychiatry, 57*(4), 152–157.

Wagner, K. D., & Berenson, A. B. (1994). Norplant-associated major depression and panic disorder. *Journal of Clinical Psychiatry, 55*(11), 478–480.

Yonkers, K. A., & Bradshaw, K. D. (1999). Hormone replacement and oral contraceptive therapy: Do they induce or treat mood symptoms? In J. O. Oldham & M. D. Riba (Series Eds.) & E. Leibenluft (Vol. Ed.), *Review of psychiatry series: Vol. 18. Gender differences in mood and anxiety disorders: From bench to bedside*. Washington, DC: American Psychiatric Press.

7

Psychiatric Aspects of Menopause

Depression

INEKE AYUBI-MOAK
BARBARA L. PARRY

Women appear to be at increased risk of experiencing a depressive episode during times of hormonal change, as evidenced by oral-contraceptive-induced dysphoria, premenstrual dysphoric disorder, and postpartum depression. Menopause is another time in the reproductive cycle that is marked by hormonal change and depression has long been theorized to accompany menopause as well. Although the nature of the depression–menopause relationship remains debatable, it is a question of increasing importance. As the U.S. population ages, the number of women living postmenopausally has increased to 35 million. Women are also living up to a third of their lifetimes during menopause, making it a very significant part of a woman's life. Data from the Cross-National Epidemiologic Study (Weissman 1995, 1996) suggest that there is an increase in new onset of depressive illness in women aged 45–50 years (during the perimenopause). Though not all research supports this linkage, it does seem clear that women with a prior history of depression are at increased risk for depression at menopause. This chapter reviews the literature pertaining to menopause, depression, and the effectiveness of estrogen replacement therapy (ERT).

PHYSIOLOGY OF MENOPAUSE

Menopause, the cessation of ovulation, is due to the depletion of responsive ovarian oocytes, and generally occurs at about age 50. The hypoestrogenism that ensues can lead to hot flushes, sleep disturbances, vaginal atrophy and dryness, and cognitive and affective disturbances; it can also predispose a woman to osteoporosis and cardiovascular disease. Menopause is generally heralded by 5–10 years of erratic ovarian function, revealed by irregular uterine bleeding. Prior to the 1800s, menopause tended to occur just before death. Previous negative associations may reflect the nearly coincident timing of menopause and death in earlier centuries; today's women, however, must adjust to the challenge of life after the loss of endogenous reproductive capacity.

A "surgical menopause" occurs when the ovaries are removed. This removal is often done in women older than age 35 years who are also receiving a hysterectomy, in an effort to protect them from future ovarian carcinoma. Prophylactic oophorectomy is a controversial procedure, and the symptoms that follow this surgical procedure before the age of natural menopause can be more pronounced than those that follow the timing of natural menopause. In natural menopause, the ovaries remain intact and continue to secrete androgens, including testosterone and androstenedione. In surgical menopause, there is an abrupt and complete loss of the ovarian secretion of androgens, estrogens, and progesterone; often this loss of ovarian function occurs well before the age of natural menopause, which typically happens between ages 47 and 53 years.

HISTORY OF VIEWS ON MENOPAUSE AND ITS RELATIONSHIP TO DEPRESSION

Menopause is a time of change for women not only in their endocrine and reproductive systems, but also in their social and psychological circumstances. Health status changes; roles evolve as children leave the home and parents become elderly and die; and fertility comes to an end. It has long been thought that menopause is accompanied by depression and other mental disturbances. Such noted 19th-century physicians as Merson (1876), Conklin (1889), Warnock (1890) and Kraepelin (1896) held this view. Kraepelin's (1896) concept of "involutional melancholia"—described as a form of depression beginning at menopause and characterized by a rigid personality, agitation but no episodes of mania, nihilistic or hypochondriac delusions, and a varying outcome—remained influential well into the 1900s. Indeed, involutional melancholia was part of the diagnostic nomenclature as late as the second edition of the *Diagnostic and Statistical Manual of Mental Disorders* (DSM-II; American Psychiatric Association, 1968), and even in the 1970s practitioners in England described menopausal women as "neurotic, depressed, and unable to cope with emotional crises" (Roberts, 1985). A survey in 1983 discovered that 90% of the general population in Canada (Kaufert et al., 1992) and high percentages of women in Massachusetts (Avis & McKinlay, 1991) agreed with the statement that "many women become depressed and irritable at menopause."

Even though interest in menopause-induced mood disorders goes back to the 19th century, scientists have not been able to conclude whether or not such disorders actually exist. Weissman (1979) in an article titled "The Myth of Involutional Melancholia," concluded from a review of epidemiological and clinical studies that there was no support for such a melancholia as a distinct diagnostic entity, and that the prevalence of depression around the menopausal years was not increased. In 1980, the diagnosis of involutional melancholia was removed from DSM-III. More recent data from the Cross-National Epidemiologic Study, however, (Weissman 1995, 1996), indicate an increase in new onsets of major depressive illness in the perimenopausal years as noted earlier. Angst (1978) reported a bimodal distribution of age in the onset of bipolar illness in women, with a second peak between the ages of 45 and 49 (the average age during the perimenopausal years). Studies by Reich and Winokur (1975) also indicated an increase in affective episodes around the age of 50 years. Allgulander (1994) reported that the number of observed suicides was highest in women between 45 and 64 years of age.

Other research, by contrast, does not indicate an increased incidence of mood disorders at this time. Winokur and Cadoret (1975) reported that first-admission rates for women with depression in England and Wales, and suicide rates of American women showed no peak in the decade from 45 to 54 years of age. Winokur (1973) studied women with a previous diagnosis of depression and found that the risk of being hospitalized was the same in peri- and postmenopausal women as it was in all other age groups. He concluded that the association between menopause and an episode of an affective disorder was chance. Data from the National Comorbidity Survey indicated that there was no significant sex difference in the average age at onset of major depression (Kessler et al., 1993). A North American study (Smith, 1971) found that of women admitted to psychiatric institutions, fewer of them were menopausal than in the general population. Studies of Norwegian (Holte, 1992), English (Hunter, 1992), and Canadian (McKinlay & Jefferys, 1974) women failed to find an increase in the incidence of depression in menopausal women. Australian women were found to have an increase in minor psychological symptoms but not major depression (Dennerstein et al., 1993).

Still other studies, however, indicate that a previous history of depression does put women at an increased risk of experiencing an episode of depression during menopause (McKinlay et al., 1987). Stewart and Boydell (1993) found that women who reported high psychological distress while attending a menopause clinic were more likely to have experienced depression in the past, both independent of and related to menses, oral contraception, and pregnancy. Tam and Parry (1999a) found that 75% of women attending a university or community menopause clinic with Beck Depression Inventory (BDI) scores over 10, met criteria for recurrent major depressive disorder. Perimenopausal compared with premenopausal women had a statistically significant ($p < .005$) increase in BDI scores.

Clearly, menopausal depression is a difficult subject to study, as there are multiple methodological problems and confounding factors that need to be considered. The very definition of "menopause" varies from study to study. The World Health Organization defines menopause as 12 months without menses, but some researchers use 6 months without menses or simply study women in the 45–55 age group, as 51 years is the median age of onset for menopause. Hormonal status is rarely used to confirm menopause. Other researchers have studied women during the perimenopause (defined as the period in which women are having irregular menses), during which time hormonal levels undergo the greatest change, theoretically putting women at greater risk for mood disturbances. In addition, the definition and determination of depression vary from study to study. Some women are given formal testing or standardized psychiatric interviews; others complete questionnaires or respond to phone interviews. Categorical diagnoses and syndromes are not always differentiated from a wide range of depressive symptoms. Moreover, choice of the patient population can affect the outcome of a study. Some researchers have studied women who are self-referred to menopause clinics; these women are more likely to suffer from emotional or physical complaints during the climacteric period that bring them into the clinic. Community-based patient populations are not without their problems, including lack of objective, professional determination of mood status. Denial is an issue when relying on community members to fill out questionnaires about depressed mood. Finally, there are multiple variables to consider when asking women about their experiences during menopause. These include a woman's personal expectations of menopause, cultural beliefs about menopause, concurrent stressful life events, hysterectomy status, and history of depression.

HYPOTHESES DEVELOPED: ESTROGEN DEFICIENCY VERSUS SOCIAL CIRCUMSTANCES

There are different hypotheses to explain the perceived relationship between menopause and depression. The biochemical hypothesis directly associates the fall in estrogen levels with depression. Estrogen is known to affect levels of serotonin, dopamine, and norepinephrine, all of which are theorized to be low in persons with depression. There are estrogen receptors in many parts of the brain, including the cerebral cortex, hypothalamus, hippocampus, amygdala, and limbic forebrain (McEwen, 1980). In the suprachiasmatic nucleus, estrogen metabolites competitively inhibit the breakdown of norepinephrine by catechol-o-methyl transferase (Ball et al., 1972). Estrogen also induces the release of endogenous catecholamines within the hypothalamus (Paul et al., 1979). Estrogen decreases monoamine oxidase activity in rat hypothalamus and in human platelets and brain (Luin et al., 1983), thereby increasing the amount of serotonin available. It enhances the transport of serotonin and increases the amount of free tryptophan that reaches the brain by displacing it from plasma albumin (Aylward, 1973). Klaiber et al. (1979) found that menopausal women had increased monoamine oxidase activity and decreased serotonin levels compared with premenopausal women. Estrogen therapy may reverse these effects. Halbreich et al. (1995) examined the effects of meta-chlorophenyl-piperazine (m-CPP), a serotonin agonist, on prolactin and cortisol levels in premenopausal and postmenopausal women with and without ERT. They found that without estrogen, postmenopausal women's response to m-CPP was blunted; with estrogen, the response was enhanced. Halbreich's group also studied the platelet binding of imipramine, which reflects the brain's serotonin uptake capacity, and found that all postmenopausal women had decreased binding compared with premenopausal women. Binding was increased with administration of estradiol.

Women who undergo surgical menopause have an increased risk of depression (Sherwin & Gelfand, 1985; McKinlay et al., 1987). The theoretical basis of this finding may be that these women undergo a sudden and total withdrawal of estrogen. Women with intact ovaries produce androgens that are aromatized into estrogens (Bäckström, 1995). Oophorectomized women lack even this small source of estrogen. It appears that the brain is an estrogen-dependent organ, and that dysfunctions of mood, cognition, and memory ensue if estrogen levels fall below some set point (Arpels, 1996).

Estrogen not only affects the limbic system, but also appears to play a role in circadian rhythms and quality of sleep. In animals, estrogen shortens the circadian period, advances activity onset, and lengthens and consolidates the rest phase (Albers, 1981; Morin et al., 1977; Thomas & Armstrong, 1989). Leibenluft (1993) hypothesized that the fall in estrogen at menopause may disrupt hormonal circadian systems, which in turn destabilize mood. Erlik et al. (1981) found that hot flushes and waking episodes were related to one another. These researchers observed that women awoke slightly before measurable increases in skin temperature occurred. These findings suggested that waking episodes are related to central events similar to those leading to hot flushes, rather than to the discomfort of the hot flushes per se. Erlich et al. theorized that hot flushes occur due to a downward shift in the central thermostat. The nuclei that regulate temperature are in close proximity to hypothalamic nuclei containing gonadotropin-releasing hormone. Erlik's group found that estrogen therapy reduced both the number of hot flushes and waking episodes. Baker et al. (1997) studied 28 women, none of whom had previous psychiatric problems. They found that mood and sleep were significantly related in the perimenopausal group but not in the premenopausal group. Perimenopausal women reported poorer sleep, drowsiness during the day, increased anxiety, and decreased vigor. They concluded that the degree of sleep disruption a perimenopausal woman experiences predicts the degree of mood change she experiences.

In contrast to the biochemical hypothesis, the symptom hypothesis claims that the vasomotor events that occur due to estrogen decline, such as hot flushes and night sweats, cause depressed symptoms and insomnia. Researchers have found that the incidence of hot flushes ranges from 39% in Australia (Dennerstein et al., 1993), to 55% in southeast England (Hunter, 1992) to 74% in Rancho Bernardo, California (Goldani von Muhlen et al., 1995). In some of these studies, the risk of suffering from troubling hot flushes appears to be related to previous premenstrual complaints (Hunter, 1992; Dennerstein et al., 1993). The increase in discomfort felt with sweating and feeling hot may in fact be what leads directly to depression. The Seattle Mid-Life Women's Health Study (Woods & Mitchell, 1996) found that vasomotor symptoms differentiated women who were consistently depressed from those recovering from a depressed mood. In other words, women who experienced more vasomotor symptoms were more likely to be depressed during the first and second years of the study. Avis et al. (1994) found that experiencing a long perimenopausal period (27 months long) was "moderately associated" with increased risk of transitory depression, which was explained by increased menopausal symptoms rather than menopause itself. Goldani von Muhlen et al. (1995) found that the California women in their study who complained of two or more vasomotor symptoms were more likely to complain of psychological symptoms than other women.

Insomnia is a common complaint during the menopause and may be caused by what some researchers term the "domino effect." That is, a woman who experiences hot flushes is then likely to experience poor sleep and subsequently a decreased feeling of well-being (Hunter, 1992; Shaver et al., 1988; Campbell & Whitehead, 1977). Campbell and Whitehead (1977) treated women with ERT and found that the women complaining of hot flushes (which were relieved with therapy) also reported significant improvements in insomnia. Women who did not suffer from hot flushes reported no improvement in insomnia.

A social circumstances perspective theorizes that the social, rather than endocrine, changes occurring during menopause lead to depression. Midlife can be a tumultuous time for some women. Roles are changing as children leave the home, and as parents or husbands become sick and dependent or die. These changes can challenge a woman's self-identity and lead to worry, stress, and possibly depression. Family dynamics are changing, and women are faced not only with a loss of fertility, but also with negative social stereotypes of aging women losing their beauty and appeal. On the other hand, some women may relish their newfound freedom from children and unwanted pregnancy, and feel happy about their new position as mature members of society.

McKinlay et al. (1987) questioned a Massachusetts cohort of 2,565 women aged 45–55 about depression and factors contributing to depression. The one factor that had no effect on the risk of depression was nonsurgical menopausal status. McKinlay's group found that clinical depression was related to "person-induced worry." A woman who was worried about her husband or two other family members was more likely to score above 16 (significant for clinical depression) on the Center for Epidemiologic Studies Depression Scale. These researchers also found a correlation between the risk for clinical depression and educational and marital status. Women who had only a high-school education and who were either divorced, separated, or widowed had an increased risk of depression; never-married women of any educational status were least likely to be depressed. Finally, women who complained about health changes (including physical symptoms, activity restriction or diagnosis of a chronic condition) had an increased incidence of depression. Avis et al. (1994) later published a longitudinal follow up of McKinlay's cross-sectional study and concluded that a history of depression was most predictive of subsequent depression.

Hunter (1992) followed 56 premenopausal women for 3 years and determined that there was an increase in depression in the women who went through menopause. The predicting factors were a history of premenopausal depression, negative stereotyped beliefs about menopause, and being unemployed. The Manitoba Project in Canada (Kaufert et al., 1992) showed similar results. Researchers interviewed 477 women six times over 3 years and concluded that mood was affected by health, changes in family life, and relationship stressors. The Seattle Mid-Life Women's Health Study (Woods & Mitchell, 1996) included in-depth interviews with 347 women, who also kept symptom diaries and provided mailed health updates. Patterns of depressed mood were related to stressful life context, past or present health status, and social learning about midlife. Menopausal status did not differentiate women with depressed mood from those without depressed mood.

A woman's expectations of menopause can greatly affect her experience during menopause. The menopause is seen by some as a relief, as they no longer have to worry about unwanted pregnancy. For other women, it represents the loss not only of fertility, but also of youth and beauty. Wilbur et al. (1995) found that both African American and European American women of different socioeconomic backgrounds in Chicago generally had neutral views about menopause. However, those women who suffered from depression had more negative views about menopause, regardless of their age or menopausal status. This finding led the authors to believe that these women would experience a more difficult menopausal transition.

During perimenopause and postmenopause, lower overall well-being, depressive symptoms, and major clinical depression can be explained by multiple psychosocial factors. It would be a disservice to women if clinicians did not consider all aspects of women's circumstances during the midlife period to help understand their changes in mood. Clinicians need to consider the effects of hormonal change, history of depressive illness, social circumstances, physical symptoms, and significant relationships on women's affect.

ESTROGEN REPLACEMENT THERAPY

The relationship between ERT and depression during menopause is not clear. The decision to start ERT is a complex one and the risks and benefits need to be assessed for each woman. It is theorized that if altered estrogen levels contribute to depression (either as a direct result of physiological changes in the brain or secondary to disturbing vasomotor

American Psychiatric Association. (1968). *Diagnostic and statistical manual of mental disorders* (2nd ed.). Washington, DC: Author.

Angst, J. (1978). The course of affective disorders: II. Typology of bipolar manic–depressive illness. *Archiv für Psychiatrie und Nervenkrankheiten, 226,* 65–73.

Arpels, J. C. (1996). The female brain hypoestrogenic continuum from the premenstrual syndrome to menopause: A hypothesis and review of supporting data. *Journal of Reproductive Medicine, 41*(9), 633–639.

Avis, N. E., Brambilla, D., McKinlay, S. M., et al. (1994). A longitudinal analysis of the association between menopause and depression. Results from the Massachusetts Women's Health Study. *Annals of Epidemiology, 4,* 214–220.

Avis, N. E., & McKinlay, S. M. (1991). A longitudinal analysis of women's attitudes toward menopause: Results from the Massachusetts Women's Health Study. *Maturitas, 13,* 65–79.

Aylward, M. (1973). Plasma tryptophan levels and mental depression in postmenopausal subjects: Effects of oral piperazine–oestrone sulphate. *IRCS Med Sci, 1,* 30–34.

Bäckström, T. (1995). Symptoms related to the menopause and sex steroid treatments. *Ciba Foundation Symposium, 191,* 171–186.

Baker, A., Simpson, S., & Dawson, D. (1997). Sleep disruption and mood changes associated with menopause. *Journal of Psychosomatic Research, 43*(4), 359–369.

Ball, P., Knuppen, R., Haupt, M., et al. (1972). Interactions between estrogens and catecholamines: III. Studies on the methylation of catechol estrogens, catecholamines and other catechols by the catechol-o-methyltransferase of human liver. *Journal of Clinical Endocrinology and Metabolism, 34,* 736–746.

Campbell, S., & Whitehead, M. (1977). Oestrogen therapy and the menopausal syndrome. *Clinics in Obstetrics and Gynecology, 4*(1), 31–47.

Conklin, W. J. (1889). Some neuroses of the menopause. *Transactions of the American Association for Obstetrics and Gynecology, 2,* 301–311.

Coope, J. (1981). Is oestrogen therapy effective in the treatment of menopausal depression? *Journal of the Royal College of General Practitioners, 31*(224), 134–140.

Dennerstein, L., Smith, A., Morse, C., et al. (1993). Menopausal symptoms in Australian women. *Medical Journal of Australia, 159,* 232–236

Ditkoff, E. C., Crary, W., Cristo, M., et al. (1991). Estrogen improves psychological function in asymptomatic post-menopausal women. *Obstetrical Gynecology, 78*(6), 991–995.

Erlik, Y., Tataryn, I., Meldrum, D., et al. (1981). Association of waking episodes with menopausal hot flushes. *Journal of the American Medical Association, 245*(17), 1741–1744.

Goldani von Muhlen, D., Kritz-Silverstein, D., & Barrett-Connor, E. (1995). A community-based study of menopause symptoms and estrogen replacement in older women. *Maturitas, 22,* 71–78.

Holte, A. (1992). Influences of natural menopause on health complaints: A prospective study of healthy Norwegian women. *Maturitas, 14,* 127–141.

Hunter, M. (1992). The South-East England longitudinal study of the climacteric and post-menopause. *Maturitas, 14,* 117–116.

Kaufert, P., Gilbert, P., & Tate, R. (1992). The Manitoba project: A re-examination of the link between menopause and depression. *Maturitas, 14,* 143–155.

Kendall, D., Stancel, G., & Enna, S. (1981a). The influence of sex hormones on antidepressant-induced alterations in neurotransmitter receptor binding. *Journal of Neuroscience, 2*(3), 354–360.

Kendall, D., Stancel, G., & Enna, S. (1981b). Imipramine: Effect of ovarian steroids on modifications in serotonin receptor binding. *Science, 211,* 1183–1185.

Kessler, R., McGonagle, K., Swartz, M., et al. (1993). Sex and depression in the National Comorbidity Survey: I. Lifetime prevalence, chronicity and recurrence. *Journal of Affective Disorders, 29,* 85–96.

Klaiber, E., Broverman, D., Vogel, W., et al. (1979). Estrogen therapy for severe persistent depressions in women. *Archives of General Psychiatry, 36*, 550–555.

Kraepelin, E. (1896). *Psychiatrie: Ein lehrbuch fur studierende und aerzte* (5 vols.). Leipzig: Abel.

Kripke, D. F., Elliott, J., Youngstedt, S., et al. (1998). Melatonin: Marvel or marker? *Annals of Medicine, 30*(1), 81–87.

Leibenluft, E. (1993). Do gonadal steroids regulate circadian rhythms in humans? *Journal of Affective Disorders, 29*, 175–181.

Linkowski, P., Mendlewicz, I., Kerkhofs, M., et al. (1987). 24-hour profiles of adrenocorticotropin, cortisol and growth hormone in major depressive illness: Effect of antidepressant treatment. *Journal of Clinical Endocrinology and Metabolism, 65*(1), 141–152.

Luin, V. N., Khylcheoskaya, R. I., & McEwen, B. S. (1975). Effect of gonadal steroids on activities of monoamine oxidase and choline acetylase in rat brain. *Brain Research, 86*, 273–306.

McEwen, B. S. (1980). The brain as a target organ of endocrine hormones. *Neuroendocrinology*, 33–42.

McEwen, B. S., & Rhodes, J. C. (1983). Gonadal hormone regulation of MAO and other enzymes in hypothalamic areas. *Neuroendocrinology, 36*, 235–238.

McKinlay, J. B., McKinlay, S., & Brambilla, D. (1987). The relative contributions of endocrine changes and social circumstances of depression in mid-aged women. *Journal of Health and Social Behavior, 28*(4), 345–53.

McKinlay, S., & Jefferys, M. (1974). The menopausal syndrome. *British Journal of Preventive Social Medicine, 28*, 108–115.

Meyers, B. S., & Moline, M. (1997). The role of estrogen in late-life depression: Opportunities and barriers to research. *Psychopharmacology Bulletin, 33*(2), 289–291.

Morin, L. P., Fitzgerald, K. M., & Zucker, I. (1977). Estradiol shortens the period of hamster circadian rhythms. *Science, 196*, 305–307.

Nicol-Smith, L. (1996). Causality, menopause, and depression: A critical review of the literature. *British Medical Journal, 313*, 1229–1232.

Nordin, B. E. C., Jones, M., Crilly, R., et al. (1980). A placebo-controlled trial of ethinyl oestradiol and norethisterone in climacteric women. *Maturitas, 2*, 247–251.

Oppenheim, G. (1983). Estrogen in the treatment of depression: Neuropharmacological mechanisms. *Biological Psychiatry, 18*(6), 721–725.

Oppenheim, G. (1984). A case of rapid mood cycling with estrogen: Implications for therapy. *Journal of Clincial Psychiatry, 45*(1), 34–35.

Palinkas, L., & Barrett-Connor, E. (1992). Estrogen use and depressive symptoms in postmenopausal women. *Obstetrics and Gynecology, 80*, 30–36.

Pariser, S. (1993). Women and mood disorders: Menarche to menopause. *Annals of Clinical Psychiatry, 5*, 249–254.

Paul, S., Axelrod, J., Saavedra, J., et al. (1979). Estrogen-induced efflux of endogenous catecholamines from the hypothalamus in vitro. *Brain Research, 178*, 499–505.

Pearce, J., Hawton, K., & Blake, F. (1995). Psychological and sexual symptoms associated with the menopause and the effects of hormone replacement therapy. *British Journal of Psychiatry, 167*, 163–173.

Pearlstein, T. (1995). Hormones and depression: What are the facts about premenstrual syndrome, menopause, and hormone replacement therapy? *American Journal of Obstetrics and Gynecology, 172*, 646–653.

Pearlstein, T., Rosen, K., & Stone, A. (1997). Mood disorders and menopause. *Endocrinology and Metabolism Clinics of North America, 26*(2), 279–294.

Polo-Kantola, P., Erkkola, R., Helenius, H., et al. (1998). When does estrogen replacement therapy improve sleep quality? *American Journal of Obstetrics and Gynecology, 187*(5), 1002–1009.

Prange, A. J., Wilson, I. C., & Alltop, L. B. (1972). Estrogen may well affect response to antide-pressant. *Journal of the American Medical Association, 219*(2), 143–144.

Reich, T., & Winokur, G. (1975). Postpartum psychoses in patients with manic depressive disorder. *Journal of Nervous Mental Disease, 151*, 60–68.

Reiter, R. (1994). Pineal function during aging: Attenuation of the melatonin rhythm and its neuro-biological consequences. *Acta Neurobiologiae Experimentalis, 54*, 31–39.

Roberts, H. (1985). *The patient patients: Women and their doctors.* London: Pandora Press.

Rubin, R., Heist, E., McGeoy, S., et al. (1992). Neuroendocrine aspects of primary endogenous de-pression. *Archives of General Psychiatry, 49*, 558–781.

Rubinow, D., Schmidt, P., & Roca, C. (1998). Hormone measures in reproductive endocrine-related mood disorders: Diagnostic issues. *Psychopharmacology Bulletin, 34*(3), 289–290.

Schiff, I., Regestein, Q., Tulchinsky, D., et al. (1979). Effects of estrogen on sleep and psychological state of hypogonadal women. *Journal of the American Medical Association, 242*, 2405–2407.

Schneider, L. S., Small, G., Hamilton, S. M., et al. (1997). Estrogen replacement and response to fluoxetine in a multicenter geriatric depression trial. *American Journal of Geriatric Psychiatry, 5*, 97–106.

Schneider, M. A., Brotherton, P. I., & Hailes, J. (1977). The effect of exogenous oestrogens on de-pression in menopausal women. *Medical Journal of Australia, 2*, 162–163.

Shapira, B., Oppenheim, G., Zohar, J., et al. (1985). Lack of efficacy of estrogen supplementation to imipramine in resistant female depressives. *Biological Psychiatry, 20*, 570–583.

Shaver, J., Giblin, E., Lentz, M., et al. (1988). Sleep patterns and stability in perimenopausal women. *Sleep, 11*(6), 556–561.

Sherwin, B., & Gelfand, M. (1985). Sex steroid and affect in the surgical menopause: A double-blind, cross-over study. *Psychoneuroendocrinology, 10*, 325–335.

Smith, W. G. (1971). Critical life-events and prevention strategies in mental health. *Archives of General Psychiatry, 25*, 103–109.

Stahl, S. (1998). Augmentation of antidepressants by estrogen. *Psychopharmacology Bulletin, 34*(3), 319–321.

Stewart, D. E., & Boydell, K. (1993). Psychologic distress during menopause: Associations across the reproductive life cycle. *International Journal of Psychiatry in Medicine, 23*(2), 157–162.

Tam, L., & Parry, B. L. (1999a). *New findings in the treatment of depression at menopause.* Manu-script submitted for publication.

Tam, L., & Parry, B. L. (1999b). *Does estrogen enhance the antidepressant effects of fluoxetine?* Manuscript submitted for publication.

Thomas, E. M., & Armstrong, S. M. (1989). Effect of ovariectomy and estradiol on unity of female rat circadian rhythms. *American Journal of Physiology, 257*, 1241–1250.

Thomson, J., & Oswald, I. (1997). Effects of oestrogen on the sleep, mood, and anxiety of meno-pausal women. *British Medical Journal, ii*, 1317–1319.

Warnock, J. (1890). On some of the relationships between menstruation and insanity. *North Amer-ican Practitioner, 2*, 49–59.

Weissman, M. M. (1979). The myth of involutional melancholia. *Journal of the American Medical Association, 242*(8), 742–744.

Weissman, M. M. (1995, May). Paper presented at the 148th Annual Convention of the American Psychiatric Association, Miami, FL.

Weissman, M. M. (1996, May). *Epidemiology of major depression in women: Women and the con-troversies in hormonal replacement therapy.* Paper presented at the 148th Annual Convention of the American Psychiatric Association, New York.

Wilbur, J., Miller, A., & Montgomery, A. (1995). The Influence of demographic characteristics, menopausal status, and symptoms on women's attitudes toward menopause. *Women and Health, 23*(3), 19–39.

Winokur, G. (1973). Depression in the menopause. *American Journal of Psychiatry, 130*(1), 92–93.

Winokur, G., & Cadoret, R. (1975). The irrelevance of the menopause to depressive disease. In E. J. Sachar (Ed.), *Topics in psychoendocrinology*. New York: Grune & Stratton.

Woods, N. F., & Mitchell, E. S. (1996). Patterns of depressed mood in mid-life women: Observations from the Seattle Mid-Life Women's Health Study. *Research in Nursing and Health, 19*, 111–123.

Part II

Assessment and Treatment of Psychiatric Disorders in Women

8

Depression

SUSAN G. KORNSTEIN
BARBARA A. WOJCIK

Women are at greater risk for depression than are men, especially during the reproductive years. In addition to the difference in prevalence, recent studies show gender differences in both clinical presentation and treatment response. This chapter provides an overview of the literature on gender differences in depression, focusing on special considerations in the evaluation and treatment of depression in women. Epidemiological data are presented, as well as vulnerability factors that contribute to women's greater predisposition to depression. Gender issues in presentation are discussed, including differences in symptoms, comorbid disorders, course of illness features, and triggers of episodes. Studies that have examined gender differences in response to various treatments for depression, including antidepressant medications, psychotherapy, and electroconvulsive therapy (ECT), are reviewed. The chapter concludes with directions for future research.

PREVALENCE DATA

Epidemiological studies have consistently shown that depression is about twice as common in women as in men. This finding has been noted in both of the major community-based surveys of psychiatric disorders in the United States, the Epidemiologic Catchment Area (ECA) study (Regier et al., 1988) and the National Comorbidity Survey (NCS; Kessler et al., 1993). For major depressive disorder (MDD), the NCS demonstrated a lifetime prevalence rate of 21.3% in women versus 12.7% in men—a female-to-male relative risk of 1.7. The lifetime prevalence rates of dysthymia showed a similar sex ratio, with rates of 8.0% in women and 4.8% in men (Kessler et al., 1994).

Cross-national studies have also found rates of MDD to be higher in women; however, the sex ratio has varied among countries, ranging from 1.6 in Beirut and Taiwan to 3.5 in Munich (Weissman et al., 1996). In the most recent large-scale worldwide study, the World Health Organization (WHO) gathered data from 14 countries on gender differences in psychological problems in primary care (Maier et al., 1999). The female-to-male prevalence ratio for current, remitted, first-episode, and lifetime MDD remained nearly constant at 2:1. A similar sex ratio has been found among Korean immigrants to Canada (Noh et al., 1992), Laotian and Vietnamese refugees (Chung & Kagawa-Singer, 1993), and Israelis living in a kibbutz (Levav et al., 1991).

The gender difference in depression varies across the life cycle, with the female-to-male predominance beginning in early adolescence and persisting through midlife (Kessler et al., 1993). Longitudinal studies have demonstrated that the gender difference emerges by the age of 13 (Choi et al., 1997; Hankin et al., 1998). By age 15, lifetime prevalence rates are 4.5% in boys and 6.9% in girls; by age 18, they are 14.1% and 27.5%, similar to those in adults. The gender gap appears to be generated from an increase in the rates of depression in girls that far exceeds the rise in prevalence among boys (Cyranowski et al., 2000; Hankin et al., 1998).

There is conflicting evidence as to whether the gender difference in rates of depression disappears after midlife. The Netherlands Mental Health Survey and Incidence Study found the prevalence of mood disorders to be lowest among the 55–64 age group; however, the 1-month, 12-month, and lifetime prevalence rates for MDD and dysthymia in this group continued to approximate 2:1 in women versus men (Bijl et al., 1998). Similarly, a prevalence ratio of 2.5:1 was found to exist among elderly women and men in Spain (Zunzunegui et al., 1998). In contrast, data from the British National Survey of Psychiatric Morbidity showed the female preponderance to be evident only before the age of 55, with the fall in the sex ratio being due to a decline in female prevalence after menopause. In support of this finding, a study of African Americans over age 65 and a study of octo- and nonagenerians revealed no gender difference in prevalence rates of depression (Brown et al., 1992; Meller et al., 1997).

VULNERABILITY FACTORS FOR DEPRESSION IN WOMEN

Artifact Theories

Some researchers have questioned whether the sex difference in prevalence rates of depression are real or artifactual. For example, women's tendency to seek help more than men could lead to an overreporting of depression in women (Kessler et al., 1981); however, the higher rates among women found in community-based surveys refute this theory (Kessler et al., 1993; Regier et al., 1988; Weissman et al., 1993). Other artifactual theories propose that the female predominance is explained by differences in symptom reporting or differential recall in men and women, or suggest that the diagnostic criteria for depression are biased by sex (Angst & Dobler-Mikola, 1984; Ernst & Angst, 1992). However, studies that have varied the method of evaluation and symptom threshold for depression have found that such factors do not account for the observed gender differences (Kessler, 2000; Young et al., 1990)

Hormonal Factors

Hormonal factors related to the reproductive cycle may play a role in women's increased vulnerability to depression (Parry, 2000). Estrogen and progesterone have been shown to affect neurotransmitter, neuroendocrine, and circadian systems that have been implicated in mood disorders (Young et al., see Chapter 1, this volume). For example, they have been shown to influence the synthesis and release of both serotonin and norepinephrine. Prenatal exposure to estrogen-like substances, specifically diethylstilbestrol, may increase the lifetime risk of depression in both genders (Blehar & Oren, 1995).

Pubertal status (specifically, Tanner Stage III) has been shown to be superior to chronological age at predicting risk for depression in adolescent girls (Angold et al., 1998; Patton et al., 1997). One possible explanation involves oxytocin, which increases fivefold at puberty and appears to be related to an increase in both sexual behavior and pair bonding in females (Frank & Young, 2000). Girls may be at risk for developing depression when their increased desire for affiliation interacts with interpersonal and romantic disappointments (Cyranowski et al., 2000; Brown et al., 1995).

The luteal phase of the menstrual cycle, which is a period of estrogen and progesterone withdrawal, is frequently associated with dysphoric mood changes as well as the onset or worsening of a major depressive episode (Endicott, 1993; Kornstein et al., 1996b). Approximately 5% of women meet criteria for a severe form of premenstrual syndrome known as premenstrual dysphoric disorder (Kornstein, 1997a; see Steiner & Born, Chapter 3, this volume). The similarity of this disorder to MDD may indicate a hormonally based vulnerability to depression in some women (Halbreich & Endicott, 1985; Parry, 1995).

The postpartum period is also a common trigger for the onset of depressive symptoms (Nonacs & Cohen, 1998; see Arnold et al., Chapter 5, this volume). Up to 80% of women experience minor mood symptoms during this period, commonly known as the "postpartum blues." Postpartum depression occurs in 10–15% of new mothers, and the rates are considerably higher in those with a prior history of mood disorder. A woman who has experienced a postpartum depression is at risk for future episodes of depression, both in association with and independent of reproductive events. The risk of a subsequent postpartum episode may exceed 50%.

Although the onset of menopause marks a time of decreased risk for depression in women, minor depressive symptoms are common during the perimenopausal period (Avis et al., 1994; see Ayubi-Moak & Parry, Chapter 7, this volume). In addition, data from the NCS demonstrate that the number of recurrent depressive episodes during a 12-month period is higher in females than in males of the 45–54 age group, suggesting that the perimenopausal period is a time of increased risk for recurrence in women with a history of MDD (Kessler et al., 1993). Also of note is a possible association between depression and premature menopause (Harlow et al., 1995).

Other hormonal factors that may contribute to women's vulnerability to mood disorders include sex differences related to the hypothalamic–pituitary–adrenal (HPA) axis and to thyroid function. The possible role of the HPA axis in female depression has been discussed extensively by Young et al. in Chapter 1. Thyroid axis abnormalities are much more prevalent in women than in men and have been closely linked to depression. In addition, thyroid dysfunction may play a possible role in both postpartum mood disorders and premenstrual syndrome (Reus, 1989; Whybrow, 1995).

Genetic Factors

Family and twin studies have investigated genetic factors as an explanation for higher rates of depression in women (Merikangas et al., 1985; Kendler & Prescott, 1999). Although genetic transmission plays an important role in the etiology of depression, researchers have generally found similar heritability in men and women. Recently, Kendler and Prescott (1999) studied the relative contributions of genetic and environmental factors to depression and found no differences by gender. The authors note, however, that specific genetic risk factors may differ between the sexes. For example, genetic susceptibility to premenstrual symptoms has been shown to account for about 17% of the genetic risk for lifetime MDD in women (Kendler et al., 1998).

Preexisting Anxiety

Breslau et al. (1995) have asserted that the greater prevalence rate of depression in women is explained by the effect of preexisting anxiety disorders, which are approximately twice as common in females as in males beginning in childhood. In their study, the risk of MDD was higher at all ages and in both genders for those with a history of anxiety disorders, with the gender difference in depression decreasing when prior anxiety was controlled for. This finding was refuted by data from the NCS (Kessler, 2000). When prior anxiety disorders as well as substance use disorders and conduct disorder were controlled for in the NCS data, the sex ratio for first onset of MDD remained 2:1, identical to the ratio for those subjects without preexisting comorbid disorders.

Gender-Specific Socialization and Coping Styles

Gender differences in early developmental socialization processes have been described extensively (Ruble et al., 1993). Parents and teachers tend to have different expectations of girls and boys, which may result in girls' becoming more nurturing and more concerned with the evaluations of others, and in boys' developing a greater sense of mastery and independence. Such stereotypical gender socialization is hypothesized to lead to differences in self-concept and vulnerability to depression.

Nolen-Hoeksema (1995) has demonstrated a self-focused, ruminative style of coping in women in response to feelings of sadness; men, in contrast, tend to use distracting strategies. This observation is consistent with the results of a positron emission tomography study that indicated sex differences in the processing of emotional stimuli (George et al., 1996). Nolen-Hoeksema (1995) hypothesizes that this difference in coping styles may contribute to longer and more severe depressive episodes in women. In addition, the interaction of a ruminative coping style with gender-specific challenges during adolescence may contribute to the emergence of the female predominance in depression.

Stressful Life Events

Across the life cycle, women may experience more stressful life events than men and may be more sensitive to their effects. Adolescent girls tend to report a greater number of negative life events, particularly those related to parent–child and peer relationships (Rudolph & Hammen, 1999), than adolescent boys, and to experience higher levels of associated distress (Cyranowski et al., 2000). A significant relationship has been demonstrated between the number of life stressors and depressive symptoms in adolescent girls (Ge et al., 1994). Girls have been shown to be more susceptible than boys to depressive symptoms in response to family discord and maternal depression (Davies & Windle, 1997).

Studies of adults have also shown women to be more likely than men to experience the onset of depression following a stressful life event, particularly in response to stressors that involve children, housing, and reproductive problems (Nazroo et al., 1997). They are also more likely to report a stressful life event in the 6 months preceding a major depressive episode (Bebbington et al., 1988; Karp & Frank, 1995). Moreover, the stressors that may precipitate depression in women may involve events not only in their own lives but also in the lives of those around them (Dohrenwend, 1976; Kessler & McLeod, 1984).

Major Life Trauma

Sex differences in major life trauma may also contribute to increased vulnerability to depression in women (see Brand, Chapter 32, this volume). A history of sexual abuse is more common in women than in men and is a major risk factor for depression and other psychiatric disorders (Bifulco et al., 1991; Weiss et al., 1999). As many as 69% of abused women develop depression (Carmen et al., 1984). On the other hand, Kessler (2000) asserts that gender differences in the incidence of life trauma do not explain the difference in prevalence rates of depression. He controlled for more than 24 types of life trauma in the NCS data and found that the sex ratio remained 2:1, identical to the ratio for those subjects without preexisting trauma.

Social Status and Roles

The socioeconomic status of women has been proposed as another possible factor leading to higher rates of depression. More women than men live in poverty, and many are single mothers (Brown & Moran, 1997). Women achieve lower educational attainment than men and face fewer opportunities and salary inequities in the workplace (see Shrier, Chapter 31, this volume). In addition, women struggle with more limited resources for obtaining health care.

Although marriage was once considered a risk factor for depression in women, it is now understood as merely being less protective for women than for men (see Lasswell, Chapter 30, this volume). A good marriage, in which support is forthcoming at times of stress, can decrease the risk of depression in both genders; however, married women continue to experience higher rates of depression, and in unhappy marriages women are much more likely than men to become depressed (Wu & DeMaris, 1996). Women's unique need for extensive social support is reflected in their decreased incidence of depression when they seek support outside marriage during stressful times. This observation stands in contrast to the increased rate of depression in men forced to seek outside support, which suggests men's greater dependence on spousal support (Edwards et al., 1998). Women are more sensitive than men to the effects of divorce, demonstrating higher rates of depression, whereas men report more alcohol problems (Horwitz et al., 1996).

In addition to marital status, both occupational status and children may influence the risk of depression in women. A satisfying job may help to decrease a woman's risk of depression, but only if she has chosen to work rather than being forced to do so by financial pressures. The presence of young children at home is also a risk factor for depression in women, especially if a woman works outside the home and has difficulty finding child care (Bebbington et al., 1998; Ross & Mirowsky, 1988). In the WHO study discussed earlier, the gender difference in prevalence was decreased by 50% when men and women were matched for marital status, occupational status, and children (Maier et al., 1999). This finding is consistent with an earlier study showing few gender differences in depression rates among college students (Stangler & Printz, 1980). With the progressive changes in environmental stressors and gender roles, some argue that the magnitude of the gender gap may be decreasing as a result of higher rates of depression among men (Weissman et al., 1993).

GENDER DIFFERENCES IN PRESENTATION

Symptoms and Severity

Although depressive symptoms in men and women have generally been found to be similar overall, women are more likely to present with atypical or "reverse vegetative" symptoms, such as increased appetite and weight gain (Benazzi, 1999; Blehar & Oren, 1997; Kornstein, 1997b; Thase et al., 2000; Young et al., 1990). In the only study using actual patient weights, a trend for weight gain in depressed women and an associated trend for weight loss in depressed men was demonstrated (Stunkard et al., 1990). Women also have higher reporting rates of disturbed sleep, psychomotor retardation, expressed anger, anxiety, and somatization (Angst & Dobler-Mikola, 1984; Frank et al., 1988; Kornstein et al., 1996a, 2000b; Perugi et al., 1990; Young et al., 1990).

Women tend to report a greater number of depressive symptoms than men (Angst & Dobler-Mikola, 1984). The difference in number of depressive symptoms appears to begin in adolescence (Avison & McAlpine, 1992; Compas et al., 1997). As the number of symptoms required to make the diagnosis of depression is increased, so does the female preponderance (Ernst & Angst, 1992; Kessler et al., 1993; Maier et al., 1999). In the WHO study discussed earlier, the highest proportion of women was found when a somatic syndrome similar to melancholia was required for a depression diagnosis (Maier et al., 1999).

Most studies have found no gender difference in severity of depressive symptoms or functional impairment, although higher scores in women have been noted on self-report measures and on depression scales that include atypical symptoms (Frank et al., 1988; Young et al., 1990). A recent study of chronically depressed patients found a greater severity of illness in women across several measures, as well as greater functional impairment, a younger age of illness onset, and greater family history of mood disorder (Kornstein et al., 2000b). These findings suggest that chronicity of depression may affect women more seriously than men. A study by Berndt et al. (2000) demonstrating that early onset of chronic MDD adversely affects the educational attainment and expected lifetime earnings of women, but not of men, supports this conclusion.

Suicide

Although women are three times more likely than men to attempt suicide, men account for 65% of completed suicides (Isometsa et al., 1994; Moscicki, 1997). In addition, women are significantly more likely than men to have received psychiatric treatment and to have related their suicidal ideation to their families or to medical professionals prior to their attempts (Isometsa et al., 1994). Men tend to choose more violent means of suicide, such as guns or hanging, whereas women more often take overdoses or drown.

Gender differences in suicidal behavior and predictors of suicide appear to emerge in the child and adolescent population. Even in this age group, girls report more frequent suicidal ideation (Andrews & Lewinsohn, 1992; Bettes & Walker, 1986) and account for a higher proportion of suicide attempts, whereas boys account for a greater percentage of completed suicides (Shaffer et al., 1988). Although depression has been demonstrated to be a strong predictor of suicidal behavior in both sexes, comorbid substance abuse or conduct disorder results in higher rates of suicidality among girls (Wannan & Fombonne, 1998).

Comorbidity

The presence of a comorbid disorder tends to complicate diagnosis and generally predicts a worse outcome in the treatment of depression (Keitner et al., 1991). The ECA study and the NCS both demonstrated that depressed women have higher rates of psychiatric comorbidity than do depressed men, with notable differences in the comorbid diagnoses (Blazer et al., 1994; Regier et al., 1990). Specifically, depressed women are more likely to have comorbid phobias, generalized anxiety disorder, panic disorder, and eating disorders (Carter et al., 1999; Ernst & Angst, 1992; Fava et al., 1996; Kendler et al., 1993; Regier et al., 1990; see Pigott & Ferguson, Chapter 11, and Powers, Chapter 13, this volume). In contrast, depressed men are more likely to have a comorbid substance use disorder (Regier et al., 1990). However, women have been shown to be more likely than men to develop alcoholism once they are depressed (Hanna & Grant, 1997), and depression has been associated with a relapse of alcohol abuse or dependence primarily in women (Schutte et al., 1997; see Canterbury, Chapter 12, this volume).

Comorbid personality disorders in depressed patients may also affect assessment and treatment outcome. Data from the National Institute of Mental Health (NIMH) Treatment of Depression Collaborative Research Program showed no gender difference in overall prevalence rates of comorbid personality disorders (Shea et al., 1987), although differences may exist with regard to specific personality disorders. Golomb et al. (1995) reported a greater prevalence of narcissistic, antisocial, and obsessive–compulsive personality disorders in men compared to women outpatients with MDD. Consistent with these findings, a recent study of chronically depressed patients also revealed no difference in overall frequency of comorbid personality disorder by gender, but obsessive–compulsive, passive–aggressive, and narcissistic personality disorders were diagnosed significantly more often in men (Kornstein et al., 1996). Grilo et al. (1996) found that among depressed adolescent inpatients, girls were more likely then boys to be diagnosed with borderline personality disorder.

With regard to general medical comorbidity, depressed women show a greater prevalence of thyroid disease (Reus, 1989; Whybrow, 1995; see Brasch et al., Chapter 29, this volume) and migraine headaches (Moldin et al., 1993; see Field & Brackin, Chapter 27) than do depressed men. Thyroid screening is recommended for depressed women aged 45 and older, or for women with a personal or family history of thyroid disease (Whybrow, 1995). Migraine headaches in women are often influenced by reproductive hormonal changes associated with menarche, the menstrual cycle, pregnancy, and oral contraceptive use (Kornstein & Parker, 1997). Other comorbid general medical disorders common in depressed women include chronic fatigue syndrome, fibromyalgia (see Staropoli & Stotzko, Chapter 22), chronic pelvic pain (see Dell, Chapter 20), and irritable bowel syndrome (see Wise & Crone, Chapter 25). The increased risk of myocardial infarction among those with a history of depression should also be borne in mind by clinicians treating depressed women patients (Pratt et al., 1996; see Hansen-Grant, Chapter 24).

Course of Illness

Studies that have examined course features of MDD generally have shown no sex differences in age at onset (Burke et al., 1990; Frank et al., 1988; Kessler et al., 1993; Thase et al., 1994; Weissman et al., 1993), although a recent study has found an earlier age of onset in women in a chronically depressed sample (Kornstein et al., 2000b). Similarly, most studies have not shown differences by gender in the number, duration, chronicity, or recurrence of major depressive episodes (Eaton et al., 1997; Frank et al., 1988; Keller et al., 1986; Kessler et al., 1993; Simpson et al., 1997; Thase et al., 1994). Evidence from several longitudinal studies, however, suggests that women have longer episodes of depression and are more likely than men to develop a chronic or recurrent course (Aneshensel, 1985; Ernst & Angst, 1992; Keitner et al., 1991; Sargeant et al., 1990; Winokur et al., 1993).

Precipitating Factors

Gender differences exist with regard to precipitating factors for depressive episodes. As mentioned earlier, women have been shown to be more sensitive than men to becoming depressed following a stressful life event (Bebbington et al., 1988). The type of stressor may be of significance, with women being more sensitive to family events and men to financial difficulties (Kessler & McLeod, 1984). Seasonal changes are also more likely to trigger depressive episodes in women than in men. Of those who suffer from seasonal affective disorder, nearly 80% are women (Leibenluft et al., 1995). In addition, many women experience depressive symptoms in relation to reproductive cycle events, such as premenstrually, during the postpartum period, and during the perimenopause. Hormonal therapies, including hormonal contraceptives, hormone replacement therapy, and infertility medications, may also be associated with depressive symptoms (Kornstein, 1997b). The assessment and management of reproductive-cycle-related mood disorders have been discussed extensively in preceding chapters of this volume (see Steiner & Born, Chapter 3; Nonacs et al., Chapter 4; Arnold et al., Chapter 5; Warnock & Blake, Chapter 6; and Ayubi-Moak & Parry, Chapter 7).

It is important to consider the influence of a patient's menstrual cycle on the course of her depression. This information is essential in order to accurately assess diagnosis, severity of depression, suicide risk, and response to treatment (Kornstein, 1997b). The patient's menstrual cycle day should be noted at the time of assessment and at subsequent visits. Prospective charting of symptoms over several cycles may be useful to clarify the symptom pattern. A depression occurring on a regular basis only during the premenstrual period would warrant a diagnosis of premenstrual dysphoric disorder (see Steiner & Born, Chapter 3). On the other hand, the presence of depressive symptoms throughout the cycle with worsening prior to menses is indicative of premenstrual exacerbation of depression. Data by Kornstein et al. (1996b) suggest that this phenomenon is reported by over 50% of chronically depressed premenopausal women, and over 25% demonstrate a pattern of premenstrual excerbation of depression with prospective charting.

A woman patient's menopausal status should also be noted in evaluating her depression, and if she is peri- or postmenopausal, the clinician should inquire whether she is taking hormone replacement therapy. As with the menstrual cycle, this clarification is important for both accurate diagnosis and treatment planning. For example, a middle-aged woman patient presenting with symptoms of insomnia, depressed mood, and concentration difficulties may be experiencing perimenopausal changes rather than a primary depressive disorder.

GENDER ISSUES IN TREATMENT

Treatment of depression requires special considerations with regard to gender (Kornstein & Wojcik, 2000). Sex differences in pharmacokinetics and pharmacological treatment response have been noted, as well as differences with regard to medication tolerability. In addition, gender differences in response to psychotherapy, combination treatment, and ECT have been reported. Such differences should be considered in choosing a treatment strategy for depressed women patients.

Pharmacotherapy

Pharmacokinetics

There is a growing literature demonstrating sex differences in pharmacokinetics, including differences in drug absorption and bioavailability, drug distribution, and drug metabolism and elimination (see Brawman-Mintzer & Book, Chapter 2). For example, women have a slower gastric emptying time, lower gastric acid secretion, higher percentage of body fat, decreased hepatic metabolism, and lower renal clearance compared to men (Hamilton & Yonkers, 1996). Such differences in pharmacokinetics may lead to higher plasma levels and longer half-lives of drugs, as well as a greater sensitivity to side effects in women. In addition, medication levels in women may be altered by hormonal changes associated with the menstrual cycle, pregnancy, or menopause, as well as by the use of exogenous hormones, such as oral contraceptives or hormone replacement therapy (Kornstein & Wojcik, 2000).

Treatment Response

Sex differences in treatment response to antidepressant medications have been described (Hamilton et al., 1996; Kornstein & Wojcik, 2000; Thase et al., 2000; see Brawman-Mintzer & Book, Chapter 2). Several researchers have noted that women respond more poorly than men to tricyclic antidepressants (TCAs) and appear to respond more favorably to selective serotonin reuptake inhibitors (SSRIs) or monoamine oxidase inhibitors (MAOIs) (Davidson & Pelton, 1985; Kornstein et al., 2000a; Old Age Depression Interest Group, 1993; Raskin, 1974; Steiner et al., 1993). A meta-analysis by Hamilton et al. (1996) of 35 studies that had reported imipramine response rates separately by gender showed significantly higher response rates in men. Davidson and Pelton (1985) found that among patients with atypical depression and panic attacks, men responded preferentially to TCAs and women to MAOIs. Steiner et al. (1993) compared paroxetine with imipramine and placebo in patients with major depression, and found that women responded significantly better to paroxetine than to imipramine. In contrast, Lewis-Hall et al. (1997) reported similar response rates to fluoxetine and TCAs in women with MDD.

The largest study to date comparing antidepressant response rates by gender is that by Kornstein et al. (2000a), who examined response rates to sertraline and imipramine in the treatment of chronic MDD and double depression. The results showed a significant gender × treatment interaction, with women responding more favorably to sertraline and men to imipramine. Response rates to the two medications in the study group as a whole were similar (Keller et al., 1998a), demonstrating the importance of analyzing data by gender. Tolerability differences were also noted, with women discontinuing their participation in the study more frequently on imipramine than on sertraline. In addition, an interaction between treatment response and menopausal status was found: Premenopausal women responded significantly better to sertraline than to imipramine, whereas there was no difference in response rates to the two drugs among postmenopausal women (Kornstein et al., 2000a). Thus the poor responsiveness to TCAs occurs predominantly in premenopausal women, as suggested in an earlier study by Raskin (1974). The positive response of chronically depressed women to SSRIs was also noted by Yonkers et al. (1996) in dysthymic patients.

Differences in response rates by gender and by age group in women were also reported by Martenyi et al. (2001). In their comparison of fluoxetine and the norepinephrine reuptake inhitibor maprotiline in depressed inpatients, women responded significantly better to fluoxetine than to maprotiline, whereas men responded similarly to the two drugs. Moreover, the difference in response rates was again noted only in younger (< 44 years) women. Older (≥ 44 years) women showed no responsivity to the two antidepressants, nor did men of either age group.

A recent meta-analysis compared response rates to nefazodone, imipramine, and placebo for the treatment of major depression (Kornstein & McEnany, 2000). No sex difference in nefazodone efficacy was found; differences in imipramine response were consistent with other studies. Men responded as well to imipramine as to nefazodone, whereas response rates to imipramine in women were no greater than placebo.

Another meta-analysis compared response rates to bupropion (sustained-release), sertraline, and placebo by gender in patients with recurrent MDD (Kornstein & Wojcik, 2000). In both men and women, bupropion and sertraline were equally effective and superior to placebo. There were no significant sex differences in response rates to any of the three treatments.

A recent study examined the effect of gender on response to venlafaxine, SSRIs (fluoxetine, fluvoxamine, or paroxetine), and placebo in patients with MDD. In both men and women, response and remission rates to venlafaxine and SSRIs were superior to placebo after 8 weeks of treatment. A more rapid response and higher remission rates were noted with venlafaxine compared to the SSRIs in both genders (Entsuah et al., in press).

Very few studies have addressed sex differences in recurrence rates during maintenance antidepressant treatment. The Old Age Depression Interest Group (1993) in Britain conducted a 2-year maintenance-phase trial of the TCA dothiepin versus placebo in elderly patients with MDD who had responded to acute-phase treatment with dothiepin. They found that in both the dothiepin and placebo groups, women were significantly more likely to experience a recurrence than men, again suggesting that women are generally at greater risk for recurrence of depression.

Similar results were seen in a recent 18-month study of sertraline versus placebo in preventing recurrence among patients with chronic MDD or double depression who had responded to sertraline during 7 months of acute- and continuation-phase treatment. Regardless of gender, the rate of recurrence of major depression was about four times higher in patients on placebo than in those who remained on sertraline (Keller et al., 1998b). For both sertraline and placebo, however, rates of recurrence were higher in women than in men, although the differences were not statistically significant (Kornstein et al., 1999).

Augmentation

Several augmentation strategies to enhance antidepressant response have shown possible advantages in women (Kornstein & Wojcik, 2000). For example, augmentation with triiodothyronine may be more beneficial in women than in men (Coppen et al., 1972; Prange et al., 1969; Frye et al., 1997). Two preliminary studies, one with fluoxetine (Schneider et al., 1997) and one with sertraline (Schneider et al., 1998), suggest that estrogen replacement therapy may enhance response to SSRIs in postmenopausal women, whereas testosterone augmentation may be a useful strategy in men (Seidman & Rabkin, 1998). In addition, there is some suggestion that lithium (Dallal et al., 1990) and stimulants (Askinazi et al., 1986) may be more effective as augmenting agents in women.

Psychotherapy

Few studies have examined gender differences in response to psychotherapy for depression. Sex was not a predictor of response to cognitive-behavioral therapy (CBT) or interpersonal psychotherapy (IPT) in the NIMH Treatment of Depression Collaborative Research Program (Sotsky et al., 1991). Thase et al. (1994) also found similar response rates in men and women treated with CBT; however, in the subgroup with more severe depression, women showed a significantly poorer response to CBT than men. A similar study using IPT found comparable results in men and women, including those with severe depression (Thase et al., 1997a).

Frank et al. (1988) explored sex differences in response to combined treatment with imipramine and IPT in recurrent MDD. They found that men were more likely than women to achieve a rapid and sustained clinical response and to be classified as "normal responders." During the 3-year placebo-controlled maintenance trial, no sex-related differences in recurrence rates were noted (Frank et al., 1990) although the study was not statistically powered to detect such differences. In a meta-analysis of the University of Pittsburgh data set, Thase et al. (1997b) compared psychotherapy alone (either IPT or CBT) to combination treatment with IPT plus a TCA (either imipramine or nortriptyline). Men showed a greater response to combined treatment than to psychotherapy alone across all age groups. In women under 40 years of age, there was no advantage of combined treatment over psychotherapy alone, whereas women over age 50 responded to combined treatment as well as did men. The use of TCAs as the medication component in these studies may be an important factor in these results, given the poorer response of younger women to TCAs.

A recently completed study by Keller et al. (2000) compared combination treatment using nefazodone and the Cognitive Behavioral Analysis System of Psychotherapy (McCullough, 2000) with both monotherapies in chronically depressed patients. A preliminary analysis of these results by gender (Kornstein, 1999) suggests equal benefit of combination treatment in men and women.

Phototherapy

Only one study has examined sex differences in response to phototherapy. Leibenluft et al. (1995) reported no differences in phototherapy response between men and women with seasonal affective disorder.

Electroconvulsive Therapy

Some studies have reported that women require lower electrical stimulus doses than men during ECT, indicating that they have lower seizure thresholds (Coffey et al., 1995; McCall et al., 1993; Sackheim et al., 1987). Differences in cognitive side effects of ECT have also been noted. One study found less cognitive impairment from right unilateral ECT in women than in men—a finding that may be explained by sex differences in the lateralization of brain functions (Sackheim et al., 1986). Several studies that reported outcome by gender suggest that women have a more favorable acute-phase response to ECT than men (Coryell & Zimmerman, 1984; Greenblatt et al., 1962; Herrington et al., 1974; Medical Research Council, 1965); however, recent data by Thase et al. (2000) indicate a higher risk of relapse in women following ECT.

SUMMARY AND FUTURE DIRECTIONS

Women show a greater risk for depression than men, particularly during the childbearing years; this appears to result from the interaction of biological, psychological, and social factors. In addition to the well-established difference in prevalence rates, other significant gender-related differences in depression have been demonstrated with regard to both clinical presentation and treatment response. The assessment of depression in women should include attention to reverse vegetative symptoms, course of illness features, comorbid psychiatric and general medical disorders, and precipitating factors (such as seasonal changes, psychosocial stressors, and reproductive cycle events). Treatment of depressed women should consider the growing evidence of sex differences in pharmacokinetics, medication tolerability, and response rates.

Clearly, there is a need for further research in this area. One important goal would be to achieve a more comprehensive understanding of the basis for women's increased vulnerability to depression. Current theories have tended to be either purely biological or purely psychosocial; a more integrated theoretical approach is warranted to account for the full complexity of gender differences in depression. There is a need for additional studies examining gender differences in clinical features of depression and differences in response to various types of pharmacotherapy, psychotherapy, and combination treatment, as well as issues of tolerability and treatment strategies for nonresponders and patients with comorbid disorders. More research is likewise necessary on gender-related issues in the long-term management of depression, including the optimum duration of treatment and the efficacy of various treatment options in preventing relapse and recurrence. Further study of the effects of reproductive cycle events, such as the menstrual cycle and menopause, on the course and treatment of depression is also in order. Finally, there is a need for research on prevention and early detection of depression in young women. A particular focus on the dramatic rise in female depression during the early adolescent years may allow for targeted interventions to prevent, or at least to lessen the burden of, this often chronic and recurrent disorder.

REFERENCES

Andrews, J. A., & Lewinsohn, P. M. (1992). Suicidal attempts among older adolescents: Prevalence and co-occurrence with psychiatric disorders. *Journal of the American Academy of Child and Adolescent Psychiatry, 32,* 655–662.

Aneshensel, C. S. (1985). The natural history of depressive symptoms. *Research in Community Mental Health, 5,* 45–74.

Angold, A., Costello, E. F., & Worthman, C. M. (1998). Puberty and depression: The roles of age, pubertal status, and pubertal timing. *Psychological Medicine, 28,* 51–61.

Angst, J., & Dobler-Mikola, A. (1984). Do the diagnostic criteria determine the sex ratio in depression? *Journal of Affective Disorders, 7,* 189–198.

Askinazi, C., Weintraub, R. J., & Karamouz, N. (1986). Elderly depressed females as a possible subgroup of patients responsive to methylphenidate. *Journal of Clinical Psychiatry, 47*(9), 467–469.

Avis, N. E., Brambilla, D., McKinley, S. M., et al. (1994). A longitudinal analysis of the association between menopause and depression. *Annals of Epidemiology, 4,* 214–220.

Avison, W. R., & McAlpine, D. D. (1992). Gender differences in symptoms of depression among adolescents. *Journal of Health and Social Behavior, 33,* 77–96.

Bebbington, P. E., Brugha, T., MacCarthy, B., et al. (1988). The Camberwell Collaborative Depression Study: I. Depressed probands: adversity and the form of depression. *British Journal of Psychiatry, 152,* 754–765.

Bebbington, P. E., Dunn, G., Jenkins, R., et al. (1998). The influence of age and sex on the prevalence of depressive conditions: Report from the National Survey of Psychiatric Comorbidity. *Psychological Medicine, 28,* 9–19.

Benazzi, F. (1999). Gender differences in bipolar II and unipolar depressed outpatients: A 557–case study. *Annals of Clinical Psychiatry, 11*(2), 55–59.

Berndt, E. R., Koran, L. M., Finkelstein, S. N., et al. (2000). Lost human capital from early-onset chronic depression. *American Journal of Psychiatry, 157,* 940–947.

Bettes, B. A., & Walker, E. (1986). Symptoms associated with suicidal behaviour in childhood and adolescence. *Journal of Abnormal Child Psychology, 14,* 591–604.

Bifulco, A., Brown, G. W., & Adler, Z. (1991). Early sexual abuse and clinical depression in adult life. *British Journal of Psychiatry, 159,* 115–122.

Bijl, R. V., Ravelli, A., & van Zessen, G. (1998). Prevalence of psychiatric disorder in the general population: Results of the Netherlands Mental Health Survey and Incidence Study (NEMESIS). *Social Psychiatry and Psychiatric Epidemiology, 33,* 587–595.

Blazer, D. G., Kessler, R. C., McGonagle, K. A., et al. (1994). The prevalence and distribution of major depression in a national community sample: The National Comorbidity Survey. *American Journal of Psychiatry, 151,* 979–986.

Blehar, M. C., & Oren, D. A. (1995). Women's increased vulnerability to mood disorders: Integrating psychobiology and epidemiology. *Depression, 3,* 3–12.

Breslau, N., Schultz, L., & Peterson, E. (1997). Sex differences in depression: The role of preexisting anxiety. *Psychiatry Research, 58,* 1–12.

Brown, D. R., Milburn, N. G., & Gary, L. E. (1992). Symptoms of depression among older African-Americans: An analysis of gender differences. *The Gerontologist, 32*(6), 789–795.

Brown, G. W., Harris, T. O., & Hepworth, C. (1995). Loss, humiliation and entrapment among women developing depression: A patient and non-patient comparison. *Psychological Medicine, 25,* 7–21.

Brown, G. W., & Moran, P. M. (1997). Single mothers, poverty, and depression. *Psychological Medicine, 27,* 21–33.

Burke, K. C., Burke, J. D., Regier, D. A., et al. (1990). Age at onset of selected mental disorders in five community populations. *Archives of General Psychiatry, 47,* 511–518.

Carmen, E., Rieker, P. P., & Mills, T. (1984). Victims of violence and psychiatric illness. *American Journal of Psychiatry, 141,* 378–383.

Carter, J. D., Joyce, P. R., Mulder, R. T., et al. (1999). Gender differences in the rate of comorbid Axis I disorders in depressed outpatients. *Depression and Anxiety, 9,* 49–53.

Choi, W. S., Patten, C. A., Gillin, J. C., et al. (1997). Cigarette smoking predicts development of depressive symptoms among U.S. adolescents. *Annals of Behavioral Medicine, 19*(1), 42–50.

Chung, R. C., & Kagawa-Singer, M. (1993). Predictors of psychological distress among Southeast Asian refugees. *Social Science and Medicine, 36*(5), 631–639.

Coffey, C. E., Lucke, J., Weiner, R. D., et al. (1995). Seizure threshold in electroconvulsive therapy: I. Initial seizure threshold. *Biologocal Psychiatry, 37,* 713–720.

Compas, B. E., Oppedisano, G., Connor, J. K., et al. (1997). Gender differences in depressive symptoms in adolescence: Comparison of national samples of clinically referred and nonreferred youths. *Journal of Consulting and Clinical Psychology, 65*(4), 617–626.

Coppen, A., Whybrow, P., Noguera, R., et al. (1972). The comparative antidepressant value of L-tryptophan and imipramine with and without attempted potentiation by liothyronine. *Archives of General Psychiatry, 26,* 234–241.

Coryell, W., & Zimmerman, M. (1984). Outcome following ECT for primary unipolar depression: A test of newly proposed response predictors. *American Journal of Psychiatry, 141,* 862–867.

Cyranowski, J. M., Frank, E., Young, E., et al. (2000). Adolescent onset of the gender difference in lifetime rates of major depression: A theoretical model. *Archives of General Psychiatry, 57,* 21–27.

Dallal, A., Fontaine, R., Ontiveros, A., et al. (1990). Lithium carbonate augmentation of desipramine in refractory depression. *Canadian Journal of Psychiatry, 35,* 608–611.

Davidson, J., & Pelton, S. (1985). Forms of atypical depression and their response to antidepressant drugs. *Psychiatry Research, 17,* 87–95.

Davies, P. T., & Windle, M. (1997). Gender-specific pathways between maternal depressive symptoms, family discord, and adolescent adjustment. *Developmental Psychology, 33,* 657–668.

Dohrenwend, B. S. (1976, April). *Anticipation and control of stressful life events: An explanatory analysis.* Paper presented at the 47th Annual Convention of the Eastern Psychological Association, New York.

Eaton, W. W., Anthony, A. C., Gallo, J., et al. (1997). Natural history of Diagnostic Interview Schedule DSM-IV major depression. *Archives of General Psychiatry, 54,* 993–999.

Edwards, A. C., Nazroo, J. Y., & Brown, G. W. (1998). Gender differences in marital support following a shared life event. *Social Science and Medicine, 46*(8), 1077–1085.

Endicott, J. (1993). The menstrual cycle and mood disorders. *Journal of Affective Disorders, 29,* 193–200.

Entsuah, R., Huang, H., & Thase, M. E. (in press). Response and remission rates in different subpopulations with major depressive disorder administered venlafaxine, selective serotonin reuptake inhibitors, or placebo. *Journal of Clnical Psychiatry.*

Ernst, C., & Angst, J. (1992). The Zurich study: XII. Sex differences in depression: Evidence from longitudinal epidemiological data. *European Archives of Psychiatry and Clinical Neuroscience, 241,* 222–230.

Fava, M., Abraham, M., Alpert, J., et al. (1996). Gender differences in Axis I comorbidity among depressed outpatients. *Journal of Affective Disorders, 38,* 129–133.

Frank, E., Carpenter, L. L., & Kupfer, D. J. (1988). Sex differences in recurrent depression: Are there any that are significant? *American Journal of Psychiatry, 145,* 41–45.

Frank, E., Kupfer, D. J., Perel, J. M., et al. (1990). Three-year outcomes for maintenance therapies in recurrent depression. *Archives of General Psychiatry, 47,* 1093–1099.

Frank, E., & Young, E. (2000). Pubertal changes and adolescent changes: Why do rates of depression rise precipitously for girls between ages 10 and 15 years? In E. Frank (Ed.), *Gender and its effects on psychopathology* (pp. 85–101). Washington, DC, American Psychiatric Press.

Frye, M. A., Denicoff, K. D., Luckenbaugh, D. A., et al. (1997, May). *Thyroid potentiation in affective illness.* Paper presented at the 150th Annual Convention of the American Psychiatric Association, San Diego, CA.

Ge, X., Lorenz, F. O., Conger, R. D., et al. (1994). Trajectories of stressful life events and depressive symptoms during adolescence. *Developmental Psychology, 30,* 467–483.

George, M. S., Ketter, T. A., Parekh, P. I., et al. (1996). Gender differences in regional cerebral blood flow during transient self-induced sadness or happiness. *Biological Psychiatry, 40,* 859–871.

Golomb, M., Fava, M., Abraham, M., et al. (1995). Gender differences in personality disorders. *American Journal of Psychiatry, 152,* 579–582.

Greenblatt, M., Grosser, G. H., & Wechsler, H. (1962). A comparative study of selected antidepressant medications and ECT. *American Journal of Psychiatry, 119,* 144–153.

Grilo, C. M., Becker, D. F., Walker, M. L., et al. (1996). Gender differences in personality disorders in psychiatrically hospitalized young adults. *Journal of Nervous and Mental Disease, 184,* 754–757.

Halbreich, U., & Endicott, J. (1985). Relationship of dysphoric premenstrual changes to depressive disorders. *Acta Psychiatrica Scandinavica, 71,* 331–338.

Hamilton, J. A., Grant, M., & Jensvold, M. F. (1996). Sex and treatment of depression: When does it matter? In M. F. Jensvold, U. Halbreich, & J. A. Hamilton (Eds.), *Psychopharmacology and women: Sex, gender, and hormones* (pp. 241–257). Washington, DC: American Psychiatric Press.

Hamilton, J. A., & Yonkers, K. A. (1996). Sex differences in pharmacokinetics of psychotropic medications: Part I. Physiological basis for effects. In M. F. Jensvold, U. Halbreich, & J. A. Hamilton (Eds.), *Psychopharmacology and women: Sex, gender, and hormones* (pp. 11–42). Washington, DC: American Psychiatric Press.

Hankin, B. L., Abramson, L. Y., Moffitt, T. E., et al. (1998). Development of depression from preadolescence to young adulthood: Emerging gender differences in a 10–year longitudinal study. *Journal of Abnormal Psychology, 107*(1), 128–140.

Hanna, E. Z., & Grant, B. F. (1997). Gender differences in DSM-IV alcohol use disorders and major depression as distributed in the general population: Clinical implications. *Comprehensive Psychiatry, 38,* 202–212.

Harlow, B. L., Cramer, D. W., & Annis, K. M. (1995). The association of medically treated depression and age at natural menopause. *American Journal of Epidemiology, 141,* 1170–1176.

Herrington, N., Bruce, A., & Johnstone, E. C. (1974). Comparative trial of l-tryptophan and ECT in severe depressive illness. *Lancet, ii,* 731–734.

Horwitz, A. V., White, H. R., & Howell-White, S. (1996). The use of multiple outcomes in stress research: A case study of gender differences in responses to marital dissolution. *Journal of Health and Social Behaviour, 37,* 278–291.

Isometsa, E. T., Henriksson, M. M., Aro, H., et al. (1994). Suicide in major depression. *American Journal of Psychiatry, 151,* 530–536.

Karp, J. F., & Frank, E. (1995). Combination therapy and the depressed women. *Depression, 3,* 91–98.

Keitner, G. I., Ryan, C. E., Miller, I. W., et al. (1991). 12–month outcome of patients with major depression and comorbid psychiatric or medical illness (compound depression). *American Journal of Psychiatry, 148,* 345–350.

Keller, M. B., Gelenberg, A. J., Hirschfeld, R. M. A., et al. (1998). The treatment of chronic depression, part 2: A double-blind randomized trial of sertraline and imipramine. *Journal of Clinical Psychiatry, 59,* 598–607.

Keller, M. B., Kocsis, J. H., & Thase, M. E. (1998b). Maintenance phase efficacy of sertraline for chronic depression: A double-blind, placebo-controlled study. *Journal of the American Medical Association, 280,* 1665–1672.

Keller, M. B., Lavori, P. W., Rice, J., et al. (1986). The persistent risk of chronicity in recurrent episodes of nonbipolar major depressive disorder: A prospective follow-up. *American Journal of Psychiatry, 143,* 24–28.

Keller, M. B., McCullough, J. P., Klein, D. N., et al. (2000). A comparison of nefazodone, Cognitive Behavioral Analysis System of Psychotherapy, and their combination for the treatment of chronic depression. *New England Journal of Medicine, 342,* 1462–1470.

Kendler, K. S., Karkowski, L. M., & Neale, M. C. (1998). A longitudinal population-based twin study of retrospectively reported premenstrual symptoms and lifetime major depression. *American Journal of Psychiatry, 155,* 1234–1240.

Kendler, K. S., Neale, M. C., Kessler, R. C., et al. (1993). Major depression and phobias: The genetic and environmental sources of comorbidity. *Psychological Medicine, 23,* 361–371.

Kendler, K. S., & Prescott, C. A. (1999). A population-based twin study of lifetime major depression in men and women. *Archives of General Psychiatry, 56,* 39–44.

Kessler, R. C. (2000). Gender differences in major depression: Epidemiological findings. In E. Frank (Ed.), *Gender and its effects on psychopathology* (pp. 61–84). Washington, DC: American Psychiatric Press.

Kessler, R. C., Brown, R. L., & Broman, C. L. (1981). Sex differences in psychiatric help-seeking: Evidence from four large-scale surveys. *Journal of Health and Social Behavior, 22,* 49–64.

Kessler, R. C., McGonagle, D. A., Swartz, M., et al. (1993). Sex and depression in the National Comorbidity Survey: I. Lifetime prevalence, chronicity, and recurrence. *Journal of Affective Disorders, 29,* 77–84.

Kessler, R. C., McGonagle, K. A., Zhao, S., et al. (1994). Lifetime and 12–month prevalence of DSM-III-R psychiatric disorders in the United States: Results from the National Comorbidity Survey. *Archives of General Psychiatry, 51,* 8–19.

Kessler, R. C., & McLeod, J. D. (1984). Sex differences in vulnerability to undesirable life events. *American Sociological Review, 49,* 620–631.

Kornstein, S. G. (1996, May). *Gender differences in chronic depression.* Paper presented at the 149th Annual Convention of the American Psychiatric Association, New York, NY.

Kornstein, S. G. (1997a). Premenstrual syndrome: An overview. *Primary Psychiatry, 4,* 56–60.

Kornstein, S. G. (1997b). Gender differences in depression: Implications for treatment. *Journal of Clinical Psychiatry, 58*(Suppl. 15), 12–18.

Kornstein, S. G., & McEnany, G. (2000). Enhancing pharmacologic effects in the treatment of depression in women. *Journal of Clinical Psychiatry, 61*(Suppl. 11), 18–27.

Kornstein, S. G., & Parker, A. J. (1997). Menstrual migraines: Pathophysiology, treatment, and relationship to premenstrual syndrome. *Current Concepts in Obstetrics and Gynecology, 9,* 154–158.

Kornstein, S. G. (July, 2000). *Longterm treatment of mood disorders.* Paper presented at XXVth Collegium Internationale Neuro-Pharmacologicum Congress, Brussels, Belgium.

Kornstein, S. G., Schatzberg, A. F., Thase, M. E., et al. (2000a). Gender differences in treatment response to sertraline and imipramine in chronic depression. *American Journal of Psychiatry, 157,* 1445–1452.

Kornstein, S. G., Schatzberg, A. F., & Thase, M. E. (2000b). Gender differences in chronic major and double depression. *Journal of Affective Disorders, 60,* 1–11.

Kornstein, S. G., Schatzberg, A. F., Yonkers, K. A., et al. (1996). Gender differences in presentation of chronic major depression. *Psychopharmacology Bulletin, 31,* 711–718.

Kornstein, S. G., & Wojcik, B. A. (2000). Gender effects in the treatment of depression. *Psychiatric Clinics of North America Annual of Drug Therapy, 7,* 23–57.

Kornstein, S. G., Yonkers, K. A., Schatzberg, A. F., et al. (1996b, May). *Premenstrual exacerbation of depression.* Paper presented at the 149th Annual Convention of the American Psychiatric Association, New York.

Leibenluft, E., Hardin, T. A., & Rosenthal, N. E. (1995). Gender differences in seasonal affective disorder. *Depression, 3,* 13–19.

Lewis-Hall, F. C., Wilson, M. G., Tepner, R. G., et al. (1997). Fluoxetine vs. tricyclic antidepressants in women with major depressive disorder. *Journal of Women's Health, 6,* 337–343.

Levav, I., Gilboa, S., & Ruiz, F. (1991). Demoralization and gender differences in a kibbutz. *Psychological Medicine, 21,* 1019–1028.

Maier, W., Gansicke, M., Gater, R., et al. (1999). Gender differences in the prevalence of depression: A survey in primary care. *Journal of Affective Disorders, 53,* 241–252.

Martenyi, F., Dossenbach, M., Mraz, K., et al. (2001). Gender differences in the efficacy of fluoxetine and maprotiline in depressed patients: A double-blind trial of antidepressants with serotonergic or norepinephrinergic reuptake inhibition profile. *European Neuropsychopharmacology, 11,* 227–232.

McCall, W. V., Shelp, F. E., Weiner, R. D., et al. (1993). Convulsive threshold differences in right unilateral and bilateral ECT. *Biological Psychiatry, 34,* 606–611.

McCullough, J. P. (2000). *Treatment for chronic depression: Cognitive behavioral analysis system of psychotherapy (CBASP).* New York: Guilford Press.

Medical Research Council. (1965). Clinical trial of the treatment of depressive illness. *British Medical Journal, i,* 881–886.

Meller, I., Fichter, M. M., & Schroppel, H. (1997). Risk factors and psychosocial consequences in depression of octo- and nonagenerians: Results of an epidemiological study. *European Archives of Psychiatry and Clinical Neuroscience, 247,* 278–287.

Merikangas, K. R., Weissman, M. M., & Pauls, D. L. (1985). Genetic factors in the sex ratio of major depression. *Psychological Medicine, 15,* 63–69.

Moldin, S. O., Scheftner, W. A., Rice, J. P., et al. (1993). Association between major depressive disorder and physical illness. *Psychological Medicine, 23,* 755–761.

Moscicki, E. K. (1997). Identification of suicide risk factors using epidemiologic studies. *Psychiatric Clinics of North America, 20,* 499–517.

Nazroo, J. Y., Edwards, A. C., & Brown, G. W. (1997). Gender differences in the onset of depression following a shared life event: A study of couples. *Psychological Medicine, 27,* 9–19.

Noh, S., Wu, Z., Speechley, M., et al. (1992). Depression in Korean immigrants in Canada: II. Correlates of gender, work, and marriage. *Journal of Nervous and Mental Disease, 180,* 578–582.

Nolen-Hoeksema, S. (1995). Gender differences in coping with depression across the lifespan. *Depression, 3,* 81–90.

Nonacs, R., & Cohen, L. S. (1998). Postpartum mood disorders: Diagnosis and treatment guidelines. *Journal of Clinical Psychiatry, 59*(Suppl. 2), 34–40.

Old Age Depression Interest Group. (1993). How long should the elderly take antidepressants?: A double-blind placebo-controlled study of continuation/prophylaxis therapy with dothiepin. *British Journal of Psychiatry, 162,* 175–182.

Parry, B. L. (1995). Sex hormones, circadian rhythms and depressive vulnerability. *Depression, 3,* 43–48.

Parry, B. L. (2000). Hormonal basis of mood disorders in women. In E. Frank (Ed.), *Gender and its effects on psychopathology* (pp. 61–84). Washington, DC: American Psychiatric Press.

Patton, G. C., Hibbert, M. E., Carlin, J., et al. (1997). Menarche and the onset of depression and anxiety in Victoria, Australia. *Journal of Epidemiology and Community Health, 50,* 661–666.

Perugi, G., Musetti, L., Simonini, E., et al. (1990). Gender-mediated clinical features of depressive illness: The importance of temperamental differences. *British Journal of Psychiatry, 157,* 835–841.

Prange, A. F., Wilson, I. C., Rabon, A. M., et al. (1969). Enhancement of imipramine antidepressant activity by thyroid hormone. *American Journal of Psychiatry, 126*(4), 457–469.

Pratt, L. A., Ford, D. E., Crum, R. M., et al. (1996). Depression, psychotropic medication, and the risk of myocardial infarction: Prospective data from the Baltimore ECA follow-up. *Circulation, 96,* 3123–3129.

Raskin, A. (1974). Age-sex differences in response to antidepressant drugs. *Journal of Nervous and Mental Disease, 159,* 120–130.

Regier, D. A., Boyd, J. H., Burke, J. D., et al. (1988). One-month prevalence of mental disorders in the United States. *Archives of General Psychiatry, 45,* 977–986.

Regier, D. A., Burke, J. D., & Burke, K. C. (1990). Comorbidity of affective and anxiety disorders in the NIMH Epidemiologic Catchment Area Program. In J. D. Maser & C. R. Cloninger (Eds.), *Comorbidity of mood and anxiety disorders* (pp. 113–122). Washington, DC: American Psychiatric Press.

Reus, V. I. (1989). Behavioral aspects of thyroid disease in women. *Psychiatric Clinics of North America, 12,* 153–165.

Ross, C. E., & Mirowsky, J. (1988). Child care and emotional adjustment to wives' employment. *Journal of Health and Social Behavior, 29,* 127–138.

Ruble, D. N., Greulich, F., Pomerantz, E. M., et al. (1993). The role of gender-related processes in the development of sex differences in self-evaluation and depression. *Journal of Affective Disorders, 29,* 97–128.

Rudolph, K. D., & Hammen, C. (1999). Age and gender as determinants of stress exposure, generation, and reactions in youngsters: A transactional perspective. *Child Development, 70*(3), 660–677.

Sackheim, H., Decina, P., Prohovnik, I., et al. (1987). Seizure threshold in electroconvulsive therapy: Effects of sex, age, electrode placements, and number of treatments. *Archives of General Psychiatry, 14,* 355–360.

Sackheim, H. A., Portnoy, S., Neeley, P., et al. (1986). Cognitive consequences of low-dosage electroconvulsive therapy. *Annals of the New York Academy of Sciences, 462,* 326–340.

Sargeant, J. K., Bruce, M. L., Florio, L. P., et al. (1990). Factors associated with 1–year outcome of major depression in the community. *Archives of General Psychiatry, 47,* 519–526.

Schneider, L. S., Small, G. W., Hamilton, S., et al. (1997). Estrogen replacement and response to fluoxetine in a multicenter geriatric depression trial. *American Journal of Geriatric Psychiatry, 5*(2), 97–106.

Schneider, L. S., Small, G., & Clary, C. (1998, May). *Estrogen replacement therapy status and antidepressant response to sertraline.* Paper presented at the 151st Annual Convention of the American Psychiatric Association, Toronto.

Schutte, K. K., Seable, J. H., & Moos, R. H. (1997). Gender differences in the relations between depressive symptoms and drinking behavior among problem drinkers: A three-wave study. *Journal of Consulting and Clinical Psychology, 65,* 392–404.

Seidman, S. N., & Rabkin, J. G. (1998). Testosterone replacement therapy for hypogonadal men with SSRI-refractory depression. *Journal of Affective Disorders, 48,* 157–161.

Shaffer, D., Garland, A., Gould, M., et al. (1988). Preventing teenage suicide: A critical review. *Journal of the American Academy of Child and Adolescent Psychiatry, 27,* 675–687.

Shea, M. T., Glass, D. R., Pilkonis, P. A., et al. (1987). Frequency and implications of personality disorders in a sample of depressed outpatients. *Journal of Personality Disorders, 1,* 27–42.

Simpson, H. B., Nee, J. C., & Endicott, J. (1997). First-episode major depression: Few sex differences in course. *Archives of General Psychiatry, 54,* 633–639.

Sotsky, S. M., Glass, D. R., Shea, M. T., et al. (1991). Patient predictors of response to psychotherapy and pharmacotherapy: Findings in the NIMH Treatment of Depression Collaborative Research Program. *American Journal of Psychiatry, 148,* 997–1008.

Stangler, R. S., & Printz, A. M. (1980). DSM-III: Psychiatric diagnoses in a university population. *American Journal of Psychiatry, 137,* 937–940.

Steiner, M., Wheadon, D. E., Kreider, M. S., et al. (1993, May). *Antidepressant response to paroxetine by gender.* Paper presented at the 146th Annual Convention of the American Psychiatric Association, San Francisco.

Stunkard, A. F., Fernstrom, M. H., Price, A., et al. (1990). Direction of weight change in recurrent depression: Consistency across episodes. *Archives of General Psychiatry, 47,* 857–860.

Thase, M. E., Buysse, D. J., Frank, E., et al. (1997a). Which depressed patients will respond to interpersonal psychotherapy? *American Journal of Psychiatry, 154,* 502–509.

Thase, M. E., Frank, E., Kornstein, S. G., et al. (2000). Sex-related differences in response to treatments of depression. In E. Frank (Ed.), *Gender and its effects on psychopathology* (pp. 103–129). Washington, DC: American Psychiatric Press.

Thase, M. E., Greenhouse, J. B., Frank, E., et al. (1997b). Treatment of major depression with psychotherapy or pharmacotherapy–psychotherapy combinations. *Archives of General Psychiatry, 54,* 1009–1015.

Thase, M. E., Reynolds, C. F., Frank, E., et al. (1994). Do depressed men and women respond similarly to cognitive behavioral therapy? *American Journal of Psychiatry, 151,* 500–505.

Wannan, G., & Fombonne, E. (1998). Gender differences in rates and correlates of suicidal behaviour among child psychiatric outpatients. *Journal of Adolescence, 21,* 371–381.

Weiss, E. L., Longhurst, J. G., & Mazure, C. M. (1999). Childhood sexual abuse as a risk factor for depression in women: Psychosocial and neurobiological correlates. *American Journal of Psychiatry, 156,* 816–828.

Weissman, M. M., Bland, R., Canino, G. J., et al. (1996). Cross-national epidemiology of major depression and bipolar disorder. *Journal of the American Medical Association, 276,* 293–299.

Winokur, G., Coryell, W., Keller, M., et al. (1993). A prospective follow-up of patients with bipolar and primary unipolar affective disorder. *Archives of General Psychiatry, 50,* 457–465.

Whybrow, P. C. (1995). Sex differences in thyroid axis dysfunction: Relevance to affective disorder and its treatment. *Depression, 3,* 33–42.

Wu, X., & DeMaris, A. (1996). Gender and marital status differences in depression: The effects of chronic strains. *Sex Roles, 34,* 299–319.

Yonkers, K. A., Halbreich, U., Rush, A. J., et al. (1996). *Sex differences in response to pharmacotherapy among early onset dysthymics.* Paper presented at the annual meeting of the Society of Biological Psychiatry.

Young, M. A., Scheftner, W. A., Fawcett, J., et al. (1990). Gender differences in the clinical features of unipolar depressive disorder. *Journal of Nervous and Mental Disease, 178,* 200–203.

Zunzunegui, M. V., Beland, F., Llacer, A., et al. (1998). Gender differences in depressive symptoms among Spanish elderly. *Social Psychiatry and Psychiatric Epidemiology, 33,* 195–205.

9

Bipolar Disorder

MARLENE P. FREEMAN
LESLEY M. ARNOLD
SUSAN L. McELROY

The presentation of bipolar disorder in women differs from that in men in clinically significant ways. This chapter reviews gender differences in the clinical features, course, and treatment of bipolar disorder and discusses the effects of bipolar disorder on the female reproductive cycle.

EPIDEMIOLOGY

Women have higher prevalence rates of mood episodes and disorders than men, with the exception of manic episodes, for which there is no sex difference (Kessler et al., 1994). A lifetime history of mania occurs in about 1.6% of the general population (Kessler et al., 1994). Bipolar I disorder, characterized by episodes of mania and depression, occurs equally in both sexes. Bipolar II disorder, characterized by episodes of hypomania and depression, occurs more frequently in women than in men (Dunner, 1998).

Gender Differences in Clinical Features and Course

The clinical features of bipolar disorder differ between men and women. Women may be more prone to a depressive diathesis of bipolar disorder, even during mania, compared with men (Leibenluft, 1996). Support for this hypothesis comes from evidence that "mixed mania," defined as mania accompanied by syndromal major depression, is more common in women (Arnold et al., 2000). Further evidence comes from reports that women with bipolar disorder have more frequent episodes of depression than men (Angst, 1978; Roy-Byrne et al., 1995a; Rybajowski et al., 1980; Taschev, 1973). The depressive episodes experienced by women are also more likely to be lengthy and resistant to treatment (Goodwin & Jamison, 1990; Kessler et al., 1993). Suicidality is associated with the number of depressive symptoms occurring during mania, but there are no gender differences in the rates of suicide in patients with mixed mania (Strakowski et al., 1996).

The course of bipolar disorder in women differs from that in men in several ways. First, women generally have a later age of onset, with onset during the fifth decade of life being more common in women (Leibenluft, 1996). Second, "rapid cycling," defined as four or more mood episodes in a year, is about three times more common in women than in men. In studies of rapid cycling, the percentage of female patients has ranged from 58% to 92%, with a mean of approximately 71% (Leibenluft, 1997). Finally, women appear to experience a seasonal pattern of mood disturbances more often than men. In women, depressive episodes occur more commonly in the fall and winter than in the spring and summer (Faedda et al., 1993). A bimodal peak of hospital admissions for bipolar disorder in the spring and fall has also been observed in female patients with bipolar disorder (D'Mello et al., 1995).

COMORBIDITY

Several psychiatric disorders, including substance use disorders, anxiety disorders, and eating disorders are commonly comorbid with bipolar disorder. Comorbidity is more common in women than in men and adversely affects recovery from mania more often in women (Black et al., 1988; Blehar et al., 1998; Strakowski et al., 1992).

Medical disorders that are frequently comorbid with bipolar disorder include migraine headaches and thyroid disease, both of which are also more common in women with bipolar disorder than in men (Blehar et al., 1998). Hypothyroidism may contribute to the elevated rates of rapid cycling in women, since hypothyroidism is more common in women, and 30–90% of patients with rapid-cycling bipolar disorder have hypothyroidism (Bauer et al., 1990; Cho et al., 1979; Cowdry et al., 1983; Tunbridge et al., 1997).

TREATMENT

Gender does not appear to affect treatment response to mood stabilizers. In a retrospective study of lithium prophylaxis in bipolar disorder, gender had no impact overall morbidity (Berghofer et al., 1996). In another study of lithium treatment of bipolar disorder, the response to lithium and effects of lithium discontinuation did not differ between women and men (Tondo et al., 1997).

The management of two presentations of bipolar disorder that are more common in women—rapid cycling and mixed states—is challenging, in part because treatment of depressive symptoms may precipitate increased cycling, especially in women that receive tricyclic antidepressants (Parry, 1989). Studies of the treatment of rapid cycling are limited, but evidence suggests that the anticonvulsants carbamazepine and valproate may be superior to lithium in reducing the frequency of episodes in rapid-cycling bipolar disorder (Leibenluft, 1997). There are increasing reports of the potential role of atypical antipsychotic medications, such as clozapine and olanzapine, as monotherapy or adjunctive therapy in the treatment of patients with rapid cycling (Leibenluft, 1997). The addition of levothyroxine to medication regimens also improves mood stabilization in some patients with rapid-cycling bipolar disorder (Bauer et al., 1990; Bauer & Whybrow, 1990). A number of studies have reported that mixed mania is less responsive to treatment with lithium than is "pure" mania (Cohen et al., 1989; Dilsaver et al., 1993; Freeman et al., 1992; Himmelhoch et al., 1976; Himmelhoch & Garfinkel, 1986; Post et al., 1987; Prien et al., 1988; Secunda et al., 1985; Swann et al., 1997). The presence of depressive symptoms during mania predicts a better response to valproate compared with lithium (Freeman et al., 1992; Swann et al., 1997). Carbamazepine also shows a better response rate than lithium in mixed mania (Post et al., 1987). Among one group of patients with mixed mania, gender did not predict response to valproate or carbamazepine (Arnold et al., 2000).

There are limited data on the utility of hormonal treatment in women with bipolar disorder. The induction of mania (Zohar et al., 1985) and rapid cycling (Oppenheim, 1984) have been reported after the use of exogenous estrogen, suggesting an antidepressant effect of estrogen. Progesterone has not been found to be effective in the treatment of postpartum mania (Meakin & Brockington, 1990). There are two case reports of mood stabilization with a combination of estrogen and progesterone in women with bipolar disorder (Chouinard et al., 1987).

The use of typical antipsychotic medications and the novel antipsychotic risperidone is associated with hyperprolactinemia, which may result in galactorrhea, amenorrhea and menstrual cycle irregularities, anovulation and infertility, and sexual dysfunction. The atypical agents clozapine, olanzapine, and quetiapine are less frequently associated with hyperprolactinemia and are better tolerated by women (Dickson et al., 2000).

There are important drug interactions to consider in treating women with bipolar disorder. First, carbamazepine induces the metabolism of oral contraceptives via the CYP3A4 cytochrome isoenzyme, hence lowering the efficacy of this method of birth control (Spina et al., 1996). Valproate and lithium do not interfere with the efficacy of oral contraceptives (Shenfield et al., 1993). Second, the putative mood stabilizer topiramate may lower levels of ethinyl estadiol in oral contraceptives, potentially interfering with efficacy (Rosenfeld et al., 1997). The other putative mood stabilizers, gabapentin and lamotrigine, lack interactions with oral contraceptives (Eldon et al., 1998; Elwes & Binnie, 1996). The relationship between polycystic ovary disease (PCO) and the use of valproate in the treatment of bipolar disorder is unclear. Polycystic ovaries, hyperandrogenism, and obesity have been associated with valproate use in patients with epilepsy, who are known to be at increased risk for PCO (Isojarvi et al., 1993, 1996). In a recent study of women with bipolar disorder, there was no evidence of PCO in patients treated with either lithium ($N = 10$), valproate ($N = 10$), or both ($N = 2$), although menstrual irregularity and obesity were prominent in all groups (Rasgon et al., 2000). There is a debate about whether weight gain from the use of valproate, rather than the drug itself, is responsible for the development of polycystic ovaries and endocrine abnormalities (Eberle, 1998). Until there are more data, it is prudent to use valproate with caution in young women with bipolar disorder (Garland & Behr, 1996; Johnston, 1999).

BIPOLAR DISORDER AND THE REPRODUCTIVE CYCLE

The Menstrual Cycle

Although data are limited, there is some evidence that symptoms of bipolar disorder worsen during the premenstrual phase of the menstrual cycle (Blehar et al., 1998;

Hendrick et al., 1996; Price & DiMarzio, 1986). About 66% of a sample of women with bipolar disorder reported regularly occurring menstrual or premenstrual exacerbation of mood symptoms (Blehar et al., 1998). One-fourth of women with bipolar disorder have been found to experience premenstrual depression (Roy-Byrne et al., 1985b). In addition, women with bipolar disorder report elevated rates of anxiety in the premenstrual phase (Roy-Byrne et al., 1985b). Interestingly, a relationship between the menstrual cycle and rapid cycling has not been found (Diamond et al., 1976; Price & DiMarzio, 1986; Wehr et al., 1988). It may be difficult to distinguish premenstrual dysphoric disorder (PMDD) from premenstrual worsening of bipolar disorder, and more data are needed to assess the rate of PMDD in women with bipolar disorder. PMDD responds to treatment with serotonergic antidepressants taken throughout the menstrual cycle or intermittently during the luteal phase (Freeman et al., 1999; Yonkers, 1997). The use of antidepressants for the treatment of mood symptoms during the premenstrual phase is problematic in women with bipolar disorder because of the risk of precipitating mania (Benazzi, 1997; Berk et al., 1996; Chouinard & Steiner, 1986; Goodman & Charney, 1987; Grubbs, 1997; Landry, 1997; McIvor & Sinanan, 1991; Oldroyd, 1997; Vesely et al., 1997). Lithium and valproate have been found to be ineffective in open studies of premenstrual syndrome (Jacobsen, 1993; Steiner et al., 1980).

Pregnancy

The treatment of women with bipolar disorder during the childbearing years includes education of the woman and her partner (with permission) about family planning, the heritability of bipolar disorder, and the course of illness and treatment options during pregnancy. Family planning in women with bipolar disorder involves individualized risk–benefit assessments. Women should be informed about the heritability of bipolar disorder, as this may affect the decision to have children. Children of women with bipolar disorder are at increased risk for developing the disorder, and the risk is estimated to be between 1.5% and 10.2% (Dunner, 1983; Gershon, 1990; Packer, 1992; Palmour, 1989; Rice et al., 1987). Planned pregnancies maximize treatment options, and it is important to advise careful family planning in all women with bipolar disorder. The importance of advocating for planned pregnancies is demonstrated by the results of a study of women with chronic psychiatric disorders, including bipolar disorder, in which about one-third of women who did not want to become pregnant failed to use contraception during their last episode of sexual intercourse (Coverdale & Aruffo, 1989). The psychiatrist should also educate women about the course of the illness during pregnancy, as well as the risks and benefits of treatment during pregnancy. The psychiatrist must determine a woman's ability to consent to treatment during pregnancy, and must document the informed consent discussions in the medical record. If there is uncertainty about a treatment approach for a particular patient, a second opinion or consultation with experts in reproductive psychiatry is recommended (Llewellyn et al., 1998). The psychiatrist should also routinely collaborate with the obstetrician in the care of women with bipolar disorder.

When a clinician is developing a treatment plan for a woman with bipolar disorder who wishes to become pregnant, the teratogenic risks of psychotropic medications must be weighed against the impact of untreated bipolar disorder on the pregnant woman and the fetus. Pregnancy appears to be "risk-neutral" in women with bipolar disorder, in that it neither protects against nor increases the risk of relapse (Viguera & Cohen, 1998).

There is a risk of relapse in pregnant and nonpregnant women who abruptly discontinue maintenance mood stabilizers, and the risk is highest for women with four or more prior depressive or manic episodes (Viguera & Cohen, 1998). Although there are no data on the effects of untreated bipolar disorder on fetal development, poor self-care and lack of prenatal care may result from a relapse in symptoms and adversely affect fetal outcome. Furthermore, impulsivity and suicidality may occur during a relapse and put the mother and her fetus at risk (Cohen & Rosenbaum, 1998). Repeated relapses of bipolar disorder may also lead to treatment resistance and chronicity in the mother (Post, 1992).

When a clinician is advising a woman about the risks and benefits of psychotropic treatment during pregnancy and possible treatment alternatives, the first step is to carefully review her psychiatric history, course and severity of symptoms, and previous response to psychotropic medications. Based on this review, an individualized treatment plan that promotes the health of the woman and avoids or limits exposure of the fetus to potential teratogens constitutes an important treatment goal. Women with mild symptoms, defined as one past manic episode or long periods of affective stability, may elect to taper and discontinue medication prior to conception because of the relatively low risk of relapse (Viguera & Cohen, 1998). Because rapid discontinuation of maintenance psychotropic medications increases the risk of relapse, a gradual taper of all mood stabilizers appears to be a more prudent approach (Viguera & Cohen, 1998). Women with moderate illness (e.g., two to three episodes of mania or depression) may also choose to taper and discontinue medications prior to conception. As the risk of relapse is greater in this group, however, they may elect to continue medication until early confirmation of pregnancy, prolonging the period of time on preventative medication. Once a woman is pregnant, a medication can be tapered in the 2 weeks prior to the establishment of the placental–fetal circulation, before the fetus is susceptible to teratogens (Viguera & Cohen, 1998). However, this strategy requires a more rapid taper and may increase the risk of relapse. Women with mild to moderate illness who elect to discontinue medications should be educated about identifying early signs of relapse and followed closely for recurrence of target symptoms. Medication treatment can be instituted for any recurrence of significant symptoms. Women with severe illness (e.g., four or more episodes of mania or depression) have a high rate of relapse, and the risks to a mother and fetus from the disorder may exceed the risk of medication treatment. In many cases, these women may not be able to safely discontinue medication treatment during pregnancy (Altshuler et al., 1996; Viguera & Cohen, 1998).

Any woman who continues psychotropic treatment for bipolar disorder during pregnancy, or who has an unplanned pregnancy, must evaluate the risk of specific medications to the fetus. The mood stabilizers used in the treatment of bipolar disorder—lithium, valproic acid, and carbamazepine—all have potential teratogenic effects. The risk estimate of cardiovascular malformations (particularly Epstein's anomaly) after first-trimester exposure to lithium is between 0.05% and 0.1%, or 10–20 times the risk in the general population (Cohen & Rosenbaum, 1998). The risk of spina bifida after first-trimester exposure to the anticonvulsants carbamazepine and valproic acid is 15 times or greater the risk in the general population (Altshuler et al., 1996). The risk estimate of spina bifida after first-trimester exposure to carbamazepine is 0.5–1.0% (Rosa, 1991) and after first-trimester exposure to valproic acid is 1–5% (Lammer et al., 1987; Lindhout et al., 1992; Omtzigt et al., 1992). The use of higher doses of anticonvulsants and multiple anticonvulsants may increase the risk of neural tube defects (Battino et al.,

cause the patient had a history of moderate bipolar illness (3 episodes of mania or depression) there would likely be a considerable risk of relapse when she stopped her medication. She was therefore advised to continue medication until she was ready to conceive. Fortunately her cycles were regular, and she was able to track them and predict the time of ovulation. During the 2-week period after presumed conception she tapered and discontinued both the lithium and sertraline. Her pregnancy was successful, and she was followed closely off of medication throughout the pregnancy. Although she experienced mild depression, she responded to cognitive psychotherapy alone and did not require resumption of medication. She delivered a healthy baby at term with no complications. Immediately after the birth of her baby, she started lithium at 300 mg/day for two days and then increased to 600 mg/day. Sertraline was restarted 3 months later with the emergence of more significant depression. Because of the use of lithium she elected not to breastfeed the baby.

Menopause

Although data about the relationship of bipolar disorder and the menopause are limited (Pariser, 1993), in one study 19.3% of 56 postmenopausal women with bipolar disorder reported worsening of their mood symptoms, mostly depression, following menopause (Blehar et al., 1998). In another retrospective study, the dose of antipsychotic medication was found to be higher in a group of women with bipolar disorder older than 40 years than in a group of younger women (D'Mello & McNeil, 1990). This was hypothesized to be related to declining estrogen levels in the older women and the subsequent loss of estrogen's purported antidopaminergic effects (D'Mello & McNeil, 1990).

EVALUATION

Before a diagnosis of bipolar disorder is made, other possible causes of mood disorder symptoms should be ruled out. The medical differential diagnosis in women includes endocrine disorders (e.g., thyroid disease), neurological disorders (e.g., multiple sclerosis), central nervous system lesions (e.g., stroke), immunological disorders (e.g., systemic lupus erythematosis), infectious diseases (e.g., HIV/AIDS), and metabolic disorders (e.g., vitamin deficiencies). Many medications may also cause or worsen mood symptoms in women, most notably oral contraceptives, corticosteroids, antihypertensives, and benzodiazepines. Although substance use disorders are more common in men, it is important to evaluate women for the presence of these disorders, as substance use may exacerbate mood disorders.

A complete assessment of women with bipolar disorder includes a psychiatric and medical history, family history, mental status exam, with a focus on mood, psychotic, anxiety, substance use, and eating disorder signs and symptoms. When indicated, medical evaluations include physical examination, laboratory tests (e.g., thyroid function tests and metabolic screens), and toxicology screen. Assessment also includes the menstrual and reproductive history, as well as the history of menstrual, pregnancy/postpartum, or menopausal mood or psychotic symptoms. The history of hormonal treatments and the effects of the treatment on mood are also important. Finally, a discussion of plans about pregnancy and contraception is a critical component of the evaluation.

CONCLUSION

Gender differences in bipolar disorder are clinically important and require more study. Improved treatments are needed for rapid affective cycling and mixed states—two presentations of bipolar disorder that are more common in women than in men. The treatment of pregnant and postpartum women is challenging, because the data about the use of psychotropic medications during pregnancy and lactation are limited. However, a careful, individualized risk–benefit assessment that promotes the health of a woman and avoids or limits exposure of a fetus or infant to potential adverse effects of medication constitutes an important treatment goal.

REFERENCES

Altshuler, L. L., Burt, V. K., McMullen, M., et al. (1995). Breast-feeding and sertraline: A 24-hour analysis. *Journal of Clinical Psychiatry, 56,* 243–245.

Altshuler, L. L., Cohen, L., Szuba, M. P., et al. (1996). Pharmacologic management of psychiatric illness during pregnancy: Dilemmas and guidelines. *American Journal of Psychiatry, 153,* 592–606.

American Academy of Pediatrics, Committee on Drugs. (1994). The transfer of drugs and other chemicals into human milk. *Pediatrics, 93,* 137–150.

Angst, J. (1978) The course of affective disorders: II. Typology of bipolar manic–depressive illness. *Archives für Psychiatrie und Nervenkrankheiten, 226,* 65–73.

Arnold, L. M., Suckow, R. F., & Lichtenstein, P. K. (2000). Fluvoxamine concentrations in breast milk and maternal and infant serum. *Journal of Clinical Psychopharmacology, 20,* 491–493.

Arnold, L. M., McElroy, S. L., & Keck, P. E., Jr. (2000) The role of gender in mixed mania. *Comprehensive Psychiatry, 41,* 83–87.

Battino, D., Binelli, S., Caccamo, M. L., et al. (1992). Malformation in offspring of 305 epileptic women: A prospective study. *Acta Neurologica Scandinavica, 85,* 204–207.

Bauer, M. S., & Whybrow, P. C. (1990). Rapid cycling bipolar affective disorder: II. Treatment of refractory rapid cycling with high-dose levothyroxine: A preliminary study. *Archives of General Psychiatry, 47,* 435–440.

Bauer, M. S., Whybrow, P. C., & Winokur, A. (1990). Rapid cycling bipolar affective disorder: I. Association with grade I hypothyroidism. *Archives of General Psychiatry, 47,* 427–432.

Benazzi, F. (1997). Antidepressant-associated hypomania in outpatient depression: A 203-case study in private practice. *Journal of Affective Disorders, 46,* 73–77.

Berghofer, A., Kossmann, B., & Muller-Oerlinghausen, B. (1996). Course of illness and pattern of recurrences in patients with affective disorders during long-term lithium prophylaxis: A retrospective analysis over 15 years. *Acta Psychiatrica Scandinavica, 93,* 349–354.

Berk, M., Koopowitz, L. F., & Szabo, C. P. (1996). Antidepressant induced mania in obsessive compulsive disorder. *European Neuropsychopharmacology, 6,* 9–11.

Birnbaum, C. S., Cohen, L. S., Bailey, J. W., et al. (1999). Serum concentrations of antidepressants and benzodiazepines in nursing infants: A case series. *Pediatrics, 104,* e11.

Black, D. W., Winokur, G., Bell, S., et al. (1988). Complicated mania: Comorbidity and immediate outcome in the treatment of mania. *Archives of General Psychiatry, 45,* 232–236.

Blehar, M. C., DePaulo, J. R., Jr., Gershon, E. S., et al. (1998). Women with bipolar disorder: Findings from the NIMH genetics initiative sample. *Psychopharmacology Bulletin, 34,* 239–243.

Cho, J., Bone, S., Dunner, D., et al. (1979). The effect of lithium treatment on thyroid function in patients with primary affective disorder. *American Journal of Psychiatry, 136,* 115–116.

Chouinard, G., Steinberg, S., & Steiner, W. (1987). Estrogen–progesterone combination: Another mood stabilizer? *American Journal of Psychiatry, 144*, 826.

Chouinard, G., & Steiner, W. (1986). A case of mania induced by high-dose fluoxetine treatment. *American Journal of Psychiatry, 143*, 686.

Cohen, L. S., & Rosenbaum, J. F. (1998). Psychotropic drug use during pregnancy: Weighing the risks. *Journal of Clinical Psychiatry, 59*, 18–28.

Cohen, L. S., Sichel, D. A., Robertson, L. M., et al. (1995). Postpartum prophylaxis for women with bipolar disorder. *American Journal of Psychiatry, 152*, 1641–1645.

Cohen, S., Kahn, A., & Cox, G. (1989). Demographic and clinical features predictive of recovery in acute mania. *Journal of Nervous and Mental Disease, 177*, 638–642.

Coverdale, J. H., & Aruffo, J. A. (1989). Family planning needs of female chronic psychiatric outpatients. *American Journal of Psychiatry, 146*, 1489–1491.

Cowdry, R., Wehr, T., Zis, A., et al. (1983). Thyroid abnormalities associated with rapid cycling bipolar illness. *Archives of General Psychiatry, 40*, 414–420.

Delgado-Escueta, A. V., & Janz, D. (1992). Consensus guidelines: Preconception counseling, management, and care of the pregnant woman with epilepsy. *Neurology, 42*, 149–160.

Diamond, S. B., Rubinstein, A. A., Dunner, D. L., et al. (1976). Menstrual problems in women with primary affective illness. *Comprehensive Psychiatry, 17*, 541–548.

Dickson, R. A., Seeman, M. V., & Corenblum, B. (2000). Hormonal side effects in women: Typical versus atypical antipsychotic treatment. *Journal of Clinical Psychiatry, 61*[Suppl. 3], 10–15.

Dilsaver, S. C., Swann, A. C., Shoaib, A. M., et al. (1993). Depressive mania associated with nonresponse to antimanic agents. *American Journal of Psychiatry, 54*, 37–42.

D'Mello, D. A., & McNeil, J. A. (1990). Sex differences in bipolar affective disorder: Neuroleptic dosage variance. *Comprehensive Psychiatry, 31*, 80–83.

D'Mello, D. A., NcNeil, J. A., & Msibi, B. (1995). Seasons and bipolar disorder. *Annals of Clinical Psychiatry, 7*, 11–18.

Dunner, D. L. (1983). Recent genetic studies of bipolar and unipolar depression. In J. M. Davis & J. W. Maas (Eds.), *The affective disorders* (pp. 183–191). Washington, DC: American Psychiatric Press.

Dunner, D. L. (1998). Bipolar disorders in DSM-IV: Impact of inclusion of rapid cycling as a course modifier. *Neuropsychopharmacology, 19*, 189–193.

Eberle, A. J. (1998). Valproate and polycystic ovaries. *Journal of the American Academy of Child and Adolescent Psychiatry, 37*, 1009.

Eldon, M. A., Underwood, B. A., Randinitis, E. J., et al. (1998). Gabapentin does not interact with a contraceptive regimen of norethindrone acetate and ethinyl estradiol. *Neurology, 50*, 1146–1148.

Elwes, R. D. C., & Binnie, C. D. (1996). Clinical pharmacokinetics of newer antiepileptic drugs: Lamotrigine, vigabatrin, gabapentin, and oxcarbazepine. *Clinical Pharmacokinetics, 30*, 403–415.

Faedda, G. L., Tondo, L., Teicher, M. H., et al. (1993). Seasonal mood disorders: Patterns of seasonal recurrence in mania and depression. *Archives of General Psychiatry, 50*, 17–23.

Freeman, E. W., Rickels, K., Sondheimer, S. J., et al. (1999). Differential response to antidepressants in women with premenstrual syndrome/premenstrual dysphoric disorder. *Archives of General Psychiatry, 56*, 932–939.

Freeman, T. W., Clothier, J. L., Pazzaglia, P., et al. (1992). A double-blind comparison of valproate and lithium in the treatment of acute mania. *American Journal of Psychiatry, 149*, 108–111.

Frey, B., Schubiger, G., & Musy, J. P. (1990). Transient cholestatic hepatitis in a neonate associated with carbamazepine exposure during pregnancy and breastfeeding. *European Journal of Pediatrics, 150*, 136–138.

Gaily, E., & Granstrom, M. L. (1992). Minor anomalies in children of mothers with epilepsy. *Neurology, 42*, 128–131.

Garland, E. J., & Behr, R. (1996). Hormonal effects of valproic acid? *Journal of American Academy of Child and Adolescent Psychiatry, 35,* 1424–1425.

Gershon, E. S. (1990). Genetics. In F. K. Goodwin & K. R. Jamison (Eds.), *Manic–depressive illness* (pp. 373–401). New York: Oxford University Press.

Goldstein, D. J., Corbin, L. A., & Fung, M. C. (2000). Olanzapine-exposed pregnancies and lactation: Early experience. *Journal of Clinical Psychopharmacology, 20,* 399–403.

Goodman, W. K., & Charney, D. S. (1987). A case of alprazolam, but not lorazepam, inducing manic symptoms. *Journal of Clinical Psychiatry, 48,* 117–118.

Goodwin, F. K., & Jamison, K. R. (Eds.). (1990). *Manic–depressive illness.* New York: Oxford University Press.

Grubbs, J. H. (1997). SSRI-induced mania. *Journal of the American Academy of Child and Adolescent Psychiatry, 36,* 445.

Hendrick, V., Altshuler, L. L., & Burt, V. K. (1996). Course of psychiatric disorders across the menstrual cycle. *Harvard Review of Psychiatry, 4,* 200–207.

Himmelhoch, J. M., Mulla, D., Neil, J. F., et al. (1976). Incidence and significance of mixed affective states in a bipolar population. *Archives of General Psychiatry. 33,* 1062–1066.

Himmelhoch, J., & Garfinkel, M. E. (1986). Sources of lithium resistance in mixed mania. *Psychopharmacology Bulletin, 22,* 613–620.

Hunt, N., & Trevor, S. (1995). Does puerperal illness distinguish a subgroup of bipolar patients? *Journal of Affective Disorders, 34,* 101–107.

Isojarvi, J. I. T., Laatikainen, T. J., Knip, M., et al. (1996). Obesity and endocrine disorders in women taking valproate for epilepsy. *Annals of Neurology, 39,* 579–584.

Isojarvi, J. I. T., Laatikainen, T. J., Pakarinen, A. J., et al. (1993). Polycystic ovaries and hyperandrogenism in women taking valproate for epilepsy. *New England Journal of Medicine, 329,* 1383–1388.

Jacobsen, F. M. (1993). Low-dose valproate: A new treatment for cyclothymia, mild rapid cycling disorders, and premenstrual syndrome. *Journal of Clinical Psychiatry, 54,* 229–234.

Jager-Roman, E., Deichl, A., Jakob, S., et al. (1986). Fetal growth, major malformation, and minor anomalies in infants born to women receiving valproic acid. *Journal of Pediatrics, 108,* 997–1004.

Johnston, H. F. (1999). More on valproate and polycystic ovaries. *Journal of the American Academy of Child and Adolescent Psychiatry, 38,* 354.

Jones, I., & Craddock, N. (2001). Familiarity of the puerperal trigger in bipolar disorder: Results of a family study. *American Journal of Psychiatry, 158,* 913–917.

Jones, K. L., Lacro, R. V., Johnson, K. A., et al. (1989). Pattern of malformations in the children of women treated with carbamazepine during pregnancy. *New England Journal of Medicine, 320,* 1661–1666.

Kasper, S., & Wehr, T. A. (1992). The role of sleep and wakefulness in the genesis of depression and mania. *Encephale, 18,* 45–50.

Kendell, R. E., Chalmers, J. C., & Platz, C. (1987). Epidemiology of puerperal psychoses. *British Journal of Psychiatry, 150,* 662–673.

Kessler, R. C., McGonagle, K. A., Swartz, M., et al. (1993). Sex and depression in the National Comorbidity Survey: I. Lifetime prevalence, chronicity and recurrence. *Journal of Affective Disorders, 29,* 85–96.

Kessler, R., McGonagle, K. A., Zhao, S., et al. (1994). Lifetime and 12-month prevalence of DSM-III-R psychiatric disorders in the United States. *Archives of General Psychiatry, 51,* 8–19

Kirchheiner, J., Berghofer, A., & Bolk-Weischedel, D. (2000). Healthy outcome under olanzapine treatment in a pregnant woman. *Pharmacopsychiatry, 33,* 78–80.

Koch, K., Hartman, A., Jager-Roman, E., et al. (1982). Major malformations of children of epileptic parents—due to epilepsy or its therapy? In D. Janz, L. Bossi, M. Dam, et al. (Eds.), *Epilepsy, pregnancy, and the child* (pp. 313–316). New York: Raven Press.

Koch, S., Losche, G., Jager-Roman, E. J., et al. (1992). Major and minor birth malformations and antiepileptic drugs. *Neurology, 42*, 83–88.

Kubacki, A. (1986). Male and female mania. *Canadian Journal of Psychiatry, 31*, 70–72.

Lammer, E. J., Sever, L. E., & Oakley, G. P. (1987). Teratogen update: valproic acid. *Teratology, 35*, 465–473.

Landry, P. (1997). Withdrawal hypomania associated with paroxetine. *Journal of Clinical Psychopharmacology, 17*, 60–61.

Leibenluft, E. (1996). Women with bipolar illness: Clinical and research issues. *American Journal of Psychiatry, 153*, 163–173.

Leibenluft, E. (1997). Issues in the treatment of women with bipolar illness. *Journal of Clinical Psychiatry, 58*, 5–11.

Linden, S., & Rich, C. L. (1983). The use of lithium during pregnancy and lactation. *Journal of Clinical Psychiatry, 44*, 358–361.

Lindhout, D., Meinardi, H., Meijer, J. W., et al. (1992). Antiepileptic drugs and teratogenesis in two consecutive cohorts: Changes in prescription policy paralleled by changes in pattern of malformations. *Neurology, 42*, 94–110.

Llewellyn, A., & Stowe, Z. N. (1998). Psychotropic medications in lactation. *Journal of Clinical Psychiatry, 59*, 41–52.

Llewellyn, A., Stowe, Z. N., & Strader, J. R. (1998). The use of lithium and management of women with bipolar disorder during pregnancy and lactation. *Journal of Clinical Psychiatry, 59*, 57–64.

McIvor, R. J., & Sinanan, K. (1991). Buspirone-induced mania. *British Journal of Psychiatry, 158*, 592.

Meakin, C., & Brockington, I. F. (1990). Failure of progesterone treatment in puerperal mania. *British Journal of Psychiatry, 156*, 910.

Medical Research Council Vitamin Study Research Group. (1991). Prevention of neural-tube defects: Results of the Medical Research Council Vitamin Study. *Lancet, 338*, 131–137.

Merlob, P., Mor, N., & Litwin, A. (1992). Transient hepatic dysfunction in an infant of an epileptic mother treated with carbamazepine during pregnancy and breastfeeding. *Annals of Pharmacotherapy, 26*, 1563–1565.

Nakane, Y., Okuma, T., Takahashi, R., et al. (1980). Multi-institutional study on the teratogenicity and fetal toxicity of antiepileptic drugs: A report of a collaborative study group in Japan. *Epilepsia, 21*, 663–680.

Oldroyd, J. (1997). Paroxetine-induced mania. *Journal of the American Academy of Child and Adolescent Psychiatry, 36*, 721–722.

Omtzigt, J. G. C., Los, F. J., Grobbee, D. E., et al. (1992). The risk of spina bifida aperta after first trimester exposure to valproate in a prenatal cohort. *Neurology, 42*, 119–125.

Oppenheim, G. (1984). A case of rapid mood cycling with estrogen: Implications for therapy. *Journal of Clinical Psychiatry, 45*, 34–35.

Packer, S. (1992). Family planning for women with bipolar disorder. *Hospital and Community Psychiatry, 43*, 479–482.

Palmour, R. M. (1989). Genetic counselling for affective disease. *Psychiatric Journal of the University of Ottowa, 14*, 323–327.

Pariser, S. F. (1993). Women and mood disorders: Menarche to menopause. *Annals of Clinical Psychiatry, 5*, 249–254.

Parry, B. L. (1989). Reproductive factors affecting the course of affective illness in women. *Psychiatric Clinics of North America, 12*, 207–219.

Piontek, C. M., Baab, S., Peindel, K. S., et al. (2000). Serum valproate levels in 6 breastfeeding mother–infant pairs. *Journal of Clinical Psychiatry, 61*, 170–172.

Post, R. M. (1992). Transduction of psychosocial stress into the neurobiology of recurrent affective disorder. *American Journal of Psychiatry, 149*, 999–1010.

Post, R. M., Uhde, T. W., Roy-Byrne, P. P., et al. (1987). Correlates of antimanic response to carbamazepine. *Psychiatry Research, 21*, 71–83.

Price, W. A., & DiMarzio, L. (1986). Premenstrual tension syndrome in rapid-cycling bipolar affective disorder. *Journal of Clinical Psychiatry, 47*, 415–417.

Prien, R. F., Himmelhoch, J. M., & Kupfer, D. J. (1988). Treatment of mixed mania. *Journal of Affective Disorders, 15*, 9–15.

Rasgon, N. L., Altshuler, L. L., Gudeman, D., et al. (2000). Medication status and polycystic ovary syndrome in women with bipolar disorder. *Journal of Clinical Psychiatry, 61*, 173–178.

Rice, J., Reich, T., Andreasen, N. C., et al. (1987). The familial transmission of bipolar illness. *Archives of General Psychiatry, 44*, 441–447.

Robert, E., & Guibaud, P. (1982). Maternal valproic acid and congenital neural tube defects [Letter to the editor]. *Lancet, ii*, 937.

Rosa, F. (1991). Spina bifida in infants of women treated with carbamazepine during pregnancy. *New England Journal of Medicine, 324*, 674–677.

Rosenfeld, W. E., Doose, D. R., Walker, S. A., et al. (1997). Effect of topiramate on the pharmacokinetics of an oral contraceptive containing norethindrone and ethinyl estradiol in patients with epilepsy. *Epilepsia, 38*, 317–323.

Roy-Byrne, P., Rubinow, D. R., Hoban, M. C., et al. (1985). Premenstrual changes: A comparison of five populations. *Psychiatry Research, 17*, 77–85.

Roy-Byrne, P., Post, R. M., Uhde, T. W., et al. (1985). The longitudinal course of recurrent affective illness: Life chart data from research patients at the NIMH. *Acta Psychiatrica Scandinavica, 71*(Suppl. 317), 1–34.

Rybakowski, J., Chlopocka-Wosniak, M., Kapelski, Z., et al. (1980). The relative prophylactic efficacy of lithium against manic and depressive recurrences in bipolar patients. *International Pharmacopsychiatry, 15*, 86–90.

Schou, M. (1976). What happened to the lithium babies?: A follow-up study of children born without malformations. *Acta Psychiatrica Scandinavica, 54*, 193–197.

Schou, M., & Amdisen, A. (1973). Lithium and pregnancy: III. Lithium ingestion by children breast-fed by women on lithium treatment. *British Medical Journal, 2*, 138.

Schou, M., & Amdisen, A. (1975). Lithium and the placenta [Letter to the editor]. *American Journal of Obstetrics and Gynecology, 122*, 541.

Scolnik, D., Nulman, I., Rovet, J., et al. (1994). Neurodevelopment of children exposed in utero to phenytoin and carbamazepine monotherapy. *Journal of the American Medical Association, 271*, 767–770.

Secunda, S. K., Katz, M. M., Swann, A., et al. (1985). Mania diagnosis, state measurement and prediction of treatment response. *Journal of Affective Disorders, 8*, 113–121.

Shenfield, G. M. (1993). Oral contraceptives: Are drug interactions of clinical significance? *Drug Safety, 9*, 21–37.

Skausig, O. B., & Schou, M. (1977). Diegivning under lithiumbehandling. *Ugeskrift for Læger, 139*, 400–401.

Spina, E., Pisani, F., & Perucca, E. (1996). Clinically significant pharmacokinetic drug interactions with carbamazepine: An update. *Clinical Pharmacokinetics, 31*, 198–214.

Stahl, M. M., Neiderud, J., & Vinge, E. (1997). Thrombocytopenic purpura and anemia in a breast-fed infant whose mother was treated with valproic acid. *Journal of Pediatrics, 130*, 1001–1003.

Steiner, M., Haskett, R. F., Osmun, J. N., et al. (1980). Treatment of premenstrual tension with lithium carbonate: A pilot study. *Acta Psychiatrica Scandinavica, 61*, 96–102.

Stowe, Z. N., Owens, M. J., Landry, J. C., et al. (1997). Sertraline and desmethylsertraline in human breast milk and nursing infants. *American Journal of Psychiatry, 154*, 1255–1260.

Strakowski, S. M., McElroy, S. L., Keck, P. E., Jr, et al. (1996). Suicidality in mixed and manic bipolar disorder. *American Journal of Psychiatry, 153,* 674–676.

Strakowski, S. M., Tohen, M., Stoll, A. L., et al. (1992). Comorbidity in mania at first hospitalization. *American Journal of Psychiatry, 149,* 554–556.

Suri, R. A., Altshuler, L. L., Burt, V. K., et al. (1998). Managing psychiatric medications in the breast-feeding woman. *Medscape Women's Health, 3,* 1.

Swann, A. C., Bowden, C. L., Morris, D., et al. (1997). Depression during mania: Treatment response to lithium or divalproex. *Archives of General Psychiatry, 54,* 37–42.

Sykes, P. A., Quarrie, J., & Alexander, F. W. (1976). Lithium carbonate and breast feeding. *British Medical Journal, 2,* 1299.

Taschev, T. (1973). The course and prognosis of depression on the basis of 652 patients deceased. In J. Angst (Ed.), *Classification and prediction of outcome of depression* (pp. 157–172). Stuttgart, Germany: Shattaner Verlag.

Tondo, L., Baldessarini, R. J., Floris, G., et al. (1997). Effectiveness of restarting lithium treatment after its discontinuation in bipolar I and bipolar II disorders. *American Journal of Psychiatry, 154,* 548–550.

Tunbridge, W., Evered, D., Hall, R., et al. (1997). The spectrum of thyroid disease in a community: The Whickham Survey. *Clinical Endocrinology, 7,* 481–493.

Tunnessen, W. W., & Hertz, C. G. (1972). Toxic effects of lithium in newborn infants: A commentary. *Journal of Pediatrics, 81,* 804–807.

Vesely, C., Fischer, P., Goessler, R., et al. (1997). Mania associated with serotonin selective reuptake inhibitors. *Journal of Clinical Psychopharmacology, 58,* 88.

Videbech, P., & Gouliaev, G. (1995). First admission with puerperal psychosis: 7–14 years of follow-up. *Acta Psychiatrica Scandinavica, 91,* 167–173.

Viguera, A. C., & Cohen, L. S. (1998). The course and management of bipolar disorder during pregnancy. *Psychopharmacology Bulletin, 34,* 339–346.

Wehr, T. A., Sack, D. A., Rosenthal, N. E., et al. (1988). Rapid cycling affective disorder: Contributing factors and treatment responses in 51 patients. *American Journal of Psychiatry, 145,* 179–184.

Weinstein, M. R., & Goldfield, M. (1969). Lithium carbonate treatment during pregnancy. *Diseases of the Nervous System, 30,* 828–832.

Wisner, K. L., & Perel, J. M. (1996). Psychopharmacological treatment during pregnancy and lactation. In M. F. Jensvold & U. Halbreich (Eds.), *Psychopharmacology and women: Sex, gender, and hormones* (191–224). Washington, DC: American Psychiatric Press.

Wisner, K. L., & Perel, J. M. (1998). Serum levels of valproate and carbamazepine in breastfeeding mother–infant pairs. *Journal of Clinical Psychopharmacology, 18,* 167–169.

Wisner, K. L., Perel, J. M., & Findling, R. L. (1996). Antidepressant treatment during breast-feeding. *American Journal of Psychiatry, 153,* 1132–1137.

Woody, J. N., London, W. L., & Wilbanks, G. D. (1971). Lithium toxicity in a newborn. *Pediatrics, 47,* 94–96.

Yonkers, K. A. (1997). The association between premenstrual dysphoric disorder and other mood disorders. *Journal of Clinical Psychiatry, 58,* 19–25.

Zohar, J., Shapira, B., Oppenheim, G., et al. (1985). Addition of estrogen to imipramine in female resistant depressives. *Psychopharmacology Bulletin, 21,* 705–706.

10

Schizophrenia

JEAN S. GEARON
JILL A. RACHBEISEL

Schizophrenia is perhaps the most devastating of all psychiatric disorders. It typically strikes in young adulthood and has a lifelong episodic course with considerable outcome heterogeneity. Its treatment requires continuous medication and periodic hospitalizations for acute exacerbations of the illness. Treatment is often incomplete and fails to fully eradicate either "positive" symptoms (such as delusions and hallucinations) or "negative" symptoms, which include apathy (low motivation) and blunted affect (restricted range of emotions). The human tragedy of the illness cannot be overemphasized, as these lingering symptoms often rob people of their ability to care for themselves, work, or develop lasting and meaningful relationships.

Individuals with schizophrenia are vulnerable to a number of pernicious outcomes. Painful awareness of their disability often leads to suicide in the early phase of the illness (Goldstein et al., 1993; Harkavy-Friedman & Nelson, 1997). The rate of suicide among young patients with schizophrenia is between 10% and 30%, which is as high as for patients with mood disorders (Caldwell & Gottesman, 1990). In comparison to their peers, they have higher rates of medical comorbidity and earlier mortality rates (Simpson & Tsuang, 1996). They are also at increased risk for HIV and hepatitis C infection (Cournos, 1996; Rosenberg et al., 2001). Furthermore, women with schizophrenia are especially vulnerable to sexual and physical abuse (Gearon & Bellack, 1999; Goodman et al., 1995). The psychological and economic price families pay is remarkable as well. Parents and siblings often harbor their own sadness, fear, anger, and frustration over adult children, who cannot live independently, who drain financial resources, and who periodically become verbally or physically disruptive to the household (Bellack et al., 2000).

Although the incidence of schizophrenia is equal between women and men, there are impressive gender differences in the expression of the illness, its course, psychosocial outcome, and treatment response. That these gender differences may reflect different aspects of the underlying biology of schizophrenia has captured researchers' attention and kept a rather constant focus on the investigation of gender differences in schizophrenia. The importance of better understanding differences in disease manifestation by gender lies not only in its potential to shed light on the pathophysiology of schizophrenia; more practically, these differences demand distinct treatment considerations. This chapter assembles recent findings on gender in schizophrenia, emphasizing timely, representative, and methodologically attentive studies.

DEFINITION AND PHENOMENOLOGY

Schizophrenia is marked by a variety of symptoms that manifest themselves similarly across cultures and over time, even though the presentation and pattern of these symptoms can vary widely among people. Characteristic symptoms fall into two categories—positive and negative. As illustrated in Table 10.1, positive symptoms represent behavioral excesses, whereas negative symptoms reflect behavioral deficits or loss of normal functions.

The acute stage of the illness is defined by extreme thought disorder and severe behavioral disorganization, more commonly referred to as "florid psychosis." Many of these symptoms, however, remain present in milder forms during prodromal periods, occurring prior to acute episodes as well as during residual stages after the episodes subside. As there is no "gold standard" or biological test by which to identify the illness, and few people with schizophrenia exhibit all the characteristic symptoms, the diagnostic criteria defining the disorder have to be derived by consensus. The most widely accepted definition in the United States appears in the *Diagnostic and Statistical Manual of Mental Disorders*, fourth edition (DSM-IV; American Psychiatric Association, 1994). This definition requires that two or more positive or negative symptoms persist for at least 1 month, and

TABLE 10.1. The Positive and Negative Symptoms of Schizophrenia

Positive symptoms	
Delusions	Disturbances in content of thought evidenced by erroneous beliefs that usually involve a misinterpretation of perceptions or experiences.
Hallucinations	Sensory perceptions that are not based on real stimuli—most commonly experienced are auditory hallucinations, better known as "voices."
Formal thought disorder	Disorganized speech as evidenced by tangentiality, loosening of associations, neologisms, or perseverations.
Psychomotor behavior	Grossly disorganized behavior characterized by bizarre or excessive mannerisms, posture, or excitability. Person may also appear disheveled, dress inappropriately (e.g., multiple overcoats in the summer), or have trouble with any goal-directed behaviors.
Negative symptoms	
Affective flattening	Restrictions in the range and intensity of emotional expression.
Alogia	Decreased fluidity and productivity of thought and speech.
Avolition/apathy	Difficulty with the initiation of goal-directed activity, or decreased motivation, interest, or energy.

that continuous signs of the illness (e.g., a prodrome) be present for at least 6 months before a diagnosis can be made. Only one symptom, however, is required if delusions are bizarre or if hallucinations consist of a voice keeping up a running commentary on a person's behaviors or thoughts, or two or more voices conversing with each other. In addition, the DSM-IV definition requires that after illness onset, one or more major areas of functioning (such as work, interpersonal relations, or self-care) be markedly below the level achieved premorbidly.

GENDER DIFFERENCES IN SYMPTOMATOLOGY

Although the symptoms of schizophrenia during *acute* psychotic episodes, whether at first break (Szymanski et al., 1995) or at relapse (Haas et al., 1990; Perry et al., 1995), do not differ between women and men in either type or severity, several studies have reported gender differences in predominant symptom clusters outside of acute stages. Specific positive symptoms (such as paranoia, persecutory delusions, and auditory hallucinations), and some affective symptoms (e.g., dysphoria), are more common in women. Negative symptoms, including affective flattening and social withdrawal, tend to be more severe in men.

In an analysis of 332 outpatients with schizophrenia (171 men and 161 women), Goldstein et al. (1990) found that although both genders expressed positive and negative symptoms, men were at differential risk for affective flattening (negative symptoms), whereas women were differentially vulnerable to dysphoria and persecutory delusions. In another study of 85 consecutively admitted psychiatric outpatients (53 men, 32 women), 41% of the women in comparison to 13% of the men met diagnostic criteria for paranoid schizophrenia (Andia et al., 1990). In a study of patients with first-break schizophrenia, Szymanski et al. (1995) found a significantly lower proportion of primary negative symptoms in female patients (7%) than in males (21%). Finally, in an investigation of unmedicated patients with schizophrenia, men received more severe ratings of negative symptoms than women did (Shtasel et al., 1992). The fact that these studies (consistently and across different patient samples and treatment settings) found women more likely to express a paranoid form of the illness and men more likely to endure negative symptoms speaks to the strength and validity of this gender difference in the expression of the illness.

PREVALENCE AND COURSE OF ILLNESS

The lifetime prevalence rate of schizophrenia is estimated to be 1.3% of the population, or approximately 1.5 million people in the United States (Rosenstein et al., 1989). A precipitous drop in psychosocial functioning during the first several years after the onset of the illness characterizes the course of illness. Following these often devastating and tumultuous early years, however, is a relatively flat or stable course of illness (Childers & Harding, 1990; Tamminga, 1997). In later years (in individuals over 50 years old), significant improvement is often evident in symptoms and function.

Although the lifetime prevalence rate of schizophrenia is equal for women and men, clear and replicated gender differences exist in age of onset and in characteristics of disease course. Women consistently demonstrate a later age of illness onset than men do. Whereas the peak age of onset for women is between 25 and 35, the illness typically strikes men between the ages of 18 and 25 (Angermeyer & Kuhn, 1988; Goldstein et al., 1990). In addition, women have higher premorbid functioning and overall social functioning across illness course than men (Andia et al., 1990; Childers & Harding, 1990; McGlashan & Bardenstein, 1990).

In a follow-up study of chronic inpatients (83 women and 80 men), women consistently ranked higher in premorbid sexual and social functioning than men (McGlashan & Bardenstein, 1990). Moreover, women were twice as likely as men to be married (32% vs. 15%). Men, on the other hand, were more aggressive, antisocial, and self-destructive than were women. In terms of outcome, women spent less time in a psychotic state and had less substance misuse, higher social functioning, greater work competence, and higher global outcome than their male counterparts.

In a study of people with schizophrenia living in a community setting (Test et al., 1990), women were more often parenting children, living with a partner, and heterosexually active then men, indicating higher social functioning. Moreover, they spent less time in jail and committed suicide less frequently. Similar findings were obtained by Andia et al. (1990): Women were more likely to have been married (37% vs. 9%), to live independently (56% vs. 24%), and to be employed (56% vs. 15%). Finally, research from a large patient sample ($n = 603$) showed fewer hospitalization days annually and a lower risk for rehospitalization for women with schizophrenia than men (Angermeyer et al., 1990).

Collectively, these findings suggest that the virulence of schizophrenia is different for women and men, with women having a more benign course of illness. Women manifest their disease later than men and exhibit higher overall functioning. Although social factors may contribute to this higher level of functioning in women, it is unlikely that this profound difference can be explained solely on this basis (Haas et al., 1990; Tamminga, 1997). Consequently, the identification of biological contributors needs to be pursued.

NEUROCOGNITIVE FUNCTIONING

The empirically derived agreement that women with schizophrenia have a less severe disease course than men do has led to the hypothesis that women are also less neurocognitively impaired. Determining the presence or absence of gender differences in neurocognitive functioning is important, as they may reflect different pathophysiologies for female and male patients (Goldstein et al., 1998). Findings from studies of gender differences in neurocognitive functioning, however, are inconsistent. Although some studies have found men more impaired than women in sustained attention, verbal memory, language, executive functions, and intelligence (Goldstein et al., 1994, 1998), others have failed to find gender differences or found the relationship to be complicated. For example, Haas et al. (1990) found no gender differences in neurocognitive functioning in the early phase of the illness, but greater impairment in men over time, possibly reflecting a more deteriorating course of illness in men than in women. Still other studies have found women to perform more poorly than men on tasks of verbal memory, spatial memory, and visual processing (Lewine et al., 1996). Many argue that these inconsistent findings result from different sampling strategies and inadequate sample sizes to test for gender effects (Goldstein, 1993; Walker & Lewine, 1993; Goldstein et al., 1998). Due to these inconsistencies in findings, however, a lack of consensus remains concerning whether gender differences actually exist in neurocognitive functioning in schizophrenia.

PSYCHOSOCIAL OUTCOME

Although research suggests a more benign and forgiving course of illness for women with schizophrenia, their risk for negative psychosocial outcomes such as exposure to traumatic events, particularly sexual and physical violence and the deleterious effects of substance use, is greatly magnified.

Trauma: Physical and Sexual Violence

Evidence documents clearly that women are at increased risk for sexual and physical violence in comparison to men (Breslau et al., 1991; Kessler et al., 1995). In a national survey of 5,877 people, the lifetime prevalence rates for sexual abuse (child and adult) for women were seven times that of men (21% vs. 3.5%; Kessler et al., 1995). Although the gender discrepancy in prevalence rates for childhood physical abuse are not as remarkable, women are still at greater risk. In Kessler et al.'s national survey, 4.8% of women in contrast to 3.2% of men reported a history of childhood physical abuse.

Women with schizophrenia are not exempt from this differential risk for interpersonal violence (Gearon & Bellack, 1999). Indeed, the prevalence rates for sexual and physical abuse of women with serious mental illnesses are twice those observed in the general population of women. Studies indicate that between 34% and 52% report childhood sexual abuse, while lifetime prevalence rates for adult sexual abuse range between 38% and 63% (Goodman et al., 1995; Mueser et al., 1998). The statistics for physical abuse are just as alarming. Between 16% and 20% of women with serious mental illnesses report childhood physical abuse (Mueser et al., 1998; Ross et al., 1994), while 37% to 64% report adult physical abuse (Hutchings & Dutton, 1993; Jacobson, 1989; Mueser et al., 1998).

Not surprisingly, trauma has been linked to a variety of adverse outcomes in people with schizophrenia. Women reporting traumatic experiences, such as sexual and physical abuse, tend to have more severe psychiatric symptoms, are more likely to have substance use disorders, are hospitalized more frequently, and are retraumatized more often (Mueser et al., 1998). Although these findings suggest the importance of understanding the effects of trauma on women with serious mental illnesses and their treatment needs, few studies have focused on investigating the impact of trauma and its manifestation in this population. Three studies, however, have observed high rates of posttraumatic stress disorder (PTSD) in women with schizophrenia and other serious mental illnesses. Craine et al. (1988) found that 34% of women admitted to state psychiatric hospitals had PTSD related to childhood sexual abuse. Other research revealed that 29% of newly admitted psychiatric inpatients experiencing domestic violence had PTSD (Cascardi et al., 1996). In a more recent study, Mueser et al. (1998) examined lifetime exposure of severely mentally ill patients to a variety of traumatic events, and found that 43% of the women self-reported symptoms of PTSD. These estimates of PTSD are clearly higher than the 18% of women estimated to have PTSD in the general population (Breslau et al., 1998). Although these studies of PTSD in people with schizophrenia are thought-provoking and provocative, they have not used standardized structured diagnostic interviews to assess PTSD, and thus their findings must be interpreted cautiously until additional research is completed.

Substance Use Problems

Substance use by people with schizophrenia is a serious public health problem. The lifetime prevalence rate of substance abuse among individuals with schizophrenia is close to 50% (Mueser et al., 1995; Regier et al., 1990), with anecdotal evidence suggesting rates as high as 65% (Drake et al., 1989; Mueser et al., 1992). Even in small amounts, substance use can lead to symptom exacerbation, relapse, rehospitalization, treatment non-compliance, and unstable housing situations (Ziedonis & Fisher, 1994). Indeed, the effective prevention and treatment of substance use is currently one of the biggest challenges facing mental health professionals treating this population (Bellack & Gearon, 1998). Although women and men both suffer from many of the same adverse social, health, psychological, and economic consequences, research suggests that women may be particularly vulnerable to the deleterious effects of substance use.

Studies of both alcohol and illicit drug use show that women become intoxicated become addicted, and develop substance-related disorders sooner than men (Lex, 1995; Schuckit et al., 1995). Because of body weight and metabolic differences between women and men, women who drink roughly half of what men drink will have the same amount of alcohol in their blood as men. Consequently, they develop alcohol-related health problems (including liver damage, hypertension, anemia, malnutrition, peptic ulcers, brain damage, and heart damage) more rapidly than men (Schuckit et al., 1995). According to the National Institute on Alcohol Abuse and Alcoholism (1993), the risk for liver cirrhosis becomes significant for men who drink more than six drinks per day (80 g of pure alcohol), but that risk becomes significant for women at less than two drinks per day (20 g).

The consequences of illicit drug use affect women with particular force as well. Because women may develop dependence on drugs sooner than men, they may experience drug-related health problems (such as heart attacks, strokes, pulmonary disorders, seizures, tremors, motor and visual problems, malnutrition, and infections from intravenous injection sites) more quickly (Trachtenberg & Fleming, 1994). Women with drug addiction are also more vulnerable to contracting HIV and hepatitis C than men—not only because of the easier transmission of the virus from a man to a woman, but because they are more likely to have a drug-using partner with whom they have unprotected sex or share dirty needles, and to have unprotected sex with multiple partners in order to finance their habit (Centers for Disease Control, 1995). Although parallel studies of women and men with schizophrenia have not been conducted, there is no reason to believe that this population of women escapes the increased vulnerability to substance use. Indeed, a recent study by Gearon and Bellack (2000) provides preliminary data indicating that the clinical impact of substance use is more severe for women with schizophrenia than for men.

In this study of 67 outpatients with schizophrenia, effect sizes measuring the magnitude of difference generated by comparisons of substance-misusing and non-substance-misusing women for age of illness onset, number of previous hospitalizations, general level of functioning, and positive and general symptoms were twice as large as those observed for parallel comparisons in men (Gearon & Bellack, 2000). The possibility that substance use may affect women with schizophrenia more swiftly and severely than men demands the development of more effective engagement and treatment interventions. The importance of this goal is underscored by the fact that women with schizophrenia are underrepresented in substance use treatment (Alexander, 1996; Gearon & Bellack, 1999) and that substance use is on the rise in women (Center for Substance Abuse Treatment, 1994; Wilsnack et al., 1991).

TREATMENT RESPONSE

The treatment of schizophrenia requires continuous medication and is often incomplete. In the vast majority of cases, medication is only partially effective at controlling the symptoms of the illness and is accompanied by prominent and uncomfortable side effects. Although the same medications are used to treat women and men with schizophrenia, substantial gender differences exist in treatment response.

Many studies have demonstrated that women with schizophrenia require lower doses of "typical" antipsychotic drugs and have a better and more rapid treatment response than men do (Glick et al., 1993; Szymanski et al., 1995). Szymanski et al. (1995) studied a cohort of patients experiencing their first-break episode of schizophrenia and found that women responded to treatment sooner than men (12.1 weeks vs. 42.1 weeks) and required lower doses. Women are also less likely to relapse into an acute psychotic state than men (2% vs. 18%). A faster response to medication with lower doses may enable women to suffer less "backslide" from an acute episode, with fewer losses (relationships, family support), and may in part explain why women achieve higher levels of functioning and independence.

These gender differences in dose requirements, however, tend to disappear or even to reverse themselves as women get older (Seeman, 1986). One explanation for this is that the antidopaminergic properties of estrogen help modulate dopamine in a similar fashion to antipsychotic medication (Lindamer et al., 1997). Support for this hypothesis is provided by the many studies that have found women with schizophrenia to have fewer symptoms during high-estrogen states (premenopausal and pregnancy) and more symptoms during low-estrogen states (premenstrual and postmenopausal) (Gattaz et al., 1994; Vogel et al., 1992; Seeman, 1996).

GENDER SPECIFIC MEDICATION SIDE EFFECTS

The positive influence of estrogen on psychiatric symptomatology in women is slightly undermined by the presence of gender-specific side effects of medication. "Typical" antipsychotic medications, such as haloperidol, phenothiazines, and thiothixene, as well as the "atypical" antipsychotic medication risperidone, are known to elevate levels of prolactin (a protein hormone linked to sex hormone secretion) (Dickson et al., 1995). As a result, many women with schizophrenia experience antipsychotic-induced hyperprolactinemia, which can result in galactorrhea and irregular menses (Marken et al., 1992; Dickson et al., 1995). Additional negative consequences associated with chronically elevated prolactin levels are sexual dysfunction, infertility, and possibly an increased vulnerability to osteoporosis (Halbreich & Palter, 1996).

With the traditional antipsychotics and risperidone, the prolactin concentrations rise quickly and peak within the first week. The degree of elevation, however, is dose-dependent, and the level at which side effects occur is unpredictable and very individualized (Marken et al., 1992). Kleinberg et al. (1999) reviewed two double-blind studies in which baseline and postbaseline prolactin levels were measured in haloperidol- and risperidone-treated subjects. Ten percent of women reported amenorrhea or galactorrhea as a result of prolactin elevations. The presence of these side effects, however, was not associated with a specific level of prolactin or drug dose. There were no differences in side effects between haloperidol and risperidone.

The management of symptomatic hyperprolactinemia has included dose reduction; bromocriptine, a dopamine receptor agonist (Smith, 1992); and amantadine, an anti-parkinsonian drug (Jann et al., 1993; Correa et al., 1987)—all of which can produce partial to no results and exacerbate psychotic symptoms. More recently, switching women from "typical" "atypical" antipsychotics has provided a more promising alternative, because the "atypical" antipsychotics (e.g., clozapine, olanzapine, and quetiapine) produce modest, if any, prolactin elevations. Olanzapine has been found to have only a transient increase in prolactin, with normalization occurring after several weeks. Similarly, clozapine causes minimal brief elevations in serum prolactin (Gazzola & Olper, 1998; Crawford et al., 1997). These two agents show promise when clinicians are dealing with reproductive dysfunction in women.

FERTILITY AND SEXUALITY

Perhaps an even more important issue in the treatment of schizophrenia in women is the effect of infertility and lack of sexual expression on their self-image. Currier and Simpson (1998) discuss the tendency of clinicians over time to consider antipsychotic-induced amenorrhea as a convenient form of contraception in a population unwilling or unable to comply with standard forms of contraception. For some women, the resulting infertility and absence of menses have a serious impact on self-esteem, with feelings of worthlessness and a loss of sense of purpose (Sullivan & Lukoff, 1990).

The importance of sexuality to many women with schizophrenia is often heightened by the improved quality of life that "atypical" antipsychotics can provide to such women. The switch from a "typical" to an "atypical" medication may help a woman stabilize her symptoms, clear her mind, and enhance her ability to think and feel. As a result, core self-issues such as sexuality may emerge, as well as her struggle with her identity as a woman. Although atypical antipsychotics provide greater choices for the individual and clinician, they also create new challenges, as fewer side effects mean greater freedom of thought and choice. Clinicians must discuss with patients the consequences of switching antipsychotic medications, including the implication of the return of menses and fertility. Furthermore, clinicians must be sensitive to the patients' new awareness of themselves and the world around them. The coordination of psychopharmacological and psychosocial interventions is crucial. For example, eventual social skills training focusing on relationship and dating skills, ways to protect oneself from dangerous and perhaps unwanted situations, and safe-sex education is warranted as the behavioral limitations induced by traditional antipsychotics are eliminated.

CONCLUSION

Gender differences in schizophrenia have been consistently documented in phenomenology, course, psychosocial characteristics, and treatment response. The prominence of these differences highlights the importance of gender-specific interventions for optimal treatment response, as well as ongoing examination of the role of gender in studies of schizophrenia. Evidence indicates that women with schizophrenia should have lower doses of medication over a shorter span of time and psychosocial interventions specifically targeting areas such as abuse prevention, safe-sex education, and parenting skills development. On the other hand, more aggressive psychiatric drug treatment regimens and psychosocial interventions aimed at modulating interpersonal aggression are more clearly indicated for men with schizophrenia.

Challenges for the future include obtaining a deeper understanding of the risk factors linked with gender-specific negative outcomes such as interpersonal trauma and violence. Longitudinal studies are needed to identify behavioral and clinical factors associated with the increased vulnerability of women with schizophrenia to abuse and other trauma. For example, the potential contribution of illness-related neurocognitive deficits to this vulnerability should be investigated, as well as the contribution of psychiatric symptomatology. Attentional deficits may interfere with the ability of women with schizophrenia to perceive danger in the environment or in interpersonal situations. Moreover, women with a greater number of negative symptoms may be at decreased risk for victimization than those with fewer negative symptoms.

The clinical impact of trauma on the course of illness and phenomenology needs to be examined as well. Women with histories of trauma may have additional comorbid diagnoses or complex symptom pictures, which complicate the treatment of schizophrenia. Furthermore, women who have been traumatized may be less likely to engage in treatment and/or to remain treatment-compliant as a result of trust issues arising from sustained interpersonal trauma.

The issue of PTSD also needs to be further addressed. Although studies indicate that the prevalence of PTSD is greater in populations of people with schizophrenia and other serious mental illnesses than in the general community, these studies are preliminary. Because of the overlap in diagnostic criteria between PTSD and schizophrenia (difficulties with concentration and sleep, social and occupational impairment, anhedonia, and restricted affect, to name a few), and the number of factors potentially threatening the validity of self-reported symptoms of PTSD (e.g., neurocognitive deficits and delusional thinking), more thorough and diagnostically sensitive studies are required to achieve accurate understanding of the incidence of PTSD in this population. Moreover, the phenomenon of PTSD in schizophrenia needs to be examined. For example, schizophrenia-related neurocognitive deficits, particularly deficits in memory, may influence how traumatic events are recalled by people with schizophrenia; this may then influence the frequency, severity, and pattern of particular PTSD symptoms, such as the reexperiencing of the traumatic event.

Other areas of future research include the investigation of gender differences in substance use behavior and consequences. Do women with schizophrenia use drugs and alcohol for similar reasons as men do, or as women without schizophrenia do? How do women with schizophrenia gain access to drugs? How does substance use affect the symptom expression and course of illness in women with schizophrenia? Finally, more research needs to focus on the negative outcomes linked with use of atypical antipsychotics in women, such as the increased risk for osteoporosis secondary to the suppression of estrogen in the presence of hyperprolactinemia. In addition, while studies demonstrate that women have a better response to typical antipsychotics than men, few studies have carefully examined the possible differential treatment response of women with schizophrenia to the atypical antipsychotics (Canuso et al., 1998).

In summary, gender differences and gender-specific problems in schizophrenia remain rich and important areas for research. Findings from gender studies in schizophrenia can potentially contribute to our understanding of the pathophysiology of schizophrenia and enable us to develop more accurate and effective interventions.

ACKNOWLEDGMENT

Preparation of this chapter was supported in part by National Institute on Drug Abuse Grant No. DA11199-01.

REFERENCES

Alexander, M. J. (1996). Women with co-occurring addictive and mental disorders: An emerging profile of vulnerability. *American Journal of Orthopsychiatry, 66*(1), 61–70.

American Psychiatric Association. (1994). *Diagnostic and statistical manual of mental disorders* (4th ed.). Washington, DC: Author.

Angermeyer, M. C., & Kuhn, L. (1988). Gender differences in age of onset of schizophrenia. *European Archives of Psychiatry and Clinical Neurosciences, 237*, 351–664.

Angermeyer, M. C., Kuhn, L., & Goldstein, J. M. (1990). Gender and the course of schizophrenia: Differences in treatment outcomes. *Schizophrenia Bulletin, 16*, 293–307.

Andia, A. M., Zisook, S., Heaton, R. K., et al. (1990). Gender differences in schizophrenia. *Journal of Nervous and Mental Disease, 183*, 522–528.

Bellack, A. S., & Gearon, J. S. (1998). Substance abuse treatment for people with schizophrenia. *Addictive Behaviors, 23*(6), 749–766.

Bellack, A. S., Gearon, J. S., & Blanchard, J. J. (2000). Schizophrenia: Psychopathology. In A. S. Bellack & M. Hersen (Eds.), *Psychopathology in adulthood* (2nd ed.). Boston: Allyn & Bacon.

Breslau, N., Davis, G. C., Andreski, P., et al. (1991). Traumatic events and posttraumatic stress disorder in an urban population of young adults. *Archives of General Psychiatry, 48*, 216–222.

Breslau, N., Kessler, R. C., & Chilcoat, H., et al. (1998). Trauma and posttraumatic stress disorder in the community: The 1996 Detroit Area Survey of Trauma. *Archives of General Psychiatry, 55*(7), 626–632.

Caldwell, C. B., & Gottesman, I. I. (1990). Schizophrenics kill themselves too: A review of risk factors for suicide. *Schizophrenia Bulletin, 16*, 571–589.

Canuso, C. M., Goldstein, J. M., & Green, A. I. (1998). The evaluation of women with schizophrenia. *Psychopharmacology Bulletin, 34*(2), 271–277.

Cascardi, M., Mueser, K. T., De Girolomo, J., et al. (1996). Physical aggression against psychiatric inpatients by family members and partners: A descriptive study. *Psychiatric Services, 47,* 531–533.

Center for Substance Abuse Treatment. (1994). *Practical approaches in the treatment of women who abuse alcohol and other drugs.* Rockville, MD: Substance Abuse and Mental Health Services Administration.

Centers for Disease Control. (1995). Update: AIDS among women—United States, 1994. *Morbidity and Mortality Weekly Report, 44*(5), 81–84.

Childers, S. E., & Harding, C. M. (1990). Gender, premorbid social functioning, and long-term outcome in DSM-III schizophrenia. *Schizophrenia Bulletin, 16,* 309–318.

Correa, N., Opler, L., & Kay, S. (1987). Amantadine in the treatment of neuroendocrine side effects of neuroleptics. *Journal of Clinical Psychopharmacology, 7,* 91–95.

Cournos, F. (1996). Epidemiology of HIV. In F. Cournos & N. Bakalar (Eds.), *AIDS and people with severe mental illness* (pp. 3–16). New Haven, CT: Yale University Press.

Craine, L. S., Hensen, C. E., Colliver, J. A., et al. (1988). Prevalence of a history of sexual abuse among female psychiatric patients in a state hospital system. *Hospital of Community Psychiatry, 39,* 300–304.

Crawford, A., Beasley, C., & Tollefson, G. (1997). The acute and long-term effect of olanzapine compared with placebo and haloperidol on serum prolactin concentration. *European Neuropsychopharmacology, 7,* S199.

Currier, G., & Simpson, G. (1998). Antipsychotic medications and fertility. *Psychopharmacology, 49*(2), 175–176.

Dickson, R., Dalby, J., Williams, R., et al. (1995). Risperidone-induced prolactin elevations in premenopausal women with schizophrenia. *American Journal of Psychiatry, 152*(7), 1102–1103.

Drake, R. E., Osher, F. C., & Wallach, M. A. (1989). Alcohol use and abuse in schizophrenia: A prospective community study. *Journal of Nervous and Mental Disease, 177,* 408–414.

Gattaz, W., Vogel, P., Riecher-Rossler, A., et al. (1994). Influence of the menstrual cycle phase on the therapeutic response in schizophrenia. *Biological Psychiatry, 36*(2), 137–139.

Gazzola, L., & Olper, L. (1998). Return of menstruation after switching from risperidone to olanzapine. *Journal of Clinical Psychopharmacology, 18*(6), 486–487.

Gearon, J. S., & Bellack, A. S. (1999). Women with schizophrenia and co-occurring substance use disorders: An increased risk for violent victimization and HIV. *Journal of Community Mental Health, 35*(5), 401–419.

Gearon, J. S., & Bellack, A. S. (2000). Sex differences in illness presentation, course, and level of functioning in substance abusing schizophrenia patients. *Schizophrenia Research.*

Glick, M., Mazure, C. M., Bowers, M. B., et al. (1993). Premorbid social competence and the effectiveness of early neuroleptic treatment. *Comprehensive Psychiatry, 34,* 396–401.

Goldstein, J. M. (1993). Sampling biases in studies of gender and schizophrenia: A reply. *Schizophrenia Bulletin, 19*(1), 9–14.

Goldstein, J. M., Santangelo, S. L., Simpson, J. C., et al. (1990). The role of gender in identifying subtypes of schizophrenia: A latent class analytic approach. *Schizophrenia Bulletin, 16,* 263–275.

Goldstein, J. M., Santangelo, S. L., Simpson, J. C., et al. (1993). Gender and mortality in schizophrenia: Do women act like men? *Psychological Medicine, 23,* 941–948.

Goldstein, J. M., Seidman, L. J., Goodman, J. M., et al. (1998). Are the sex differences in neuropsychological functions among patients with schizophrenia? *American Journal of Psychiatry, 155*(10), 1358–1364.

Goldstein, J. M., Seidman, L. J., Santangelo, S., et al. (1994). Are schizophrenic men at higher risk for developmental deficits than schizophrenic women? Implications for adult neurological functions. *Journal of Psychiatric Research, 28,* 483–498.

Goodman, L., Dutton, M. A., & Harris, M. (1995). Episodically homeless women with serious mental illness: Prevalence of physical and sexual assault. *American Journal of Orthopsychiatry, 65*(4), 468–478.

Haas, G. L., Glick, I. D., Clarkin, J. F., et al. (1990). Gender and schizophrenia outcome: A clinical trial of an inpatient family intervention. *Schizophrenia Bulletin, 16,* 277–292.

Halbreich, U., & Palter, S. (1996). Accelerated osteoporosis in psychiatric patients: Possible pathophysiological processes. *Schizophrenia Bulletin, 22*(3), 447–454.

Harkavy-Friedman, J. M., & Nelson, E. (1997). Management of the suicidal patient with schizophrenia. *Psychiatric Clinics of North America, 20*(3), 625–640.

Hutchings, P. S., & Dutton, M. A. (1993). Sexual assault history in a community mental health center clinical population. *Community Mental Health Journal, 29,* 59–63.

Jacobson, A. (1989). Physical and sexual assault histories among psychiatric outpatients. *American Journal of Psychiatry, 146*(6), 755–758.

Jann, M., Grimsley, D., Gray, E., et al. (1993). Pharmacokenetics and pharmacodynamics of clozapine. *Clinical Pharmacokinetics, 24,* 161–176.

Kessler, R. C., Sonnega, A., Bromet, E., et al. (1995). Posttraumatic stress disorder in the National Comorbidity Survey. *Archives of General Psychiatry, 144,* 508–513.

Kleinberg, D., Davis, J., DeCoster, R., et al. (1999). Prolactin levels and adverse events in patients treated with risperidone. *Journal of Clinical Psychopharmacology, 19*(1), 57–61.

Lewine, R. R. J., Walker, E. F., Shurett, R., et al. (1996). Sex differences in neuropsychological functioning among schizophrenic patients. *American Journal of Psychiatry, 153,* 1178–1184.

Lex, B. W. (1995). Alcohol and other psychoactive substance dependence on women and men. In M. V. Seeman (Ed.), *Gender and psychopathology* (pp. 311–358). Washington, DC: American Psychiatric Press.

Lindamer, L., Lohr, J., Harris, M., et al. (1997). Gender, estrogen, and schizophrenia. *Psychopharmacology Bulletin, 33*(2), 221–228.

Marken, P., Haykal, R., & Fisher, J. (1992). Therapy review: Management of psychotropic-induced hyperprolactinemia. *Clinical Pharmacy, 11*(10), 851–856.

McGlashan, T. H., & Bardenstein, K. K. (1990). Gender differences in affective, schizoaffective, and schizophrenic disorders. *Schizophrenia Bulletin, 16,* 319–329.

Mueser, K. T., Bennett, M., & Kushner, M. G. (1995). Epidemiology of substance use disorders among persons with chronic mental illnesses. In A. F. Lehman & L. B. Dixon (Eds.), *Double jeopardy: Chronic mental illness and substance use disorders* (Vol. 3, pp. 9–25). Langhorne, PA: Harwood Academic.

Mueser, K. T., Goodman, L., Trumbetta, S., et al. (1998). Trauma and posttraumatic stress disorder in severe mental illness. *Journal of Consulting and Clinical Psychology, 66,* 493–499.

Mueser, K. T., Yarnold, P. R., & Bellack, A. S. (1992). Diagnostic and demographic correlates of substance abuse in schizophrenia and major affective disorder. *Acta Psychiatrica Scandinavica, 85,* 48–55.

National Institute on Alcohol Abuse and Alcoholism. (1993). *Eighth special report to the U. S. Congress on alcohol and health.* Alexandria, VA: Author.

Perry, W., Moore, D., & Braff, D. (1995). Gender differences on thought disturbance measures among schizophrenia patients. *American Journal of Psychiatry, 152,* 1298–1301.

Rosenberg, S., Goodman, L. A., Osher, F. C., et al. (2001). Prevalence of HIV, hepatitis B and hepatitis C in people with severe mental illness. *American Journal of Public Health, 91*(1), 31–37.

Rosenstein, M. J., Milazzo-Sayre, L. J., & Manderscheid, R. W. (1989). Care of persons with schizophrenia: A statistical profile. *Schizophrenia Bulletin, 15,* 45–58.

Ross, C. A., Anderson, G., & Clark, P. (1994). Childhood abuse and the positive symptoms of schizophrenia. *Hospital and Community Psychiatry, 45,* 489–491.

Schuckit, M. A., Anthenelli, R. M., Bucholz, K. K., et al. (1995). The time course of development of alcohol-related problems in men and women. *Journal of Studies on Alcohol, 56*(2), 218–225.

Seeman, M. (1996). The role of estrogen in schizophrenia. *Journal of Psychiatry and Neuroscience,* *21*(2), 123–127.

Shtasel, D. L., Gur, R. E., Gallacher, F., et al. (1992). Gender differences in the clinical expression of schizophrenia. *Schizophrenia Research, 7,* 255–231.

Simpson, J. C., & Tsuang, M. T. (1996). Mortality among patients with schizophrenia. *Schizophrenia Bulletin, 22*(3), 485–499.

Smith, S. (1992). Neuroleptic-associated hyperprolactinemia: Can it be treated with bromocriptine? *Journal of Reproductive Medicine, 37*(8), 737–740.

Sullivan, G., & Lukoff, D. (1990). Sexual side effects of antipsychotic medication: Evaluation and interventions. *Hospital and Community Psychiatry, 41*(11), 1238–1241.

Szymanski, S., Lieberman, J. A., Alvir, J. M., et al. (1995). Gender differences in onset of illness, treatment response, course, and biologic indexes in first-episode schizophrenic patients. *American Journal of Psychiatry, 152,* 698–703.

Tamminga, C. A. (1997). Gender and schizophrenia. *Journal of Clinical Psychiatry, 58,* 33–37.

Test, M. A., Burke, S. S., & Wallisch, L. S. (1990). Gender differences of young adults with schizophrenic disorders in community care. *Schizophrenia Bulletin, 16,* 331–344.

Trachtenberg, A. I., & Fleming, M. F. (1994). *Diagnosis and treatment of drug abuse in family practice.* Kansas City, MO: American Academy of Family Physicians.

Vogel, P., Soddu, B., Riecher, A., et al. (1992). Effects of the menstrual cycle of the therapeutic response in schizophrenic patients. *Psychopharmacology, 58,* 92.

Walker, E. F., & Lewine, R. R. J. (1993). Sampling biases in studies of gender and schizophrenia. *Schizophrenia Bulletin, 19*(1), 1–14.

Wilsnack, S. C., Klassen, A. F., Schur, B. E., et al. (1991). Predicting onset and chronicity of women's problem drinking: A five-year longitudinal analysis. *American Journal of Public Health, 81,* 305–318.

Ziedonis, D. M., & Fisher, W. (1994). Assessment and treatment of comorbid substance abuse in individuals with schizophrenia. *Psychiatric Annals, 24,* 447–493.

11

Anxiety Disorders

TERESA A. PIGOTT

ANXIETY DISORDERS: A GENERAL INTRODUCTION

Though the findings are rarely appreciated, population surveys suggest that nearly one out of four Americans will meet criteria for an anxiety disorder during their lifetimes, with females having a much higher risk in comparison to males. In fact, almost one-third of females will meet lifetime criteria for an anxiety disorder. Estimates based on data from the Epidemiologic Catchment Area (ECA) study and the National Comorbidity Survey suggest that lifetime prevalence rates in females for panic disorder (3.4% vs. 0.9%), agoraphobia (9.0% vs. 3.0%), specific phobia (formerly called specific phobia; 13.9% vs. 7.2%), generalized anxiety disorder (GAD; 7.7% vs. 2.9%), and posttraumatic stress disorder (PTSD; 11.3% vs. 6.0%) are two to three times greater than those demonstrated in males (Kessler et al., 1994; Regier et al., 1988; Robins et al., 1984; Yonkers et al., 1996; Boyd et al., 1990; Breslau et al., 1997a; Joyce et al., 1989). Although the gender difference is less pronounced, females in the United States are also more likely to meet lifetime criteria for obsessive–compulsive disorder (OCD; 3.1% vs. 2.0%) and social anxiety disorder (also known as social phobia; 16.4% vs. 11.2%) (Karno et al., 1988; Kessler et al., 1994; Regier et al., 1988; Robins et al., 1984; Bourdon et al., 1988; Magee et al., 1996). Results from epidemiological surveys conducted on an international basis also indicate that anxiety disorders are common and occur predominantly in females (Lindal & Stefansson, 1993; Dick et al., 1994a, 1994b; Weissman et al., 1994).

Females are more frequently afflicted with anxiety disorders at every age, although the overall incidence decreases with advancing age. There is a narrowing in the gender difference for anxiety disorder prevalence rates after the age of 65 (Krasucki et al., 1998). This finding may be explained by several factors, including the cumulative effects of anxiety-related mortality, the difficult task of accurately differentiating an anxiety disorder from cognitive impairment in elderly individuals, and the relative absence of the female reproductive hormone cycle in elderly females (Krasucki et al., 1998).

The presence of an anxiety disorder has been linked to several unfavorable outcomes (Leon et al., 1995). Patients with anxiety disorders are reported to have increased functional impairment, reduced educational and occupational opportunities, and elevated morbidity and mortality rates in comparison to individuals without anxiety disorders (Kessler et al., 1998; Katerndahl & Realini, 1997; Leon et al., 1995; Rogers et al., 1994; Schneier et al., 1994). Increased utilization rates for emergency medical and mental health services have also been linked to an anxiety disorder diagnosis (Wittchen et al., 1994; Roy-Byrne, & Katon, 1997). The onset of anxiety disorders during childhood or adolescence may have particularly serious implications (Regier et al., 1998). Adolescents with an anxiety disorder have an increased risk for teenage pregnancy and parenthood (Kessler et al., 1997). Despite these consequences, relatively few anxiety sufferers receive appropriate treatment (Dick et al., 1994a, 1994b; Kessler et al., 1994; Schneier et al., 1994; Lecrubier & Weiller, 1997; Hollander et al., 1998; Boyd et al., 1990).

Recognition rates for anxiety disorders remain low, and this represents a significant obstacle in preventing effective treatment. Prominent somatic complaints such as heart palpitations, shortness of breath, shaking, sweating, numbness, headaches, and chest pain are common features associated with anxiety disorders. Since these symptoms may also herald the presence of a serious medical condition, a psychiatric condition is often not considered until all other diagnoses have been effectively excluded. This often results in the performance of unnecessary laboratory tests, needless invasive procedures, and considerable delays in treatment and/or referral to mental health professionals. Gender differences in the presentation, attribution, and expression of anxiety symptoms may contribute to further delays in the recognition and treatment of patients with anxiety disorders (Breslau et al., 1997a; Fredrikson et al., 1996; Hantouche & Lancrenon, 1996; Turgeon et al., 1998; Yonkers & Ellison, 1996; Hohmann, 1989). Recent investigations also indicate that primary care physicians are more likely to diagnose patients with primary anxiety disorders as depressed, even in the absence of a mood disorder (Bisserbee et al., 1996; Lecrubier & Weiller, 1997).

Anxiety disorders have extensive comorbidity with other psychiatric disorders. Patients with an anxiety disorder have an increased risk of developing another anxiety disorder during their lifetimes. For example, 40% of patients with OCD will develop an additional anxiety disorder diagnosis during their lifetimes (Rasmussen & Eisen, 1992; Pigott et al., 1994). Lifetime prevalence estimates also suggest that more than two-thirds of patients with an anxiety disorder will subsequently develop a mood disorder, particularly major depressive disorder (Kessler et al., 1994; Regier et al., 1998). The finding of a substantial risk for comorbid mood disorders is likely to further complicate the prompt and accurate recognition of anxiety disorders.

Genetic, biological, developmental, and environmental factors are all routinely implicated, but it remains unclear why anxiety disorders are so much more common in women than in men. Since depressive disorders also occur more frequently in females than in males, a similar underlying genetic diathesis has been proposed. As will be reviewed in this chapter, results from female twin studies provide some evidence that similar or shared genetic components may be involved in the pathophysiology of depression and anxiety disorders, especially GAD (Kendler et al., 1992c, 1995; Kendler, 1996). However, there appears to be considerable genetic heterogeneity, so that the relative contributions of hereditary factors within the specific anxiety disorders may have considerable variance (Kendler et al., 1992c, 1995; Black et al., 1995; Kessler et al., 1998; Stein et al., 1998a).

Developmental and environmental factors may also be important in the pathogenesis of anxiety disorders. Although a history of childhood trauma is associated with an increased risk for subsequent anxiety disorder development in both sexes, females may be particularly sensitive to adverse consequences associated with childhood abuse (Young et al., 1997). Breslau et al. (1997a) have extensively investigated potential gender differences in PTSD. Their findings suggest that even when trauma exposure rates are similar between males and females, females are significantly more likely to develop PTSD. Moreover, a history of childhood trauma is a much more reliable predictor for the presence of adult PTSD in women than in men (Breslau et al., 1997a, 1997b). There is also evidence of gender differences in response to chronic environmental circumstances. For example, Galbaud-du-Fort et al. (1998) investigated the potential association in psychiatric diagnoses between spouses. They reported that the presence of depression, drug addiction, or antisocial personality disorder in one spouse, regardless of gender, increased the risk that the other spouse would meet criteria for an anxiety disorder. However, there were gender differences in the type of anxiety disorder that was likely to be present in the other spouse. For example, drug addiction in one spouse was likely to be associated with GAD in men, but with PTSD in women (Galbaud-du-Fort et al., 1998).

Recently considerable attention has been focused on the potential role of female reproductive hormones, especially estrogen and progesterone, in the pathogenesis of anxiety and mood disorders (Altshuler et al., 1998; Noshirvani et al., 1991; Weiss et al., 1995; Yonkers & Ellison, 1996). Both estrogen and progesterone can produce potent biological actions within the central nervous system (CNS) (Stahl, 1997; McEwen & Parsons, 1987; Seeman, 1997; Shear, 1997). The neurobiological effects associated with estrogen and progesterone may provide critical modulating influences that contribute to the significant gender differences identified in the anxiety disorders.

Moreover, the female reproductive cycle is characterized by periodic fluctuations in these hormone concentrations throughout life, which are likely to have some influence on the subsequent course of anxiety disorders in women. As will be discussed later in this chapter, there is some evidence that anxiety sensitivity may be influenced by the presence of the menstrual cycle as well as by its specific phase. For example, increased anxiety sensitivity has been reported to occur in the luteal, in comparison to the follicular, phase of the menstrual cycle (Stein et al., 1999; Fishman et al., 1994). Elevated rates of anxiety symptoms are also reported during the perimenopause; the presence of very high levels of follicle-stimulating hormone during this period may be helpful in distinguishing women who have depression or anxiety disorders from those who are merely perimenopausal (Huerta et al., 1995).

Pregnancy and the postpartum period have also been linked to substantial changes in anxiety symptoms, including the onset of an anxiety disorder, as well as significant changes in the severity of preexisting anxiety disorders. Although psychological distress and somatic symptoms are frequent complaints during pregnancy and the postpartum period, their presence does not necessarily herald the onset of psychiatric disturbance. In fact, Fava et al. (1990) demonstrated that hypochondriac concerns were quite common in pregnant women and they often increased in severity as the pregnancy progressed. Anxiety complaints such as fear of dying were also found to be frequent, especially during the third trimester in pregnant women. However, these symptoms failed to predict the subsequent development of a psychiatric illness in the pregnant women evaluated during the study (Fava et al., 1990).

Since they have a relatively early onset and are often chronic in clinical course, anxiety disorders are present during the years associated with childbearing capacity in women. There are relatively few data, however, concerning the potential impact of pregnancy and the postpartum period on preexisting anxiety disorders. Given these issues, this chapter provides an overview of the anxiety disorders, with a special focus on potential gender differences that may exist. In addition, available information concerning the potential impact of the female reproductive cycle (menstruation, menopause, and pregnancy) on the clinical presentation and course of anxiety disorders is summarized.

GENERALIZED ANXIETY DISORDER

Epidemiology and Clinical Overview

GAD is one of the most common of the anxiety disorders, with most estimates suggesting a lifetime prevalence rate between 5% and 6% (Kessler et al., 1994; Boyd et al., 1990). Most studies report a two- to threefold greater lifetime risk for GAD in females than in males. The onset of GAD is typically during late adolescence or early adulthood, and most studies suggest that a chronic, persistent course is most common (Kessler et al., 1994; Boyd et al., 1990; Wittchen et al., 1994; Woodman et al., 1999). In contrast to prevalence estimates suggesting that anxiety disorder prevalence decreases with increasing age, the prevalence of GAD remains constant throughout life (Krasucki et al., 1998).

A diagnosis of GAD is associated with elevated rates of functional impairment, higher rates of medically unexplained symptoms, and overutilization of health care resources (Roy-Byrne & Katon, 1997; Kennedy & Schwab, 1997; Wittchen et al., 1994). These findings may reflect the tendency for patients with GAD to present in a primary care, rather than a behavioral health care, setting. Available evidence indicates that GAD increases health care utilization by an indirect route. That is, the presence of GAD appears to modify the presentation and course of other coexisting psychiatric conditions that directly result in increased health care costs (Roy-Byrne & Katon, 1997). Patients with GAD are also more likely to be prescribed psychotropic medication than are patients with other anxiety disorders (Wittchen et al., 1994; Hohmann, 1989).

In addition to the association of GAD with an elevated risk of disability and morbidity, remission rates are also apparently fairly low. In fact, preliminary results from the large, prospective Harvard Anxiety Research Project (HARP) study indicate that only 8% of the patients with GAD were considered symptom-free at the time of the 2-year follow-up assessment (Yonkers et al., 1996). A systematic comparison of patients with GAD and panic disorder provides more support for the contention that GAD is often associated with a grave clinical course. In this comparative study, GAD had an earlier age of onset and a longer duration of illness than panic disorder. In addition, significantly lower remission rates were reported for the patients with GAD (18%) than for the patients with panic disorder (45%) throughout the 5-year study (Woodman et al., 1999).

GAD and Gender

Much of the disability associated with GAD may be attributable to the frequent co-occurrence of other psychiatric conditions. Large-scale population surveys suggest that 85–90% of patients with GAD will develop a comorbid psychiatric disorder during their lifetimes (Wittchen et al., 1994). Despite the extremely high occurrence of comorbid conditions in GAD, some important gender differences have been identified. Complicated GAD (GAD with a coexisting psychiatric disorder) is much more likely to occur in females than in males. Moreover, depressive disorders such as dysthymia coexist more frequently in females with GAD (Wittchen et al., 1994; Yonkers et al., 1996). Females are also more likely to seek treatment for GAD than males, especially when comorbid diagnoses are present (Bland et al., 1997b).

In addition to potentially modifying the clinical features and presentation of GAD, gender may have an important impact on the clinical course and ultimate outcome of GAD. Results from population surveys and prospective studies indicate that complicated GAD has a worse prognosis and reduced chance of remission than GAD alone does (Yonkers et al., 1996; Wittchen et al., 1994). Coexisting GAD and depression, in particular, have been linked to a number of unfavorable consequences, including greater functional impairment and an elevated risk of suicide (Bakish, 1999; Wittchen et al., 1994; Robins et al., 1984; Breslau et al., 1995). Given the finding that they are more likely to have complicated GAD as well as comorbid depression, it is not surprising that greater symptom severity and a more chronic course are reported for GAD in females than in males (Yonkers et al., 1996).

The identified gender differences may have additional ramifications besides their apparent impact on clinical course and outcome in GAD. The frequent occurrence of depression in females with GAD may represent an important clue in understanding its underlying pathophysiology. That is, their more common coexistence in females may reflect an enhanced vulnerability that is in part mediated by gender-specific factors. Whereas earlier investigations tended to emphasize sociocultural and environmental influences in the preponderance of females with anxiety disorders, more recent research has focused on the potential contribution of genetic factors in this finding. Kendler and colleagues (Kendler et al., 1992a, 1995; Kendler, 1996) have analyzed data obtained from bivariate female twin pairs to investigate the potential genetic basis of GAD. Their findings suggest that genetic factors are more important than environment factors in mediating the expression of GAD. Moreover, their findings suggest that a shared genetic basis (genotype) may determine the risk for subsequent development of GAD and depression. That is, GAD and depression may represent separate expressions (phenotypes) of the same underlying genotype in females. Kendler (1996) hypothesizes that a confluence of environmental and biological factors may ultimately determine whether GAD or depression is expressed when the genotype is present within an individual.

Patients with GAD exhibit evidence of several underlying biological abnormalities. Dysfunction within the central serotonin (5-HT) and γ-aminobutyric acid (GABA) pathways has been demonstrated in patients with GAD versus control subjects (Brawman-Mintzer & Lydiord, 1997). Evidence of dysregulation within the complex modulation of the locus ceruleus–norepinephrine–sympathetic nervous system and the hypothalamic–pituitary–adrenocortical (HPA) axis has also been demonstrated in patients with GAD in comparison to control subjects (Brawman-Mintzer & Lydiard, 1997). Results from neuroimaging studies also provide support for the presence of altered CNS function in GAD. Patients with GAD are reported to have a significantly more homogeneous pattern of distribution of benzodiazepine receptors within the brain than control subjects have. This finding implies that patients with GAD may have relatively less heterogeneity in their cerebral blood flow and metabolism than control subjects have. Although the clinical relevance of this finding may seem obscure, it may represent a finding analogous to the discovery that patients with ischemic heart disease exhibit reduced myocardial blood flow heterogeneity in comparison to subjects with normal cardiac function (Tiihonen et al., 1997). It is not clear, however, whether these findings are substantially influenced by gender. Further systematic studies of potential gender differences are currently lacking in GAD.

GAD and the Female Reproductive Cycle

In addition, little is known about the impact of the female reproductive cycle on the development or course of GAD. There is some evidence that GAD symptoms become more severe during the premenstrual period in females with GAD and coexisting premenstrual syndrome (McLeod et al., 1993). However in the same report, there was no significant correlation between GAD symptoms and menstrual cycle phase in the patients with GAD who did not have coexisting premenstrual syndrome.

Medications generally considered first-line treatments for GAD include buspirone, venlafaxine, high-potency benzodiazepines, and selective serotonin reuptake inhibitor (SSRI) antidepressants (Brawman-Mintzer & Lydiard, 1997). In animal models, gender may have a substantial impact on the anxiolytic effects associated with benzodiazepine administration. In particular, anxiolytic response in female rodents may differ according to the phase of the estrous cycle (Fernandez-Guasti & Picazo, 1990). Unfortunately, the potential impact of gender and the menstrual cycle on the therapeutic response of medication in GAD has yet to be reported.

PANIC DISORDER

Epidemiology and Clinical Overview

Epidemiological surveys suggest that 15–20% of people will endorse panic symptoms and that approximately 4–8% experience symptoms consistent with a panic attack. Lifetime prevalence estimates indicate that 2.5–5.0% will meet criteria for panic disorder (Joyce et al., 1989; Dick et al., 1994a; Kessler et al., 1994; Eaton et al., 1991). Interestingly, panic attacks, even in the absence of panic disorder, may represent a significant development, especially in females. For example, 63% of females and 40% of males with panic attacks subsequently developed an additional psychiatric disorder in one report (Reed & Wittchen, 1998).

Data from epidemiological surveys also indicate that females are two to three times more likely than males to develop panic disorder (Joyce et al., 1989; Kessler et al., 1994; Eaton et al., 1991; Weissman et al., 1997). Most reports suggest that panic disorder typically emerges in the mid-20s (Eaton et al., 1991; Robins et al., 1984; Kessler et al., 1994), although some reports have suggested additional peaks of onset during adolescence (Weissman et al., 1997; Reed & Wittchen, 1998) and between 30 and 40 years of age (Dick et al., 1994a). A diagnosis of panic disorder has been linked to several unfavorable outcome measures, including increased utilization of medical and mental health services (Hollifield et al., 1997; Katerndahl & Realini, 1997; Katerndahl, 1990) and an increased risk of suicide (Weissman et al., 1989). Keller and Hanks (1993) estimate that 40% of patients with panic disorder may need treatment for 1 year and that 20–40% will require continued maintenance treatment. Preliminary results from an ongoing, 12-site naturalistic long-term study of patients with panic disorder, the HARP study, also confirm that many patients treated for panic will require long-term or chronic treatment.

Despite the adverse consequences associated with panic disorder, however, surprisingly few patients seek treatment for it. In a report by Katerndahl (1990), 44% of patients with prominent symptoms of either "nervousness" or "panic attacks" failed to seek medical care for those complaints. Certain factors such as race (white), educational level (higher), and access to health care (easier access and closer proximity) were found to correlate with increased health-care-seeking behaviors. The presence of panic-related symptoms, as well as the patients' belief that they could freely discuss panic symptoms, was also linked to increased use of health-care-related services. Gender and other variables, such as age, marital status, and panic-related symptoms or behaviors, failed to predict health-seeking behavior in these patients (Katerndahl, 1990).

Patients with panic disorder are more likely than other anxiety disorder sufferers to present to an emergency department for treatment of anxiety-related symptoms. In fact, a recent report (Fleet et al., 1998) found that 25% (108/441) of patients presenting to an emergency department with chest pain were subsequently diagnosed with panic disorder. Factors more likely to predict panic-related chest pain were younger age (37 vs. 52 years), female gender (63% vs. 39%), and the presence of a comorbid psychiatric disorder (especially agoraphobia, social anxiety disorder, or PTSD) (Fleet et al., 1998). High rates of comorbid panic disorder have also been linked to the presence of a functional gastrointestinal disorder such as irritable bowel syndrome (Walker et al., 1993).

Panic Disorder and Gender

Several gender differences have been identified in panic disorder. Females with panic disorder report more individual panic-related symptoms and a greater level of phobic avoidance than males (Dick et al., 1994a; Turgeon et al., 1998). Females with panic disorder are also more likely to report situations such as leaving home or using public transportation as precipitants for panic attacks (Starcevic et al., 1998). These findings may explain the greater levels of dependence and functional impairment detected when panic disorder occurs in females in comparison to males.

Most patients with panic disorder (80–90%) will also have a coexisting psychiatric diagnosis. Depression (60–80%), substance use disorders (40–50%), and phobic disorders (40–50%) are the most common comorbid diagnoses in panic disorder (Marshall, 1996; Kessler et al., 1994; Reed & Wittchen, 1998; Andrade et al., 1996; Yonkers et al., 1998). In general, females with panic disorder have a greater risk for comorbid psychiatric disorders than males with panic disorder do. Agoraphobia occurs more frequently in females with panic disorder. This finding has important implications, since the presence of agoraphobia in panic disorder is associated with a less favorable outcome than the presence of panic disorder alone. Females who have panic disorder with agoraphobia report greater phobic avoidance, more catastrophic thoughts, and a heightened awareness of body sensations than do males who have panic disorder with agoraphobia. Panic disorder with agoraphobia is more likely to be complicated by social phobia or PTSD in females (Turgeon et al., 1998).

Comorbid psychiatric disorders such as depression, GAD, specific phobia, and somatization disorder also occur more frequently in females with panic disorder (Yonkers

& Ellison, 1996; Yonkers et al., 1998; Marshall, 1996; Andrade et al., 1996). These findings may help to explain why the course of panic disorder in females is reported to be more chronic and severe. They may also account for the increased risk of recurrence in panic after a period of remission occurs in females with panic disorder (Yonkers et al., 1998). Coexisting alcohol abuse is more common in males with panic disorder, but females with panic disorder also have an increased risk for alcohol abuse and dependence (Cox et al., 1993; Kessler et al., 1994). Two reports (Kendler et al., 1995; Battaglia et al., 1995) suggest that the relatives of females with panic disorder may also have an increased risk for alcohol dependence. Although further research and replication is indicated, this finding has been interpreted as evidence of a possible genetic link between panic disorder and alcohol use disorder in females.

These findings indicate that a diagnosis of panic disorder in females is associated with a more complicated course and an overall poorer outcome than in males. Since the etiology of panic disorder remains obscure, it is difficult to explain why females have a greater risk and a more malevolent course for panic disorder than males. Numerous neurobiological and psychological theories have been proposed for panic disorder. Most psychological theories emphasize the importance of cognitive misinterpretation and "false threat alarms" as the basis for the subsequent development of panic disorder (Windmann, 1998). Biological theories, in contrast, implicate altered brain function and an abnormal ventilatory response in the pathophysiology of panic (Nutt et al., 1998). Neural circuits within the amygdala and its ascending cortical pathways are most often speculated to represent the functional neuroanatomy of panic disorder. Altered dysregulation of the ventilatory response and associated neurovascular instability may also be important factors in the pathophysiology of panic disorder (Coplan & Lydiard, 1998). Both physiological (e.g., carbon dioxide [CO_2] sensitivity) and psychological (anxiety sensitivity) factors have been suggested as predisposing factors in the development of panic disorder (Stein et al., 1999; Coplan & Lydiard, 1998). Despite the striking gender differences identified in the prevalence and clinical features associated with panic disorder, evidence of significant gender differences in the purported pathophysiology of panic disorder have not been detected.

Results from covariate female twin studies suggest that genetic or familial factors play a role in panic disorder, although their contribution is estimated to be relatively modest (Kendler et al., 1993). There is some evidence that genetic factors may be particularly critical in determining risk for panic disorder in females. That is, the presence of a specific genetic polymorphism in females may convey an increased risk for panic disorder. Females with panic disorder had a higher occurrence of a novel repeat genetic polymorphism on chromosome X than control subjects in one report (Deckert et al., 1999). This genetic polymorphism is thought to mediate expression of monoamine oxidase (MAO) A. Since MAO inhibitor (MAOI) antidepressants are known to be effective antipanic agents, this finding has been interpreted as evidence that altered MAO activity may be a risk factor for panic disorder in females (Deckert et al., 1999). These results are very interesting, but require replication and further study.

Panic Disorder and the Female Reproductive Cycle

Estrogen and progesterone have complex effects on the CNS. Estrogen is generally considered a facilitator of neurotransmission via its ability to reduce MAO enzyme activity and enhance serotonergic tone. Estrogen's biological actions are thought to convey some mood enhancing or antidepressant effects. In contrast, progesterone increases MAO enzyme activity. Allopregnanolone, a major metabolite of progesterone, enhances GABA tone via its effects as an allosteric modulator at the GABA–benzodiazepine receptor complex. Since GABA represents one of the major inhibitors of neurotransmission within the CNS, progesterone's biological effects may convey an anxiolytic action (Stahl, 1997; Warnock & Bundren, 1997; Shear, 1997).

The female reproductive cycle (menstruation, pregnancy, and menopause) is characterized by relatively dramatic fluctuations in estrogen and progesterone concentrations. These hormonal fluctuations may have a role in determining the overall risk for panic disorder and may also have a substantial impact on the clinical course of panic disorder in women. The dramatic decline in estrogen and progesterone levels that characterizes the midluteal phase of the menstrual cycle has been linked to the emergence or worsening of anxiety symptoms in female subjects (Yonkers & Ellison, 1996). Several reports, primarily retrospective in nature, confirm that females with panic disorder report an increase in their anxiety and panic symptoms during the midluteal or premenstrual phase of the menstrual cycle (Cook et al., 1990; Griez et al., 1990). This finding, however, has not been replicated in studies conducted on a prospective basis. Instead, prospective studies reported to date in females with panic disorder have failed to detect any significant correlation between menstrual cycle phase and ratings of panic or anxiety symptoms (Cook et al., 1990; Stein et al., 1989a; McLeod et al., 1993).

However, biological challenge paradigms conducted in females with panic disorder have detected evidence of changes in anxiety sensitivity across the menstrual cycle. Acute ingestion of CO_2 is often used as a provocative challenge to precipitate anxiety and panic attacks in experimental conditions (Griez et al., 1990). Females with panic disorder appear to have menstrual cycle phase (follicular vs. luteal) changes in anxiety sensitivity (Fishman et al., 1994). That is, females with panic disorder who were administered CO_2 had greater anxiety responses during the midluteal phase in comparison to the earlier follicular phase of the menstrual cycle. In contrast, there was no correlation between CO_2-induced anxiety response and phase of the menstrual cycle in the female control subjects (Perna et al., 1995). Alprazolam treatment was reported to subsequently "normalize" the CO_2-induced anxiety response in females with panic disorder (Fishman et al., 1994).

Precipitous estrogen withdrawal, whether physiological or induced by medication or surgical intervention, has been linked to the subsequent emergence of panic disorder. In a large study ($n = 390$) of perimenopausal women with new-onset but "ill-defined" psychological and somatic symptoms, 7% were found to meet criteria for panic disorder (Ushiroyama & Sugimoto, 1994). Moreover, results from another report indicate that a diagnosis of panic disorder should be considered in perimenopausal women with hot flushes that fail to attenuate during hormone replacement therapy (Van der Feltz-Cornelis, 1999). Medical interventions that have primary progesterone-like effects, such as birth control pills or Norplant implants, have also been associated with the acute development of panic disorder (Wagner & Berenson, 1994). Ovarian suppressants utilized for the treatment of endometriosis, such as leuprolide, may elicit panic attacks and other psychiatric disturbances (Warnock & Bundren, 1997).

Pregnancy and the postpartum period are marked by particularly dramatic fluctuations in gonadal hormone concentrations. Pregnancy is characterized by two- to threefold increases in estrogen and a dramatic elevation (80- to 100-fold) in progesterone concentration (Altshuler et al., 1998). Progesterone is a potent stimulant for oxygen drive, and (as previously noted) its metabolite, allopregnanolone, has GABA-enhancing effects. Given these actions, women with preexisting panic disorder might be expected to experience a substantial attenuation or remission in panic during pregnancy. Available data, however, suggests a more variable course for preexisting panic disorder during pregnancy. It appears from available data that about half (40–45%) will not have a significant change in their panic symptoms, whereas 30–35% will experience improvement and a substantial worsening in panic will occur in 20–30% of patients with preexisting panic disorder during the course of a first pregnancy (Northcott & Stein, 1989; Cohen et al., 1994a). Interestingly, the course of panic disorder during successive pregnancies is often markedly different (Northcott & Stein, 1989; Cohen et al., 1994a; Villeponteaux et al., 1992).

Postpartum worsening (35–63%) is a much more consistent finding demonstrated in women with preexisting panic disorder (Northcott & Stein, 1994; Beck, 1998; Cohen et al., 1994b; Sholomskas et al., 1993). The postpartum period may also be associated with an increased risk for the onset of panic disorder. According to available data, 11–29% of women with panic disorder report onset during the postpartum period (Wisner et al., 1996; Sholomskas et al., 1993). Since this rate is significantly greater than the expected age-corrected rate for panic onset in females, it is unlikely to represent a coincidental event (Sholomskas et al., 1993).

In patients with preexisting panic disorder, pregnancy does not appear to increase the likelihood that medication for panic can be successfully discontinued (Cohen et al., 1994a). Instead, there is some rationale for continuing or restarting pharmacotherapy during the latter part of pregnancy. Cohen et al. (1994b) demonstrated that pregnant women with preexisting panic disorder who received antipanic medication were significantly less likely to experience a postpartum exacerbation than those who did not receive treatment during pregnancy.

SSRIs, MAOIs, and tricyclic antidepressants (TCAs) have all demonstrated efficacy in the treatment of panic disorder (Sheehan, 1999). High-potency benzodiazepine medications, such as lorazepam, alprazolam, and clonazepam are also effective antipanic agents. Each of the antipanic medications classes (SSRIs, MAOIs, TCAs, and benzodiazepines) is associated with a similar rate of improvement (60–70%) in panic symptomatology. However, buspirone and other medications with primary serotonergic effects do not appear to be more effective than placebo for panic disorder (Bell & Nutt, 1998). Males had a poorer response than females during treatment with the TCA desipramine in one study conducted in patients with panic disorder (Kalus et al., 1991). However, very few studies have specifically focused on the potential impact of gender on medication or treatment response in patients with panic disorder.

SPECIFIC PHOBIA

Epidemiology and Clinical Overview

Large population surveys conducted in the United States have established specific phobia as one of the most common of the psychiatric disorders (20% lifetime prevalence) (Kessler et al., 1994; Eaton et al., 1991). Specific phobia occurs twice as often in females as in males. Such phobias encompass a wide range of situations and "feared" objects. Several authors have suggested that three primary types of specific phobias exist: (1) situational phobias (e.g., claustrophobia, acrophobia); (2) animal phobias (e.g., fear of spiders, insects, snakes, etc.); and (3) health-related phobias (e.g., fear of injections, blood, dental procedures, etc.). The most common of these categories appears to be situational phobias, followed by animal phobias and health-related phobias, respectively (Boyd et al., 1990; Bourdon et al., 1988; Dick et al., 1994b).

Comorbid disorders frequently occur in specific phobia. Depressive disorders, substance use disorders, and OCD are reported to be the most common comorbid conditions in primary specific phobia (Bourdon et al., 1988; Eaton et al., 1991; Kessler et al., 1994; Regier et al., 1990; Magee et al., 1996). Although specific phobias tend to persist, they are rarely associated with significant disability or functional impairment. It is not surprising, therefore, that relatively few (20–25%) patients present for treatment of these phobias (Lindal & Stefansson, 1993; Boyd et al., 1990). Bivariate twin studies suggest that specific phobia is much more likely to arise from environmental than from genetic factors (Kendler et al., 1992b).

Specific Phobia and Gender

Population surveys indicate that females are two to three times more likely than males to have the situational type of specific phobia. Similarly, lifetime prevalence estimates suggest that animal phobias are two to three times more common in females. In contrast, no gender difference occurs in prevalence rates for the health-related type of specific phobia (Fredrikson et al., 1996). Some reports have suggested that females may have a significantly earlier age of onset for specific phobia (Dick et al., 1994b). Additional data concerning potential gender differences or the possible influence of reproductive cycles on specific phobia are currently lacking.

SOCIAL ANXIETY DISORDER

Epidemiology and Clinical Overview

Although results from the ECA study suggested that social anxiety disorder is a relatively rare condition, the National Comorbidity Survey reported much higher (13%) prevalence rates (Schneier et al., 1992; Kessler et al., 1994). Both studies, however, confirmed that social anxiety disorder is associated with significant disability and functional impairment (Schneier et al., 1994; Boyd et al., 1990; Kessler et al., 1994; Stein et al., 1998a). Lifetime prevalence estimates suggest that females have a slightly higher lifetime prevalence risk for social anxiety (1.5 times) than males (Kessler et al., 1994; Dick et al., 1994b). The onset of social anxiety disorder is typically during childhood or adolescence. According to the ECA data, the mean age of onset for social anxiety disorder is 12 years (Regier et al., 1998).

According to the *Diagnostic and Statistical Manual of Mental Disorders*, fourth edition (DSM-IV), social anxiety disorder can be generalized or nongeneralized (American Psychiatric Association, 1994). The generalized and nongeneralized subtypes of social anxiety disorder are reported to be similar in ages of onset, family histories, and certain sociodemographic correlates (Kessler et al., 1998; Stein & Chavira, 1998). Considerable differences, however, exist in the course and outcome associated with the generalized versus the nongeneralized subtype of social anxiety disorder. The nongeneralized subtype is usually episodic in course and rarely results in significant functional impairment (Stein & Chavira, 1998). Generalized social anxiety disorder, in contrast, is chronic in course and associated with significant dysfunction in a wide range of educational, occupational, and familial arenas (Kessler et al., 1998; Westenberg, 1998; Stein & Chavira, 1998; Schneier et al., 1992, 1994).

Despite these adverse consequences, relatively few people with social anxiety disorder receive adequate treatment (Kessler et al., 1994; Boyd et al., 1990; Essau et al., 1998). This may in part result from the poor recognition rate associated with the diagnosis of social anxiety disorder. In one report (Bisserbee et al., 1996), 5% of patients assessed in a primary care setting met criteria for social anxiety disorder. However, according to their primary treating physicians, fewer than half of these patients were considered to have a "psychiatric condition." The primary care physicians correctly identified only 15% of the patients with social anxiety disorder (Lecrubier & Weiller, 1997; Bisserbee et al., 1996).

Comorbid disorders occur frequently (80–90%) and may also obscure or delay recognition of social anxiety disorder. Since the onset is very early, these comorbid disorders generally represent secondary phenomena (Schneier et al., 1992; Stein & Chavira, 1998; Kessler et al., 1998). Agoraphobia is the most common coexisting illness (odds ratio = 10.4), but patients with generalized social anxiety disorder may also have an elevated risk for major depressive episodes and substance use disorders (Kessler et al., 1994, 1998; Dick et al., 1994b; Regier et al., 1998; Bisserbee et al., 1996; Lecrubier & Weiller, 1997). Available data also indicate that most patients (70–90%) with generalized social anxiety disorder also meet criteria for avoidant personality disorder (Alpert et al., 1997). Although some of this comorbidity is attributable to an extensive overlap in diagnostic criteria, the coexistence of avoidant personality disorder and social anxiety disorder may convey some prognostic significance. That is, patients with social anxiety disorder and avoidant personality may have greater functional impairment and an elevated risk for subsequently developing depressive disorder than patients with social anxiety disorder alone (Alpert et al., 1997). Patients with coexisting social anxiety and panic disorder may also have a substantially increased risk for depression (Stein et al., 1989b).

Childhood behavioral inhibition is implicated as a nonspecific risk factor for the development of an anxiety disorder in adults. However, social anxiety disorder in particular is most strongly associated with a history of behavioral inhibition during childhood (Mick & Telch, 1998). Childhood selective mutism may represent a precursor to the development of social anxiety disorder. In fact, 70% of the first-degree relatives of children with selective mutism were reported to have social anxiety disorder in one study (Black & Uhde, 1995).

The neurobiology of social anxiety disorder is poorly understood, although preliminary research has identified evidence of several different biological abnormalities. Challenge paradigms comparing patients with social anxiety disorder and control subjects after acute administration of CO_2, cholecystokinin, or caffeine have detected evidence of enhanced sensitivity and potential cardiovascular and adrenergic abnormalities in the patients. Serotonergic dysfunction is implicated by pharmacological challenge results as well as by the efficacy of the SSRI antidepressants in the treatment of social anxiety disorder (Nutt et al., 1998; Davidson, 1998). Patients with social anxiety disorder who are administered serotonergic probes demonstrate evidence of altered neuroendocrine and behavioral responses in comparison to control subjects. Functional neuroimaging studies also reveal evidence of altered dopaminergic function in patients with social anxiety disorder. In particular, a significant reduction in striatal dopamine reuptake has been detected in patients versus control subjects (Nutt et al., 1998).

Results from bivariate female twin studies and family studies conducted in patients with generalized social anxiety disorder also support the importance of genetic factors (Kendler et al., 1992b; Stein et al., 1998a, 1999). Relatives of patients with generalized social anxiety disorder have a ten times greater risk for social anxiety disorder than relatives of control subjects do. In contrast, results from family and twin studies of nongeneralized social anxiety disorder fail to detect evidence that supports an essential role for genetic or familial factors in the transmission of this subtype (Stein et al., 1998a).

A number of pharmacological treatments, including MAOIs, ß-blockers, high-potency benzodiazepines, and SSRIs, have all demonstrated efficacy in the treatment of social anxiety disorder (Davidson, 1998; Pollack, 1999; Ballenger et al., 1998). In the largest multicenter, placebo-controlled trial reported to date, paroxetine was more effective than placebo in both moderate and severe social anxiety disorder (Stein et al., 1998b). According to the International Consensus Treatment Guidelines for Mood and Anxiety Disorders, SSRI antidepressants are considered first-line therapy for social anxiety disorder. These guidelines also advocate long-term treatment (>12 months) for patients with generalized social anxiety disorder who have (1) persistent symptoms despite treatment, (2) a comorbid psychiatric condition, (3) a history of relapse after treatment discontinuation, or (4) a very early onset of social anxiety disorder (Ballenger et al., 1998). However, little information is available concerning the potential impact of gender on treatment response in social anxiety disorder.

Social Anxiety Disorder and Gender

Although data are limited, some significant gender differences have been identified in social anxiety disorder. Lifetime prevalence rates, as previously noted, are slightly higher in women than in men (15.5% vs. 11.1%) However, men may seek treatment significantly more often than women when social anxiety disorder is present (Weinstock, 1999). In an exploratory investigation (Turk et al., 1998), no gender differences were detected in the course or subtype of social anxiety disorder. Males and females with this disorder also had similar rates of comorbidity for additional anxiety disorders, mood disorders, and avoidant personality disorder. The women with social anxiety disorder did exhibit more severe social fears. Gender differences were also detected in self-report measures of fear in certain social situations. For example, the women reported significantly greater fear in association with a wide range of activities, including talking to authority figures, acting/performing/speaking/working in front of others or while being observed, being the center of attention, expressing disagreement or disapproval to people they did not know very well, or giving a party. In contrast, the men reported significantly more fear than women regarding urinating in public bathrooms and returning goods to a store (Turk et al., 1998). Although gender differences in comorbid conditions were not detected in this study, other reports have suggested that agoraphobia may co-occur at a greater rate in females than in males with social anxiety disorder (Dick et al., 1994b; Lecrubier & Weiller, 1997).

Preliminary evidence also suggests that the presence of social anxiety disorder during pregnancy may be particularly problematic since depression, panic, and substance use disorders are frequent complications of untreated social anxiety disorder (Weinstock, 1999). Unfortunately, further information concerning the potential impact of gender, as well as the possible effects of the female reproductive cycle on social anxiety disorder, is currently lacking.

OBSESSIVE-COMPULSIVE DISORDER

Epidemiology and Clinical Overview

Estimates derived from the ECA study and the Cross-National OCD Group Study suggest a 2–3% lifetime prevalence rate for OCD. Prevalence rates for OCD are slightly higher in females (1.5:1) than in males (Karno et al., 1988; Weissman et al., 1994). Baer (1994) has demonstrated that OCD symptoms can be subdivided into three primary symptom factors: "symmetry/hoarding," "contamination/cleaning," and "pure obsessions." Population surveys indicate that the mean age of onset for OCD is significantly earlier in males (20 vs. 25 years) than in females (Karno et al., 1988; Weissman et al., 1994). Although data from clinical samples suggest a much earlier age of onset, males with OCD continue to exhibit a much earlier onset than females with OCD (Rasmussen & Eisen, 1990, 1992).

About two-thirds of patients with OCD experience substantial psychosocial and occupational impairment (Koran et al., 1996; Hollander et al., 1998). An OCD diagnosis is also associated with elevated utilization of medical and mental health services (Hollander et al., 1998; Kennedy & Schwab, 1997). Results from a survey of patients with OCD suggest that the average time between symptom onset and initial treatment contact in OCD exceeds 10 years (Hollander et al., 1998). OCD has historically been considered to be chronic in course, but recent data suggest that the course may be more variable than previously appreciated. An episodic clinical course may occur in as many as one-third of patients with OCD (Perugi et al., 1998; Antony et al., 1998; Steketee et al., 1997; Thomsen & Mikkelsen, 1995). Factors reported to be associated with an episodic course of OCD include lower rates of checking rituals and an increased risk of relatives with mood disorders (Perugi et al., 1998). Sustained remission, however, appears to be fairly rare in OCD with either an episodic or a chronic clinical course (Perugi et al., 1998; Hollander et al., 1996a, 1996b; Bland et al., 1997a).

Most patients with OCD will have comorbid psychiatric disorders. Major depressive disorder appears to be the most common comorbid diagnosis, with a 60–80% lifetime prevalence rate. Additional anxiety disorder diagnoses (40%) also frequently coexist in OCD, especially panic disorder and social anxiety disorder (Antony et al., 1998; Pigott et al., 1994; Weissman et al., 1994; Rasmussen & Eisen, 1992). Other conditions that frequently occur in OCD include substance use disorders, schizophrenia, body dysmorphic disorder, hypochondriasis, Tourette's syndrome, anorexia nervosa, and bipolar disorder (Pigott et al., 1994; Rasmussen & Eisen, 1992; Antony et al., 1998; Weissman et al., 1994; Perugi et al., 1998). Most studies suggest that the presence of comorbid mood or anxiety disorders in OCD does not convey any additional burden in terms of clinical course or prognosis (Steketee et al., 1997; Demal et al., 1993). Certain OCD symptoms may have some prognostic significance, however. For example, the presence of prominent "symmetry/hoarding" compulsions in OCD has been linked to an elevated risk of certain comorbid conditions, including obsessive–compulsive personality disorder and chronic tic disorders such as Tourette's syndrome (Baer, 1994).

The SSRI antidepressants and the TCA clomipramine remain the cornerstones of pharmacological treatment for OCD (Stein et al., 1995; Jefferson et al., 1995; Orloff et al., 1994). Although these medications effectively reduce OCD symptoms, the average improvement is fairly modest (30–40%). Analyses of a large multicenter clinical trial of clomipramine in the treatment of OCD (Ackerman et al., 1994) failed to detect a significant relationship between therapeutic response and a host of variables, including baseline measures of OCD severity, type of OCD symptoms, and demographic factors (such as age, race, or sex). Only age of onset was a strong predictor of response to clomipramine: Patients who developed OCD later in life had a better chance of response than did those who became ill earlier, regardless of length of illness (Ackerman et al., 1994). Reanalysis of data from a multicenter, placebo-controlled, fixed-dose trial of fluoxetine in OCD revealed that response rates and overall improvement were greatest for patients with histories of remission, lack of previous drug treatment, and more severe OCD (especially with greater interference and distress from obsessions) (Ackerman et al., 1998). Nonresponse to either clomipramine or fluoxetine treatment has been linked to the presence of (1) concomitant schizotypal personality disorder, (2) prominent compulsions, and (3) a longer illness length (Ravizza et al., 1995).

Numerous challenge studies with 5-HT probes have revealed evidence of altered behavioral or neuroendocrine responses in patients with OCD versus control subjects. In contrast, patients with OCD do not appear to exhibit evidence of altered norepinephrine function in comparison to control subjects during challenge paradigms (Pigott, 1996; Goodman et al., 1990; Zohar & Insel, 1987). The preferential efficacy of serotonin-selective medications for OCD, coupled with the evidence of selective serotonergic dysfunction in challenge studies provides fairly compelling evidence for the importance of serotonin in OCD.

OCD and Gender

As previously noted, males typically have an earlier onset of OCD than females. In fact, three times as many boys as girls meet diagnostic criteria for OCD. Several investigations have identified a potential variant of OCD designated as "early-onset OCD." This variant is characterized by the onset of OCD before the age of 10, occurs predominantly in boys, and is strongly associated with tic disorder and a positive family history (Leonard et al., 1992; Pauls et al., 1995). Males are much more likely to have OCD with a comorbid tic disorder, as well as an earlier onset of illness. This finding also suggests that gender differences may exist in the pathophysiological mechanisms that underlie OCD. Dopamine dysregulation may be more prominent in males with OCD, whereas female gonadal steroid hormones and their complex interactions with serotonin may be more critical to the development of OCD in females. The dramatic shift that occurs in gender prevalence rates for OCD after the onset of puberty provides support for the importance of female reproductive hormones. Females begin to develop OCD at a much greater rate than males after menarche; the increase is sufficiently robust that the overall prevalence rate in OCD is greater for females (1.5:1) than males (Weissman et al., 1994; Karno et al., 1988).

Gender differences have also been identified in the phenomenology and clinical course of OCD. Aggressive obsessions and cleaning compulsions may occur more frequently in females with OCD (Noshirvani et al., 1991; Lensi et al., 1996; Castle et al., 1995). In a systematic assessment of adolescents with OCD, the females endorsed a greater amount of compulsive rituals, whereas obsessions were more common in the males with OCD (Valleni-Basile et al., 1994). Women with OCD may also have a more episodic clinical course and less severe symptoms (Hantouche & Lancrenon, 1996; Thomsen & Mikkelsen, 1995).

Females with OCD may also have a greater risk of certain comorbid conditions than males with OCD. Comorbid panic disorder, anorexia nervosa, and bulimia nervosa are reported to occur more frequently in females than in males with OCD (Rubenstein et al., 1992; Yaryura-Tobias et al., 1995; Kendler et al., 1995; Noshirvani et al., 1991; Tamburrino et al., 1994; Lensi et al., 1996; Castle et al., 1995). Since anorexia nervosa and bulimia nervosa are associated with marked alterations in female reproductive hormone function, the frequent association of OCD with eating disorders provides indirect evidence for the importance of the female reproductive cycle in the course of OCD.

Gender differences have also been found in response to serotonergic probes during challenge studies conducted in patients with OCD. Females with OCD who were administered the serotonergic probe fenfluramine had an attenuated cortisol response, in comparison to males with OCD and control subjects (Monteleone et al., 1997). Males with OCD experienced an increase in symptoms during intravenous clomipramine challenge, another probe of 5-HT function, whereas no substantial change was detected in females with OCD (Mundo et al., 1999). The females also demonstrated a better antiobsessional response during a subsequent 10-week trial with either clomipramine or fluvoxamine. Interestingly, the gender difference detected in antiobsessional response was more pronounced after clomipramine than fluvoxamine treatment (Mundo et al., 1999). Potential gender differences in treatment response to clomipramine or fluoxetine were not demonstrated in other studies (Ackerman et al., 1994, 1998). Future studies should explore the potential relationship between distinct OCD subgroups and medication response.

OCD and the Female Reproductive Cycle

There are numerous reports suggesting that the female reproductive cycle may have a substantial influence on OCD. The striking increase in prevalence rates for OCD that occurs in females after the onset of puberty has already been reviewed. Several reports suggest a relationship between the menstrual cycle and OCD. Undergraduate females without demonstrable OCD have been reported to engage in more OCD-like behaviors (such as "excessive cleaning or cleaning of things not usually cleaned") during the luteal phase than at any other time during the menstrual cycle (Dillon & Brooks, 1992). Moreover, the premenstrual period (late luteal phase) may be associated with an exacerbation in symptoms in females with OCD (Yaryura-Tobias et al., 1995; Williams & Koran, 1997). In the largest study to date, the impact of the menstrual cycle on the course of their OCD symptoms was retrospectively examined in 57 women with OCD. Nearly half (42%) of the women reported premenstrual worsening in their OCD symptoms, and a substantial number (21%) also noted premenstrual dysphoria (Williams & Koran, 1997).

Several case series suggest that a substantial portion (13–36%) of females with OCD report the onset of their illness during pregnancy or the postpartum period (Sichel et al., 1993; Williams & Koran, 1997; Neziroglu et al., 1994; Altshuler et al., 1998; Buttolph

& Holland, 1990). A number of case reports suggest that women with pre-existing OCD will experience a worsening in symptomatology during pregnancy (Altshuler et al., 1998; Brandt & Mackenzie, 1987; Buttolph & Holland, 1990; Chelmow & Halfin, 1997; Neziroglu et al., 1994; Weiss et al., 1995; Stein et al., 1993). However, in the largest reported study to date concerning the impact of pregnancy on OCD (Williams & Koran, 1997), most of the women with preexisting OCD (69%) reported no significant change in symptoms during pregnancy. Relatively few patients reported a significant worsening (17%) or a substantial improvement (14%) in OCD symptoms during pregnancy, and relatively few (13%) reported the onset of OCD during pregnancy. Substantial changes in OCD symptoms, however, were likely to occur during the postpartum period. Postpartum worsening of OCD (29%) and postpartum depression (37%) were frequent findings in the women with OCD (Williams & Koran, 1997). The exacerbation noted during the postpartum period is a fairly consistent finding in women with preexisting OCD. Most studies have reported that 20–30% of females with OCD will experience a significant postpartum worsening in OCD symptoms (Buttolph & Holland, 1990; Williams & Koran, 1997; Sichel et al., 1993; Altshuler et al., 1998).

These results provide further evidence that changes in female reproductive hormone concentrations can substantially influence the severity and course of OCD. Pregnancy and the postpartum period may represent a time of increased vulnerability for the initial emergence of OCD or for significant worsening in women with preexisting OCD.

POSTTRAUMATIC STRESS DISORDER

Epidemiology and Clinical Overview

Although many individuals are exposed to trauma, most investigations reveal that only one out of four will develop PTSD (Breslau et al., 1990). Estimates from the National Comorbidity Survey suggest that the lifetime prevalence rate for PTSD is approximately 8% (Kessler et al., 1995). PTSD is reported to be twice as common in females (10.4%) as in males (5%). The most common causes of trauma leading to PTSD in men are combat exposure or witnessing someone being injured or killed. In contrast, women are most likely to develop PTSD as a consequence of sexual assault, sexual molestation, or childhood physical abuse (Kessler et al., 1995). PTSD can occur at any age, but certain traumatic events are associated with an especially high risk of subsequent PTSD development. For example, Foa (1997) reported that 95% of rape survivors and 75% of survivors of nonsexual assaults developed PTSD symptoms within 2 weeks of the traumatic event.

Although exposure to life-threatening traumatic events is fairly common, a number of studies confirm that PTSD is poorly recognized in a variety of clinical settings. For example, Davidson and Smith (1990) found that 81% of new patient referrals to an outpatient psychiatric clinic had a positive history of significant trauma. Although almost 30% of the patients with exposure to trauma met criteria for PTSD, only 8% were correctly diagnosed with PTSD. Unfortunately, the low rates of recognition typically associated with PTSD can have catastrophic consequences. Comorbid conditions are extremely common in PTSD, especially mood and substance use disorders. In fact, the presence of PTSD has been associated with an elevated risk for major depression, dysthymia, and mania. According to the National Comorbidity Survey, comorbid alcohol and other substance abuse occur twice as often in patients with PTSD as in patients without PTSD (Kessler et al., 1995; Breslau et al., 1997b).

Cumulative evidence indicates that the SSRI antidepressants constitute first-line pharmacotherapy for PTSD (Connor et al., 1993; Davidson & Connor, 1999; Klein et al., 1994; Marshall & Pierce, 2000; Marshall et al., 1998; Nagy et al., 1993; Rothbaum et al., 1996). TCAs and MAOIs are also effective for PTSD and should be considered for patients with PTSD who fail to respond to SSRI treatment (Davidson & Connor, 1999). The SSRI antidepressants appear to have a broad spectrum of activity in PTSD. Many common PTSD symptoms—such as anxiety, insomnia, an exaggerated startle response, intrusive trauma-related recollections, feelings of emotional numbing, and avoidance behaviors—are reported to improve during SSRI treatment (Davidson & Connor, 1999). Pharmacotherapy for PTSD should be initiated at a relatively low dose and maintained for at least 12 months before discontinuation is considered.

PTSD and Gender

The gender difference in prevalence of PTSD has been linked to a differential rate of exposure to trauma. However, this assumption may be incorrect. In a sample of over 1,000 young adults, Breslau et al. (1997a) found similar rates of exposure to traumatic events, but substantially more females than males met criteria for PTSD. Potential confounding factors (such as the increased prevalence of preexisting anxiety disorders or major depressive disorder in females) were examined, but failed to account for the observed gender difference noted in the prevalence of PTSD. Instead, females appeared to have a markedly increased susceptibility for PTSD development, especially if the trauma occurred prior to age 15 (Breslau et al., 1990, 1995, 1997a; Kessler et al., 1994). Results from the National Comorbidity Survey also implicated multiple factors in the elevated risk of PTSD in women. However, there was substantial overlap between factors that predicted an increased risk for trauma exposure and development of PTSD. Once the overlapping risk factors were excluded, only one risk factor (history of mood disorder) predicted PTSD in women, whereas two factors (history of anxiety disorder and parental mental disorder) were associated with an increased risk of PTSD in men (Bromet et al., 1998). These findings suggest that most variables identified as predictive of PTSD are actually more indicative of trauma exposure than of PTSD.

Preexisting depression appears to convey an increased risk for subsequent exposure to traumatic events, as well as for the development of PTSD once trauma occurs (Breslau et al., 1997b). Certain traumatic experiences are more likely to precipitate PTSD. Females who are sexually assaulted are at extremely high risk for subsequent development of PTSD. For example, Foa (1997) found that 3 months after the trauma, female rape survivors were twice as likely as female survivors of nonsexual crimes (48% vs. 25%) to have PTSD. Females may be particularly susceptible to the long-term complications of childhood abuse. In fact, women with histories of childhood abuse are reported to have a level of functional impairment commensurate with that of women with recent abuse (McCauley et al., 1997). Female survivors of domestic violence are more likely to develop anxiety symptoms as well as PTSD, whereas male survivors of domestic violence are at greater risk of developing substance use disorders. An elevated risk of depression and an increased number of physical and psychological health problems have also been reported in women exposed to ongoing domestic violence; this finding appears to be independent of the severity of domestic violence or the presence of injuries sustained (Sutherland et al., 1998). Although this finding may seem counterintuitive, it many reflect the importance of "perceived threat" in the formation of PTSD. That is, the perception of danger or possibility of death during an assault or exposure to trauma may be more important for subsequent risk for PTSD than more objective or realistic assessments of life-threatening events may be. These findings suggest that sexual assault, childhood abuse, and individual assessment of threat during the occurrence of trauma may represent the strongest predictors of PTSD development in females.

PTSD and the Female Reproductive Cycles

Gender differences may also occur in the biological alterations identified in PTSD. An elevated norepinephrine-to-cortisol ratio has been reported in males with PTSD, whereas females with PTSD have demonstrated significantly elevated levels of urinary norepinephrine, epinephrine, dopamine, and cortisol on a daily basis (Lemieux & Coe, 1995). The HPA axis has strong, multilevel inhibitory effects on the female reproductive hormones (Chrousos et al., 1998). Since HPA axis alterations are implicated in PTSD, the marked fluctuations in estrogen and progesterone levels that characterize the female reproductive cycle may well have a significant impact on the course of PTSD. The relative hypercortisolism that occurs during the third trimester of pregnancy is speculated to cause a transient suppression of the adrenals during the postpartum period (Chrousos et al., 1998). This finding suggests that women with preexisting PTSD may experience substantial changes in symptomatology during pregnancy or the postpartum period. Unfortunately, very little systematic information is available concerning the potential impact of the reproductive cycle on PTSD.

REFERENCES

Ackerman, D., Greenland, S., & Bystritsky, A. (1998). Clinical characteristics of response to fluoxetine treatment of obsessive–compulsive disorder. *Journal of Clinical Psychopharmacology, 18*(3), 185–192.

Ackerman, D., Greenland, S., Bystritsky, A., et al. (1994). Predictors of treatment response in obsessive–compulsive disorder: Multivariate analyses from a multicenter trial of clomipramine. *Journal of Clinical Psychopharmacology, 14*(4), 247–254.

Alpert, J. E., Uebelacker, L. A., McLean, N. E., et al. (1997). Social phobia, avoidant personality disorder and atypical depression: Co-occurrence and clinical implications. *Psychological Medicine, 27*(3), 627–633.

Altshuler, L., Hendrick, V., & Cohen, L. S. (1998). Course of mood and anxiety disorders during pregnancy and the postpartum period. *Journal of Clinical Psychiatry, 2*, 29–33.

American Psychiatric Association. (1994). *Diagnostic and statistical manual of mental disorders* (4th ed.). Washington, DC: Author.

Andrade, L., Eaton, W. W., & Chilcoat, H. D. (1996). Lifetime co-morbidity of panic attacks and major depression in a population-based study: Age of onset. *Psychological Medicine, 26*, 991–996.

Antony, M., Downie, F., & Swinson, R. (1998). Diagnostic issues and epidemiology in OCD. In R. Swinson, M. Antony, S. Rachman, & M. Richter (Eds.), *Obsessive–compulsive disorder: Theory, research, and treatment* (pp. 3–32). New York: Guilford Press.

Baer, L. (1994). Factor analysis of symptom subtypes of obsessive-compulsive disorder and their relation to personality and tic disorders. *Journal of Clinical Psychiatry, 55,* 18–23.

Bakish, D. (1999). The patient with comorbid depression and anxiety: The unmet need. *Journal of Clinical Psychiatry, 60*(6), 20–24.

Ballenger, J., Davidson, J., Lecrubier, Y., et al. (1998). Consensus statement on social anxiety disorder from the International Consensus Group on Depression and Anxiety. *Journal of Clinical Psychiatry, 59*(17), 54–60.

Battaglia, M., Bernardeschi, L., Politi, E., et al. (1995). Comorbidity of panic and somatization disorder: A genetic–epidemiological approach. *Comprehensive Psychiatry, 36*(6), 411–420.

Beck, C. (1998). Postpartum onset of panic disorder. *Image—The Journal of Nursing Scholarship, 30*(2), 131–135.

Bell, C., & Nutt, D. (1998). Serotonin and panic. *British Journal of Psychiatry, 172,* 465–471.

Bisserbee, J. C., Weiller, E., Boyer, P., et al. (1996). Social phobia in primary care: Level of recognition and drug use. *International Journal of Clinical Psychopharmacology, 3,* 25–28.

Black, B., & Uhde, T. (1995). Psychiatric characteristics of children with selective mutism: A pilot study. *Journal of the American Academy of Child and Adolescent Psychiatry, 34*(7), 847–856.

Black, D. W., Goldstein, R. B., Noyes, R., Jr., et al. (1995). Psychiatric disorders in relatives of probands with obsessive–compulsive disorder and co-morbid major depression or generalized anxiety. *Psychiatric Genetics, 5*(1), 37–41.

Bland, R., Newman, S., & Orn, H. (1997a). Age and remission of psychiatric disorders. *Canadian Journal of Psychiatry, 42*(7), 722–729.

Bland, R., Newman, S., & Orn, H. (1997b). Help-seeking for psychiatric disorders. *Canadian Journal of Psychiatry, 42*(9), 935–942.

Bourdon, K., Boyd, J., Rae, D., et al. (1988). Gender differences in phobias: Results of the ECA community survey. *Journal of Anxiety Disorders, 2,* 227–241.

Boyd, J. H., Rae, D. S., Thompson, J. W., et al. (1990). Phobia: Prevalence and risk factors. *Social Psychiatry and Psychiatric Epidemiology, 25*(6), 314–323.

Brandt, K. R., & Mackenzie, T. B. (1987). Obsessive–compulsive disorder exacerbated during pregnancy: A case report. *International Journal of Psychiatry in Medicine, 17*(4), 361–366.

Brawman-Mintzer, O., & Lydiard, R. (1997). Biological basis of generalized anxiety disorder. *Journal of Clinical Psychiatry, 58*(3), 16–25.

Breslau, N., Davis, G. C., & Andreski, P. (1990). Traumatic events and traumatic stress disorder in an urban population of young adults. *Archives of General Psychiatry, 48,* 218–222.

Breslau, N., Davis, G. C., Andreski, P., et al. (1997a). Sex differences in posttraumatic stress disorder. *Archives of General Psychiatry, 54*(11), 1044–1048.

Breslau, N., Davis, G. C., Peterson, E. L., et al. (1997b). Psychiatric sequelae of posttraumatic stress disorder in women. *Archives of General Psychiatry, 54*(1), 81–87.

Breslau, N., Schultz, L., & Peterson, E. (1995). Sex differences in depression: A role for pre-existing anxiety. *Psychiatry Research, 58,* 1–12.

Bromet, E., Sonnega, A., & Kessler, R. (1998). Risk factors for DSM-III-R posttraumatic stress disorder: Findings from the National Comorbidity Survey. *American Journal of Epidemiology, 147*(4), 353–361.

Buttolph, M., & Holland, A. (1990). OCD in pregnancy and childbirth. In M. Jenike, L. Baer, & W. Minichiello (Eds.), *Obsessive–compulsive disorders: Theory and management* (pp. 89–97). Chicago: Year Book Medical.

Castle, D. J., Deale, A., & Marks, I. M. (1995). Gender differences in obsessive compulsive disorder. *Australian and New Zealand Journal of Psychiatry, 29*(1), 114–117.

Chelmow, D., & Halfin, V. P. (1997). Pregnancy complicated by obsessive–compulsive disorder. *Journal of Maternal and Fetal Medicine, 6*(1), 31–34.

Chen, Y. W., & Dilsaver, S. C. (1995). Comorbidity for obsessive–compulsive disorder in bipolar and unipolar disorders. *Psychiatry Research, 59*(1–2), 57–64.

Chrousos, G. P., Torpy, D. J., & Gold, P. W. (1998). Interactions between the hypothalamic–pituitary–adrenal axis and the female reproductive system: Clinical implications. *Annals of Internal Medicine, 129*(3), 229–240.

Cohen, L. S., Sichel, D. A., Dimmock, J. A., et al. (1994a). Impact of pregnancy on panic disorder: A case series [see comments]. *Journal of Clinical Psychiatry, 55*(7), 284–288.

Cohen, L. S., Sichel, D. A., Dimmock, J. A., et al. (1994b). Postpartum course in women with pre-existing panic disorder [see comments]. *Journal of Clinical Psychiatry, 55*(7), 289–292.

Connor, K. M., Sutherland, S. M., Tupler, L. A., et al. (1999). Fluoxetine in posttraumatic stress disorder: Randomised, double-blind study. *British Journal of Psychiatry, 175*, 17–22.

Cook, B., Noyes, R., Garvey, M., et al. (1990). Anxiety and the menstrual cycle in panic disorder. *Journal of Affective Disorders, 19*(3), 221–226.

Cook, E., & Leventhal, B. (1992). Neuropsychiatric disorders of childhood and adolescence. In S. C. Yudovsky & R. E. Jales (Eds.), *Neuropsychiatry* (2nd ed., pp. 639–661). Washington, DC: American Psychiatric Association.

Coplan, J., & Lydiard, R. (1998). Brain circuits in panic disorder. *Biological Psychiatry, 44*(12), 1264–1276.

Cox, B. J., Swinson, R. P., Shulman, I. D., et al. (1993). Gender effects and alcohol use in panic disorder with agoraphobia. *Behaviour Research and Therapy, 31*(4), 413–416.

Davidson, J. (1998). Pharmacotherapy of social anxiety disorder. *Journal of Clinical Psychiatry, 59*(17), 47–53.

Davidson, J., & Smith, R. (1990). Treatment of posttraumatic stress disorder with amitriptyline and placebo. *Archives of General Psychiatry, 47*(3), 259–266.

Davidson, J. R., & Connor, K. M. (1999). Management of posttraumatic stress disorder: Diagnostic and therapeutic issues. *Journal of Clinical Psychiatry, 60*(Suppl. 18), 33–38.

Deckert, J., Catalano, M., Syagailo, Y., et al. (1999). Excess of high activity monoamine oxidase A gene promoter alleles in female patients with panic disorder. *Human Molecular Genetics, 8*(4), 621–624.

Demal, U., Lenz, G., Mayrhofer, A., et al. (1993). OCD and depression: A retrospective study on course and interaction. *Psychopathology, 26*, 145–150.

Dick, C. L., Bland, R. C., & Newman, S. C. (1994a). Epidemiology of psychiatric disorders in Edmonton: Panic disorder. *Acta Psychiatrica Scandinavica*, (Suppl. 376), 45–53.

Dick, C. L., Sowa, B., Bland, R. C., et al. (1994). Epidemiology of psychiatric disorders in Edmonton: Phobic disorders. *Acta Psychiatrica Scandinavica*, (Suppl. 376), 36–44.

Dillon, K., & Brooks, D. (1992). Unusual cleaning behavior in the luteal phase. *Psychological Reports, 70*(1), 35–39.

Eaton, W., Dryman, A., & Weissman, M. (1991). Panic and phobia. In L. Robins & D. Regier (Eds.), *Psychiatric disorders in America: The Epidemiologic Catchment Area study* (pp. 53–80). New York: Free Press.

Essau, C., Conradt, J., & Petermann, F. (1998). Frequency and comorbidity of social anxiety and social phobia in adolescents: Results of a Bremen adolescent study. *Fortschritte der Neurologie–Psychiatrie, 66*(11), 524–530.

Fava, G. A., Grandi, S., Michelacci, L., et al. (1990). Hypochondriacal fears and beliefs in pregnancy. *Acta Psychiatrica Scandinavica, 82*(1), 70–72.

Fernandez-Guasti, A., & Picazo, O. (1990). The actions of diazepam and serotonergic anxiolytics vary according to the gender and the estrous cycle phase. *Pharmacology, Biochemistry and Behavior, 37*(1), 673–677.

Fishman, S., Carr, D., Beckett, A., et al. (1994). Hypercapneic ventilatory response in patients with panic disorder before and after alprazolam treatment and in pre- and postmenstrual women. *Journal of Psychiatric Research, 28*(2), 165–170.

Fleet, R., Marchand, A., Dupuis, G., et al. (1998). Comparing emergency department and psychiatric setting patients with panic disorder. *Psychosomatics, 39*(6), 512–518.

Foa, E. B. (1997). Trauma and women: Course, predictors, and treatment. *Journal of Clinical Psychiatry, 9,* 25–28.

Fredrikson, M., Annas, P., Fischer, H., et al. (1996). Gender and age differences in the prevalence of specific fears and phobias. *Behaviour Research and Therapy, 34*(1), 33–39.

Galbaud-du-Fort, G., Bland, R., Newman, S., et al. (1998). Spouse similarity for lifetime psychiatric history in the general population. *Psychological Medicine, 28*(4), 789–802.

Goodman, W., McDougle, C., Price, L., et al. (1990). Beyond the serotonin hypothesis: A role for dopamine in some forms of obsessive–compulsive disorder? *Journal of Clinical Psychiatry, 51*(8), 36–43.

Hantouche, E. G., & Lancrenon, S. (1996). [Modern typology of symptoms and obsessive–compulsive syndromes: Results of a large French study of 615 patients]. *Encephale, 22*(1), 9–21.

Hohmann, A. A. (1989). Gender bias in psychotropic drug prescribing in primary care. *Medical Care, 27*(5), 478–490.

Hollander, E., Greenwald, S., Neville, D., et al. (1996a). Uncomplicated and comorbid obsessive–compulsive disorder in an epidemiological sample. *Depression and Anxiety, 4*(3), 111–119.

Hollander, E., Kwon, J. H., Stein, D. J., et al. (1996b). Obsessive–compulsive and spectrum disorders: Overview and quality of life issues. *Journal of Clinical Psychiatry, 8,* 3–6.

Hollander, E., Stein, D., Kwon, J., et al. (1998). Psychosocial function and economic costs of obsessive–compulsive disorder. *CNS Spectrums, 3*(5), 48–58.

Hollifield, M., Katon, W., Skipper, B., et al. (1997). Panic disorder and quality of life: Variables predictive of functional impairment. *American Journal of Psychiatry, 154*(6), 766–772.

Huerta, R., Mena, A., Malacara, J., et al. (1995). Symptoms at perimenopausal period: Its association with attitudes toward sexuality, life-style, family function, and FSH levels. *Psychoneuroendocrinology, 20*(2), 135–148.

Jefferson, J. W., Altemus, M., Jenike, M. A., et al. (1995). Algorithm for the treatment of obsessive–compulsive disorder (OCD). *Psychopharmacology Bulletin, 31*(3), 487–490.

Joyce, P. R., Bushnell, J. A., Oakley Browne, M. A., et al. (1989). The epidemiology of panic symptomatology and agoraphobic avoidance. *Comprehensive Psychiatry, 30*(4), 303–312.

Kalus, O., Asnis, G., Rubinson, E., et al. (1991). Desipramine treatment in panic disorder. *Journal of Affective Disorders, 21*(4), 239–244.

Karno, M., Golding, J., Sorenson, S., et al. (1988). The epidemiology of obsessive–compulsive disorder in five U.S. communities. *Archives of General Psychiatry, 45,* 1094–1099.

Katerndahl, D. (1990). Factors associated with persons with panic attacks seeking medical care. *Family Medicine, 22*(6), 462–466.

Katerndahl, D. A., & Realini, J. P. (1997). Quality of life and panic-related work disability in subjects with infrequent panic and panic disorder. *Journal of Clinical Psychiatry, 58*(4), 153–158.

Keller, M. B., & Hanks, D. L. (1993). Course and outcome in panic disorder. *Progress in Neuropsychopharmacology and Biological Psychiatry, 17*(4), 551–570.

Kendler, K. S. (1996). Major depression and generalized anxiety disorder: Same genes, (partly) different environments—revisited. *British Journal of Psychiatry, 22*(Suppl. 30), 68–75.

Kendler, K. S., Neale, M. C., Kessler, R. C., et al. (1992a). Generalized anxiety disorder in women: A population-based twin study. *Archives of General Psychiatry, 49*(4), 267–272.

Kendler, K. S., Neale, M. C., Kessler, R. C., et al. (1992b). The genetic epidemiology of phobias in women: The interrelationship of agoraphobia, social phobia, situational phobia, and specific phobia. *Archives of General Psychiatry, 49*(4), 273–281.

Kendler, K. S., Neale, M. C., Kessler, R. C., et al. (1992c). Major depression and generalized anxiety disorder: Same genes, (partly) different environments? *Archives of General Psychiatry, 49*(9), 716–722.

Kendler, K. S., Neale, M. C., Kessler, R., et al. (1993). Panic disorder in women: A population-based twin study. *Psychological Medicine, 23*(2), 397–406.

Kendler, K. S., Walters, E. E., Neale, M. C., et al. (1995). The structure of the genetic and environmental risk factors for six major psychiatric disorders in women: Phobia, generalized anxiety
disorder, panic disorder, bulimia, major depression, and alcoholism. *Archives of General Psychiatry, 52*(5), 374–383.

Kennedy, B., & Schwab, J. (1997). Utilization of medical specialists by anxiety disorder patients.
Psychosomatics, 38(2), 109–112.

Kessler, R., Berglund, P., Foster, C., et al. (1997). Social consequences of psychiatric disorders: II.
Teenage parenthood. *American Journal of Psychiatry, 154*(10), 1405–1411.

Kessler, R., McGonagle, K., Zhao, S., et al. (1994). Lifetime and 12–month prevalence of DSM-III-
R psychiatric disorders in the United States: Results from the National Comorbidity Survey.
Archives of General Psychiatry, 51, 8–19.

Kessler, R. C., Sonnega, A., Bromet, E., et al. (1995). Posttraumatic stress disorder in the National
Comorbidity Survey. *Archives of General Psychiatry, 52*(12), 1048–1060.

Kessler, R. C., Stein, M. B., & Berglund, P. (1998). Social phobia subtypes in the National Comorbidity Survey. *American Journal of Psychiatry, 155*(5), 613–619.

Kline, N. A., Dow, B. M., Brown, S. A., et al. (1994). Sertraline efficacy in depressed combat veterans with posttraumatic stress disorder [letter]. *American Journal of Psychiatry, 151*(4), 621.

Koran, L., Thieneman, M., & Davenport, R. (1996). Quality of life for patients with obsessive–
compulsive disorder. *American Journal of Psychiatry, 153*, 783–788.

Krasucki, C., Howard, R., & Mann, A. (1998). The relationship between anxiety disorders and
age. *International Journal of Geriatric Psychiatry, 13*(2), 79–99.

Lecrubier, Y., & Weiller, E. (1997). Comorbidities in social phobia. *International Journal of Clinical Psychopharmacology, 12*(6), 1268–1315.

Lemieux, A., & Coe, C. (1995). Abuse-related posttraumatic stress disorder: Evidence for chronic
neuroendocrine activation in women. *Psychosomatic Medicine, 57*(2), 105–115.

Lensi, P., Cassano, G., Correddu, G., et al. (1996). Obsessive–compulsive disorder: Familial–developmental history, symptomatology, comorbidity and course with special reference to gender-
related differences. *British Journal of Psychiatry, 169*(1), 101–107.

Leon, A., Portera, L., & Weissman, M. (1995). The social costs of anxiety disorders. *British Journal of Psychiatry, 4*(27), 19–22.

Leonard, H., Lenane, M., Swedo, S., et al. (1992). Tics and Tourette's syndrome: A two to seven
year follow-up of 54 OCD children. *American Journal of Psychiatry, 149*, 1244–1251.

Lindal, E., & Stefansson, J. G. (1993). The lifetime prevalence of anxiety disorders in Iceland as estimated by the US National Institute of Mental Health Diagnostic Interview Schedule. *Acta
Psychiatrica Scandinavica, 88*(1), 29–34.

Magee, W., Eaton, W., Wittchen, H., et al. (1996). Agoraphobia, specific phobia, and social phobia
in the National Comorbidity Survey. *Archives of General Psychiatry, 53*(2), 159–168.

Marshall, J. R. (1996). Comorbidity and its effects on panic disorder. *Bulletin of the Menninger
Clinic, 60*(2, Suppl. A), 39–53.

Marshall, R. D., & Pierce, D. (2000). Implications of recent findings in posttraumatic stress disorder and the role of pharmacotherapy. *Harvard Review of Psychiatry, 7*(5), 247–256.

Marshall, R. D., Schneier, F. R., Fallon, B. A., et al. (1998). An open trial of paroxetine in patients
with noncombat-related chronic posttraumatic stress disorder. *Journal of Clinical Psychopharmacology, 18*(1), 10–18.

McCauley, J., Kern, D. E., Kolodner, K., et al. (1997). Clinical characteristics of women with a history of childhood abuse: Unhealed wounds. *Journal of the American Medical Association,
277*(17), 1362–1368.

McEwen, B., & Parsons, B. (1987). Gonadal steroid action on the brain: Neurochemistry and
neuropharmacology. *Annual Review of Pharmacology and Toxicology, 22*, 555–598.

McLeod, D., Hoehn-Saric, R., Foster, G., & Hipsley, P. (1993). The influence of premenstrual syndrome on ratings of anxiety in women with generalized anxiety disorder. *Acta Psychiatrica Scandinavica, 88*(4), 248–251.

Mick, M., & Telch, M. (1998). Social anxiety and history of behavioral inhibition in young adults. *Journal of Anxiety Disorders, 12*(1), 1–20.

Monteleone, P., Catapano, F., Torttorella, A., et al. (1997). Cortisol response to D-fenfluramine in patients with obsessive–compulsive disorder and in healthy subjects: Evidence for a gender-related effect. *Neuropsychobiology, 36*(1), 8–12.

Mundo, E., Bareggi, S., Pirola, R., & Bellodi, L. (1999). Effect of acute intravenous clomipramine and antiobsessional response to proserotonergic drugs: Is gender a predictive variable? *Biological Psychiatry, 45*(3), 290–294.

Nagy, L. M., Morgan, C. A., Southwick, S. M., et al. (1993). Open prospective trial of fluoxetine for posttraumatic stress disorder. *Journal of Psychopharmacology, 13*(2), 107–113.

Neziroglu, F., Yaryura-Tobias, J., Lemli, J., et al. (1994). Demographic study of obsessive compulsive disorder. *Acta Psiquiatrica Psicologica America Latina, 40*(3), 217–223.

Northcott, C. J., & Stein, M. B. (1994). Panic disorder in pregnancy. *Journal of Clinical Psychiatry, 55*(12), 539–542.

Noshirvani, H., Kasvikis, Y., Marks, I., et al. (1991). Gender-divergent aetiological factors in OCD. *British Journal of Psychiatry, 158*, 260–263.

Nutt, D., Bell, C., & Malizia, A. (1998). Brain mechanisms of social anxiety disorder. *Journal of Clinical Psychiatry, 59*(17), 4–11.

Orloff, L., Battle, M., Baer, L., et al. (1994). Long-term follow-up of 85 patients with OCD. *American Journal of Psychiatry, 151*, 441–442.

Pauls, D., Alsobrook, J., Goodman, W., et al. (1995). A family study of obsessive–compulsive disorder. *American Journal of Psychiatry, 152*, 76–84.

Perna, G., Brambilla, F., Arancio, C., et al. (1995). Carbon dioxide inhalation sensitivity in panic disorder: Effect of menstrual cycle phase. *Biological Psychiatry, 37*(8), 528–532.

Perugi, G., Akiskal, H., Gemignani, A., et al. (1998). Episodic course in obsessive–compulsive disorder. *European Archives of Psychiatry and Clinical Neuroscience, 248*(5), 240–244.

Pigott, T. A. (1996). OCD: Where the serotonin selectivity story begins. *Journal of Clinical Psychiatry, 57*(Suppl. 6), 11–20.

Pigott, T. A., L'Heureux, F., Dubbert, B., et al. (1994). Obsessive–compulsive disorder: Comorbid conditions. *Journal of Clinical Psychiatry, 55*(10), 15–27.

Pollack, M. (1999). Social anxiety disorder: Designing a pharmacologic treatment strategy. *Journal of Clinical Psychiatry, 60*(9), 20–26.

Rasmussen, S., & Eisen, J. (1990). Epidemiology and clinical features of OCD. In M. Jenike, L. Baer, & W. Minichiello (Eds.), *Obsessive–compulsive disorders: Theory and management* (pp. 10–27). St. Louis, MO: Mosby–Year Book.

Rasmussen, S., & Eisen, J. (1992). The epidemiology and differential diagnosis of OCD. *Journal of Clinical Psychiatry, 53*(Suppl.), 4–10.

Ravizza, L., Barzega, G., Bellino, S., et al. (1995). Predictors of drug treatment response in obsessive–compulsive disorder. *Journal of Clinical Psychiatry, 56*(8), 368–373.

Reed, V., & Wittchen, H. (1998). DSM-IV panic attacks and panic disorder in a community sample of adolescents and young adults: How specific are panic attacks? *Journal of Psychiatric Research, 32*(6), 335–345.

Regier, D., Boyd, J., Burke, J., et al. (1988). One-month prevalence of mental disorders in the United States: Based on five Epidemiologic Catchment Area sites. *Archives of General Psychiatry, 45*, 977–986.

Regier, D., Rae, D., Narrow, W., et al. (1998). Prevalence of anxiety disorders and their comorbidity with mood and addictive disorders. *British Journal of Psychiatry, 34*, 24–28.

Robins, L., Helzer, J., Weissman, M., et al. (1984). Lifetime prevalence of specific psychiatric disorders in three sites. *Archives of General Psychiatry, 41*, 949–958.

Rogers, M. P., White, K., Warshaw, M. G., et al. (1994). Prevalence of medical illness in patients with anxiety disorders. *International Journal of Psychiatry in Medicine, 24*(1), 83–96.

Rothbaum, B. O., Ninan, P. T., & Thomas, L. (1996). Sertraline in the treatment of rape victims with posttraumatic stress disorder. *Journal of Trauma and Stress, 9*(4), 865–871.

Roy-Byrne, P., & Katon, W. (1997). Generalized anxiety disorder in primary care: The precursor/ modifier pathway to increased health care utilization. *Journal of Clinical Psychiatry, 58*(3), 34–38.

Rubenstein, C., Pigott, T., L'Heureux, F., et al. (1992). A preliminary investigation of the lifetime prevalence rate of anorexia and bulimia nervosa in patients with OCD. *Journal of Clinical Psychiatry, 53*(9), 309–314.

Schneier, F., Heckelman, L., Garfinkel, R., et al. (1994). Functional impairment in social phobia. *Journal of Clinical Psychiatry, 55*(8), 322–331.

Schneier, F., Johnson, J., Hornig, C., et al. (1992). Social phobia: Comorbidity and morbidity in an epidemiological sample. *Archives of General Psychiatry, 49*, 282–291.

Seeman, M. V. (1997). Psychopathology in women and men: Focus on female hormones. *American Journal of Psychiatry, 154*(12), 1641–1647.

Shear, M. K. (1997). Anxiety disorders in women: Gender-related modulation of neurobiology and behavior. *Seminars in Reproductive Endocrinology, 15*(1), 69–76.

Sheehan, D. (1999). Current concepts in the treatment of panic disorder. *Journal of Clinical Psychiatry, 60*(Suppl. 18), 16–21.

Sholomskas, D., Wickamaratne, P., Dogolo, L., et al. (1993). Postpartum onset of panic disorder: A coincidental event? *Journal of Clinical Psychiatry, 54*(12), 476–480.

Sichel, D., Cohen, L., Rosenbaum, J., et al. (1993). Postpartum onset of obsessive–compulsive disorder. *Psychosomatics, 34*(3), 277–279.

Stahl, S. (1997). Reproductive hormones as adjuncts to psychotropic mediation in women. *Essential Psychopharmacology, 2*(2), 147–164.

Starcevic, V., Djordjevic, A., Latas, M., et al. (1998). Characteristics of agoraphobia in women and men with panic disorder with agoraphobia. *Depression and Anxiety, 8*(1), 8–13.

Stein, D., Hollander, E., Simeon, D., et al. (1993). Pregnancy and OCD. *American Journal of Psychiatry, 150*, 1131–1132.

Stein, D., Spadaccini, E., & Hollander, E. (1995). Meta-analysis of pharmacotherapy trials for obsessive–compulsive disorder. *International Journal of Clinical Psychopharmacology, 10*(1), 11–18.

Stein, M., Chartier, M. J., Hazen, A. L., et al. (1998a). A direct-interview family study of generalized social phobia. *American Journal of Psychiatry, 155*(1), 90–97.

Stein, M., & Chavira, D. (1998). Subtypes of social phobia and comorbidity with depression and other anxiety disorders. *Journal of Affective Disorders, 50*(1), 11–16.

Stein, M., Jang, K., & Livesley, W. (1999). Heritability of anxiety sensitivity: A twin study. *American Journal of Psychiatry, 156*(2), 246–251.

Stein, M., Liebowitz, M., Lydiard, R., et al. (1998b). Paroxetine treatment of generalized social phobia: A randomized controlled trial. *Journal of the American Medical Association, 280*(8), 708–713.

Stein, M., Schmidt, P., Rubinow, D., et al. (1989a). Panic disorder and the menstrual cycle: Panic disorder patients, healthy control subjects, and patients with premenstrual syndrome. *American Journal of Psychiatry, 146*(10), 1299–1303.

Stein, M., Shea, C., & Uhde, T. (1989b). Social phobic symptoms in patients with panic disorder: Practical and theoretical implications. *American Journal of Psychiatry, 146*(2), 235–238.

Steketee, G., Eisen, J., Dyck, I., et al. (1997). Course of Illness in OCD. In L. Dickstein, M. Riba, & J. Oldham (Eds.), *Review of psychiatry* (Vol. 16, pp. 73–95). Washington, DC: American Psychiatric Press.

Sutherland, C., Bybee, D., & Sullivan, C. (1998). The long-term effects of battering on women's health. *Women's Health, 4*(1), 41–70.

Tamburrino, M., Kaufman, R., & Hertzer, J. (1994). Eating disorder history in women with obsessive–compulsive disorder. *Journal of American Medical Women's Association, 49*(1), 24–26.

Thomsen, P. H., & Mikkelsen, H. U. (1995). Course of obsessive-compulsive disorder in children and adolescents: A prospective follow-up study of 23 Danish cases. *Journal of the American Academy of Child and Adolescent Psychiatry, 34*(11), 1432–1440.

Tiihonen, J., Kuikka, J., Rasanen, P., et al. (1997). Cerebral benzodiazpine receptor binding in GAD. *Molecular Psychiatry, 2*(6), 463–471.

Turgeon, L., Marchand, A., & Dupuis, G. (1998). Clinical features in panic disorder with agoraphobia: A comparison of men and women. *Journal of Anxiety Disorders, 12*(6), 539–553.

Turk, C., Heimberg, R., Orsillo, S., et al. (1998). An investigation of gender differences in social phobia. *Journal of Anxiety Disorders, 12*(3), 209–223.

Ushiroyama, T., & Sugimoto, O. (1994). [Correlation of ill-defined syndrome with depression in the climacterium]. *Nippon Rinsho, 52*(5), 1345–1349.

van-der Feltz-Cornelis, C. M. (1999). Hot flashes resistant to hormone replacement in menopausal women: Panic disorder? *Nederlands Tijdschrift voor Geneeskunde, 143*(6), 281–284.

Villeponteaux, V., Lydiard, R., Laraia, M., et al. (1992). The effects of pregnancy on preexisting panic disorder. *Journal of Clinical Psychiatry, 53*(6), 201–203.

Wagner, K. D., & Berenson, A. B. (1994). Norplant-associated major depression and panic disorder. *Journal of Clinical Psychiatry, 55*(11), 478–480.

Walker, A., & Bancroft, J. (1990). Relationship between premenstrual symptoms and oral contraceptive use: a controlled study. *Psychosomatic Medicine, 52*(1), 86–96.

Walker, E., Katon, W., Roy-Byrne, P., et al. (1993). Histories of sexual victimization in patients with irritable bowel syndrome or inflammatory bowel disease. *American Journal of Psychiatry, 150*(10), 1502–1506.

Warnock, J., & Bundren, J. (1997). Anxiety and mood disorders associated with gonadotropin-releasing hormone agonist therapy. *Psychopharmacology Bulletin, 33*(2), 311–316.

Weinstock, L. (1999). Gender differences in the presentation and management of social anxiety disorder. *Journal of Clinical Psychiatry, 60*(9), 9–13.

Weiss, M., Baerg, E., Wisebord, S., et al. (1995). The influence of gonadal hormones on periodicity of obsessive–compulsive disorder. *Canadian Journal of Psychiatry, 40*(4), 205–207.

Weissman, M., Bland, R., Canino, G., et al. (1994). The cross national epidemiology of obsessive–compulsive disorder. *Journal of Clinical Psychiatry, 55*, 5–10.

Weissman, M., Bland, R., Canino, G., et al. (1997). The cross-national epidemiology of panic disorder. *Archives of General Psychiatry, 54*, 305–309.

Weissman, M., Klerman, G., Markowitz, J., et al. (1989). Suicidal ideation and suicide attempts in panic disorder and attacks. *New England Journal of Medicine, 321*, 1209–1214.

Westenberg, H. (1998). The nature of social anxiety disorder. *Journal of Clinical Psychiatry, 59*(17), 20–26.

Williams, K., & Koran, L. (1997). Obsessive–compulsive disorder in pregnancy, the puerperium, and the premenstruum. *Journal of Clinical Psychiatry, 58*(7), 330–334.

Windmann, S. (1998). Panic disorder from a monistic perspective: Integrating neurobiological and psychological approaches. *Journal of Anxiety Disorders, 12*(5), 485–507.

Wisner, K. L., Peindl, K. S., & Hanusa, B. H. (1996). Effects of childbearing on the natural history of panic disorder with comorbid mood disorder. *Journal of Affective Disorders, 41*(3), 173–180.

Wittchen, H. U., Zhao, S., Kessler, R. C., et al. (1994). DSM-III-R generalized anxiety disorder in the National Comorbidity Survey. *Archives of General Psychiatry, 51*(5), 355–364.

Woodman, C., Noyes, R., Black, D., et al. (1999). A 5-year follow-up study of generalized anxiety disorder and panic disorder. *Journal of Nervous and Mental Disease, 187*(1), 3–9.

Yaryura-Tobias, J. A., Neziroglu, F. A., & Kaplan, S. (1995). Self-mutilation, anorexia, and dysmenorrhea in obsessive compulsive disorder. *International Journal of Eating Disorders,* *17*(1), 33–38.

Yonkers, K., & Ellison, J. (1996). Anxiety disorders in women and their pharmacological treatment. In M. Jensvold, U. Halbreich, & J. Hamilton (Eds.), *Psychopharmacology and women: Sex, gender, and hormones* (pp. 261–285). Washington, DC: American Psychiatric Press.

Yonkers, K. A., Warshaw, M. G., Massion, A. O., et al. (1996). Phenomenology and course of generalised anxiety disorder. *British Journal of Psychiatry, 168*(3), 308–313.

Yonkers, K. A., Zlotnick, C., Allsworth, J., et al. (1998). Is the course of panic disorder the same in women and men? *American Journal of Psychiatry, 155*(5), 596–602.

Young, E., Abelson, J., Curtis, G., et al. (1997). Childhood adversity and vulnerability to mood and anxiety disorders. *Depression and Anxiety, 5*(2), 66–72.

Zohar, J., & Insel, T. (1987). Obsessive–compulsive disorder: Psychobiological approaches to diagnosis, treatment, and pathophysiology. *Biological Psychiatry, 22,* 667–687.

12

Alcohol and Other Substance Abuse

R. J. CANTERBURY

Substance use has commonly been considered primarily a male problem, and many of the studies of both alcohol and substance abuse disorders were conducted predominantly with male subjects. For many years, women were perceived as not suffering from substance use problems to the same extent as men. This perception, coupled with the intense social stigma associated with substance abuse, has resulted in inadequate diagnosis, treatment, and investigation of substance abuse disorders in women. Researchers and clinicians who study female women with substance abuse problems find that they differ from men in many important ways that have only recently received increasing attention (Stein & Cyr, 1997). This chapter concentrates on issues regarding epidemiology, physiological differences, clinical course, psychiatric comorbidity, and treatment of alcohol and other substance abuse and dependence that are specific to women or for which there are significant male–female differences.

EPIDEMIOLOGY

The Epidemiologic Catchment Area (ECA) study showed a number of interesting gender differences in substance abuse (Regier et al., 1990). The ECA sample of five communities revealed a male-to-female ratio of 4:1 for heavy drinking, whereas other samples have yielded lower estimates at 2.3:1 (Robins et al., 1988). In all large surveys, men continue to outnumber women in problem drinking; however, male-to-female ratios are lowest among younger age groups, suggesting increasing prevalence of drinking among young women and a closure of this gender gap (Stein & Cyr, 1997). The ECA study also found that the lifetime prevalence of alcohol abuse or dependence was more than three times greater in women who reported a history of sexual assault than in women who did not have such a history. The lifetime prevalence of other substance abuse or dependence was more than four times greater in women who reported having been sexually assaulted.

Statistics related to the prevalence of alcohol dependence and abuse diagnoses in men and women were presented in the 1992 National Longitudinal Alcohol Epidemiologic Survey of the general population in the United States over age 18 (Grant & Harford, 1995; Harford & Grant, 1994). The prevalence rates for alcohol dependence were 2.1% for men and 1.2% for women. The gender differences widened when both alcohol abuse and dependence were considered: Men were three times more likely to have a diagnosis of alcohol abuse or dependence than were women.

The National Comorbidity Survey investigated the prevalence of psychiatric disorders, including substance use disorders, in a representative sample of individuals aged 15 to 54 years throughout the United States (Kessler et al., 1994). This study showed that substance use disorders were more prevalent in men than in women, although the difference for alcohol dependence was larger than that for other substance dependence. The gender difference for nicotine dependence was substantially less than any other class of drugs.

The National Household Survey on Drug Abuse (NHSDA) is an annual survey conducted by the Substance Abuse and Mental Health Services Administration (SAMHSA). This survey has been a primary source of estimates of the prevalence and incidence of illicit drug, alcohol, and tobacco use in the population since 1971. Data from the 1998 NHSDA (SAMHSA, 1999a, 1999b, 2000) revealed that approximately 40% of men and 30% of women endorsed lifetime illicit drug use. The gender difference was smaller in the younger age groups (12–17 years), which reported almost equal illicit drug use in males and females. As in prior years, men in 1998 had a higher rate of current illicit drug use than women (8.1% vs. 4.5%).

For nontherapeutic use of psychotherapeutic agents, the gender differences was also small, with 11.1% of men and 7.6% of women reporting the use of psychotherapeutic agents in a nonprescribed manner. Lifetime tranquilizer use was 2.8% for women and 4.3% for men.

According to the 1998 NHSDA data, men were much more likely than women to binge-drink (23.2% vs. 8.6%) and to drink heavily (9.7 vs. 2.4%). Males had higher rates of smoking than females (29.7% vs. 25.7%). Among youths aged 12–17, the rates for males and females were similar (18.7% vs. 17.7%).

SAMHSA (1998) has conducted the first major analysis of substance abuse in a nationally representative sample of women. Using data from the NHSDA, this report showed that in the early 1960s, about 7% of new alcohol users among girls were between the ages of 10 and 14. By the early 1990s, that percentage had increased to 31% of new alcohol users. During the periods 1961–1965 and 1986–1990, females generally initiated alcohol use at later ages than males. But in 1991–1995, the gender difference in age-specific rates of alcohol initiation became negligible. The National Center on Addiction and Substance Abuse (CASA) at Columbia University demonstrated, from a meta-analysis of over 1,700 scientific publications, similar findings with regard to tobacco and illicit drugs ("CASA Study, " 1996).

Drinking behavior differs with the age, life role, and marital status of women. In general, a woman's drinking resembles that of her husband, siblings, or close friends (R. W. Wilsnack et al., 1984). Whereas younger women (aged 18–34) report higher rates of drinking-related problems than do older women (R. W. Wilsnack et al., 1984; Williams et al., 1987), the incidence of alcohol dependence appears greater among middle-aged women (aged 35–49) (Williams et al., 1987, 1989).

Women who have multiple roles (e.g., married women who work outside the home) may have lower rates of alcohol problems than women who do not have multiple roles (R. W. Wilsnack et al., 1984). Role deprivation (e.g., loss of role as wife, mother, or worker) may increase a woman's risk for abusing alcohol (Wilsnack & Cheloha, 1987). Women who have never been married or who are divorced or separated are more likely to drink heavily and to experience alcohol-related problems than women who are married or widowed. Unmarried women living with a partner are more likely still to engage in heavy drinking and to develop drinking problems.

Drinking patterns and alcohol-related problems vary among women of different racial or ethnic groups. Women characterized as non-Hispanic European Americans are the group most likely to drink any alcohol, whereas African American and Hispanic women have the highest rates of abstention (Herd, 1989, 1991). African American women who do drink are more likely to drink heavily and experience more alcohol-related health problems (Herd, 1989; Stein & Cyr, 1997), despite the finding that the onset of heavy drinking appears to be later among African American women (45–59 years) than among European American women (25–44 years) (Lillie-Blanton et al., 1991).

Data from self-report surveys suggest that Hispanic women are more likely to drink infrequently or to abstain (Holck et al., 1984; Caetano, 1987), but this may change as they enter new social and work arenas. Gilbert (1987) has found that reports of abstention are greater among Hispanic women who have immigrated to the United States, whereas moderate or heavy drinking is more common among younger, American-born Hispanic women.

Race has not been shown to be associated with current alcohol use disorders when other variables are controlled. Low household income has been shown to correlate with heavy drinking, as have widowhood and lower levels of education. One exception is that women in college are more likely to binge-drink than women of the same age who are not in college. Women who work outside the home and have recently become unemployed are more likely to drink heavily. Class and socioeconomic status may be more important than race in delineating the epidemiology of drinking in women (Stein & Cyr, 1997).

The gender gap in drug and alcohol abuse is closing. During adolescence, girls and boys are now equally likely to drink or to use illicit drugs, so the age of first drug use essentially is the same. Historically, women have been protected by their later onset of use, but this gender difference has recently disappeared (Stein & Cyr, 1997).

BINGE-DRINKING AND DRUG ABUSE PATTERNS IN COLLEGE STUDENTS

Binge drinking is reported to be the primary substance use problem among college students today (Syre et al., 1997). Binge drinking is related to a number of negative behavioral consequences, including unsafe sex, sexual assault, violent behavior, and poor school outcomes (Hanson & Engs, 1992; Canterbury & McGarvey, 1999). Among a nonrepresentative sample of over 56,000 college students nationwide, 42% reported binge drinking in a 2-week period prior to being surveyed (Presley & Meilman, 1992). A national study found that 50% of men and 39% of women binge-drink (Wechsler et al., 1994).

Fifty percent of women in a 1999 University of Virginia sample reported engaging in binge drinking at least once in the previous 2 weeks (Canterbury & McGarvey, 1999).

Men reported consuming more drinks, on average, than women—8.4 versus 4.1 drinks. Men were significantly more likely than women to report that they engaged in binge drinking in the 2 weeks prior to the survey (58.8% vs. 49.7%), even though comparable numbers of men and women reported prior use of alcohol (89.9% of men and 91.8% of women). There were no gender differences in use of alcohol in the past year or the past month. Men and women also did not differ on self-reports of getting drunk: 59.4% of men and 51.2% of women reported that they drank until they became intoxicated on at least one occasion in the past 14 days.

The prevalence of lifetime tobacco use did not differ by gender in the University of Virginia sample (Canterbury & McGarvey, 1999): 65.7% of men and 60.7% of women reported that they had tried tobacco. European American students (67.7%) were significantly more likely to have tried tobacco than were either African American students (40%) or Asian American students (44.4%).

Almost half (45.5%) of the students in this sample reported smoking marijuana at least once in their lifetimes, with no significant gender differences (Canterbury & McGarvey, 1999). The median age of first-time use was between 16 and 17 years. Sixty-one percent first used marijuana before the age of 18, including 2.5% who started before age 14. In this sample, 56% reported first-time marijuana use occurring before age 18.

Alcohol abuse is associated with high-risk sexual behaviors. In our data (Canterbury & McGarvey, 1999), 31.3% of women and 22.3% of men reported that they engaged in sexual activity, when ordinarily they would not have, while drinking or under the influence of alcohol. Also, 3.1% of women and 7.2% of men reported that they had taken advantage of another person sexually. Female students who engaged in binge drinking at least once during the past 2 weeks were almost three times more likely than those who did not to say that their alcohol use had led them to have been taken advantage of sexually (26.7% vs. 9.2%). Both males and females who reported binge drinking were significantly more likely than students who did not binge-drink to report taking advantage of another person sexually while drinking. Females who binge-drank were 4.6 times more likely than females who did not binge-drink to report sexually exploiting their partners (4.9% vs. 0.9%). The females who binge-drank (43.3%) were also 2.5 times more likely than other females (17.0%) to report that their drinking had led them to engage in sexual activity when ordinarily they would not have.

Twenty percent of women in the University of Virginia sample (Canterbury & McGarvey, 1999) reported that they had been drinking before the last time they had sexual intercourse. Dating status was one of many related factors. Women who were dating nonexclusively (24.8%) or not dating anyone (38%) were significantly more likely than students who are dating only one person (13.9%) to report drinking before their last sexual encounter. It appears that the use of alcohol has an important role in dating and initiating sexual relations with a partner, particularly if one is not in a long-term, committed relationship with the other person. This finding is supported by another study indicating that alcohol was used at least once by 33% of men and 17% of women to facilitate a sexual encounter (Anderson & Mathieu, 1996).

Women (16.3%) were no more likely than men (14.5%) to say that they had unprotected sex while using alcohol. In 1998 15.8% of women and 15.5% of men reported having unprotected sex due to their alcohol use. However, females reporting binge drinking were 2.7 times more likely to report having had unprotected sex than other females (22.7% vs. 8.6%).

Driving while under the influence of alcohol is significantly associated with binge drinking (Duncan, 1997). Twenty-eight percent (27.7%) of students in our sample (Canterbury & McGarvey, 1999) who used alcohol reported having driven while under the influence of alcohol, but only 1.1% had been detained or arrested by the police for drunk driving. Significantly more male students (35.1%) than female students (21.3%) reported previously driving while intoxicated. Females who binge-drank were 3.8 times more likely than other females to say that they had driven while intoxicated.

ALCOHOL AND OTHER SUBSTANCE ABUSE IN OLDER WOMEN

The incidence of substance misuse among older adults in the United States is unknown. Moreover, diagnostic criteria, which were validated in samples who were younger, probably underestimate the prevalence of substance use disorders among older and elderly women (Patterson & Jeste, 1999; DeHart & Hoffmann, 1995). In a cross-sectional study of 5,065 consenting primary care patients who completed the CAGE questionnaire (a commonly used measure to screen for serious alcohol problems), 12% of women compared to 15% of men drank more than the limited recommended by the National Institute on Alcohol Abuse and Alcoholism. The study also indicated that using the CAGE alone to assess alcohol use problems was not sufficient (Adams et al., 1996).

Since the population of people 65 and older is rising rapidly, since about 10% of the general population is believed to have a substance abuse problem, and since older adults have numerous factors that place them at risk for such problems, it is reasonable to assume that substance abuse is a problem for a significant number of older women. According to a report from the House of Representatives Select Committee on Aging, about 70% of all hospitalized older adults have alcohol-related problems. However, in one study of alcohol abuse in elderly emergency room patients, physicians identified only 21% of those with current alcohol use problems (Adams et al., 1992).

Issues such as grief, isolation, shame, retirement, financial problems, and health problems make older adults especially vulnerable to substance abuse (Rozenweig et al., 1997). Older women may be at even greater risk for substance abuse problems than older men because of increased struggles with shame, stigma, and denial.

Women tend to live longer than men do, so they deal with more losses, they continue to take responsibility for children and grandchildren, and they continue to play the hostess role. Because of the gentle, caretaking, nurturing stereotype that older women are expected to play, they generally feel a greater sense of shame and guilt about their substance use problems. They and their families are often all too ready to deny a substance use problem. Depression and isolation can also be problems for older women who hide their substance abuse problems, leading to more physical complications and more depression.

As women age, their metabolism changes, making them more susceptible to the effects of alcohol. Mixing alcohol with over-the-counter or prescription drugs is still another problem for older women, and one that can be fatal (Eliason, 1998). The potential for drug interactions increases if they are taking many different prescriptions, or if they are having trouble taking them correctly. The overuse of psychoactive prescription drugs, such as tranquilizers, sedatives, and antidepressants, poses a particular threat. A recent study found that one in four women over 60 takes at least one of these drugs daily, and that some of them develop serious drug problems ("Drug Strategies 1998: Keeping Score," 1998).

FACTORS ASSOCIATED WITH SUBSTANCE ABUSE DISORDERS

A number of social factors differentiating women from men with regard to substance use have been identified (Brady & Randall, 1999). Although substance abuse disorders in general are stigmatized, women experience more social disapproval of substance use, and substance use is more stigmatized in women than in men (Blume, 1986). Women with alcoholism are more likely than men to have alcoholic role models in their nuclear families and to have spouses who are also alcoholic (Lex, 1991). Substance use for men is more likely to affect jobs or career, whereas disruptions for women are more likely to occur in family life. More females with substance use problems are separated or divorced compared with men (Lex, 1991).

In a gender comparison of childhood disorders in adults with opiate dependence, women reported significantly lower levels of conduct problems, less social deviance, and higher levels of internalizing problems (Luthar et al., 1996). Women are more likely to attribute their drinking to a traumatic event or a stressor (Lex, 1991), and women who abuse alcohol and drugs are more likely to have been sexually or physically abused than other women. In addition, women with alcoholism are more likely than men to have another mental health disorder, most often depression (Stein & Cyr, 1997).

The increasing presence of women in the workplace has afforded women more opportunities to drink away from the home, and entering the workplace in general is likely to increase drinking among women. For some women employment may actually be a protective factor, whereas for others it may be a facilitative factor (Ames & Rebhun, 1996).

The etiology of alcohol dependence is multifactorial. Currently, it is very difficult to differentiate genetic factors from psychosocial ones. There are many publications on the inheritance of alcohol dependence, and most suggest that genetics accounts for approximately 50% of the variance. In addition, metabolic factors may play an important role. Factors such as socioeconomics, parental drinking, childhood experiences, friends' drinking behaviors, and individual impulse control all play a role in enhancing susceptibility (Stein & Cyr, 1997).

Experiences in childhood have been shown to be predictors of alcohol and other substance abuse. Childhood sexual abuse has been recognized as an antecedent of problem drinking, as well as of opiate and cocaine misuse (Hurley, 1991). Women with alcoholism are twice as likely as other women to have been beaten or sexually assaulted as children. Prior sexual abuse has been associated with prostitution, injection drug use, crack use, and unsafe sex. Frequent, heavy drinking during college years has been a strong predictor of later problem drinking. Younger age of first intoxication and early smoking are also correlated with later alcohol problems (Stein & Cyr, 1997).

Mental health problems, particularly depression, suicidality, sexual dysfunction, reproductive problems (Blume, 1998), use of other drugs, a partner's use of drugs, and eating disorders have all been associated with substance abuse among women. All psychiatric diagnoses are more prevalent in females with alcoholism than in other females (Helzer & Pryzbeck, 1988). The ECA study found that 37% of women with alcohol use disorders had comorbid mental illness (Regier et al., 1990). Major depression was the most common psychiatric comorbidity among these women. The relationship between alcoholism and anxiety in women has been documented repeatedly, but it remains unclear whether the anxiety conditions are lifelong disorders or temporary conditions related to intoxication and withdrawal. When women in alcohol treatment have been asked about their reasons for seeking help, the most often cited reason is deepening depression (Turnbull & Gomberg, 1991).

Rates of depression among those with alcoholism vary, depending on the study subjects, assessment tools, and definitions of depression. The reported prevalence has ranged from 30% to 70% (Schuckit & Monteiro, 1988). Schuckit and Monteiro (1988) found that most women with major depression had either not altered or decreased their alcohol intake after beginning to experience depressive symptoms. Whether depression is a cause or consequence of drinking, screening for it is critical in primary care settings. At the same time, it should be noted that depression could mask signs of alcohol abuse (Stein & Cyr, 1997).

The combination of alcohol dependence and depression makes for high vulnerability to suicidal behavior (Blume, 1998). Women with alcoholism under age 40 are 5 times more likely to attempt suicide than nonalcoholic women (Gomberg, 1989). This suicidal risk begins in adolescence. Teenage girls who drink on more than five occasions per month are five times more likely to attempt suicide than those who never drink (26% vs. 5%) (Centers for Disease Control and Prevention, 1995). The suicide rate for women equals that for men among adults with alcoholism. Differentiating mood disorders symptoms from the pharmacological depressive effects of alcohol is difficult. Feelings of sadness can be generated by a combination of alcohol and the social and psychological consequences of heavy drinking. Many symptoms of depression (sleep disturbance, loss of appetite, irritability) are also reported during heavy alcohol use and withdrawal (Hesselbrock et al., 1985). Stein and Cyr (1997) reported that the following factors are associated with increased risk of alcohol problems in women:

- Drinking to improve psychological function (e.g., shyness, anxiety) in young adulthood
- Low self-esteem in adolescence
- Poor coping skills in adolescence
- Family history of alcoholism, particularly in the father
- Severe premenstrual syndrome
- Concomitant psychiatric diagnosis (depression, anxiety)
- Lifetime use of drugs other than alcohol
- History of rape or incest
- Fertility problems
- Heavy-drinking partner
- Sexual dysfunction
- Eating disorders
- Low utilization of prenatal care
- Domestic violence
- Suicidality

Reproductive problems also may cause heavy drinking (Blume, 1998). Infertility, miscarriage, premature delivery, and early hysterectomy are all associated with alcohol abuse. The association of problem drinking and sexual dysfunction suggests that women may use alcohol to cope with sexual dissatisfaction, or, alternatively, that the dysfunction may be a consequence of drinking (Gomberg, 1986). In either case, women who are drinking heavily are less likely to use contraceptives and more likely to engage in unsafe sexual practices (Leigh, 1990; Canterbury & McGarvey, 1999).

Females with drug addictions are usually initiated into drug use by men. Cohabiting with a partner who has alcohol or other substance dependence may contribute to the development of substance abuse in a woman. This observation has been made for females with opiate addiction, cocaine addiction, and alcoholism. There is a strong positive correlation between a woman's level of drug or alcohol consumption and that of her partner or husband. Women progress more quickly from initiation to addiction than do men (Stein & Cyr, 1997).

High rates of alcohol and other substance abuse rates were found in women with eating disorders, compared with the general female population (Beary et al., 1986: Kassett et al., 1989). Twenty to forty percent of women being treated for anorexia nervosa or bulimia nervosa abuse alcohol. Conversely, women with substance abuse disorders report higher rates of eating disorders. Although alcohol is the drug most often used by patients with eating disorders, a high prevalence of cocaine use has also been noted. Dieting, routine among high school and college women, has also been associated with alcohol and other substance use.

PHYSIOLOGICAL DIFFERENCES BETWEEN MEN AND WOMEN IN BIOLOGICAL RESPONSE TO ALCOHOL AND OTHER SUBSTANCES

Important gender differences exist in the physiological effects of alcohol. Women become intoxicated after drinking smaller quantities of alcohol compared to men (Brady & Randall, 1999; Blume, 1998; El-Guebaly, 1995). Three possible mechanisms may explain this response.

First, it may be related to the fact that women have a lower total body water content than men of comparable size (51% vs. 65%), meaning that they achieve higher blood alcohol concentrations (BACs) than men after drinking equivalent amounts of alcohol (Marshall et al., 1983). The ratio of water to fat decreases with age, so this effect is more prominent in older women. Similarly, lipid-soluble benzodiazepines will have a longer half-life in women.

Second, women have lower levels of alcohol dehydrogenase. Frezza et al. (1990) demonstrated that women have a lower concentration of gastric alcohol dehydrogenase than do men and metabolize only 25% of the alcohol metabolized by men. This enzyme is responsible for the metabolism of a substantial amount of alcohol before it enters systemic circulation, also contributing to higher BACs and probably creating a heightened vulnerability to the consequences of drinking in women. Women, in general, also have smaller livers than men and less total hepatic alcohol dehydrogenase.

Third, fluctuations in gonadal hormone levels during the menstrual cycle may affect the rate of alcohol metabolism, making a woman more susceptible to elevated BACs at different points in the cycle (Marshall et al., 1983; Sutker et al., 1987). In addition to metabolism-related differences that might explain the gender difference in response to alcohol, some investigators have suggested that basic variations in the organization and modulation of male and female brains, especially neurosteroids, influence the response to alcohol (Lancaster, 1994). Similarly, gender differences in alcohol-induced adrenocortical hormone levels may play a role in the medical consequences (Brady & Randall, 1999).

Females with alcoholism have death rates 50% to 100% higher than those of males. Furthermore, a greater percentage of females with alcoholism die from suicides, alcohol-related accidents, circulatory disorders, and cirrhosis of the liver (Sutker et al., 1987; Tuyns & Pequignot, 1984).

The effects of alcohol on the liver are more severe for women than for men. Women develop alcoholic liver disease, particularly alcoholic cirrhosis and hepatitis, after a comparatively shorter period of heavy drinking and at a lower level of daily drinking than men (Hill, 1982; Saunders et al., 1981); moreover, proportionately more women with alcoholism die from cirrhosis, as noted above. The exact mechanisms that underlie women's vulnerability to alcohol-induced liver damage are unclear. Differences in body weight and fluid content between men and women may be contributing factors. Gender-specific biochemical differences in hepatocytes may also play a role (Pascale et al., 1989). In addition, Johnson and Williams (1985) suggested that the combined effect of estrogens and alcohol may augment liver damage. Finally, women may be more susceptible to liver damage because of the diminished activity of gastric alcohol dehydrogenase and less first-pass metabolism (Julkunen et al., 1985).

Drinking may also be associated with an increased risk for breast cancer. After reviewing epidemiological data on alcohol consumption and the incidence of breast cancer, Longnecker et al. (1988) reported that risk increases when a woman consumes 1 ounce or more of absolute alcohol daily. Increased risk appears to be related directly to the effects of alcohol (Willett et al., 1987).

Menstrual disorders (e.g., painful menstruation, heavy flow, premenstrual discomfort, and irregular or absent cycles) are associated with chronic heavy drinking or drug use (S. C. Wilsnack et al., 1984; Hugues et al., 1980; Busch et al., 1986). These disorders can have adverse effects on fertility (Mendelson et al., 1983). Furthermore, continued drinking may lead to early menopause (Gavaler, 1988; Ryback, 1977). Alcohol depresses sexual function and has been shown to increase latency and decrease intensity of orgasm in women (Blume, 1986).

Cardiomyopathy and myopathy are as common in women with alcoholism as in men. The threshold dose for the development of alcoholic cardiomyopathy is considerably less in women, and the slope of decline in the left ventricular ejection fraction is steeper in women, suggesting that women are more sensitive than men to the toxic effects of alcohol on the myocardium (Stein & Cyr, 1997).

Hip fractures are associated with alcohol intake in women. Felson et al. (1988) noted an increased risk of hip fracture for women under 65 years old who consumed 2 to 6 ounces per week of alcohol. Falls and osteopenia may be contributory.

Important gender differences also exist in the physiological effects of nicotine. Women in general smoke fewer cigarettes than do men, but metabolize nicotine more slowly; therefore, nicotine levels in the body are similar in males and females who smoke (Benowitz, 1997). Women who smoke generally have earlier menopause. If women (especially after age 30) smoke cigarettes and also take oral contraceptives, they are more prone to cardiovascular and cerebrovascular diseases than other smokers.

Pregnant women who smoke cigarettes run an increased risk of having stillborn or premature infants or infants with low birthweight (Kleinman et al., 1988). Children of women who smoked while pregnant have an increased risk for developing conduct disorder (Wakschlag et al., 1999). National studies of mothers and daughters have also found that maternal smoking during pregnancy increases the probability that female children will smoke and will persist in smoking (Kandel et al., 1994).

Illicit drug use during pregnancy has been associated with poor pregnancy outcome for most substances examined. Cocaine, opiates, nicotine, and marijuana have all been shown to have adverse consequences for offspring, although the nature of the consequences varies with the substance used (Brady & Randall, 1999).

Benzodiazepines are frequently prescribed for the symptomatic treatment of anxiety and sleep disorders, especially in women. Many abused women report taking medications such as benzodiazepines to alleviate anxiety and/or insomnia. Individuals with alcohol, opioid, or polydrug dependence may be at higher risk than others for benzodiazepine abuse and dependence.

Females who use drugs are at high risk of contracting HIV disease because of the greater transmissibility from men to women, because women are more likely to have drug-using partners, and because women often have unprotected sex to finance their addiction. Seventy percent of women with AIDS have a history of illicit drug use. In addition, three-quarters of AIDS cases in women are among African Americans and Latinas (Wallace et al., 1994). Women drug users are at increased risk of acquiring other sexually transmitted diseases. Syphilis in particular has been linked to crack use. Female adolescents who use cocaine are 31 times more likely to be sexually active, 27 times more likely to have four or more partners, and twice as likely never to use condoms as other girls (Lowry et al., 1994; Stein, 1999).

SUBSTANCE USE DURING PREGNANCY

Babies whose mothers drink during pregnancy may be born with fetal alcohol syndrome (FAS), which is one of the leading known causes of mental retardation. Babies born with FAS weigh less and are shorter than normal infants. They have smaller heads, malformed facial features, abnormal joints and limbs, and poor coordination. Difficulties with learning, attention, memory, and problem solving are common. Some babies also have speech and hearing impairments and heart defects. Many of these problems persist into adulthood.

Pregnant women who use drugs such as heroin, methadone, amphetamines, phencyclidine, marijuana, or cocaine give birth to infants in double jeopardy. These drug-exposed infants may be dependent and experience drug withdrawal or have other medical problems at birth. The medical problems are worsened by poor caretaking and the stress and chaos caused by their mothers' drug-using lifestyle.

Exposure to tobacco smoke poses grave risks to babies both before and after they are born. The National Center for Health Statistics reports that babies born to smoking mothers face double the risk of low birthweight, increasing the likelihood of illness and death during infancy. Infants are three times more likely to die from sudden infant death syndrome if their mothers smoked during and after pregnancy, and twice as likely even if their mothers stopped smoking during pregnancy but started again after birth. Children, especially those under age 2, are particularly vulnerable to secondhand smoke. Secondhand smoke causes 150,000 to 300,000 respiratory infections in infants that result in 7,500 to 15,000 hospitalizations a year. Other effects on children include increased prevalence of fluid in the middle ear, irritated upper respiratory tract, increased frequency and severity of symptoms in asthmatic children, and an overall increased risk of asthma.

CLINICAL COURSE

The course of substance dependence, particularly alcohol dependence, is different for women compared to men. The interval between the age of first drinking and treatment seeking seems to be shorter for women than for men (Piazza et al., 1989). As previously mentioned, studies also suggest that women experience greater medical, physiological, and psychological impairment earlier in their drinking careers. In addition, women seem to progress between landmarks associated with the developmental course of alcoholism (e.g., regular drinking or loss of control) sooner than do men (Brady & Randall, 1999). These findings have led to the theory that a more accelerated progression of alcoholism may occur in women. This phenomenon has not been well studied in other abused substances, but one study (Griffin et al., 1989) found that women with cocaine dependence sought treatment earlier in the course of their illnesses than did men. This has also been found for women who abuse opiates (Hser et al., 1987).

PSYCHIATRIC COMORBIDITY

Many important differences between males and females with substance use disorders have been found with regard to comorbid psychiatric illness. Hesselbrock et al. (1985) reported more depression, panic disorder, and phobia among hospitalized females versus males with alcoholism. Similarly, Cornelius et al. (1995) found significantly more major depression and anxiety disorders in females with alcoholism, and more antisocial personality disorder in males with alcoholism. Helzer et al. (1987) indicate that in general, females with alcoholism have more comorbid psychiatric disorders than do their male counterparts. Helzer and Pryzbeck (1988) analyzed ECA data concerning men and women in the general population who had a lifetime diagnosis of both alcohol abuse or dependence and major depression. Major depression was primary in 66% of the women, but in only 22% of the men. Hesselbrock et al. (1985) found a similar contrast: 52% of the women in their study satisfied a lifetime diagnosis of major depression, compared with 32% of the men. In 66% of these female patients, the major depression was primary, compared with 41% of the males. Another study found that adolescent girls in addiction treatment were more likely than boys to have a history of depression. Since these patients had early onset of both depression and addiction, it is of interest that in 58% of the boys (but only 28% of the girls) with both diagnoses, the substance use disorder was clearly primary (Deykin et al., 1992).

Kessler et al. (1997) showed that women with alcohol use disorders were two to three times more likely to experience anxiety and depressive disorders than their male counterparts. Men and women with alcohol use disorders had approximately equal prevalence of concurrent substance use disorders, but men were more than twice as likely as women to have conduct disorder and antisocial personality disorder (Brady & Randall, 1999).

Studies of depressive symptoms in women suggest that these may represent a psychological condition that in some way predisposes women to increased drinking, alcohol dependence, and perhaps other substance dependence. In addition, the increased risk of substance abuse in women associated with traumatic events such as sexual assault may be mediated through such symptoms as discouragement, low self-esteem, and demoralization, often associated with depression (Blume, 1998).

Studies of comorbid psychiatric disorders in those with opiate and cocaine abusers have shown higher percentages of mood and anxiety disorders in women than in men (Brady & Randall, 1999). In a recent study of persons seeking treatment for opiate abusers (Brooner et al., 1997), lifetime psychiatric comorbidity was more than twice as common in women as in men. Major depression, social phobia, and eating disorders were much more commonly seen in women compared with men.

Rounsaville et al. (1991) found nearly equal gender distribution of mood disorder (43% for men, 47% for women), but nearly twice as much anxiety disorder in women as in men, in 298 individuals with cocaine dependence. For nicotine dependence, gender differences in comorbidity are of particular importance. An association seems to exist between depression and cigarette smoking, in that depressed individuals are more likely to smoke cigarettes and are less successful in attempts at smoking cessation than are nondepressed individuals. This association between depression and smoking seems to be stronger in women than in men (Kessler et al., 1996).

Other issues of particular importance to gender differences in psychiatric comorbidity with substance use are traumatization and violence. Several studies in both epidemiological samples and treatment-seeking populations have demonstrated a high incidence of traumatic events and subsequent development of posttraumatic stress disorder (PTSD) in individuals with substance use disorders. Estimates of lifetime PTSD prevalence rates range from 30% to 50% among treatment-seeking individuals with substance abusing (Brady & Randall, 1999).

The relationship between substance use disorders and traumatization seems to be particularly important for women. One study comparing women with alcoholism to a household comparison sample found higher rates of childhood trauma in the former group, even when demographic and family background differences were controlled (Miller et al., 1993). In a longitudinal, national study of women in the United States, Kilpatrick et al. (1997) demonstrated that the use of illicit drugs was strongly associated with both sexual and physical assault in women. In an analysis of individuals with PTSD from the ECA study, it has been found that female gender and the use of cocaine or opiates were the strongest predictors of PTSD (Regier et al., 1990).

Another gender-specific issue with regard to psychiatric comorbidity is the etiological relationship between other psychiatric disorders and substance use disorders. Kessler et al. (1996) found that the onset of psychiatric disorders preceded the onset of substance use disorders more often in women than in men. Similarly, in a study by Dunne et al. (1993) of persons seeking treatment for alcoholism, women were more likely than men to have primary anxiety and depression. These gender differences in order of onset of other psychiatric disorders and substance use disorders may have etiological significance and implications for gender-specific treatment approaches.

Special care should be taken to avoid iatrogenic drug dependence. Benzodiazepines, other sedative drugs, and analgesics capable of producing dependence should be avoided wherever possible. When these medications are necessary, their use should be kept to a minimum and closely monitored.

PROGNOSIS

The effectiveness of addiction treatment in women has received far less attention than such treatment in male populations. Generally, studies that have compared male and female patients outcomes show that men and women treated together for alcoholism and other substance dependence do about equally well when the data are corrected for demographic and clinical variables (Vannicelli, 1986; McLellan et al., 1986). A meta-analysis of 20 alcoholism treatment follow-up studies, in which data were analyzed by gender, did find some significant sex differences (Jarvis, 1992). Women did better for the first 12 months, but men showed more improvement than women in longer-term outcome.

Factors that influence treatment effectiveness for women include the presence or absence of a supportive social network and the number of life problems encountered (MacDonald, 1987). Mortality rates among women with alcohol dependence are high, both when compared with rates in the general population of women and with rates of excess mortality in men with alcoholism (Klatsky et al., 1992; Hill, 1986).

TREATMENT

Although significant progress has been made in the past decade in understanding the health-related and socioeconomic impact of substance abuse among women, treatment is still scarce. Only a small fraction of the estimated 9 million women with serious alcohol or other substance use problems are able to get treatment unless they can afford to pay. Programs that treat pregnant women with addictions are even more limited, particularly those that allow women to live with their children during treatment ("Drug Strategies 1998: Keeping Score," 1998). There has been increasing federal involvement in the issue of gender-sensitive treatment since the 1980s, as federal policy makers respond to increasing numbers of drug-exposed infants. There has been only modest growth in specialized and women-only treatment units, however, and moderate increases in the number of women receiving substance use treatment overall (Stein & Cyr, 1997).

Women are more likely to be poor and without insurance than men seeking treatment. Although men with alcohol use problems outnumber women 2:1, the ratio of males to females in treatment is 4:1 (Harford & Grant, 1994). This may be due in part to barriers, but it is also a result of case-finding systems that concentrate on convicted drunk drivers and workplace intervention programs, both of which disproportionately reach males with alcoholism. National drug and alcohol treatment statistics reveal a ratio of men to women in drug treatment of 1.8:1, compared to a drug dependence prevalence of 2.3:1 (Kessler et al., 1994).

When compared to men entering treatment, women are more likely to be depressed, to have encountered more opposition to treatment from family and friends, and to perceive higher personal psychosocial costs (Allen, 1994; Beckman & Amaro, 1986). Women are also more often divorced in the course of alcoholism treatment than men are (O'Connor et al., 1994). Other obstacles to treatment include ineffective health care provider screening, inadequate financial resources, lack of child care facilities, fear of losing children, and internal barriers (such as guilt, shame, and denial). Although pregnancy may motivate women to enter treatment, it also aggravates feelings of guilt and may discourage help seeking (Chavkin et al., 1993). The most common reason given by both sexes for delaying help seeking was the belief that their drinking was not serious enough (denial) (Hingson et al., 1982).

Treatment opportunities for pregnant women are inadequate. In 1989, of 78 drug treatment facilities in New York City, 54% refused to treat pregnant women, 67% denied treatment to women on Medicaid, and 87% denied treatment to pregnant women addicted to crack cocaine (Chavkin et al., 1993). The notion of "one-stop shopping," in which one facility provides comprehensive services for women, is appealing; it requires programs such as mental health treatment, prenatal and gynecological care, contraceptive counseling, job training, and pediatric services (Finkelstein, 1993).

Treatment personnel believe that women have a poorer prognosis than men, despite the fact that there is no supportive evidence. This belief may create yet another barrier to women seeking help for alcohol and other substance use problems. Although most treatment outcome studies do not consider gender, those that do find little difference between the sexes in short-term alcohol or drug treatment outcomes (Marzuk et al., 1992).

Alcoholics Anonymous (AA) is the treatment most frequently used by American women, and its use continues to increase. Thirty-five percent of AA members are women. For both men and women, the social consequences of drinking carry more predictive power for entering treatment than dependence symptoms do (Stein & Cyr, 1997).

Specialized treatment units for women have been developed since the late 1980s. Some report improved outcome compared to mixed-gender units in terms of decreased alcohol use and increased social functioning (Dahlgren & Willander, 1989). Some women prefer an all-female environment that eliminates the problem of sexual harassment and facilitates discussion of past physical and sexual abuse (Harvey et al., 1994).

Women with drug and alcohol problems who are parents and in a primary caregiving role face great emotional demands when attempting to remain drug-free or alcohol-free. Classes in parent–child relations, parenting skills, and vocational training have become standard offerings in many programs. Some treatment programs are now accepting mother and their children into residential programs.

The process of recovery is not the same for both genders. For instance, being married contributed in one study to relapse in women with alcoholism but not men, presumably because of spousal drinking behaviors (Schneider et al., 1995). Screening for spousal violence is necessary, because women who return to violent relations tend to relapse (Miller et al., 1989).

Women who seek treatment tend to be coping with a large number of problems and to have exhausted informal social supports before resorting to professional services (Reed, 1987). Most of their relationships are related to substance use. One beneficial effect of treatment is the increase in the number of social supports for women who are often isolated.

Those who seek treatment for illicit drug abuse are more likely than women with alcohol abuse to be involved in prostitution and to enter treatment because of legal pressure exerted by the criminal justice system (Moise et al., 1981). For women facing incarceration or the loss of children, coerced treatment has increasingly been used. The shortage of treatment in prisons is of great concern, aggravated by the rising number of incarcerated pregnant women with addictions. Two small studies of pregnant women found that enhanced methadone programs (with rewards for clean urines and group therapy) may improve the health of newborns (Chang et al., 1992).

Methodological problems limit many studies of substance use problems in women, making it difficult to draw final conclusions as to treatment efficacy or appropriateness. Most large studies of screening and treatment have been done on predominantly male populations; cohort comparisons with men rarely take baseline gender differences into account.

PREVENTION

Primary prevention designed specifically for women is a subject that has received relatively little attention. A preferred strategy would be education about women's special sensitivity to alcohol, the teratogenicity of alcohol, the risk involved in using alcohol to medicate feelings of inadequacy or other dysphoric states, the risks of mixing alcohol and sedatives, and similar issues. Such an approach should include education about the properties and appropriate use of prescription drugs, as well as the dangers of tobacco and illicit substances for women and their offspring.

In addition to generally targeted education, culturally appropriate programs are needed for high-risk special populations such as Native American women. All women can be helped to develop coping skills and self-esteem, so that they are able to negotiate stressful life events and transitions without the use of alcohol or other substances. School-based counseling; individual and group support for women involved in separation, divorce, or widowhood; supports for single parents, working mothers, and caretakers of elderly or chronically ill individuals; and other similar sources of help for women who find themselves in stressful situations have the potential to prevent addiction.

Physicians have a unique opportunity to educate patients and their families about the characteristics, properties, and dangers of the drugs they may encounter. Physicians can help with stress-reduction counseling and referral. In addition, through the identification, referral, and treatment of those with addictions and their families, physicians can help to break the chain of substance use disorders that runs through many generations of American families (Blume, 1998).

CONCLUSIONS

Despite the fact that the rates of substance abuse and dependence are higher among men than among women, recent prevalence rates indicate that substance use disorders are common in women and that the gender gap is closing rapidly. Alcohol dependence in women has a complex etiology that includes biological factors, family history, difficulties in impulse control, depression, and drinking by significant others.

Recommendations can be made regarding clinical approaches to women who abuse alcohol. Because women have a lower threshold for harmful drinking than men who drink, screening and education are important elements of care and should be done for every patient. Health care professionals must be prepared to detect substance use and provide referrals. It is critical for health care workers not to attribute a woman's alcohol problems to depression. Family problems, a partner with alcoholism, or a family history of alcoholism should serve as clues to a potential substance use problem. Educating women about gender-specific health risks and the different metabolism of alcohol in women is essential. This information, along with a risk factor assessment for problems known to be associated with alcohol abuse, allows providers to intervene appropriately with their women patients (Stein & Cyr, 1997).

Alcohol abuse and other substance abuse often coexist in women. Crime, violence, and physical and mental illness are linked with substance use. The age of first illicit drug use has dropped over the past two decades, and primary prevention must begin in the community. Finally, the spectrum of disease related to substance abuse is broad and often insidious. Health care providers must consider alcohol and other substance use actively when taking patient histories, performing physical examinations, and considering differential diagnoses, to identify substance use problems before serious complications occur (Stein, 1999). This is especially true in women because of the "compressed phenomenon," in which the window between initiation and severe complications is smaller for women than for men. The gender differences in physical and sexual abuse and other psychiatric comorbidity are evident in females seeking treatment for substance abuse. The barriers to treatment for women are being addressed in many treatment settings to encourage more women to enter treatment. Negative consequences associated with substance abuse are different for men and women, and gender-sensitive rating instruments must be used not only to measure the severity of the problem, but also to evaluate treatment efficacy.

It will be interesting to determine in the future whether gender differences observed over the past 25 years become less clearly demarcated in comparisons of younger cohorts with substance abuse. Changing societal roles and attitudes toward women—especially the increase in women entering the workplace in general, and previously male-dominated sports and professions in particular—may influence not only opportunities to drink but also drinking culture.

Future clinical studies should be directed at identifying gender differences in the risk and protective factors involved in substance abuse by girls and women, with emphasis on early identification and the full spectrum of prevention activities, as well as on the coexistence of substance abuse and dependence with other psychiatric disorders. Researchers also need to develop and evaluate the effectiveness of new substance abuse treatment models that are specific to the unique needs of females. Such models should include treatment for substance abuse or dependence as well as any coexisting psychiatric disorder, and they must be culturally relevant.

REFERENCES

Adams, W. L., Barry, K. L., & Fleming, M. F. (1996). Screening for problem drinking in older primary care patients. *Journal of the American Medical Association, 276*(24), 1964–1967.

Adams, W. L., Magruder-Habib, K., Trued, S., et al. (1992). Alcohol abuse in elderly emergency department patients. *Journal of the American Geriatrics Society, 40*(12), 1236–1240.

Alameda County Low Birth Weight Study Group. (1990). Cigarette smoking and the risk of low birth weight: A comparison in black and white women. *Epidemiology, 1*, 201–205.

Allen, K. (1994). Development of an instrument to identify barriers to treatment for addicted women from their perspective. *International Journal of the Addictions, 29*(4), 429–444.

Ames, G. M., & Rebhun, L. A. (1996). Women, alcohol and work: Interactions of gender, ethnicity and occupational culture. *Social Science and Medicine, 43*(11), 1649–1663.

Anderson, P. B., & Mathieu, D. A. (1996). College students' high-risk sexual behavior following alcohol consumption. *Journal of Sex and Marital Therapy, 22*(4), 259–264.

Beary, M. D., Lacey, J. H., & Merry, J. (1986). Alcoholism and eating disorders in women of fertile age. *British Journal on Addiction, 81*(5), 685–689.

Beckman, L. J., & Amaro, H. (1986). Personal and social difficulties faced by women and men entering alcoholism treatment. *Journal of Studies on Alcohol, 47*(2), 135–145.

Benowitz, N. L. (1997). *Gender differences in the pharmacology of nicotine addiction.* Paper presented at the College on Problems of Drug Dependence, Nashville, TN.

Blume, S. B. (1986). Women and alcohol: A review. *Journal of the American Medical Association, 256*(11), 1467–1470.

Blume, S. (1998). Understanding addictive disorders in women. In A. W. Graham & T. K. Schultz (Eds.), *Principles of addiction medicine* (pp. 1173–1190). Chevy Chase, MD: American Society of Addiction Medicine.

Brady, K. T., & Randall, C. L. (1999). Gender differences in substance use disorders. *Psychiatric Clinics of North America, 22*(2), 241–252.

Brooner, R. K., King, V. L., Kidorf, M., et al. (1997). Psychiatric and substance comorbidity among treatment-seeking opioid abusers. *Archives of General Psychiatry, 54*(1), 71–80.

Busch, D., McBride, A. B., & Benaventura, L. M. (1986). Chemical dependency in women: The link to OB/GYN problems. *Journal of Psychosocial Nursing and Mental Health Services, 24*(4), 26–30.

Caetano, R. (1987). Drinking patterns and alcohol problems in a national survey of U.S. Hispanics. In D. Spiegler, D. Tate, S. Aitken, & C. Christian (Eds). *Alcohol use among U.S. ethnic minorities* (pp. 147–162). Washington, DC: U.S. Government Printing Office.

Canterbury, R. J., & McGarvey, E. (1999). *Health behavior survey: Spring 1999.* Charlottesville: University of Virginia, Department of Psychiatric Medicine.

CASA study: *The gender gap between adolescent girls' and boys' tobacco, alcohol and drug use has closed.* (1996). Available: http://www.health.org/pressrel/casapr.htm [August 2000].

Centers for Disease Control and Prevention. (1995). Suicide among children, adolescents, and young adults—United States 1980–1992. *Morbidity and Mortality Weekly Report, 44* 289–291.

Chang, G., Carrol, K. M., Behr, H. M., et al. (1992). Improving treatment outcome in pregnant opiate-dependent women. *Journal of Substance Abuse Treatment, 9*(4), 327–330.

Chavkin, W., Paone, D., Friedmann, P., et al. (1993). Reframing the debate: Toward effective treatment for inner-city drug-abusing mothers. *Bulletin of the New York Academy of Medicine, 70*(1), 50–68.

Cornelius, J. R., Jarrett, P. J., Thase, M. E., et al. (1995). Gender effects on the clinical presentation of alcoholics at a psychiatric hospital. *Comprehensive Psychiatry, 36*(6), 435–440.

Cottler, L. B., Compton, W. M., Mager, D., et al. (1992). Posttraumatic stress disorder among substance users from the general population. *American Journal of Psychiatry, 149*(5), 664–670.

Dahlgren, L., & Willander, A. (1989). Are special treatment facilities for female alcoholics needed?: A controlled 2–year follow-up study from a specialized female unit (EWA) versus a mixed male/female treatment facility. *Alcoholism: Clinical and Experimental Research, 13*(4), 499–504.

DeHart, S. S., & Hoffmann, N. G. (1995). Screening and diagnosis of "alcohol abuse and dependence" in older adults. *International Journal of the Addictions, 30*(13–14), 1717–1747.

Deykin, E. Y., Buka, S. L., & Zeena, T. H. (1992). Depressive illness among chemically dependent adolescents. *American Journal of Psychiatry, 149*(10), 1341–1347.

Drug Strategies Organization. *Drug strategies 1998: Keeping score. Women and drugs: Looking at the federal drug control budget (1998).* (http://www.drugstrategies.org/KS1998). Washington, DC: Author.

Duncan, D. F. (1997). Chronic drinking, binge drinking and drunk driving. *Psychological Reports, 80*(2), 681–682.

Dunne, F. J., Galatopoulos, C., & Schipperheijn, J. M. (1993). Gender differences in psychiatric morbidity among alcohol misusers. *Comprehensive Psychiatry, 34*(2), 95–101.

El-Guebaly, N. (1995). Alcohol and polysubstance abuse among women. *Canadian Journal of Psychiatry, 40*(2), 73–79.

Eliason, M. J. (1998). Identification of alcohol-related problems in older women. *Journal of Gerontological Nursing, 24*(10), 8–15.

Felson, D. T., Kiel, D. P., Anderson, J. J., et al. (1988). Alcohol consumption and hip fracture: The Framingham Study. *American Journal of Epidemiology, 128*(5), 1102–1107.

Finkelstein, N. (1993). Treatment programming for alcohol and drug-dependent pregnant women. *International Journal of the Addictions, 28*(13), 1275–1309.

Frezza, M., di Padova, C., Pozzato, G., et al. (1990). High blood alcohol levels in women: The role of decreased gastric alcohol dehydrogenase activity and first-pass metabolism. *New England Journal of Medicine, 322*(2), 95–99.

Gavaler, J. S. (1988). Effects of moderate consumption of alcoholic beverages on endocrine function in postmenopausal women: Bases for hypotheses. In M. Galanter (Ed.), *Recent developments in alcoholism* (Vol. 6, pp. 229–251). New York: Plenum Press.

Gilbert, J. (1987). Alcohol consumption patterns in immigrant and later generation Mexican American women. *Hispanic Journal of Behavioral Sciences, 9*(3), 299–313.

Gomberg, E. S. L. (1986). Women and alcoholism: Psychosocial issues. In *Women and alcohol: Health-related issues* (pp. 78–120). Washington, DC: U.S. Department of Health and Human Services.

Gomberg, E. S. L. (1989). Suicide risk among women with alcohol problems. *American Journal of Public Health, 79*(10), 1363–1365.

Grant, B. F., & Harford, T. C. (1995). Comorbidity between DSM-IV alcohol use disorders and major depression: Results of a national survey. *Drug and Alcohol Dependence, 39*(3), 197–206.

Griffin, M. L., Weiss, R. D., Mirin, S. M., et al. (1989). A comparison of male and female cocaine abusers. *Archives of General Psychiatry, 46*(2), 122–126.

Hanson, D. J., & Engs, R. C. (1992). College students' drinking problems: A national study, 1982–1991. *Psychological Reports, 71*(1), 39–42.

Harford, T. C., & Grant, B. F. (1994). Prevalence and population validity of DSM-III-R alcohol abuse and dependence: The 1989 National Longitudinal Survey on Youth. *Journal of Substance Abuse, 6*(1), 37–44.

Harvey, E. M., Rawson, R. A., & Obert, J. L. (1994). History of sexual assault and the treatment of substance abuse disorders. *Journal of Psychoactive Drugs, 26*(4), 361–367.

Helzer, J. E., & Pryzbeck, T. R. (1988). The co-occurrence of alcoholism with other psychiatric disorders in the general population and its impact on treatment. *Journal of Studies on Alcohol, 49*(3), 219–224.

Helzer, J. E., Robins, L. N., & McEvoy, L. (1987). Post-traumatic stress disorder in the general population: Findings of the Epidemiologic Catchment Area survey. *New England Journal of Medicine, 317*(26), 1630–1634.

Herd, D. (1989). The epidemiology of drinking patterns and alcohol-related problems among U.S. blacks. In D. Spiegler, D. Tate, S. Aitken, & C. Christian (Eds.), *Alcohol use among U.S. ethnic minorities* (pp. 3–50). Washington, DC: U.S. Government Printing Office.

Herd, D. (1991). Drinking problems in the black population. In W. Clark & M. Hitton (Eds.), *Alcohol in America: Drinking practices and problems* (pp. 308–328). Albany: State University of New York Press.

Hesselbrock, M. N., Meyer, R. E., & Keener, J. (1985). Psychopathology in hospitalized alcoholics. *Archives of General Psychiatry, 42*(11), 1050–1055.

Hill, S. Y. (1982). Biological consequences of alcoholism and alcohol-related problems among women. In *Special populations issues* (pp. 43–73). Washington, DC: U.S. Government Printing Office.

Hill, S. Y. (1986). Physiological effects of alcohol in women. In *Women and alcohol: Health-related issues*. Washington, DC: U.S. Department of Health and Human Services.

Hingson, R., Magione, T., Meyers, A., et al. (1982). Seeking help for drinking problems: A study in the Boston metropolitan area. *Journal of Studies on Alcohol, 43*(3), 273–288.

Holck, S. E., Warren, C. W., Smith, J. C., et al. (1984). Alcohol consumption among Mexican American and Anglo women: Results of a survey along the U.S.–Mexico border. *Journal of Studies on Alcohol, 45*(2), 149–154.

Hser, Y. I., Anglin, M. D., & Booth, M. W. (1987). Sex differences in addict careers. *American Journal of Drug and Alcohol Abuse, 13*(3), 231–251.

Hugues, J. N., Coste, T., Perret, G., et al. (1980). Hypothalamo-pituitary ovarian function in thirty-one women with chronic alcoholism. *Clinical Endocrinology, 12*(6), 543–551.

Hurley, D. L. (1991). Women, alcohol and incest: An analytical review. *Journal of Studies on Alcohol, 52*(3), 253–268.

Jarvis, T. J. (1992). Implications of gender for alcohol treatment research: A quantitative and qualitative review. *British Journal of Addiction, 87*(9), 1249–1261.

Johnson, R. D., & Williams, R. (1985). Genetic and environmental factors in the individual susceptibility to the development of alcoholic liver disease. *Alcohol and Alcoholism, 20*(2), 137–160.

Julkunen, R. J. K., Tannenbaum, L., Baraona, E., et al. (1985). First pass metabolism of ethanol: An important determinant of blood levels after alcohol consumption. *Alcohol, 2*(3), 437–441.

Kandel, D. B., Wu, P., & Davies, M. (1994). Maternal smoking during pregnancy and smoking by adolescent daughters. *American Journal of Public Health, 84*(9), 1407–1413.

Kassett, J. A., Gershon, E. S., Maxwell, M. E., et al. (1989). Psychiatric disorders in the first-degree relatives of probands with bulimia nervosa. *American Journal of Psychiatry, 146*(11), 1468–1471.

Kessler, R. C., Crum, R. M., Warner, L. A., et al. (1997). Lifetime co-occurrence of DSM-III-R alcohol abuse and dependence with other psychiatric disorders in the National Comorbidity Survey. *Archives of General Psychiatry, 54*(4), 313–321.

Kessler, R. C., McGonagle, K. A., Zhao, S., et al. (1994). Lifetime and 12–month prevalence of DSM-III-R psychiatric disorders in the United States: Results from the National Comorbidity Survey. *Archives of General Psychiatry, 51*(5), 8–19.

Kessler, R. C, Nelson, C. B., McGonagle, K. A., et al. (1996). The epidemiology of co-occurring addictive and mental disorders: Implications for prevention and service utilization. *American Journal of Orthopsychiatry, 66*(1), 17–31.

Kilpatrick, D. G., Acierno, R., Resnick, H. S., et al. (1997). A 2–year longitudinal analysis of the relationships between violent assault and substance use in women. *Journal of Consulting and Clinical Psychology, 65*(5), 834–847.

Klatsky, A. L., Armstrong, M. A., & Friedman, G. D. (1992). Alcohol and mortality. *Annals of Internal Medicine, 117*(8), 646–654.

Klebe, E., & Judge, K. (1993). *Health care fact sheet on alcohol use in the U.S.* Congressional Research Service, Library of Congress.

Kleinman, J. C., Pierre, M. B., Madans, J. H., et al. (1988). The effects of maternal smoking on fetal and infant mortality. *American Journal of Epidemiology, 127*, 274–282.

Lancaster, F. E. (1994). Gender differences in the brain: Implications for the study of human alcoholism. *Alcoholism: Clinical and Experimental Research, 18*(3), 740–746.

Leigh, B. C. (1990). "Venus gets in my thinking": Drinking and female sexuality in the age of AIDS. *Journal of Substance Abuse, 2*(2), 129–145.

Lex, B. W. (1991). Some gender differences in alcohol and polysubstance users. *Health Psychology, 10*(2), 121–32.

Lillie-Blanton, M., Mackenzie, E., & Anthony, J. (1991). Black–white differences in alcohol use by women: Baltimore survey findings. *Public Health Reports, 10*(2), 124–133.

Longnecker, M. P., Berlin, J. A., Orza, M. J., et al. (1988). A meta-analysis of alcohol consumption in relation to risk of breast cancer. *Journal of the American Medical Association, 260*(5), 652–656.

Lowry, R., Holtzman, D., Truman, B. I., et al. (1994). Substance use and HIV-related sexual behaviors among U.S. high school students: Are they related? *American Journal of Public Health,* *84*(7), 1116–1120.

Luthar, S. S., Cushing, G., & Rounsaville, B. J. (1996). Gender differences among opioid abusers: Pathways to disorder and profiles of psychopathology. *Drug and Alcohol Dependence, 43*(3), 179–189.

MacDonald, J. G. (1987). Predictors of treatment outcome for alcoholic women. *International Journal of the Addictions, 22*(3), 235–248.

Marshall, A. W., Kingstone, D., Boss, M., et al. (1983). Ethanol elimination in males and females: Relationship to menstrual cycle and body composition. *Hepatology, 3*(5), 701–706.

Marzuk, P. M., Tardiff, K., Leon, A. C., et al. (1992). Prevalence of cocaine use among residents of New York City who committed suicide during a one-year period. *American Journal of Psychiatry, 149*(3), 317–375.

McLellan, A. T., Luborsky, L., & O'Brien, C. P. (1986). Alcohol and drug abuse treatment in three different populations: Is there improvement and is it predictable? *American Journal of Drug and Alcohol Abuse, 12*(1–2), 101–120.

Mendelson, J. H., Mello, N. K., Bavli, S., et al. (1983). Alcohol effects on female reproductive hormones. In T. Cicero (Ed.), *Ethanol tolerance and dependence: Endocrinological aspects* (pp. 146–161). Washington, DC: U.S. Government Printing Office.

Miller, B. A., Downs, W. R., & Gondoli, D. M. (1989). Spousal violence among alcoholic women as compared to a random household sample of women. *Journal of Studies on Alcohol, 50*(6), 533–540.

Miller, B. A., Downs, W. R., & Testa, M. (1993). Interrelationships between victimization experiences and women's alcohol use. *Journal of Studies on Alcohol, 11,* 109–117.

Moise, R., Reed, B. G., & Conell, C. (1981). Women in drug abuse treatment programs: Factors that influence retention at very early and later stages in two treatment modalities. A summary. *International Journal of the Addictions, 16*(7), 1295–1300.

O'Connor, L. E., Berry, J., Inaba, D., et al. (1994). Shame, guilt, and depression in men and women in recovery from addiction. *Journal of Substance Abuse Treatment, 11*(6), 503–510.

Office on Smoking and Health. (1980). *The health consequences of smoking for women: A report of the Surgeon General.* Rockville, MD: U.S. Department of Health and Human Services, Public Health Service.

Pascale, R., Daino, L., Garcea, R., et al. (1989). Inhibition of ethanol of rat liver plasma membrane (Na+, K+) ATPase: Protective effect of S-adenosyl-L-methionine, L-methionine, and N-acetylcysteine. *Toxicology and Applied Pharmacology, 97*(2), 216–229.

Patterson, T. L., & Jeste, D. V. (1999). The potential impact of the baby-boom generation on substance abuse among elderly persons. *Psychiatric Services, 50*(9), 1184–1188.

Perkins, K. A. (1996). Sex differences in nicotine versus non-nicotine reinforcement as determinants of tobacco smoking. *Experimental and Clinical Psychopharmacology, 4*(2), 166–177.

Piazza, N. J., Vrbka, J. L., & Yeager, R. D. (1989). Telescoping of alcoholism in women alcoholics. *International Journal of the Addictions, 24*(1), 19–28.

Presley, C., & Meilman, P. (1992, September 10). *Alcohol and drugs on American college campuses: A report to college presidents.* Carbondale: Southern Illinois University.

Reed, B. G. (1987). Developing women-sensitive drug dependence treatment services: Why so difficult? *Journal of Psychoactive Drugs, 19*(2), 151–164.

Regier, D. A., Farmer, M. E., Rae, D. S., et al. (1990). Comorbidity of mental disorders with alcohol and other drug abuse: Results from the Epidemiologic Catchment Area (ECA) study. *Journal of the American Medical Association, 264*(19), 2511–2518.

Robins, L. N., Helzer, J. E., & Przybeck, T. R. (1988). Alcohol disorders in the community: A report from the Epidemiologic Catchment Area study. In R. M. Rose & J. Barrett (Eds.), *Alcoholism: Origins and outcome* (pp. 15–29). New York: Raven Press.

Rounsaville, B. J., Anton, S. F., Carroll, K., et al. (1991). Psychiatric diagnoses of treatment seeking cocaine abusers. *Archives of General Psychiatry, 48*(1), 43–51.

Rozenzweig, A., Prigerson, H., Miller, M. D., et al. (1997). Bereavement and late-life depression: Grief and its complications in the elderly. *Annual Review of Medicine, 48,* 421–428.

Ryback, R. S. (1977). Chronic alcohol consumption and menstruation. *Journal of the American Medical Association, 238*(20), 2143.

Saunders, J. B., Davis, M., & Williams, R. (1981). Do women develop alcoholic liver disease more readily than men? *British Medical Journal, 282*(6270), 1140–1143.

Schneider, K. M., Kviz, F. J., Isola, M. L., et al. (1995). Evaluating multiple outcomes and gender differences in alcoholism treatment. *Addictive Behaviors, 20*(1), 1–21.

Schuckit, M. A., & Monteiro, M. G. (1988). Alcoholism, anxiety and depression. *British Journal of Addictions, 83*(12), 1373–1380.

Stein, M. D. (1999). Medical consequences of substance abuse. *Psychiatric Clinics of North America, 22*(2), 351–370.

Stein, M. D., & Cyr, M. G. (1997). Women and substance abuse. *Medical Clinics of North America, 81*(4), 979–998.

Substance Abuse and Mental Health Services Administration (SAMHSA). (1999a). *National Household Survey on Drug Abuse: Population estimates, 1998.* Washington, DC: U.S. Government Printing Office.

Substance Abuse and Mental Health Services Administration (SAMHSA). 1999b). *Summary of findings from the 1998 National Household Survey on Drug Abuse.* Hyattsville, MD: United States Government Printing Office. Washington, DC: U.S. Government Printing Office.

Substance Abuse and Mental Health Services Administration (SAMHSA). (2000). *National Household Survey on Drug Abuse: Main findings, 1998.* Washington, DC: U.S. Government Printing Office.

Sutker, P. B., Goist, K. C., Jr., & King, A. R. (1987). Acute alcohol intoxication in women: Relationship to dose and menstrual cycle phase. *Alcoholism: Clinical and Experimental Research, 11*(1), 74–79.

Syre, T. R., Martino-McAllister, J. M., & Vanada, L. M. (1997). Alcohol and other drug use at a university in the southeastern United States: Survey findings and implications. *College Student Journal, 31*(3), 373–381.

Turnbull, J. E., & Gomberg, E. S. L. (1991). The structure of drinking-related consequences in alcoholic women. *Alcoholism: Clinical and Experimental Research, 15*(1), 29–38.

Tuyns, A. J., & Pequignot, G. (1984). Greater risk of ascitic cirrhosis in females in relation to alcohol consumption. *International Journal of Epidemiology, 13*(1), 53–57.

Vannicelli, M. (1986). Treatment considerations. In *Women and alcohol: Health-related issues.* Washington, DC: U.S. Department of Health and Human Services.

Wakschlag, L. S., Lahey, B. B., Loeber, R., et al. (1997). Maternal smoking during pregnancy and the risk of conduct disorder in boys. *Archives of General Psychiatry, 54,* 670–676.

Wallace, R., Fullilove, M., Fullilove, R., et al. (1994). Will AIDS be contained within U.S. minority urban populations? *Social Science and Medicine, 39*(18), 1051–1062.

Wechsler, H., Davenport, A., Dowdall, G., et al. (1994). Health and behavioral consequences of binge drinking in college: A national survey of students at 140 campuses. *Journal of the American Medical Association, 272*(2), 1672–1677.

Weissman, M. M., Warner, V., Wickramaratne, P. J., et al. (1999). Maternal smoking during pregnancy and psychopathology in offspring followed to adulthood. *Journal of the American Academy of Child and Adolescent Psychiatry, 38*(7), 892–899.

Willett, W. C., Stampfer, M. J., Colditz, G. A., et al. (1987). Moderate alcohol consumption and the risk of breast cancer. *New England Journal of Medicine, 316*(19), 1174–1180.

Williams, G. D., Grant, B. F., Harford, T. C., et al. (1989). Population projections using DSM-III criteria: Alcohol abuse and dependence, 1990–2000. *Alcohol Health and Research World,* *13*(4), 366–370.

Williams, G. D., Stinson, F. S., Parker, D. A., et al. (1987). Demographic trends, alcohol abuse and alcoholism, 1985–1995. *Alcohol Health and Research World, 11*(3), 80–83, 91.

Wilsnack, R. W., & Cheloha, R. (1987). Women's roles and problem drinking across the lifespan. *Social Problems, 34*(3), 231–248.

Wilsnack, R. W., Wilsnack, S. C., & Klassen, A. D. (1984). Women's drinking and drinking problems: Patterns from a 1981 national survey. *American Journal of Public Health, 74*(11), 1231–1238.

Wilsnack, S. C., Klassen, A. D., Wilsnack, R. W. (1984). Drinking and reproductive dysfunction among women in a 1981 national survey. *Alcoholism: Clinical and Experimental Research, 8*(5), 451–458.

13

Eating Disorders

PAULINE S. POWERS

Anorexia nervosa (AN) has fascinated physicians since its earliest clinical descriptions in the mid-1800s. Even today, Louis-Victor Marcé's (1860) astute description of AN is revealing:

> We see . . . young girls, who at the period of puberty and after a precocious physical development, become subject to inappetency carried to utmost limits. Whatever the duration of their abstinence they experience a distaste for food, which the most pressing want is unable to overcome; . . . these patients arrive at a delirious conviction that they cannot or ought not to eat . . . the affective sentiments undergo alteration . . . these unhappy patients only regain some amount of energy in order to resist attempts at alimentation, and very often the physician beats a retreat before their desperate resistance. (Quoted in Silverman, 1989, pp. 833–834)

In the last 30 years, bulimia nervosa (BN) has also been described as a distinct clinical entity. Since 1994, eating disorders have been codified in the fourth edition of the *Diagnostic and Statistical Manual of Mental Disorders* (DSM-IV; American Psychiatric Association, 1994) as a separate category.

Etiological theories of eating disorders have swung from a purely biological viewpoint of AN in the 1920–1940s to a model emphasizing the role of culture, family communication styles, and psychological vulnerabilities of the patient. Now the importance of biological factors—including genetic vulnerability, abnormalities in neurotransmitters, and the potential for new medications to modify underlying physiological abnormalities—is fostering the development of a new etiological model of eating disorders. This comprehensive biopsychosocial model is likely to lead to new, more effective, treatments.

The purpose of this chapter is to emphasize the benefit of early identification and treatment of patients with eating disorders. The knowledge base required by physicians in all specialties and by mental health practitioners to achieve early identification of patients with eating disorders and facilitate their entry into the appropriate level of care is described. Special issues related to female patients, including menstrual irregularities, infertility, and pregnancy, are emphasized. The major evidence-based treatment modalities are described.

DIAGNOSTIC CRITERIA

Anorexia Nervosa

The DSM-IV criteria for AN (American Psychiatric Association, 1994) include the following:

1. Refusal to maintain body weight at or above a minimal normal weight for age and height (that is, weight less than 85% of that expected, or failure to make expected weight gain during a period of growth leading to a body weight less than 85% of that expected).
2. Intense fear of gaining weight or becoming obese, even though the person is underweight.
3. Disturbed experience of the person's own body weight or shape.
4. In females who have experienced menarche, absence of three or more consecutive menstrual cycles, or the occurrence of periods only after hormone administration.

In addition, the type of AN is specified. In the restricting type the person has not regularly engaged in binge-eating or purging and utilizes dieting, fasting, and/or exercise to lose weight. In the binge-eating/purging type, the person regularly engages in binge eating or purging (i.e., self-induced vomiting, or misusing laxatives, enemas, or diuretics).

Bulimia Nervosa

The DSM-IV criteria for BN (American Psychiatric Association, 1994) include the following:

1. Recurring episodes of binge eating (characterized by consumption of large quantities of food in a discrete time period *and* a sense of losing control over eating during the episode).
2. Recurring compensatory behaviors to prevent weight gain including self-induced vomiting; misusing laxatives, enemas, or diuretics, or other medications; fasting; or exercising excessively.
3. The binge eating and compensatory behaviors both occur at least twice weekly for 3 months, on average.
4. Self-evaluation is excessively influenced by body weight and shape.
5. The disorder does not occur exclusively during episodes of AN.

There are two types of BN: the purging type (in which self-induced vomiting or misuse of medications occurs) and the nonpurging type (in which other inappropriate compensatory methods are used, such as overexercise or fasting).

Eating Disorder Not Otherwise Specified

The DSM-IV classification system has resulted in identification of groups which meet strict criteria for AN or BN and research has been advanced by identifying these specific diagnostic entities. However, this classification system does not take into account the course of the illness. For example, many patients with AN have a past history of BN, and at least a fourth of patients with BN have a past history of AN (Sullivan et al., 1996). Furthermore, many patients with eating disorder symptoms do not meet the full criteria for either AN or BN, but have subsyndromal or atypical eating disorders and are therefore diagnosed as having "eating disorder not otherwise specified" (ED NOS) (Sullivan et al., 1998; Garfinkel et al., 1995, 1996). Myra Hornbacher has wryly commented on this in her (1999) book *Wasted: A Memoir of Anorexia and Bulimia*: "I became bulimic at the age of nine, anorexic at the age of fifteen. I couldn't decide between the two and veered back and forth from one to the other until I was twenty, and now, at twenty-three, I am an interesting creature, an Eating Disorder Not Otherwise Specified" (p. 2). Garfinkel et al. (1995, 1996) have found that patients with ED NOS are as severely ill, with the same vulnerability to co-morbid psychiatric disorders, as patients who meet the full criteria for AN or BN. These and other findings have led to the proposal that eating disorders should be conceptualized as lying on a continuum. Figure 13.1 is a Venn diagram illustrating the overlap of various eating disorder symptoms in AN, BN, and Binge Eating Disorder (Beumont et al., 1994).

Binge-Eating Disorder and Night-Eating Syndrome

Included in the ED NOS category is a newly proposed disorder called "binge-eating disorder" (BED) for which provisional criteria are described in Appendix B of DSM-IV (Ameri-

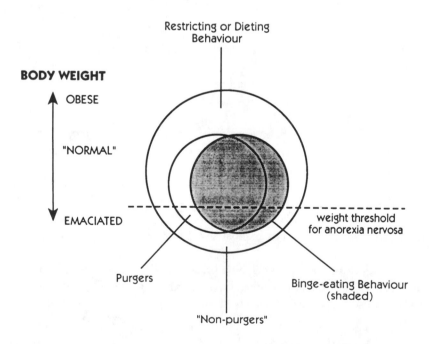

FIGURE 13.1. A Venn diagram illustrating the overlap of eating disorder symptoms: restricting or dieting behavior, binge-eating behavior, purging behavior, and body weight. From Beumont et al. (1994). Copyright 1994 by John Wiley & Sons, Inc. Reprinted by permission.

can Psychiatric Association, 1994). BED is characterized by episodes of binge eating which are not followed by compensatory behavior to prevent weight gain; most patients with BED are overweight or obese as a consequence. This new category is important for several reasons. BED has similarities to BN: it is more common in females, and it is often associated with depression (Robertson & Palmer, 1997). Also as in BN, body image disturbances and cognitive distortions (e.g., dichotomous, all-or-none thinking) are common (Powers et al., 1999). Perhaps more importantly, the diagnosis of BED represents the first formal diagnostic link between eating disorders and obesity. Patients with BED may be more amenable to treatment than patients with obesity in general (Stice, 1999).

There are other conditions that bridge the gap between eating and weight disorders. For example, "night-eating syndrome" (NES) occurs in a subgroup of patients with difficult-to-treat obesity (Stunkard, 1959; Rand et al., 1997). It is characterized by morning anorexia, consumption of 25% or more of the daily calories after the evening meal, initial insomnia (inability to fall asleep), and evening tension. Cognitive distortions are also associated with NES (Powers et al., 1999).

The Female Athlete Triad

The "female athlete triad" refers to the disordered eating, amenorrhea, and osteoporosis that frequently occur in elite female athletes (Nattiv et al., 1994). Although this term does not appear in the formal nomenclature, it is being increasingly used by athletic personnel and would conceptually belong in the ED NOS category of DSM-IV.

During the last decade, several studies have found that elite athletes appear to be at greater risk of eating disorders. Certain sports also increase risk for female athletes, including gymnastics and distance running. One important factor that may increase risk for eating disorders among athletes is the widespread (unproven) belief that weight loss and decrease in fat content will invariably improve performance. It has been hypothesized that this performance-related drive for thinness (in addition to the culture-wide drive for appearance-related thinness) increases the risk of eating disorders among female athletes (Powers & Johnson, 1996). Van DeLoo and Johnson (1995) have devised a brief questionnaire designed to elicit symptoms of eating disorders among young female athletes.

EPIDEMIOLOGY

Incidence/Prevalence

At least 5 million people in the United States have AN or BN, and another 5 million suffer from closely related conditions (often diagnosed as ED NOS). Estimates of the prevalence of AN have ranged from 0.5% for a narrowly defined version of the disorder (Walters & Kendler, 1995) to 3.7% for more broadly defined AN (Garfinkel et al., 1996). The prevalence of BN in the United States has been estimated to be between 1.1% and 4.2% (Kendler et al., 1991; Garfinkel et al., 1995).

There is some evidence that the prevalence of BN may have decreased slightly in recent years (Heatherton et al., 1995). This is difficult to believe from the perspective of tertiary care providers, but differences in detection and reporting may account for what appears to be an increase in prevalence. Sonja van 't Hof (1994) makes a convincing argument that the incidence of AN has remained constant for at least a century.

BED appears to increase in prevalence with an increase in weight. The current National Heart, Lung and Blood Institute (1998) classification of overweight and obesity by body mass index (BMI) is shown in Table 13.1. A study of females with Class II obesity (BMI = 35.0–39.9) in a weight reduction program found that BED occurred in 7.6% of patients (Stunkard et al., 1996). In another study of male and female patients with Class IV obesity (BMI > 40) being evaluated for bariatric surgery, 16% had BED (Powers et al., 1999).

Among the general population, NES occurs in 1.5% (Rand et al., 1997), but the prevalence among patients being evaluated for bariatric surgery is much higher—between 10% (Powers et al., 1999) and 27% (Rand et al., 1997).

Sex Distribution

Eating disorders are more common in women than in men (Andersen & Holman, 1997; Striegel-Moore et al., 1998). About 95–97% of patients with AN and about 80% patients with BN are female. Probably 60–70% of patients with BED are female. Most patients thus far reported with NES are female (Powers et al., 1999). The reasons for the difference in sex distribution are unknown but several theories have been advanced. Women may be more susceptible than men to weight and eating problems than men for several reasons. These reasons include the following: (1) physiological vulnerabilities (e.g., women's bodies normally have a greater fat content than men's); (2) cultural pressures (emphasis on a thin body physique is greater for women than for men); (3) greater vulnerability to psychiatric disorders (most types of mental illness are more common in women than in men); and (4) increased risk related to sexual abuse which occurs more often to females than males (for a review see Vanderlinden & Vandereycken, 1997).

Age of Onset

AN and BN usually begin in adolescence but may begin in childhood or much later in life. Frequently patients who present with a later onset report eating problems earlier in life, often of a similar type. Age of onset of BED appears to be related to whether binge eating or dieting begins first (Abbott et al., 1998): Patients who begin binge eating first usually develop BED in adolescence whereas patients who diet first and then begin to binge usu-

TABLE 13.1. Classification of Overweight and Obesity by BMI

	Obesity class	BMI (kg/m^2)
Normal		18.5–24.9
Overweight		25.0–29.9
Obesity	I	30.0–34.9
	II	35.0–39.9
Extreme obesity	III	> 40

Note. BMI, body mass index (weight in kilograms/height in meters squared). Adapted from National Heart, Lung and Blood Institute (1998).

ally develop BED in young adulthood. The onset of NES appears to occur in young adulthood, but little information on this topic is available.

KEY ELEMENTS OF INITIAL ASSESSMENT

The key factors to be evaluated in order to establish the diagnosis of an eating disorder include weight history, eating behavior, history of binge-eating or purging behavior, diet history, use of diet aids, exercise patterns, body image, and (in females) menstrual history. An initial assessment includes a psychiatric history, mental status examination, and physical examination (including weight and height). In eating disorder specialty clinics, an anthropometric evaluation may be performed; this includes various body measurements aimed at determining body composition, especially body fat content. Specialized psychological tests may also be administered, including the well-known Eating Attitudes Test (Garner et al., 1982) or the Eating Disorders Inventory—2 (Garner, 1991). The Yale–Brown–Cornell Eating Disorders Scale (Sunday et al., 1995) is often used to assess the severity of obsessive–compulsive symptoms in patients with eating disorders.

Screening Questions

The following screening questions usually elicit sufficient information to determine whether a patient has an eating disorder (adapted from Powers, 1996):

> What is your current weight and height?
> Has there been any change in your weight?
> What have been your highest and lowest weights since achieving your current height?
> What did you eat yesterday?
> Do you ever binge?
> Have you ever used self-induced vomiting, laxatives, diuretics, or enemas to lose weight or compensate for overeating?
> How much do you exercise in a typical week?
> How do you feel about how you look?
> (For females) Are your menstrual periods regular?

Differential Diagnosis

Although some conditions may masquerade as eating disorders, this is typically easy to detect. The most common cause of significant weight loss in adolescent girls *is* AN. Less common causes of weight loss in teenage girls include diabetes mellitus, cancer, and various endocrine conditions (Root, 1994).

BN may be confused with psychogenic vomiting but in the latter there is typically no binge eating or prominent preoccupation with weight, size, and shape. Overeating episodes may occur in a variety of situations (including nonpathological ones), but to qualify as a "binge," an episode must be associated with a feeling of loss of control. In a recent study (Johnson et al., 1999), male National Collegiate Athletic Association Division 1 athletes were frequently found to overeat large quantities of food; compared to females, however, they were less likely to feel out of control during these episodes. Hence, by definition, most of the male athletes were not binge-eating.

Common Diagnostic Dilemmas

Failure to Gain Weight during Adolescent Growth Spurt

Since AN usually starts during adolescence, the disorder may begin before or during the adolescent growth spurt. The adolescent may not initially lose weight, but rather fail to gain weight as expected; therefore, detection may be delayed. This situation is shown graphically in Figure 13.2. The patient illustrated (Powers, 1996) had primary amenorrhea and had been ill a year longer than was initially realized. She also had severe osteoporosis of her lumbar spine by the time treatment was initiated at age 14.

Comorbid Psychiatric Disorders

Comorbid psychiatric disorders are common among patients with eating disorders. The most common conditions associated with AN are mood disorders (Casper, 1998) and ob-

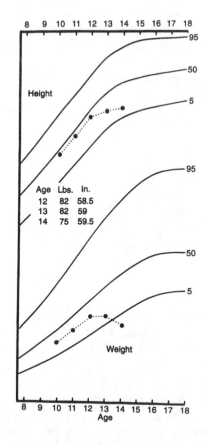

FIGURE 13.2. Failure to gain weight as expected in an adolescent with AN. From Powers (1996). Copyright 1996 by W. B. Saunders Company. Reprinted by permission.

sessive–compulsive conditions (Kaye, 1997). Nearly half of patients with BN have depressive disorders (Casper, 1998), and Bulik et al. (1997) found that 47% of patients with BN have a lifetime prevalence of alcohol use disorders. Obsessions and compulsions about food, weight, and eating are also common in BN.

Physiological Complications

AN and BN are both associated with multiple physiological complications arising from semistarvation and the effects of binge eating and purging. Since many patients with eating disorders (and sometimes their families) deny their condition or disavow the implications of their behavior, detection of and explanation of these physiological complications can be therapeutic.

The three most important physiological complications among patients with AN are osteoporosis, cardiac complications, and renal abnormalities. Osteoporosis (decreased bone mineral density associated with the risk of nonstress fractures) occurs in over 60% of patients with AN and may develop after as brief a period as 6 months of semistarvation (for reviews, see Grinspoon et al., 1997; Powers, 1999). The osteoporosis that occurs in AN is more severe than postmenopausal osteoporosis; it is associated with both decreased bone formation and increased bone resorption. The hip and lumbar spine are the areas most likely to be affected. Neither estrogen treatment nor calcium supplementation has been shown to correct or prevent this osteoporosis, unlike postmenopausal osteoporosis. Males with AN are just as likely to develop osteoporosis (Powers & Spratt, 1994). Weight history is the most important predictor of the presence of osteoporosis, and with weight restoration, there is improvement but not normalization of bone mineral density (Hotta et al., 1998).

Cardiac and renal complications probably account for at least half the deaths that occur in patients with AN but this is difficult to determine because of the imprecise way in which deaths related to eating disorders are reported (Neumarker, 1997; Emborg, 1999). Electrolyte disturbances (notably hypokalemia) may cause dangerous or lethal cardiac arrhythmias (Powers et al., 1995). Prolonged QT interval on the electrocardiogram is associated with semistarvation and perhaps with sudden death (Cooke & Chambers, 1995; Swenne & Larson, 1999). Mitral valve prolapse occurs in one-third to two-thirds of patients (Alvin et al., 1993; de Simone et al., 1994). Renal complications are the result of repeated episodes of dehydration and prerenal azotemia (Alvin et al., 1993).

Patients with BN are prone to some of the same physiological complications because they may also be underweight (or have a past history of semistarvation). Electrolyte disturbances are common and may result in cardiac arrhythmias. Many dangerous purge methods may be utilized including use of ipecac that has direct cardiac toxicity (Schiff et al., 1986). In addition, dental complications (including erosion of dental enamel on the lingual surfaces of the teeth) are common among patients who utilize self-induced vomiting (Milosevic, 1999). Parotid gland enlargement and associated salivary isoenzyme amylase elevations are common (Anderson et al., 1999).

Recommended Laboratory Testing

All patients with eating disorders should have a complete blood count; assessments of serum electrolytes, blood urea nitrogen, and creatinine levels; and thyroid function tests (T_4

and T_3 by radioimmune assay, thyroid-stimulating hormone and free thyroxine calculated from T_4 and T_3 resin uptake). Malnourished patients should also have calcium, magnesium, liver function tests, and albumin test; an electrocardiogram; and a 24-hour urine collection for creatinine clearance. C3 (a complement protein of the alternate pathway) is low in AN and returns to normal with weight gain (Pomeroy et al., 1997). C3 is a useful clinical measure of the severity of semistarvation. Certain laboratory tests have been shown to correlate with a fatal or chronic course in AN (Herzog et al,, 1997). Low serum albumin levels and a low weight ($\leq 60\%$ of average body weight) at initial evaluation were best able to predict a lethal course. High serum creatinine and uric acid levels predict a chronic course.

Patients who have been underweight for more than 6 months should have an assessment for osteopenia and osteoporosis. This assessment includes dual energy X-ray absorptiometry, as well as estradiol levels for females and testosterone levels for males.

Multiple other tests may be indicated in specific circumstances. For example, an echocardiogram may be needed for patients who have significant semistarvation and a click or systolic murmur on physical examination. Underweight patients with significant mental status changes may need brain magnetic resonance imaging. Katzman et al. (1997) have shown decreased white and gray matter volumes and increased cerebral spinal fluid volumes in underweight patients with AN. Only the white matter volumes fully returned to normal with weight restoration.

APPROPRIATE LEVEL OF CARE AND REQUIRED TREATMENT PERSONNEL

Level of Care

In recent years, strides have been made in determining the intensity of care required for patients with eating disorders. Most patients with BN do not require structured inpatient or residential treatment whereas many (if not most) patients with AN do require structured treatment at some point in the recovery process.

Guidelines for determining the appropriate level of care for a patient with AN have recently been devised (La Via et al., 1998; Yager et al., 2000). For example, a patient with AN who is medically stable, is less than 15% below ideal body weight, is motivated to recover, is not suicidal, has adequate emotional and environmental support, and lives near the treatment center can usually be treated as an outpatient. However, a patient with AN who has a heart rate less than 40, who is more than 25% below ideal body weight, and whose motivation to recover is poor will require inpatient hospitalization for initial treatment. There is now evidence that patients who reach an ideal body weight prior to leaving a structured treatment program are less likely to relapse than those who leave prematurely (Baran et al., 1995). Recent studies have shown that long-term outpatient treatment (up to 9 years) is required for many patients who have required inpatient hospitalization, but that if this is provided, prognosis for a full and lasting recovery occurs in over three-fourths of patients (Strober et al., 1997).

Treatment Personnel

Patients with BN who do not have any associated co-morbid conditions and who are committed to treatment may only require brief cognitive-behavioral therapy provided in a group or individual format of 12–20 sessions by trained personnel. There is some evidence that self-administered manual-based treatment guided by ancillary staff can be effective for some in this group of patients (Fairburn & Carter, 1997). Most patients with BN, however, have comorbid psychiatric disorders as well as physiological complications that require treatment by several professionals working in a team effort with the patient. Such a team might include an internist, a psychiatrist, a psychotherapist, and a registered dietician.

Most patients with AN require an experienced treatment team, including a psychiatrist, an individual and a family therapist, a primary care physician, and a registered dietician. Patients who require inpatient structured treatment usually need treatment in a specialized eating disorder treatment program.

SPECIAL ISSUES RELATED TO FEMALES

Menstrual Irregularities

Amenorrhea is a key symptom in females with AN and is associated with the development of osteoporosis (for a review, see Powers, 1999). Many patients with BN also have irregular menses (perhaps because many are also underweight but do not meet formal criteria for AN). Many partially recovered patients with AN also have irregular menses. Since menses can be affected by many factors, including weight, body composition, exercise, stress, and dietary composition, assessment of menstrual irregularities can be challenging.

Perhaps the most important lesson of the studies from the last decade is that menstrual irregularities should not be dismissed as unimportant. The cause of the irregularities must be determined and, if possible, corrected. Use of hormone replacements, without serious efforts to determine the etiology of the menstrual irregularities, is inappropriate. Return of regular menses following weight gain in AN is a positive prognostic factor. These patients have fewer psychological characteristics of eating disorders and are much less likely to relapse than similarly weight-restored patients with AN who do not have a return of menses (Meyer et al., 1986).

Infertility

Most, but not all, underweight patients with AN are infertile. Absence of menses does not mean that a patient is unable to conceive, and this needs to be considered when medications are prescribed. Among patients with AN who have been ill for many years, body fat content may increase even if weight is not gained, and thus the patients may become fertile.

Several studies from infertility clinics have found that a significant percentage of the patients attending have eating disorders. For example, Stewart et al. (1990) found that 17% of women aged 21–39 who presented to an infertility clinic had eating disorders. Bates et al. (1982) found that among underweight women with eating disorders who presented to an infertility clinic willing to gain weight, 73% were able to conceive.

Pregnancy

Although most patients with AN do not become pregnant, those who do usually have a very difficult course. Several reports have shown that there is either a maternal or a fetal complication in most cases (for a review, see Powers, 1997). Bulik et al. (1999) found that compared to controls, women with a history of AN had more miscarriages and cesarean deliveries, and the babies of women with AN were more likely to be born prematurely and were of lower birthweight than the infants of control women.

Most patients with BN are able to conceive. Some patients with BN are able to suspend binge eating and purging during pregnancy, but the symptoms often recur following delivery. There is also a high rate of maternal and/or fetal complications among patients with BN (Blais et al., 2000; Morgan et al., 1999).

When possible, it is wise to advise patients to receive treatment and be in remission prior to contemplating pregnancy. Often, however, a physician first sees a patient when she is already pregnant. In this situation, it is important to assess her current symptoms and medications to determine possible teratogenic effect. It is helpful to remember that semistarvation and purging behavior may be more dangerous to the fetus than various medications utilized to treat the eating disorder or comorbid conditions. For example, several large-scale studies of fluoxetine have found no teratogenic effects related to the use of fluoxetine in the first trimester (Addis & Koren, 2000). For a patient with BN who is in remission on fluoxetine, it may be wise to continue the medication. Pregnant patients with eating disorders need a team approach that includes a psychiatrist, a high-risk obstetrician, and a neonatologist.

EVIDENCE-BASED TREATMENT MODALITIES

AN: Weight Restoration in a Structured Setting

Most adult patients with AN who are more than 25% below ideal body weight will require treatment within a structured treatment setting with a specialized multidisciplinary treatment team. Inpatient programs can usually achieve a weight gain of 2–3 pounds per week safely. It is often estimated that a minimum goal weight is 90% of ideal weight for height according to standard tables; at that weight, 86% of patients resume menstruation (although not necessarily ovulation) within 6 months (Golden et al., 1997). However, a more accurate method of determining when ideal body weight is achieved is utilization of pelvic ultrasound to demonstrate the return of a dominant follicle, which indicates that ovulation has returned (Treasure et al., 1988).

Different methods have been used to facilitate weight gain including various forms of contracting for weight gain, with privileges contingent upon weight gain. Tube feeding may be necessary, and for many patients may actually be a relief, since the need to choose whether or not to eat is lessened. Individual therapy and family therapy are usually key aspects of treatment in structured treatment settings. With weight restoration, there is often some decrease in other eating disorder symptoms, but abnormal eating habits do not necessarily improve simply as a function of weight gain. Body image disturbances may be the last symptom to resolve (Rosen, 1996).

AN: Outpatient Family Therapy for Children and Adolescents

Robin and colleagues (Robin et al., 1994, 1995, 1998; Robin & Siegel, 1999) have recently described a working model for outpatient treatment of young patients with AN living in intact nuclear families. A basic tenet of Robin et al.'s behavioral–family systems model is that the appropriate hierarchy of "parent in charge of adolescent" is reversed in the area of eating at the time of presentation for treatment. The aim of the treatment is to place parents clearly in charge of their adolescent's eating in order to return the hierarchy to normal and restart eating, overcoming the momentum of starvation. Several treatment models are combined in this strategy including behavior modification, cognitive therapy, psychodynamic techniques, and family systems techniques. This treatment includes three phases: assessment (4–8 sessions), weight gain (4–12 months), and weight maintenance and termination (3–8 months). Treatment lasts 1–2 years. Two-thirds of the subjects in a long-term study utilizing this treatment (Robin et al., 1994) attained target weight at the end of treatment, and weight gain continued after treatment ended.

BN: Cognitive-Behavioral Therapy

Cognitive-behavioral therapy (CBT) is a brief treatment intervention typically provided in a group format on a weekly basis over 2–4 months. It has been found to be effective in reducing (but usually not eliminating) episodes of binge eating and purging (Agras et al., 1991; Garner et al., 1993; Fairburn et al., 1993b). CBT is based on the premise that the fundamental psychopathology in BN is the attempt to compensate for deficits in self-esteem by defining and evaluating oneself excessively in terms of weight and shape. Thus the pursuit of thinness becomes the central organizing principle for the patient's life. A number of cognitive distortions facilitate the maintenance of disturbed behavior including restrictive dieting, binge eating, and purging. The focus of treatment is on the present and the future rather than on the past and various etiological factors.

There are typically three phases of treatment. In the first stage the cognitive view on maintenance of BN is presented, and behavioral techniques to replace binge eating with a stable eating pattern are introduced. In the second phase there is an emphasis on elimination of dieting while maintaining a stable eating pattern. During this phase, the cognitive distortions (thoughts, beliefs and values) that maintain the problematic behavior are identified. Various additional behavioral strategies are introduced. Stimulus control methods are taught; these include eating in one place and at certain times, and limiting the amount of food available in the house. Response prevention techniques to decrease purge behavior may be used: for example, a patient might ask a family member to accompany her an hour after eating in order to help her avoid vomiting. In the final phase, the maintenance of change following treatment is addressed. Manuals are available which provide specific details needed to implement each phase of treatment (Agras, 1991; Fairburn et al., 1993b)

BN: Interpersonal Psychotherapy Compared to CBT

Interpersonal psychotherapy (IPT) for BN was developed by Fairburn et al (1991) and is a type of focal psychotherapy aimed at addressing underlying interpersonal problems thought to be etiologically related to the emergence of bulimic symptoms. This treatment is also usually provided in a time-limited group format. The focus is to identify relationships among interpersonal functioning, self-esteem, mood, the occurrence of significant life events, and the onset and maintenance of eating problems. There are specific goals with written contracts to address the underlying issues, but no direct focus on binge eating, dieting, or purging.

CBT has been shown to be more effective than IPT at the end of 3–4 months of treatment (Fairburn et al., 1993a). However, at long-term follow-up (5.8 years) patients in the IPT group had "caught up" in terms of improvement in binge eating, purging, restrictive dieting, and attitudes toward shape and weight (Fairburn et al., 1995).

Although both CBT and IPT have been shown to have benefits, neither is a panacea. Most patients continue to have episodes of binge eating and purging (although the frequency and intensity is often reduced); there is a high dropout rate before the end of the prescribed treatment; and relapse after treatment is common (Waller, 1997; Wilson, 1996).

Medications for BN

The only medication currently approved by the U.S. Food and Drug Administration for the treatment of eating disorders is fluoxetine. Fluoxetine has been shown to reduce binge-eating and purging episodes compared to placebo (Fluoxetine Bulimia Nervosa Collaborative Study Group, 1992). This effect is independent of the presence or absence of depressive symptoms. The most effective dose is 60 mg per day. Most patients do not have a full remission of symptoms. Side effects are generally not troublesome. Although a study has been undertaken to determine how long fluoxetine should be continued, the results of this study are not yet available. Other antidepressants studied have also been found to reduce binge eating and purging, but many of these medications have unacceptable side effects, such as weight gain. These studies have also usually been conducted at only one site, have had few subjects, or have had no placebo controls. Naltrexone, an opiate antagonist, has been shown to reduce episodes of binge eating and purging (Marrazzi et al., 1995). Although this was a placebo-controlled study, it was a small study that utilized a crossover design, and much larger doses were used than have yet been demonstrated to be safe.

Two other medications are promising in the treatment of BN. Feris et al. (2000) have shown that ondansetron, compared to placebo, resulted in a significant reduction of binge/vomit frequencies over the course of 4 weeks. Ondansetron is a peripherally active antagonist of the serotonin receptor 5-HT3; it is currently marketed for the prevention of vagally-mediated emesis caused by cancer chemotherapeutic agents. A second promising medication for BN is topiramate, a new antiepileptic drug which is associated with a decrease in appetite (Knable, 2001).

Bupropion has been found to be associated with a higher incidence of seizures in patients with BN, and hence is contraindicated in patients with eating disorders (Horne et al., 1988). In general, it is advisable to avoid use of buproprion even in recovered patients, since there is no information available on when, or whether, it is safe to use this medication in patients with eating disorders.

Medications for AN

Cyproheptadine is the only medication found to be useful in a controlled study for the weight gain treatment phase of AN (Halmi et al., 1986). However, the design of this study makes it difficult to be sure that the cause of the weight gain was the medication. Fluoxetine has been found to be useful in decreasing relapse rate in weight-restored patients with AN (Kaye et al., 1998), but it is not useful during the weight gain phase (Attia et al., 1998).

Several case reports have noted improvements in weight and less resistance to treatment with olanzapine (La Via et al., 2000; Hansen, 1999; Jensen & Mejlhede, 2000). Olanzapine is an atypical antipsychotic associated with weight gain and a minimal risk of movement disorders. Powers et al. (2001) have reported an outpatient open label study of olanzapine that resulted in a weight gain of 8.75 lbs. in 10 weeks in half of the patients who enrolled. Patients who gained weight also had a reduction in symptoms associated with eating disorders as well as a reduction in symptoms typically associated with psychotic disorders.

Medications: Complexities Related to Comorbid Conditions

Since psychiatric and medical comorbidities are common among patients with eating disorders, many other medications may be needed. In these circumstances, the effect of malnutrition or electrolyte imbalance on possible side effects of the medication needs to be considered. For example, a patient with AN who also has bipolar I disorder may need lithium. During the underweight and dehydrated phase of treatment, lithium may need to be discontinued or careful monitoring may be needed in the hospital.

OUTCOME

Untreated AN is associated with the highest mortality rate of any psychiatric disorder. Without treatment 15–18% of patients with AN have a premature mortality rate after 20 years (Ratnasuriya et al., 1991). However, with appropriate treatment, most patients can achieve a full and lasting recovery. The studies by Robin et al. (1994, 1995, 1998) demonstrate the benefit of early intervention: Two-thirds of patients receiving behavioral–family systems treatment were able to attain target weight, usually without treatment in a structured residential or hospital-based program. Most of these patients had been ill less than a year, were in intact nuclear families and were adolescents living at home. This group constitutes a subset known to have a better prognosis and this intervention is less intense than has been required in the past for more severely ill patients with a chronic course. Nonetheless, Strober et al. (1997) have shown that with appropriate inpatient treatment and long-term outpatient treatment, 76% of severely chronically ill patients with AN can recover fully.

The untreated premature mortality rate of BN is less well understood, but is probably about 2–5% after 5–10 years (Crow et al., 1999). Similarly, the recovery rate from BN with treatment is not well known. Keel et al. (1999) found that more than 10 years after initial presentation, about 30% of one group of patients, continued to have recurrent binge-eating or purging behaviors.

CONCLUSIONS AND FUTURE DIRECTIONS

Recent advances in the diagnosis and treatment of eating disorders are likely to significantly improve the prognosis for a full and lasting recovery for some patients. However, relapse continues to be common, and improved treatment methods are needed. The etiology of these disorders is still poorly understood, and until the causes of these conditions are clarified, it is unlikely that prevention efforts will be successful. As with other mental disorders, discrimination against patients is very common, and many patients cannot access appropriate treatment. The development of treatment guidelines and treatment algorithms is likely to have some impact on this problem.

REFERENCES

Abbott, D. W., de Zwaan, M., Mussell, M. P., et al. (1998). Onset of binge eating and dieting in overweight women: Implications for etiology, associated features and treatment. *Journal of Psychosomatic Research, 44*(3–4), 367–374.

Addis, A., & Koren, G. (2000). Safety of fluoxetine during the first trimester of pregnancy: A meta-analytic review of epidemiological studies. *Psychological Medicine, 30,* 809–894.

Agras, W. S. (1991). *Cognitive behavioral therapy treatment manual for bulimia nervosa.* Stanford, CA: Stanford University, Department of Psychiatry and Behavioral Sciences.

Alvin, P., Zogheib, J., Rey, C., et al. (1993). Severe complications and mortality in mental eating disorders in adolescence: On 99 hospitalized patients. *Archives of French Pediatrics, 50,* 755–762.

American Psychiatric Association. (1994). *Diagnostic and Statistical Manual of Mental Disorders.* Washington, DC: Author.

Andersen, A. E., & Holman, J. E. (1997). Males with eating disorders: Challenges for treatment and research. *Psychopharmacology Bulletin, 33,* 391–397.

Anderson, L., Shaw, J. M., & McCargar, L. (1997). Physiological effects of bulimia nervosa on the gastrointestinal tract. *Canadian Journal of Gastroenterology, 11,* 451–459.

Attia, E., Haiman, C., Walsh, B. T., et al. (1998). Does fluoxetine augment the inpatient treatment of anorexia nervosa? *American Journal of Psychiatry, 155,* 548–551.

Baran, S. A., Wltzin, T. E., & Kaye, W. H. (1995). Low discharge weight and outcome in anorexia nervosa. *American Journal of Psychiatry, 152,* 1070–1072.

Bates, G. W., Bates, S. R., & Whiteworth, N. S. (1982). Reproductive failure in women who practice birth control. *Fertility and Sterility, 37,* 373–378.

Beumont, P. J., Garner, D. M., & Touyz, S. W. (1994). Diagnoses of eating or dieting disorders: What may we learn from past mistakes? *International Journal of Eating Disorders, 16,* 349–367.

Blais, M. A., Becker, N. E., Burwell, R. A., et al. (2000). Pregnancy: Outcome and impact on symptomatology in a cohort of eating-disordered women. *International Journal of Eating Disorders, 27,* 140–149.

Bulik, C. M., Sullivan, P. F., Carter, F. A., et al. (1997). Lifetime comorbidity of alcohol dependence in women with bulimia nervosa. *Addictive Behavior, 22,* 437–446.

Bulik, C. M., Sullivan, P. F., Fear, J. L., et al. (1999). Fertility and reproduction in women with anorexia nervosa: A controlled study. *Journal of Clinical Psychiatry, 60,* 130–135.

Casper, R. C. (1998). Depression and eating disorders. *Depression and Anxiety, 8*(Suppl. 1), 96–104.

Cooke, R. A., & Chamber, J. B. (1995). Anorexia nervosa and the heart. *British Journal of Hospital Medicine, 54,* 313–317.

Crow, S., Praus, B., & Thuras, P. (1999). Mortality from eating disorders: A 5- to 10-year record linkage study. *International Journal of Eating Disorders, 26,* 97–101.

de Simone, G., Scalfi, L., Galderisi, M., et al. (1994). Cardiac abnormalities in young women with anorexia nervosa. *British Heart Journal, 71,* 287–292.

Emborg, C. (1999). Mortality and causes of death in eating disorders in Denmark 1970–1993: A case register study. *International Journal of Eating Disorders, 25,* 243–251.

Fairburn, C. G., & Carter, J. C. (1997). Self-help and guided self-help for binge-eating problems. In D. M. Garner & P. E. Garfinkel (Eds.), *Handbook of treatment for eating disorders* (2nd ed., pp. 494–499). New York: Guilford Press.

Fairburn, C. G., Jones, R., & Peveler, R. C. (1991). Three psychological treatments for bulimia nervosa. *Archives of General Psychiatry, 48*, 453–469.

Fairburn, C. G., Jones, R., Peveler, R. C., et al. (1993a). Psychotherapy and bulimia nervosa: Longer-term effects of interpersonal psychotherapy, behavior therapy, and cognitive behavioral therapy. *Archives of General Psychiatry, 50*, 419–428.

Fairburn, C. G., Marcus, M. D., & Wilson, G. T. (1993b). Cognitive-behavioral therapy for binge eating and bulimia nervosa: A comprehensive treatment manual. In C. G. Fairburn & G. T. Wilson (Eds.), *Binge eating: Nature, assessment, and treatment* (pp. 361–404). New York: Guilford Press.

Fairburn, C. G., Normal, P. A., Welch, S. L., et al. (1995). A prospective study of outcome in bulimia nervosa and the long-term effects of three psychological treatments. *Archives of General Psychiatry, 52*, 304–312.

Faris, P. L., Kim, S. W., Meller, W. H., et al. (2000). Effect of decreasing afferent vagal activity with ondansetron on symptoms of bulimia nervosa: A randomized double-blind trial. *Lancet, 355*, 769–770.

Fluoxetine Bulimia Nervosa Collaborative Study Group. (1992). Fluoxetine in the treatment of bulimia nervosa: A multicenter, placebo-controlled, double-blind trial. *Archives of General Psychiatry, 49*, 139–147.

Garfinkel, P. E., Lin, E., Goering, P., et al. (1995). Bulimia nervosa in a Canadian community sample: Prevalence and comparison of subgroups. *American Journal of Psychiatry, 152*, 1052–1058.

Garfinkel, P. E., Lin, E., Goering, P., et al. (1996). Should amenorrhea be necessary for the diagnoses of anorexia nervosa?: Evidence from a Canadian community sample. *British Journal of Psychiatry, 168*, 500–506.

Garner D. M. (1991). *Eating Disorder Inventory—2: Professional manual.* Odessa, FL: Psychological Assessment Resources.

Garner, D. M., Olmsted, M. P., Bohr, Y., et al. (1982). The Eating Attitudes Test: Psychometric features and clinical correlates. *Psychological Medicine, 12*, 871–878.

Garner, D. M., Rockert, W., Davis, R., et al. (1993). A comparison between cognitive-behavioral and supportive–expressive therapy for bulimia nervosa. *American Journal of Psychiatry, 150*, 37–46.

Golden, N. H., Jacobson, M. S., Schebendach, J., et al. (1997). Resumption of menses in anorexia nervosa. *Archives of Pediatric and Adolescent Medicine, 151*, 16–21.

Grinspoon, S., Herzog, D., & Klibanski, A. (1997). Mechanisms and treatment options for bone loss in anorexia nervosa. *Psychopharmacology Bulletin, 33*, 399–404.

Halmi, K. A., Eckert, E., LaDu, T. J., et al. (1986). Anorexia nervosa: Treatment efficacy of cyproheptadine and amitriptyline. *Archives of General Psychiatry, 43*, 177–181.

Hansen, L. (1999). Olanzapine in the treatment of anorexia nervosa. *British Journal of Psychiatry, 175*, 592.

Heatherton, T. F., Nichols, P., Mahamedi, F., et al. (1995). Body weight, dieting, and eating disorder symptoms among college students, 1982–1992. *American Journal of Psychiatry, 152*, 1623–1629.

Herzog, W., Deter, H. C., Fiehn, W., et al. (1997). Medical findings and predictors of long-term physical outcome in anorexia nervosa: A prospective, 12-year follow-up study. *Psychological Medicine, 27*, 269–279.

Hornbacher, M. (1999). *Wasted: A memoir of anorexia and bulimia.* New York: Harper Perennial.

Horne, R. L., Fergus, J. M., Hope, H. G. Jr., et al. (1988). Treatment of bulimia with bupropion: A multicenter controlled trial. *Journal of Clinical Psychiatry, 49*, 262–266.

Hotta, M., Shibasaki, T., Sato, K., et al. (1998). The importance of body weight history in the occurrence and recovery of osteoporosis in patients with anorexia nervosa: Evaluation by dual X-ray absorptiometry and bone metabolic markers. *European Journal of Endocrinology, 139*, 276–283.

Jensen, V. S., & Mejlhede, A. (2000). Anorexia nervosa: Treatment with olanzapine. *British Journal of Psychiatry, 177, 592.*

Johnson, C., Powers, P., & Dick, R. (1999). Athletes and eating disorders: The National Collegiate Athletic Association study. *International Journal of Eating Disorders, 26, 179–188.*

Katzman, D. K., Zipursky, R. B., Lambe, E. K., et al. (1997). A longitudinal magnetic resonance imaging study of brain changes in adolescents with anorexia nervosa. *Archives of Pediatric and Adolescent Medicine, 151, 793–797.*

Kaye, W. (1997). Anorexia nervosa, obsessional behavior, and serotonin. *Psychopharmacology Bulletin, 33, 335–344.*

Kaye, W., Gendall, K., & Strober, M. (1998). Serotonin neuronal function and selective serotonin reuptake inhibitor treatment in anorexia and bulimia nervosa. *Biological Psychiatry, 44*, 825–838.

Keel, P. K., Mitchell, J. E., Miller, K. B., et al. (1999). Long-term outcome of bulimia nervosa. *Archives of General Psychiatry, 56, 63–69.*

Kendler, K. S., MacLean, C., Neale, M., et al. (1991). The genetic epidemiology of bulimia nervosa. *American Journal of Psychiatry, 148, 1627–1637.*

Knable, M. (2001). Topiramate for bulimia nervosa in epilepsy. *American Journal of Psychiatry, 158, 322–323.*

La Via, M., Gray, N., & Kaye, W. H. (2000). Case reports of olanzapine treatment of anorexia nervosa. *International Journal of Eating Disorders, 27, 363–366.*

La Via, M., Kaye, W. H., Andersen, A., et al. (1998, November). *Anorexia nervosa: Criteria for levels of care.* Poster presented at the annual meeting of the Eating Disorder Research Society, Boston.

Marcé, L.-V. (1860). Note sur une forme de délire hypochondriaque consécutive aux dyspepsies et charactérisée principalement par le refus d'aliments. *Annales Médico-Psychologiques, 6*, 15–18.

Marrazzi, M. A., Bacon, J. P., Kinzie, J., et al. (1995). Naltrexone use in the treatment of anorexia nervosa and bulimia nervosa. *International Clinical Psychopharmacology, 10*, 163–172.

Meyer, A. E., von Holtzapfel, B., Deffnor, G., et al. (1986). Psychoneuroendocrinology of remenorrhea in the late outcome of anorexia nervosa. *Psychotherapy and Psychosomatics, 45*, 174–185.

Milosevic, A. (1999). Eating disorders and the dentist. *British Dental Journal, 86, 109–113.*

Morgan, J. F., Lacey, J. H., & Sedgwick, P. M. (1999). Impact of pregnancy on bulimia nervosa. *British Journal of Psychiatry, 174, 135–140.*

National Heart, Lung, and Blood Institute. (1998). *Clinical guidelines on the identification, evaluation, and treatment of overweight and obesity in adults: Executive summary* [Online]. Available: http://www.nhlbi.nih.gov [2000, April 7].

Nattiv, A., Agostini, R., Drinkwater, B., et al. (1994). The female athlete triad: The inter-relatedness of disordered eating, amenorrhea, and osteoporosis. *Clinics in Sports Medicine, 13, 405–418.*

Neumarker, K. J. (1997). Mortality and sudden death in anorexia nervosa. *International Journal of Eating Disorders, 21, 205–212.*

Pomeroy, C., Mitchell, J., Eckert, E., et al. (1997). Effect of body weight and caloric restriction on serum complement proteins, including Factor D/adipsin: Studies in anorexia nervosa and obesity. *Clinical and Experimental Immunology, 108, 507–515.*

Powers, P. S. (1996). Initial assessment and early treatment options for anorexia nervosa and bulimia nervosa. *Psychiatric Clinics of North America, 19, 639–655.*

Powers, P. S. (1997). Management of patients with comorbid medical conditions. In D. M. Garner

& P. E. Garfinkel (Eds.), *Handbook of treatment for eating disorders* (2nd ed., pp. 424–436). New York: Guilford Press.

Powers, P. S. (1999). Osteoporosis and eating disorders. *Journal of Pediatric and Adolescent Gynecology, 12,* 51–57.

Powers, P. S., & Johnson, C. (1996). Small victories: Prevention of eating disorders among athletes. *Eating Disorders: The Journal of Treatment and Prevention, 4,* 364–377.

Powers, P. S., Perez, A., Boyd, F., et al. (1999). Eating pathology before and after bariatric surgery: A prospective study. *International Journal of Eating Disorders, 25,* 293–300.

Powers, P. S., Santana, C. A., & Bannon, Y. (2001). *Olanzapine in the treatment of anorexia nervosa: A pilot study.* Presented at NCDEU, Phoenix, Arizona, May 29, 2001.

Powers, P. S., & Spratt, E. G. (1994). Males and females with eating disorders. *Eating Disorders: The Journal of Treatment and Prevention, 2,* 197–214.

Powers, P. S., Tyson, I. B., Stevens, B. A., et al. (1995). Total body potassium and serum potassium among eating disorder patients. *International Journal of Eating Disorders, 18,* 269–276.

Rand, C. S., Macgregor, A. M., & Stunkard, A. J. (1997). The night eating syndrome in the general population and among post-operative obesity surgery patients. *International Journal of Eating Disorders, 22,* 65–69.

Ratnasuriya, R. H., Eisler, I., Szmukler, G. I., et al. (1991). Anorexia nervosa: Outcome and prognostic factors after 20 years. *British Journal of Psychiatry, 158,* 495–502.

Robertson, D. N., & Palmer, R. L. (1997). The prevalence and correlates of binge eating in a British community sample of women with a history of obesity. *International Journal of Eating Disorders, 22,* 323–327.

Robin, A. L., Gilroy, M., & Dennis, A. B. (1998). Treatment of eating disorders in children and adolescents. *Clinical Psychology Review, 18,* 421–446.

Robin, A. L., & Siegel, P. (1999). *Behavioral family systems therapy for treating eating disorders in children and adolescents (BFST).* (Available from A. L. Robin, Wayne State University, Detroit, MI, 48202)

Robin, A. L., Siegel, P. T., Koepke, T., et al. (1994). Family therapy versus individual therapy for adolescent females with anorexia nervosa. *Journal of Developmental and Behavioral Pediatrics, 15,* 111–116.

Robin, A. L., Siegel, P. T., & Moye, A. (1995). Family versus individual therapy for anorexia: Impact on family conflict. *International Journal of Eating Disorders, 17,* 313–322.

Root, A. (1984). Role of the medical consultant. In P. S. Powers & R. C. Fernandez (Eds.), *Current treatment of anorexia nervosa and bulimia* (pp, 208–214). Basel, Switzerland: Karger.

Rosen, J. C. (1996). Body image assessment and treatment in controlled studies of eating disorders. *International Journal of Eating Disorders, 20,* 331–343.

Schiff, R. J., Wurzel, C. L., Brunson, S. C., et al. (1986). Death due to chronic syrup of ipecac use in a patient with bulimia. *Pediatrics, 78,* 412–416.

Silverman, J. A. (1989). Louis-Victor Marcé, 1828–1864: Anorexia nervosa's forgotten man. *Psychological Medicine, 19,* 833–835.

Stice, E. (1999). Clinical implications of psychosocial research on bulimia nervosa and binge-eating disorder. *Journal of Clinical Psychology, 55,* 675–683.

Striegel-Moore, R. H., Wilson, G. T., Wilfley, D. E., et al. (1998). Binge eating in an obese community sample. *International Journal of Eating Disorders, 23,* 27–37.

Strober, M., Freeman, R., & Morrell, W. (1997). The long-term course of severe anorexia nervosa in adolescents: Survival analysis of recovery, relapse, and outcome predictors over 10–15 years in a prospective study. *International Journal of Eating Disorders, 22,* 339–360.

Stunkard, A. J. (1959). Eating patterns and obesity. *Psychiatric Quarterly, 33,* 284–294.

Stunkard, A. J., Berkowitz, R., Wadden, T., et al. (1996). Binge eating disorder and the night-eating syndrome. *International Journal of Obesity and Related Metabolic Disorders, 20,* 1–6.

Sullivan, P. F., Bulik, C. M., Carter, F. A., et al. (1996). The significance of a prior history of anorexia in bulimia nervosa. *International Journal of Eating Disorders, 20,* 253–261.

Sullivan, P. F., Bulik, C. M., & Kendler, K. S. (1998). Genetic epidemiology of bingeing and vomiting. *British Journal of Psychiatry, 173,* 75–79.

Sunday, S. R., Halmi, K. A., & Einhorn, A. (1995). The Yale–Brown–Cornell Eating Disorder Scale: A new scale to assess eating disorder symptomatology. *International Journal of Eating Disorders, 18,* 237–245.

Swenne, I., & Larsson, P. T. (1999). Heart risk associated with weight loss in anorexia nerovsa and eating disorders: Risk factors for QTc interval prolongation and dispersion. *Acta Paediatrica, 88,* 304–309.

Treasure, J. L., Wheeler, M., King, E. A., et al. (1988). Weight gain and reproductive function: Ultrasonographic and endocrine features in anorexia nervosa. *Clinical Endocrinology, 29,* 607–616.

van 't Hof, S. (1994). *Anorexia nervosa: The historical and cultural specificity: Fallacious theories and tenacious "facts."* Berwyn, PA: Swets & Zeitlinger.

VanDeLoo, D. A., & Johnson, M. D. (1995). The young female athlete. *Clinics in Sports Medicine, 14,* 687–707.

Vanderlinden, J., & Vandereycken, W. (1997). *Trauma, dissociation, and impulse dyscontrol in eating disorders.* Bristol, PA: Brunner/Mazel.

Waller, G. (1997). Drop-out and failure to engage in individual outpatient cognitive behavioral therapy for bulimic disorders. *International Journal of Eating Disorders, 22,* 35–41.

Walters, E. E., & Kendler, K. S. (1995). Anorexia nervosa and anorexic-like syndromes in population-based female twin sample. *American Journal of Psychiatry, 152,* 64–71.

Wilson, G. T. (1996). Treatment of bulimia nervosa: When CBT fails. *Behaviour Research and Therapy, 34,* 197–212.

Yager, J., Andersen, A., Devlin, M., et al. (2000). Practice guidelines for the treatment of patients with eating disorders (revision). *American Journal of Psychiatry, 157*(Suppl.), 1–36.

14

Sexual Dysfunction

ANITA H. CLAYTON

SEXUALITY

Sexuality is an important aspect of health. Sexuality includes, but is not limited to, biological, psychological/social/emotional, cognitive, and cultural experiences. Sexual behavior may be heterosexual or homosexual, cognitive or physical, and involves complex interactions of sex steroids and neurotransmitters. In women, there appears to be a relationship between the timing of sexual behavior and reproductive endocrinology. The pubertal rise in testosterone is associated with subsequent increases in female sexual interest and activity, perhaps as a causal factor mediated by relevant social variables (Halpern et al., 1997). Women who engage in sexual activity less than weekly are more likely to have aberrant-length menstrual cycles, which are more likely to be anovulatory, and to have luteal phase deficiencies or infertility, than women who engage in sexual activity at least weekly (Cutler et al., 1979, 1985). In one study, users of triphasic oral contraceptives reported more sexual thoughts, fantasies, and sexual interest than users of monophasic oral contraceptives (McCoy & Matyas, 1996). Pregnancy also influences sexuality, primarily related to the presence of dyspareunia and diminished orgasmic capacity, which contribute to a decline in coital frequency as the pregnancy progresses (Oruç et al., 1999). Restoration of sexual functioning following delivery parallels restoration of hormonal cycling, and is delayed in breastfeeding women experiencing lactational amenorrhea (Glazener, 1997; Visness & Kennedy, 1997). Menopause, with its decline in estrogen and testosterone, may lead to decreased libido (Chiechi et al., 1997), dyspareunia associated with vaginal dryness (Chiechi et al., 1997; Kingsberg, 1998), and other sexual dysfunction. Changes unrelated to menopause, such as body image, general health status, psychological issues, relationship status, and beliefs about menopause and sexuality, may also influence sexual functioning in the climacteric (Kingsberg, 1998). Sexual functioning in older, postmenopausal women may be influenced by psychological issues of aging, medication use, and illness-related factors, but a meaningful sexual relationship may be maintained through later life with a realistic understanding of the sexual changes that accompany normal aging (Meston, 1997).

Sexuality may also be influenced by such factors as fear of pregnancy, desire for pregnancy, infertility, concern about sexually transmitted diseases, partner availability, history of childhood sexual abuse, and cultural practices (such as female circumcision).

THE BIOLOGY OF THE SEXUAL RESPONSE

The current diagnostic classification of sexual dysfunctions in the *Diagnostic and Statistical Manual of Mental Disorders*, fourth edition (DSM-IV; American Psychiatric Association, 1994) utilizes a motivational/psychophysiological model based on the first three phases of the sexual response cycle: desire, arousal, and orgasm. Sexual desire includes physiological, cognitive, and behavioral components manifested by sexual thoughts and fantasies, and interest in participation in sexual activity. Testosterone appears to be the primary gonadal steroid influencing desire and may be mediated by the neurotransmitters dopamine and serotonin via the hypothalamus and associated limbic structures. Baseline levels of circulating androgen are considerably lower in women than in men, with greater fluctuations due to reproductive life events, creating difficulties in establishing hormone–behavior relationships. Although combination estrogen-plus-androgen replacement enhances desire in postmenopausal women (Sherwin, 1991), measurements of circulating testosterone in relation to sexual desire in premenopausal women have been inconclusive (Persky et al., 1978; Udry et al., 1986); these findings suggest that factors in addition to hormones, such as psychosocial context, influence desire. Conditioning may also play a role, as women in one study reported a greater increase in sexual desire after exposure to an erotic video during the follicular phase than women viewing erotica in the luteal phase reported (Slob et al., 1996).

Sexual arousal is the phase of sexual excitement, manifested in the female by pelvic vasocongestion, vaginal lubrication, and swelling of the external genitalia. Vasoactive intestinal peptide appears to mediate the autonomic effects on vaginal blood flow during sexual arousal (Levin, 1992). Schreiner-Engel et al. (1981) found increased physiological arousal during the early follicular and late luteal phases, without significant hormonal correlations. In addition, Slob et al. (1991) found an order effect, with increased arousal if exposure to erotica occurred first during the follicular phase versus during the luteal phase. In the presence of adequate estrogen levels, potential physiological mechanisms mediating arousal include central dopamine stimulation, modulation of the cholinergic–adrenergic balance, α_{-1}-adrenergic agonism, and the presence of nitric oxide (Segraves, 1989; Burnett et al., 1992).

Orgasm is the process of physiological release of sexual tension, and is associated with rhythmic contractions of perineal and reproductive organ structures with cardiovascular and respiratory changes. Women do not have a postorgasmic refractory period, and therefore have the potential to experience multiple orgasms. The underlying physiological mechanism of orgasm is poorly understood. It may be related to oxytocin, a neuropeptide hormone; positive correlations of plasma levels of oxytocin to perineal contractions and increased systolic blood pressure have been found in both men and women (Carmichael et al., 1994). Delay in achieving orgasm may occur with serotonergic effects, postulated to be due to 5-HT_2 stimulation (Watson & Gorzalka, 1992), and α-adrenergic antagonism (Segraves, 1989).

PRIMARY SEXUAL DYSFUNCTIONS

As noted above, the current diagnostic system for primary sexual dysfunctions in DSM-IV is based on the first three phases of the sexual response cycle. In women, sexual dysfunctions include hypoactive sexual desire disorder, sexual aversion disorder, female sexual arousal disorder, and female orgasmic disorder (formerly inhibited female orgasm). They also include two sexual pain disorders, dyspareunia and vaginismus. Finally, sexual dysfunctions may be due to a general medical condition or may be substance-induced. Subtypes catalog the nature of the onset (lifelong or acquired type) and the context of the sexual dysfunction (generalized or situational type). Etiology may be indicated by the descriptors "due to psychological factors" or "due to combined factors" (American Psychiatric Association, 1994).

Epidemiological data from the 1992 National Health and Social Life Survey (NHSLS) in U.S. adults (1,749 women and 1,410 men) who reported at least one partner in the prior 12-month period indicated that sexual dysfunction was more prevalent in women (43%) than in men (31%), with different patterns of sexual dysfunction between genders (Laumann et al., 1999). For women, the prevalence of sexual problems decreased with increasing age, except problems with lubrication/arousal. Younger women reported more problems with sexual desire and difficulty achieving orgasm than did older women. Nonmarried women reported orgasm problems at 1.5 times the prevalence rates in married women. Women with lower educational attainment described less pleasurable sexual experiences and higher levels of sexual anxiety than did women with higher educational attainment. Hispanic women reported lower rates of sexual problems than did either black women, who reported lower sexual desire and satisfaction, or white women, who described more sexual pain. However, Hispanic women in general may have fewer sexual experiences or may be less likely to report sexual problems. Female college students in a Spanish study to establish the validity and reliability of the Spanish version of the Changes in Sexual Functioning Questionnaire (CSFQ) reported fewer sexual experiences and less pleasure than U.S. cohorts (Bobes et al., 2000). Declining social status and/or a history of sexual trauma can also negatively affect sexual functioning. Poor physical health was correlated with sexual pain in women in the NHSLS.

Similar rates of sexual dysfunction were found in a postal questionnaire in England (Dunn et al., 1998, 1999), and lower rates, but a similar distribution, in a survey in Denmark (Ventegodt, 1998). In the Dunn et al. (1999) report, marital difficulties were associated with arousal, orgasmic, and enjoyment difficulties, as were anxiety and depression. In addition, dyspareunia was found to decrease with age. Fifty-two percent of the responders in the Dunn et al. (1998) survey stated that they would like to receive professional help for a sexual problem, but only 1 in 10 had received such assistance.

SECONDARY SEXUAL DYSFUNCTIONS

The etiology of sexual dysfunctions may be medical, psychosocial/situational, substance-induced, or a combination of these factors. Psychiatric conditions may affect sexual functioning in all phases of the sexual response cycle. For example, 70% of patients with major depressive disorder reported diminished libido (Casper et al., 1985); 41% of women with hypomania experienced increased sexual intensity (Goodwin & Jamison, 1990); and women with eating disorders had decreased sexual interest and more negative affect during sexual activity than normal subjects did (Morgan et al., 1995). Apt and Hurlbert (1994) reported lower sexual desire and greater orgasmic dysfunction in women with histrionic personality disorder, and 60% of women with schizophrenia versus 13% of normal volunteers reported having never experienced an orgasm (Friedman & Harrison, 1984).

Other medical conditions may cause sexual dysfunction, including neurological illness, endocrine disorders, genitourinary conditions, infectious processes, cardiovascular disease, and autoimmune disorders. Forty-five percent of women with multiple sclerosis reported sexual dysfunction (vs. 78% of men), unassociated with level of disability or fatigue (Mattson et al., 1995). Sexual dysfunction has been reported in women with Crohn's disease (Moody et al., 1992), in women with vaginal changes after treatment for cervical cancer (Bergmark et al., 1999), and in surgically menopausal women (Shifren et al., 1998). Schiel and Muller (1999) found that 18% of women with insulin-dependent diabetes reported sexual disorders, as opposed to 42% of women with non-insulin-dependent diabetes. Black women with diabetes described lower levels of sexual desire than nondiabetic black women, unrelated to length of illness or glucose control (Watts, 1994). However, some effects of medical conditions may be psychologically or socially mediated. Nosek et al. (1996) found that women with physical disabilities had low sexual activity, response, and satisfaction, but normal desire, compared to the sexual functioning of able-bodied female friends.

Other physiological effects may influence sexual functioning. Women with complaints of premenstrual symptoms reported less sexual desire, less frequent sexual activity, less frequent orgasms, and less satisfaction with orgasm during the late luteal phase than during other phases of the menstrual cycle (Clayton et al., 1999).

Psychological factors, such as interpersonal relationships, body image, sexual self-esteem, and prior psychosexual adjustment, may also affect sexual functioning. A meta-analysis of three studies of women with dysmenorrhea, menorrhagia, or sexual dysfunction in the general population revealed a substantially greater risk in such women (before menopause) of having a history of sexual assault than in women without gynecological complaints (Golding et al., 1999).

Psychoactive substances may affect sexual functioning, including psychotropic drugs, nonpsychotropic medications, and drugs of abuse. Alcohol is the most commonly misused substance with effects on sexual functioning—potentially increasing desire, but decreasing other aspects of sexual function. Sexual dysfunction was found in 62% of males with cocaine and alcohol use problems (Cocores et al., 1987), but no data have been published for females with substance abuse disorders. Well over 100 non-psychotropic medications may cause sexual dysfunction; the most commonly used include antihypertensives, steroids, and H_2 blockers ("Drugs That Cause Sexual Dysfunction," 1992).

Few psychotropic medications have been reported to enhance sexual functioning, although some data suggest that bupropion may be used to treat hypoactive sexual desire disorder in women (Segraves et al., 2000). Moclobemide, a reversible and selective inhibitor of monoamine oxidase A (MAO-A) not available in the United States, has been reported to induce reversible hypersexuality in two male patients with depression and neurological disease (Korpelainen et al., 1998). Gartrell (1986) reported that trazodone increased libido in women, but subsequent widespread use of trazodone has failed to replicate this effect. Clomipramine has been reported to induce spontaneous orgasm with yawning (McLean et al., 1983), but other published reports describe a high incidence of sexual dysfunction with clomipramine.

Psychotropic medications are much more likely to produce untoward effects on sexual functioning than positive effects. However, most studies of psychotropics other than antidepressants have examined effects on males only and consist of isolated case reports. Thioridazine (Kotin et al., 1976), trifluoperazine (Degen, 1982), and fluphenazine (Ghadirian et al., 1982) have been reported to induce anorgasmia in females. This effect may be mediated by dopaminergic or α-adrenergic blockade. Sangal (1985) reported inhibited female orgasm as a side effect of alprazolam, and Riley and Riley (1986) demonstrated a dose–response relationship of diazepam to difficulty achieving arousal and orgasm with masturbation in women. The inhibitory neurotransmitter γ-aminobutyric acid may produce negative effects on sexual functioning.

The effects of antidepressant medications on sexual functioning have been studied most systematically. There are prospective studies comparing effects, some with placebo controls, but few have used a validated and reliable instrument for the assessment of sexual functioning. There has been limited stratification by gender, therapeutic response, phases of the sexual response cycle, or exclusion of preexisting primary sexual disorders. Montejo-González et al. (1997) reported that 52.5% of women treated with selective serotonin reuptake inhibitors (SSRIs) experienced sexual dysfunction; the greatest effects were on orgasmic function and libido, and there was a higher severity of dysfunction in women than in men. Rates of dysfunction were similar among treatments (fluoxetine, paroxetine, fluvoxamine, and sertraline), ranging from 54% to 64% when females and males were combined, but paroxetine differed significantly from the other SSRIs in being more likely to produce anorgasmia. Tricyclic antidepressants (TCAs), MAO inhibitors (MAOIs), trazodone, and venlafaxine have all been reported to impair sexual functioning in all sexual phases (Segraves, 1992). The mechanism of these effects includes potential hormonal changes, dopamine blockade, disturbance of adrenergic–cholinergic balance, α-adrenergic antagonism, inhibition of nitric oxide, and serotoninergic activation, particularly 5-HT$_2$.

Three new antidepressants, each with a unique mechanism of action, appear to have minimal effects on sexual functioning: bupropion, mirtazapine, and nefazodone. Bupropion is a dopamine and norepinephrine reuptake inhibitor; mirtazapine is an $\alpha_2$adrenergic, 5-HT$_{2A}$, and 5-HT$_3$ antagonist, and is an antihistamine; and nefazodone is a 5-HT$_{2A}$ antagonist, a serotonin reuptake inhibitor, and a 5-HT$_{2C}$ agonist via a metabolite, meta-chlorophenylpiperazine. These actions have a limited adverse impact on sexual functioning. In double-blind, placebo-controlled studies comparing bupropion sustained-release (SR) and sertraline in patients with major depression and normal sexual functioning (except diminished libido as a symptom of depression), significantly better orgasmic function and overall sexual function were seen with bupropion, beginning at Week 1 and persisting through Week 8 (Coleman et al., 1999; Croft et al., 1999). In a 12-week open-label study of 25 outpatients with mirtazapine assessed with a validated questionnaire, females ($n = 18$) reported improved desire (41%), arousal (52%), and ease/satisfaction with orgasm (48%) (Boyarsky et al., 1999). In a study of 143 outpatients with major depression, women ($n = 82$) reported nefazodone to be superior to sertraline in ease of achieving orgasm and satisfaction with ability to achieve orgasm (Feiger et al., 1996). Fifty-one healthy volunteers (women, $n = 22$) were randomly assigned to receive moclobemide or placebo for 3 weeks, with no differences between groups on measures of sexual desire or function (Kennedy et al., 1996).

ASSESSMENT

Evaluation of sexual function in women should examine each of the four phases of the sexual response cycle: desire, arousal, orgasm, and resolution. As there are no reports of dysfunction associated with resolution, information regarding sexual satisfaction may replace this phase. Diminished libido may be seen in the desire phase. Arousal problems include inhibited sexual excitement, diminished genital sensation, and failure to achieve or maintain vaginal lubrication. Orgasm may be delayed or absent. Pain with sexual activity is not phase-specific. It is important to discuss sexual functioning with patients because of the impact on quality of life through relationships and self-esteem, and to ensure compliance with treatment so as to prevent relapse/recurrence of illness. Increasing sexual dysfunction may herald progression or inadequate treatment of underlying medical conditions.

Barriers to adequate assessment of sexual functioning include patient factors of silence due to shame, fear, or ignorance; illness effects (e.g., negative thoughts or loss of interest or pleasure associated with depression); lack of interest in or absence of an ongoing relationship; attribution to other factors (e.g., stressors, problems in interpersonal relationships); comorbidity of Axis II disorders; and the gender of the patient (women are less likely than men to spontaneously report sexual problems). Physician barriers include discomfort asking about sexual functioning, failure to ask phase- and gender-specific questions, ignorance about sexual dysfunction associated with illness and medications, and interpersonal effects (e.g., gender of the patient vs. gender of the physician, age prejudice). Another barrier is failure to use an assessment tool appropriate to the situation. An instrument to assess sexual functioning needs to be gender-specific, to assess phase-specific function, to be brief, not to be perceived as intrusive, to be able to separate illness from medication effects (monitor over time), and to assess premorbid and lifelong sexual function (Ashton et al., 1998).

Currently available assessment tools are the Arizona Sexual Experiences Scale (ASEX), the Changes in Sexual Functioning Questionnaire, Clinical version (CSFQ-C), the Derogatis Interview for Sexual Functioning—Self-Report (DISF-SR), and the Rush Sexual Inventory (RSI) (Clayton et al., 1997; Derogatis, 1997; McGahuey et al., 2000; Zajecka et al., 1997). Table 14.1 presents a comparison of these instruments.

Strategies to address barriers to assessment include the physician's normalizing the issue for the patient by broaching the subject with a discussion of how common sexual dysfunctions are in the population or with specific treatments. Baseline measures of sexual functioning should be obtained, with reassessment following any changes in the illness, treatment, or psychosocial situation. This may be done through the use of a screening tool to identify problem areas requiring further discussion, which may also serve as an introduction of the topic to the patient. Discussions may refer to sexual activity rather than specific sexual behaviors, since patients might view questions about specific behaviors as intrusive.

The evaluation for sexual dysfunction should include the following: a sexual history and assessment of the current level of sexual functioning; documentation of medical and

TABLE 14.1. Comparison of Available Assessment Tools

Characteristics	ASEX	CSFQ-C	DISF-SR	RSI
Validated?	Yes—mod.	Yes—good	Yes—good	In progress
<10 minutes?	Yes	Yes	No	Yes
Explicit/intrusive?	No	No	Yes	Yes
Gender-specific?	Yes	Yes	Yes	Yes
Measures change over time?	Yes	Yes	No	Yes
Likert Scale?	Yes	Yes	Yes	Only 5 questions

psychiatric history/diagnoses; identification of all substances that might contribute to sexual dysfunction (medications, alcohol, illicit substances); endocrine tests and measures as indicated (free and total testosterone, thyroid function, hemoglobin A_{1C}, prolactin, estradiol, follicle-stimulating hormone, and luteinizing hormone); and neurological and/or genitourinary exam, as appropriate.

TREATMENT OF SEXUAL DYSFUNCTION

Limited treatments are available for primary sexual dysfunctions, with few published studies. Psychotherapy may be helpful, particularly when there is a history of negative sexual experiences such as sexual assault. Use of erotica in sex therapy may also have a place (Striar & Bartlik, 1999). Ensuring adequate levels of hormones, particularly sex steroids, appears to be important in the desire and arousal phases. Other approaches offer some hope; in a study of 51 women with hypoactive sexual desire disorder with no change in libido after 4 weeks of single-blind placebo administration, 29% responded to 8 weeks of treatment with 300 mg/day of bupropion SR (Segraves et al., 2000). Though low, this response rate encourages further examination of medication treatment for primary sexual dysfunctions. Combining psychotherapy and medications may increase response rates.

Strategies to manage secondary sexual dysfunctions have focused primarily on antidepressant-induced sexual dysfunction, but may be generalized to some degree. Accommodation to antidepressant-induced sexual dysfunction may occur in 5–10% of patients by 6 months (Ashton & Rosen, 1998; Montejo-González et al., 1997). Reducing the dose of an antidepressant risks subtherapeutic antidepressant effects and resultant relapse. "Drug holidays" on weekends for medications with short half-lives may improve sexual functioning on the weekends (Rothschild, 1995), but have the potential for serotonin discontinuation syndrome (Rosenbaum et al., 1998), and may encourage medication noncompliance and subsequent relapse. Antidotes or adjunctive agents may be useful, particularly in women who have a history of treatment-resistant depression, and who are fearful of lack of therapeutic efficacy with a change to another antidepressant medication. Table 14.2 lists available antidotes (Rosen et al., 1999) in order of clinical utility, with notation of those medications that might have adjunctive antidepressant efficacy (Clayton et al., 2000). Replacement of the offending antidepressant with one that has few negative effects on sexual functioning—bupropion (Clayton et al., 1999; Walker et al.,

TABLE 14.2. Available Antidotes

Commonly used	Uncommonly used
Bupropion SR[a]	Psychostimulants[a]
Buspirone[a]	Mirtazapine[a]
Yohimbine	Nefazodone[a]
Amantadine	Trazodone
Sildenafil	Cyproheptadine
	Ginkgo biloba

Note. The data are from Rosen et al. (1999) and Clayton et al. (2001).
[a]Indicates potential adjunctive therapeutic agents.

1993), mirtazapine (Gelenberg et al., 1998; Koutouvidis et al., 1999), or nefazodone (Ferguson et al., 2001)—is likely to be successful in more than 50% of patients, but the transition from the SSRI to the new antidepressant must be carefully titrated to avoid serotonin discontinuation syndrome and other adverse events.

CONCLUSIONS

As yet, sexuality remains mysterious, and a knowledge gap persists in our understanding of the etiologies and treatments for primary and secondary sexual dysfunctions. Particularly in women, appropriate and systematic assessment must be performed to identify all factors contributing to sexual dysfunction in specific individuals. Multiple interventions may be needed to restore sexual functioning. But that should be the goal, as a satisfying sex life is possible throughout a lifetime.

REFERENCES

American Psychiatric Association. (1994). *Diagnostic and statistical manual of mental disorders* (4th ed.). Washington, DC: Author.

Apt, C., & Hurlbert, D. F. (1994). The sexual attitudes, behavior, and relationships of women with histrionic personality disorder. *Journal of Sex and Marital Therapy, 20*(2), 125–133.

Ashton, A. K., & Rosen, R. C. (1998). Accommodation to serotonin reuptake inhibitor-induced sexual dysfunction. *Journal of Sex and Marital Therapy, 24*, 191–192.

Ashton, A. K., Segraves, R. T., Clayton, A. H., et al. (1998). *Assessment of sexual functioning.* Paper presented at the 151st Annual Convention of the American Psychiatric Association, Toronto.

Bergmark, K., Avall-Lundqvist, E., Dickman, P. W., et al. (1999). Vaginal changes and sexuality in women with a history of cervical cancer. *New England Journal of Medicine, 340*(18), 1383–1389.

Bobes, J., Gonzalez M. P., Rico-Villandemoros, F., et al. (2000). Validation of the Spanish version of the Changes in Sexual Functioning Questionnaire (CSFQ). *Journal of Sex and Marital Therapy, 26*, 119–131.

Boyarsky, B. K., Haque, W., Rouleau, M. R., et al. (1999). Sexual functioning in depressed outpatients taking mirtazapine. *Depression and Anxiety, 9*, 175–179.

Burnett, A. L., Lowenstein, C. J., Bredt, D. S., et al. (1992). Nitric oxide: A physiologic mediator of penile erection. *Science*, *257*, 401–403.

Carmichael, M. S., Warburton, V. L., Dixen, J., et al. (1994). Relationships among cardiovascular, muscular, and oxytocin responses during sexual functioning. *Integrative Psychiatry*, *23*(1), 59–79.

Casper, R. C., Redmond, E., Jr., Katz, M. M., et al. (1985). Somatic symptoms in primary affective disorder. *Archives of General Psychiatry*, *42*, 1098–1104.

Chiechi, L. M., Granierik, M., Lobascio, A., et al. (1997). Sexuality in the climacterium. *Clinical and Experimental Obstetrics and Gynecology*, *24*(3), 158–159.

Clayton, A. H. (2000). *Sexual dysfunction associated with treatment of major depression*. Annual Convention of the American Psychiatric Association, Chicago, IL.

Clayton, A. H., Clavet, G. J., McGarvey, E. L., et al. (1999). Assessment of sexual functioning during the menstrual cycle. *Journal of Sex and Marital Therapy*, *25*, 281–291.

Clayton, A. H., McGarvey, E. L., & Clavet, G. J. (1997). The Changes in Sexual Functioning Questionnaire (CSFQ), Development, reliability, and validity. *Psychopharmacology Bulletin*, *33*(4), 731–745.

Cocores, J. A., Miller, N. S., Pottash, A. C., et al. (1988). Sexual dysfunction in abusers of cocaine and alcohol. *American Journal of Drug and Alcohol Abuse*, *14*(2), 169–173.

Coleman, C. C., Cunningham, L. A., Foster, V. J., et al. (1999). Sexual dysfunction associated with the treatment of depression: A placebo-controlled comparison of bupropion sustained release and sertraline treatment. *Annals of Clinical Psychiatry*, *11*(4), 205–215.

Croft, H., Settle, E., Jr., Houser, T., et al. (1999). A placebo-controlled comparison of the antidepressant efficacy and effects on sexual functioning of sustained-release bupropion and sertraline. *Clinical Therapeutics*, *21*(4), 643–658.

Cutler, W. B., Garcia, C. R., & Krieger, A. M. (1979). Sexual behavior frequency and menstrual cycle length in mature premenopausal women. *Psychoneuroendocrinology*, *4*, 297–309.

Cutler, W. B., Preti, G., Huggins, G., et al. (1985). Sexual behavior frequency and fertile-type menstrual cycle. *Physiology and Behavior*, *34*, 214–218.

Degen, K. (1982). Sexual dysfunction in women using major tranquilizers. *Psychosomatics*, *23*, 959–961.

Derogatis, L. R. (1997). The Derogatis Interview for Sexual Functioning (DISF/DISF-SR), An introductory report. *Journal of Sex and Marital Therapy*, *23*(4), 291–304.

Drugs that cause sexual dysfunction: An update. (1992). *Medical Letter*, *34*(876), 73–78.

Dunn, K. M., Croft, P. R., & Hackett, G. I. (1998). Sexual problems: A study of the prevalence and need for health care in the general population. *Family Practice*, *15*(6), 519–524.

Dunn, K. M., Croft, P. R., & Hackett, G. I. (1999). Association of sexual problems with social, psychological, and physical problems in men and women: A cross sectional population survey. *Journal of Epidemiology and Community Health*, *53*, 144–148.

Feiger, A., Kiev, A., Shrivastava, R. K., et al. (1996). Nefazodone versus sertraline in outpatients with major depression: Focus on efficacy, tolerability, and effects on sexual function and satisfaction. *Journal of Clinical Psychiatry*, *57*(Suppl. 2), 53–62.

Ferguson, J. M., Shrivastava, R. K., Stahl, S. M., et al. (2001). Re-emergence of sexual dysfunction in patients with major depressive disorder: Double-blind comparison of nefazodone and sertraline. *Journal of Clinical Psychiatry*, *62*, 24–29.

Friedman, S., & Harrison, G. (1984). Sexual histories, attitudes, and behavior of schizophrenic and "normal" women. *Archives of Sexual Behavior*, *13*(6), 555–567.

Gartrell, N. (1986). Increased libido in women receiving trazodone. *American Journal of Psychiatry*, *143*, 781–782.

Gelenberg, A. J., Laukes, C., McGahuey, C. A., et al. (1998). *Mirtazapine-substitution in SSRI-induced sexual dysfunction*. Paper presented at the 53rd Annual Scientific Convention and Program of the Society for Biological Psychiatry, Toronto.

Ghadirian, A. M., Chouinard, G., & Annable, A. (1982). Sexual dysfunction and plasma prolactin levels in neuroleptic-treated schizophrenic outpatients. *Journal of Nervous and Mental Disease, 170*, 463–467.

Glazener, C. M. (1997). Sexual function after childbirth: Women's experiences, persistent morbidity and lack of professional recognition. *British Journal of Obstetrics and Gynaecology, 104*(3), 330–335.

Golding, J. M., Wilsnack, S. C., & Learman, L. A. (1999). Prevalence of sexual assault history among women with common gynecologic symptoms. *American Journal of Obstetrics and Gynecology, 179*(4), 1013–1019.

Goodwin, F. K., & Jamison K. R. (Eds.). (1990). *Manic–depressive illness.* New York: Oxford University Press.

Halpern, C. T., Udry, R., & Suchindran, C. (1997). Testosterone predicts initiation of coitus in adolescent females. *Psychosomatic Medicine, 59*, 161–171.

Kennedy, S. H., Ralevski, E., Davis, C., et al. (1996). The effects of moclobemide on sexual desire and function in healthy volunteers. *European Neuropsychopharmacology, 6*, 177–181.

Kingsberg, S. A. (1998). Postmenopausal sexual functioning: A case study. *International Journal of Fertility and Women's Medicine, 43*(2), 122–128.

Korpelainen, J. T., Hiltunen, P., & Myllylä, V. V. (1998). Moclobemide-induced hypersexuality in patients with stroke and Parkinson's disease. *Clinical Neuropharmacology, 21*(4), 251–254.

Kotin, J., Wilber, D. E., & Verburg, D. (1976). Thioridazine and sexual dysfunction. *American Journal of Psychiatry, 133*, 82–85.

Koutouvidis, N., Pratikakis, M., & Fotiadou, A. (1999). The use of mirtazapine in a group of 11 patients following poor compliance to selective serotonin reuptake inhibitor treatment due to sexual dysfunction. *International Clinical Psychopharmacology, 14*, 253–255.

Laumann, E. O., Paik, A., & Rosen, R. C. (1999). Sexual dysfunction in the United States: Prevalence and predictors. *Journal of the American Medical Association, 281*(6), 537–544.

Levin, R. J. (1992). The mechanism of human female sexual arousal. *Annual Review of Sex Research, 3*, 1.

Mattson, D., Petrie, M., Srivastava, D. K., et al. (1995). Multiple sclerosis: Sexual dysfunction and response to medications. *Archives of Neurology, 52*, 862–868.

McCoy, N. L., & Matyas, J. R. (1996). Oral contraceptives and sexuality in university women. *Archives of Sexual Behavior, 25*(1), 73–90.

McGahuey, C. A., Gelenbers, A. J., Laukes, C. A., et al. (2000). The Arizona Sexual Experience Scale (ASEX), Reliability and validity. *Journal of Sex and Marital Therapy, 26*(1), 25–40.

McLean, J. D., Forsythe, R. G., & Kaplim, I. A. (1983). Unusual side effects of clomipramine associated with yawning. *Canadian Journal of Psychiatry, 28*, 569–570.

Meston, C. M. (1997). Aging and sexuality. *Western Medical Journal, 167*, 285–290.

Montajo-González, A. L., Llorca, G., Izquierdo, J. A., et al. (1997). SSRI-induced sexual dysfunction: Fluoxetine, paroxetine, sertraline, and fluvoxamine in a prospective, multicenter, and descriptive clinical study of 344 patients. *Journal of Sex and Marital Therapy, 23*(3), 176–188.

Moody, G., Probert, C. S. J., Sriastava, E. M., et al. (1992). Sexual dysfunction amongst women with Crohn's disease: A hidden problem. *Digestion, 52*, 179–183.

Morgan, C. D., Wiederman, M. W., & Pryor, T. L. (1995). Sexual functioning and attitudes of eating-disordered women: A follow-up study. *Journal of Sex and Marital Therapy, 21*(2), 67–77.

Nosek, M. A., Rintala, D. H., Young, M. E., et al. (1996). Sexual functioning among women with physical disabilities. *Archives of Physical Medicine and Rehabilitation, 77*, 107–115.

Oruç, S., Esen, A., Laçin, S., et al. (1999). Sexual behavior during pregnancy. *Australian and New Zealand Journal of Obstetrics and Gynaecology, 39*(1), 48–50.

Persky, H., Lief, H. I., Strauss, D., et al. (1978). Plasma testosterone level and sexual behavior in couples. *Archives of Sexual Behavior, 7*(3), 157–175.

Riley, A. J., & Riley, E. J. (1986). The effect of single dose diazepam on female sexual response induced by masturbation. *Sexual and Marital Therapy, 1,* 49–53.

Rosen, R. C., Lane, R. M., & Menza, M. (1999). Effects of SSRIs on sexual function: A critical review. *Journal of Clinical Psychopharmacology, 19*(1), 67–85.

Rosenbaum, J. F., Fava, M., Hoog, S. L., et al. (1998). Selective serotonin reuptake inhibitor discontinuation syndrome: A randomized clinical trial. *Biological Psychiatry, 44*(2), 77–87.

Rothschild, A. J. (1995). Selective serotonin reuptake inhibitor-induced sexual dysfunction: Efficacy of a drug holiday. *American Journal of Psychiatry, 152*(10), 1514–1516.

Sangal, R. (1985). Inhibited female orgasm as a side effect of alprazolam. *American Journal of Psychiatry, 142,* 1223–1224.

Schiel, R., & Muller, U. A. (1999). Prevalence of sexual disorders in a selection-free diabetic population (JEVIN). *Diabetes Research and Clinical Practice, 44*(2), 115–121.

Schreiner-Engel, P., Schiavari, R. C., Smith, H., et al. (1981). Sexual arousability and the menstrual cycle. *Psychosomatic Medicine, 43*(3), 199–214.

Segraves, R. T. (1989). Effects of psychotropic drugs on human erection and ejaculation. *Archives of General Psychiatry, 46,* 275–284.

Segraves, R. T. (1992). Overview of sexual dysfunction complicating the treatment of depression. *Journal of Clinical Psychiatry Monograph, 10*(2), 4–10.

Segraves, R. T., Croft, H., Kavoussi, R., et al. (2000). *Bupropion sustained release for the treatment of hypoactive sexual desire disorder in nondepressed women.* Poster presented at the 153rd Annual Convention of the American Psychiatric Association, Chicago.

Sherwin, B. (1991). The psychoendocrinology of aging and female sexuality. *Annual Review of Sex Research, 2,* 181–198.

Shifren, J. L., Nahum, R., & Mazer, N. A. (1998). Incidence of sexual dysfunction in surgically menopausal women. *Menopause, 5*(3), 189–190.

Slob, A. K., Ernste, M., & van der Werff ten Bosch, J. J. (1991). Menstrual cycle phase and sexual arousability in women. *Archives of Sexual Behavior, 29*(6), 567–577.

Slob, A. K., Bax, C. M., Hop, W. C. J., et al. (1995). Sexual arousability and the menstrual cycle. *Psychoneuroendocrinology, 21*(6), 545–558.

Striar, S., & Bartlik, B. (1999). Stimulation of the libido: The use of erotica in sex therapy. *Psychiatric Annals, 29*(1), 60–62.

Udry, J. R., Talbert, L. M., & Morris, N. M. (1986). Biosocial foundations for adolescent female sexuality. *Demography, 23*(1), 53–66.

Ventegodt, S. (1998). Sex and the quality of life in Denmark. *Archives of Sexual Behavior, 27*(3), 295–307.

Visness, C. M., & Kennedy, K. I. (1997). The frequency of coitus during breastfeeding. *Birth, 24*(4), 253–257.

Walker, P. W., Cole, J. O., Gardner, E. A., et al. (1993). Improvement in fluoxetine-associated sexual dysfunction in patients switched to bupropion. *Journal of Clinical Psychiatry, 54*(12), 459–465.

Watson, N. V., & Gorzalka, B. B. (1992). Concurrent wet dog shaking and inhibition of male rat copulation after ventromedial brainstem injection of the $5-HT_2$ agonist DOI. *Neuroscience Letters, 141,* 25–29.

Watts, R. J. (1994). Sexual functioning of diabetic and nondiabetic African American women: A pilot study. *Journal of the National Black Nurses Association, 7*(1), 50–59.

Zajecka, J., Mitchell, S., & Fawcett, J. (1997). Treatment-emergent changes in sexual function with selective serotonin reuptake inhibitors as measures with the Rush Sexual Inventory. *Psychopharmacology Bulletin, 33*(4), 755–760.

15

Sleep Disorders

RACHEL MANBER
IAN M. COLRAIN
KATHRYN A. LEE

Sleep disturbance and daytime sleepiness are commonly reported by patients seen in outpatient psychiatry clinics. At times sleep disturbance is the main presenting symptom, but most often insomnia is a symptom of the presenting psychopathology. In the latter case, symptoms of disturbed sleep may be exacerbated by some psychotropic medications and can be resistant to change with psychotherapy (Kopta et al., 1994). However, specific empirically validated treatments for sleep disturbance can produce significant improvement in disrupted sleep. Two meta-analyses of 59 and 66 studies found that short-term cognitive-behavioral therapies for insomnia (varying in length from 4 to 12 weeks) produced substantial improvement (Morin et al., 1994; Murtagh & Greenwood, 1995). These outcome studies targeted patients with primary insomnia and excluded individuals with comorbid psychopathology. Nevertheless, these existing empirically supported interventions for disturbed sleep hold promise even for insomnia that is comorbid with or secondary to psychopathology.

This chapter provides an overview of the most common sleep disorders, with an emphasis on issues specific to women. It is intended to provide information to help mental health care providers assess and treat sleep complaints; be attentive to specific factors affecting women's sleep; become knowledgeable about the potential side effects of psychotropic medications on common sleep disorders, such as sleep apnea and periodic limb movement; and determine when a referral to a sleep disorders center may be indicated. A comprehensive review of all sleep disorders is beyond the scope of this chapter. Interested readers are referred to *The International Classification of Sleep Disorders: Diagnostic and Coding Manual* (American Sleep Disorders Association [ASDA], 1997) or to *Principles and Practices of Sleep Medicine* (Kryger et al., 2000).

BASIC SLEEP PHYSIOLOGY

Human sleep is a dynamic process. It can be divided into two types: rapid-eye-movement (REM) sleep and non-rapid-eye-movement (NREM) sleep. Apart from the obvious presence of large saccadic eye movements in REM sleep, the two types of sleep differ in distribution across the night and in physiological function. NREM sleep can be further subdivided into four stages. These can be viewed as sleep depth markers, with Stage 1 the lightest and Stage 4 the deepest stage of NREM sleep.

Standardized criteria (Rechtschaffen & Kales, 1968) are used to stage sleep. These criteria are based on data from electroencephalogram (EEG), eye movement (electrooculogram, or EOG), and postural muscle tone (electromyogram, or EMG). The process of falling asleep is associated with increased synchronization of neuronal firing and a slowing of the EEG from alpha frequency prior to sleep (when the eyes are closed) to theta frequency during the first stage of sleep (Stage 1). The onset of theta is the point at which consciousness awareness is lost (Gora et al., 1999). Stage 2 sleep is also dominated by theta activity, but is defined by the presence of at least one of two distinctive EEG features: sleep spindles (a burst of synchronized sigma frequency resembling the shape of a spinning wheel's spindle) and K-complexes. Stages 3 and 4 include slower EEG frequency (delta), which take up more than 20% or more than 50% of a time epoch, respectively. Stages 3 and 4 are associated with high arousal thresholds, and together they are referred to as "slow-wave sleep" (SWS). REM sleep is dominated by theta EEG activity, but unlike Stage 1, REM sleep is associated with rapid eye movements, dreams, and a drop in EMG activity. During REM there is active hyperpolarization of spinal motor neurons, leading to hypotonicity and paralysis, which affect all major striated postural muscle groups of the body.

The organization of sleep stages follows a particular pattern or architecture organized into sleep cycles, with a cycle length of approximately 90 to 110 minutes. The first cycle contains more SWS and has less REM sleep than subsequent cycles. REM periods become longer across the night, whereas SWS occupies less time in the second cycle and may disappear completely from later cycles.

The most marked age-related change seen in the macrostructure of sleep is the decrease in SWS. This probably reflects the endpoint of a gradual reduction that may commence as early as late adolescence. Other age-related observed changes in sleep include an increase in the proportion of Stage 1 sleep; a decrease in sleep continuity; and an increase in the prevalence of sleep pathology, such as sleep-disordered breathing or periodic leg movement syndrome (PLMS) (Bliwise, 1994).

Sleep is associated with marked physiological changes. The most pronounced changes are those associated with breathing. Normal adults display a 10–20% reduction in ventilation in NREM sleep as compared to wakefulness (Phillipson & Bowes, 1986). The reduction in ventilation is rapid and occurs early in the sleep onset process (Colrain et al., 1987, 1990), and it is typically due to a reduction in tidal volume rather than to change in respiratory rate. The reduction in breathing volume is associated with an elevation in upper airway resistance (UAR) (Henke et al., 1990) and with changes in the ventilatory response to elevated levels of carbon dioxide (CO_2) (Berthon-Jones & Sullivan, 1984; Douglas et al., 1982). Falling asleep for normal humans thus represents the rapid transition into a state of relative hypoventilation, elevated airway resistance, and moderate hypercapnia relative to wakefulness. REM sleep is a period in which breathing is extremely unstable, with both tidal volume and respiratory rate showing great variability. Unlike NREM sleep, REM sleep involves paralysis of the intercostal muscles, and all breathing effort is via the diaphragm. This can lead to paradoxical breathing in which the chest moves inward with inspiration, due to the subatmospheric pressure produced by diaphragmatic contraction.

Women have been reported to maintain robust mouth occlusion pressure responses during NREM sleep, whereas men show a sleep-related reduction in this measure of central respiratory drive (White, 1986). Women also show steeper hypercapnic ventilatory responses during the luteal phase (Schoene et al., 1981) and during sleep, indicating that they are more able to respond to elevated CO_2 levels, with an increase in the volume of breathing. Nonetheless, women still reduce their breathing volume during NREM sleep (White, 1986).

Heart rate and blood pressure decrease during NREM sleep relative to wakefulness. This is associated with increased parasympathetic nervous system activity, especially during SWS (Burgess et al., 1996), but this effect may be related to circadian control factors rather than to sleep stage (Burgess et al., 1997). The effect of NREM sleep on sympathetic nervous system activity is less clear. REM sleep is associated with substantial lability of autonomic nervous system activity. Both blood pressure and heart rate show marked fluctuation relative to NREM sleep (Bonnet & Arand, 1997), and there is a marked increase in sympathetic nerve activity (Somers et al., 1993).

Effects of Estrogen and Progesterone on Sleep Physiology

There is compelling evidence that exogenous administration of sex hormones affects sleep and brain systems involved in the regulation of sleep. Progesterone affects primarily NREM sleep, whereas estrogen affects primarily REM sleep. Estrogen enhances REM sleep in humans. It increases the time spent in REM sleep and decreases the latency to REM sleep (Schiff et al., 1979).

Progesterone has a sedating effect (Selye, 1941), and it alters human and animal sleep architecture in a manner similar to benzodiazepines. Its hypnotic effects appear to be dose-dependent; they are caused primarily by nongenomic, direct action of select progesterone metabolites (particularly 5α- and 5ß-pregnanolone) on the γ-aminobutyric acid$_A$ (GABA$_A$) receptor (Gee et al., 1988), and to a lesser extent through activation of intracellular progesterone receptors. Progesterone shortens the latency to sleep onset and reduces wakefulness after sleep onset. It decreases EEG activity in the slow-frequency range (0.4–4.3 Hz) and increases activity in the higher-frequency range (>15 Hz) during NREM sleep (Friess et al., 1997).

Progesterone acts as a respiratory stimulant, probably by its action on central CO_2 receptors (Brownell et al., 1986). In addition, progesterone has an excitatory effect on the genioglossus muscle, one of the major muscles responsible for dilation of the upper airway. This muscle has elevated activity during the luteal menstrual phase in premenopausal women, and is also elevated following progesterone administration in postmenopausal women (Popovic & White, 1998).

Placebo-controlled studies of hypogonadal and perimenopausal women report improvements in sleep after the initiation of estrogen replacement therapy. These improvements include decreased latency to sleep onset, decreased wakefulness after sleep onset (e.g., Polo-Kantola et al., 1998), increased total sleep time (Schiff et al., 1979), and decreased rate of cyclic alternating patterns (Scharf et al., 1997). Two studies comparing placebo with more contemporary hormone replacement therapy (HRT) regimens consisting of combinations of estrogen and progesterone report some improvement in sleep with both placebo and active treatment, but no differential effects (Pickett et al., 1989; Purdie et al., 1995). Failure to find a significant difference between more contemporary HRT regimens and placebo might be related to sample characteristics. In the past, women who chose HRT typically reported greater prevalence of sleep disturbance before treatment initiation than women who did not choose HRT (Matthews et al., 1990). Contemporary samples include women with lower sleep disturbances at baseline compared with women in previous samples.

Effects of Menstrual Cycle on Sleep

Existing studies of sleep in relation to the menstrual cycle report significant menstrual phase effects on sleep architecture. Their results have not converged into a clear and consistent picture, perhaps because of small sample sizes and differential timing of sleep measurement relative to the menstrual cycle. One of the most consistent results is the decrease in subjective and objective measures of sleep quality. Polysomnographic studies report increase in the number of awakenings after sleep onset during the late luteal phase and during the ovulatory period (Driver et al., 1996; Parry et al., 1989). Diary-based studies report lower ratings of sleep quality, longer latencies to sleep onset, and lower sleep efficiencies during the late luteal phase than during the midfollicular phase (Manber & Bootzin, 1997). Compared to the follicular phase, the luteal phase is associated with a significantly greater percentage of NREM sleep (primarily Stage 2 sleep) and significantly greater EEG activity in the spindle frequency range that is lowest in the days preceding ovulation (Driver et al., 1996; Ishizuka et al., 1992).

However, there appear to be large individual differences in the degree to which the physiology of the menstrual cycle affects sleep. Some women experience marked changes in their sleep after ovulation, whereas others do not. Individual differences in levels, rates of change, and rates of metabolism of sex steroids may explain why some women experience more severe premenstrual sleep disruptions than others (Manber & Armitage, 1999).

There is evidence that women with and without premenstrual dysphoric disorder (PMDD) may differ on some objective and subjective sleep measures. For example, throughout the menstrual cycle, women with premenstrual symptoms have a higher percentage of Stage 2 sleep, less SWS, a lower percentage of REM sleep (Lee et al., 1990; Parry et al., 1989) and higher nocturnal body temperatures (Severino et al., 1991) than women without premenstrual symptoms. In addition, women with PMDD have an altered melatonin rhythm during the luteal phase compared with the follicular phase, whereas healthy controls do not (Parry et al., 1997). Women with premenstrual symptoms report more insomnia symptoms, increased difficulty waking up in the morning, heightened mental activity during the night, more frequent and more unpleasant dreams, and increased sleepiness during the day (e.g., Manber et al., 1997).

Sleep during Pregnancy and Lactation

Pregnancy and postpartum are times in a woman's life when sleep patterns are greatly disturbed. Poor sleep is affected by hormonal changes during the first trimester; by carrying a large fetus and by anxiety about labor and delivery during the third trimester; and by the unpredictable sleep patterns of the newborn during the postpartum period (Lee, 1998).

Shortness of breath is common for women during the third trimester, but respiratory function does not appear to be adversely affected during sleep, most likely because of progesterone's stimulant effect on breathing and its effect on respiratory muscles. Nevertheless, women who gain excessive weight and women who snore during pregnancy are at increased risk for sleep apnea and hypoxia, which can result in intrauterine growth retardation and other neonatal complications (Schutte et al., 1994).

Although less serious for the fetus, complaints of heartburn and leg cramps increase during pregnancy (Gee, Zaffke, & Baratte-Beebe, in press). These complaints need to be taken seriously because of the potential for severe sleep deprivation for the mother if heartburn progresses to severe nocturnal esophageal reflux, or if leg cramps are undifferentiated from severe restless legs syndrome (RLS) (Goodman et al., 1988; Hertz et al., 1992). Both sleep apnea and PLMS, which often coexist in patients with RLS, are associated with sleep fragmentation leading to daytime sleepiness and fatigue. Thus complaints of excessive sleepiness and fatigue during pregnancy should be pursued and evaluated because of potential harm to the fetus.

Sleep deprivation is common during the postpartum period. It is most pronounced after the first delivery, particularly during the first postpartum month, regardless of type of delivery or type of infant feeding (Lee et al., in press). Women with a psychiatric history are at increased risk for postpartum depression and postpartum psychosis, but sleep research with this population is sparse. Coble et al. (1994) studied women until 8 months postpartum and found no differences in sleep patterns between those with a history of mental health problems and controls; however, no woman developed postpartum depression in their study.

Sleep during Menopause

Many epidemiological and survey studies report an increase in the incidence of insomnia complaints from pre- to postmenopause (Lugaresi et al., 1983; Owens & Mathews, 1998). Specifically, the transition into menopause is associated with longer latencies to sleep onset, more sleep maintenance insomnia, and a greater incidence of hypnotic use; these phenomena are particularly prevalent among women with very low or very high body mass index (e.g., Asplund & Aberg, 1995; Ballenger, 1976). Women with hot flushes have more disturbed sleep (lower sleep efficiency), with a significantly greater number of intermittent awakenings and a significantly greater number of stage shifts. These findings hold even after the effect of age is controlled for (e.g., Woodward & Freedman, 1994). It is not clear, however, whether these effects are mediated by hot flushes or result directly from the unstable hormonal milieu that independently affects both hot flushes and sleep.

CIRCADIAN RHYTHMS

There is substantial evidence that sleep–wake behavior has an endogenous circadian (daily) rhythm, which under normal conditions is synchronized with other circadian rhythms, including core body temperature, cortisol, and melatonin. In day-active people, body temperature peaks in the late afternoon and reaches a minimum in the early morning hours, during sleep (Waterhouse et al., 1990). Melatonin has a marked circadian rhythm that is closely linked to the light–dark cycle and to sleep–wake, temperature, and cortisol rhythms. A late evening surge in melatonin begins shortly after darkness, and its secretion peaks about 3 A.M., when the body temperature reaches its minimum. Exposure to bright light suppresses melatonin secretion, which remains at barely detectable levels during the day. Body temperature is regulated at a lower set point during NREM sleep than during wakefulness and sleep onset is associated with a fall in temperature (Barrett et al., 1993). The normal temperature-regulating mechanisms are markedly inhibited during REM sleep, and body temperature during REM sleep is influenced more by the environment than by the hypothalamus (Glotzbach & Heller, 1994).

The time spent asleep is influenced by the phase of the circadian temperature rhythm at bedtime, since a rising temperature triggers awakening from sleep. A sleep period that begins when body temperature is low—for example, at 3 A.M.—will be relatively short, since body temperature will soon rise (Czeisler et al., 1980; Gillberg & Akerstedt, 1982). Circadian rhythm disorders occur when individuals attempt to sleep at times that are inconsistent with their underlying biological clocks. In delayed sleep phase syndrome, the sleep–wake circadian rhythm is delayed compared to bedtime. Consequently, individuals with this syndrome have difficulty falling asleep at a desired bedtime, but have normal sleep if they attempt to sleep later. This problem is often seen in adolescents and young adults. In contrast, in advanced sleep phase syndrome, sleep occurs at an earlier-than-desired time and the individual awakens earlier than desired. This problem is often seen in older adults, consistent with the documented advance in body temperature rhythm phase associated with aging (Campbell et al., 1989). Night shift workers, particularly those on rotating shift schedules who complain of insomnia, often have a circadian sleep disorder. Individuals with seasonal affective disorder also report changes in sleep quality with the changing seasons of the year.

During the menstrual cycle, body temperature is elevated after ovulation because of the thermogenic properties of progesterone secretion from the ovary. This elevation causes a temporary dampening of the amplitude of the temperature rhythm, as the temperature during sleep fails to drop as low as it normally does during the follicular (preovulatory) phase (Lee, 1988; Lee et al., 1990). Some women with PMDD may have dampened melatonin rhythms and experience an earlier peak in their daily temperature rhythm (a phase advance), while others experience a phase delay (Lee et al., 1990). These studies have involved very few women, however, and the clinical significance of these findings is not clear. Treatment of circadian phase disorder with exogenous melatonin should be cautiously considered for women, because melatonin is known to suppress ovulatory function (Voordouw et al., 1992).

PHYSIOLOGICAL CAUSES OF SLEEP FRAGMENTATION

Sleep-Disordered Breathing

Sleep-disordered breathing can cause sleep fragmentation and significant daytime sleepiness. The prevalence of undiagnosed sleep-disordered breathing is higher in women than men (Young et al., 1993), putting women at a higher risk for misdiagnosis, idiopathic hypersomnolence, and possibly chronic fatigue syndrome. Severe snoring (particularly when snorting is present), observed breathing cessation by a bed partner, an awareness of gasping for air, and excessive daytime sleepiness are the most dramatic symptoms of obstructive sleep apnea syndrome (OSAS). This disorder is characterized by the presence of repetitive apneas (total cessation of breathing during sleep of at least 10 seconds) and hypopneas (clear decrease in the volume of air flow by at least 50%, which is associated with either an oxygen desaturation of at least 3% or an arousal). The breathing cessation in OSAS is produced by collapse of the upper airway during inspiration due to low muscle tone. Central apnea is another form of apnea, in which the absence of a central respiratory command leads to cessation of breathing with no respiratory movements. In addition to hypoxemia, apneas often produce arousals, which fragment sleep. The severity of OSAS is measured by the respiratory disturbance index (RDI), which indicates the average number of apneas or hypopneas per hour of sleep. Other symptoms of OSAS include morning headaches, frequent sore throats, and (for premenopausal women) dysmenorrhea or amenorrhea (Guilleminault et al., 1995b). A referral to a sleep disorders specialist is indicated whenever sleep-disordered breathing is suspected.

OSAS is thought to be relatively rare in premenopausal women, with a prevalence rate (approximately 2% of the population) that is about half of that reported for age-matched males (Young et al., 1993). The reduced incidence of OSAS in premenopausal women has been attributed to the presence of progesterone and to gender differences in fat distribution profiles. Although obesity is a risk factor for OSAS in both genders, the upper-body fat deposition that is more typical in men seems to be related to the development of the disorder. In particular, there is evidence that increased neck circumference is a risk factor (Skomro & Kryger, 1999), and that there is more soft tissue loading of the upper airway in men (Whittle et al., 1999). There are also gender-related structural differences in the upper anatomy (Popovic & White, 1995), which may further contribute to the gender difference in the incidence of OSAS. A recent study (Ferini-Strambi et al., 1999) reports a much higher prevalence of OSAS in Italian women. The differences in the prevalence rates among epidemiological samples might be related to differences in criteria used and to differences in sample characteristics.

Another common form of sleep-disordered breathing is Upper Airway Resistance syndrome (UARS) (Guilleminault et al., 1992). The defining clinical characteristic of this syndrome is the presence of excessive daytime sleepiness. Sleepiness results from repeated arousals (Guilleminault et al., 1993), which in UARS are produced by elevations in inspiratory effort that occur before altered airflow is measurable. Thus patients with UARS have a low RDI. The severity of UARS is measured by the respiratory-related arousal index, which is the number of arousals linked to elevations in inspiratory effort per hour of sleep.

Treatment for sleep-disordered breathing typically involves the use of nasal continuous positive airway pressure (nCPAP). An appropriate titration of positive pressure can be extremely effective in relieving OSAS symptoms. Compliance can be an issue, however, because many patients find it difficult to cope with the discomfort and with nasal symptoms. Oxygenation is indicated in some cases. Other treatment approaches for OSAS include surgery, dental appliances, and medications that stimulate breathing. Many of the complex issues associated with the treatment of sleep apnea remain beyond the scope of this chapter, and the reader is referred to Berry (1995) for a comprehensive review.

Periodic Limb Movement Syndrome and Restless Legs Syndrome

Like respiratory sleep disorders, PLMS results in sleep fragmentation and excessive day-time sleepiness. PLMS involves rhythmic extensions of the big toe and dorsoflexions of the ankle, with occasional flexion of the knee and hip (Montplaisir et al., 1994). Each movement lasts between 0.5 and 5 seconds and is identified as an increase of at least 25% over the baseline EMG activity recorded from the anterior tibialis muscle (ASDA, Atlas Task Force, 1993). Periodic limb movements are often associated with EEG arousals and cluster into episodes. The prevalence of PLMS is estimated at 6% in young adults, and it increases with age (Bixler et al., 1982).

RLS is characterized by leg sensations that occur when a person attempts to rest, particularly when lying down. The sensation often interferes with sleep onset, either at the beginning of the night or upon awakening during the night. Patients describe crawling, tingling, or prickling sensations in the legs that are often relieved by leg motion. Thus RLS needs to be assessed as part of the comprehensive assessment of insomnia. Patients with RLS often also have PLMS, and when these co-occur, RLS is associated with involuntary limb movements (ASDA, 1997). Both disorders may be present as a feature of peripheral neuropathies and myelopathies, and they have also been associated with anemia due to iron or folate deficiency (Montplaisir et al., 1994). The prevalence of RLS is unknown. It has recently been estimated at between 9% and 15% (Hening et al., 1999), increasing with age (Roehrs et al., 1983) and during the third trimester of pregnancy (Hertz et al., 1992). The highest prevalence of RLS is among individuals with rheumatoid arthritis (Salih et al., 1994).

Treatment for RLS and PLMS usually involves the administration of dopamine agonist medication. A recent study has indicated that the use of slow-release L-dopa may be effective in facilitating sleep onset and improving sleep maintenance (Collado-Seidel et al., 1999). Opioids, benzodiazepines, anticonvulsants, and adrenergic antagonists have also been used to reduce arousal associated with PLMS (Hening et al., 1999).

EFFECTS OF SUBSTANCES AND THE ENVIRONMENTAL ON SLEEP

Both prescription and nonprescription substances can cause sleep disturbances. The chronic use of drugs, alcohol, and caffeine to induce or to suppress sleepiness may cause adverse effects. Furthermore, many substances taken for other health and lifestyle reasons can affect sleep, as can various factors in a person's environment.

Alcohol

Some individuals self-medicate with alcohol to induce sleep. Continued use results in tolerance to the alcohol as a sleep-inducing agent, and sleep fragmentation becomes more prominent. The amount of alcohol is then often increased, and other sedatives are added in an effort to improve sleep. Some individuals report that they have no sleep disturbance as long as they continue to take substantial amounts of alcohol nightly. Withdrawal from heavy drinking produces a REM rebound effect that is accompanied by restless sleep and nightmares. Sleep fragmentation often persists long after alcohol use is discontinued (Gillin, 1994). Alcohol, like other central nervous system (CNS) depressants, exacerbates sleep apnea and potentiates the effects of hypnotics and other depressants, thus intensifying and prolonging deleterious side effects. Women often have increased sensitivity to alcohol, and there is some evidence that female sex hormones modulate the action of alcohol on μ-opioid receptors in the brain (Carter & Soliman, 1998). Nevertheless, the pharmacokinetics of alcohol do not appear to be significantly influenced by the menstrual cycle (Mumenthaler et al., 1999).

Stimulants

Substances that have stimulating effects on the CNS include caffeine, nicotine, some prescription mediations, cocaine, and amphetamines. The effects of stimulants on sleep include an increase in sleep latency, a decrease in total sleep time, and an increase in spontaneous awakenings (ASDA, 1997; Brown et al., 1995). Caffeine, the most commonly used stimulant, has a plasma half-life of approximately 6 hours, and its effects can be felt long after it has been ingested. Reducing or eliminating the intake of caffeine, particularly in the afternoon and evening, can reduce its negative impact on sleep. For the most part, the pharmacokinetics of caffeine are not significantly influenced by the menstrual cycle (Kamimori et al., 1999), but caffeine elimination may be somewhat slowed in the late luteal (premenstrual) phase (Lane et al., 1992).

The Environment

Environmental factors such as noise level, light intensity, room temperature, and safety are important to the quality and continuity of sleep (ASDA, 1997). Sleeping in an environment that is perceived to be unsafe leads to hypervigilance, which results in lighter sleep. The sense of physical safety at night is extremely important for good sleep. Approximately 75% of battered women experience disturbed sleep and significant daytime sleepiness (Humphreys et al., 1999; Saunders, 1994).

Noise, particularly unpredictable noise (Sanchez & Bootzin, 1985), decreases both the amount of SWS and the continuity of sleep. It also increases sleep fragmentation, body movement, and number of stage shifts. In contrast, continuous white noise is often useful for masking noisy sleep environments. An uncomfortable temperature appears to have a greater negative effect on measures of sleep continuity, primarily during REM sleep, than on the ability to fall asleep at bedtime (Satinoff, 1988).

Sleep problems also need to be considered within the family context. Choices about sleep schedules, sleep environments, and other sleep behaviors may depend on the family environment. For example, some individuals with insomnia might go to bed at times that are not congruent with their own biological clocks, because it is important within their family context that they go to bed at the same time as their bed partners. Concerns about waking up their bed partners may prolong the time these individuals stay in bed worrying about their inability to fall asleep. Family issues may also influence the sleep environment itself. For example, the division of responsibilities for caring for a crying infant at night, or sharing the bed or bedroom with children, can affect parental sleep.

COGNITIVE AND BEHAVIORAL FACTORS AFFECTING SLEEP

It is helpful to consider three types of factors that contribute to insomnia: predisposing, precipitating, and maintaining factors. Predisposing factors include (but are not limited to) general hyperarousability, a tendency to worry, a history of trauma or abuse in the middle of the night, and family history of insomnia. Research has demonstrated that compared to normal controls, persons with insomnia have greater whole-body metabolic rates, body temperature, and heart rate both during the day and at night (Bonnet & Arand, 1995). Although it is not clear whether this heightened arousal is the cause or consequence of poor sleep, several investigators have raised the hypothesis that insomnia results from increased CNS activation that interferes with the sleep system (Bonnet & Arand, 1992; Stepanski et al., 1988).

Stress is one of the most common precipitants of insomnia. It is usually associated with physiological, cognitive, and emotional arousal that contribute to sleep disruptions. Pain, personal loss, and changes associated with important role transitions in life are also common precipitants. Even after the initial precipitating factor is no longer present, the insomnia often persists, in part because individuals with insomnia often adopt ineffective strategies for coping with their sleep problem. These strategies often perpetuate the problem rather than eliminate it. For example, sleeping in is a common strategy for coping with lost sleep. This strategy can lead to irregular sleep–wake schedules that may prolong the sleep difficulties by weakening the underlying sleep–wake rhythm. Insomnia patients commonly become preoccupied with sleep during the day and worry about the consequences of poor sleep at night, thus rendering the bed a cue for stressful arousal rather than for sleep (Bootzin, Epstein, & Wood, 1991). This conditioned arousal is most pronounced among patients who describe "fear" or "dread" associated with going to sleep.

TREATMENT OF PRIMARY INSOMNIA

Primary insomnia is a diagnostic category in the *Diagnostic and Statistical Manual of Mental Disorders*, fourth edition (DSM-IV). It is characterized by difficulty initiating or maintaining sleep that is not attributable solely to extrinsic factors or to other sleep disorders (American Psychiatric Association, 1994). Primary insomnia is twice as prevalent in women as in men and increases with age. Approximately 13% of menstruating women with primary insomnia experience exacerbation of the problem during the premenstrual period (Manber et al., 1997), but premenstrual sleep disturbance and premenstrual exacerbation of insomnia have not been well studied.

Sedative/hypnotics are the most common treatments for insomnia in general practice settings and in psychiatric clinics. A number of effective nonpharmacological interventions for insomnia have been designed and tested alone or in combination with these individuals. These include stimulus control instructions, sleep restriction, relaxation training, paradoxical intention, cognitive therapy, light therapy, and sleep hygiene education. Benzodiazepine hypnotics appear to be more immediately effective, but behavioral therapy can exert significant improvement within 2 weeks (McClusky et al., 1991). Most important, cognitive-behavioral treatment of insomnia is better sustained over time and is associated with greater patient satisfaction than is pharmacotherapy (Morin et al., 1999).

Pharmacological Approaches

The use of sedative/hypnotics to induce sleep is effective and indicated for short-term use (2 to 4 weeks). Tolerance increases with continued use, and as dosage is increased to offset tolerance, daytime carryover effects also increase (ASDA, 1997). Cessation of sedative/hypnotics results in withdrawal symptoms that include severe insomnia. With-drawal symptoms promote psychological dependence, as the individual becomes con-vinced that the hypnotic agent is the only solution. Both physiological and psychologi-cal dependence on medication complicate the treatment of insomnia. Patients with long-term use of hypnotic medications benefit from a gradual taper in combination with cognitive-behavioral components (Kirmil-Gray et al., 1985; Morin et al., 1994). The important cognitive-behavioral components include ample support, preparation for rebound insomnia, and an early introduction of effective cognitive-behavioral skills for improving sleep.

Beyond the intended effect of benzodiazepines to reduce sleep onset latency, decrease the number and duration of nocturnal awakenings, and increase the total sleep time, these agents also decrease REM and delta sleep, and (like all CNS depressants) depress respiration and exacerbate sleep apnea. The pharmacological effects of hypnotics depend upon dose, absorption rate, and serum half-life (Greenblatt, 1992). Hypnotics with long half-lives (e.g., flurazepam) may produce drug hangover and daytime sedation. Hypnotics with short half-lives (e.g., triazolam) may produce rebound insomnia the very same night that the medication is taken.

During the past few years, zolpidem and (more recently) zaleplon, two nonbenzo-diazepine hypnotics, have been available in the United States. To date, the data indicate little to no rebound insomnia upon withdrawal and reduced daytime residual effects (Nicholson, 1994), though some individuals do experience mild rebound insomnia with zolpidem (Nicholson, 1994). Both have very short half-lives (approximately 2.6 hours for zolpidem and approximately 1.5 hours for zaleplon) and are primarily indicated for sleep onset problems.

Given the evidence that progesterone is soporific and acts on the $GABA_A$ receptors, there is a potential for synergy between progesterone and hypnotic medication. Recent data suggest that postmenopausal women are more sensitive to triazolam-induced psy-chomotor performance impairment when progesterone is administered concomitantly (McAuley & Friedman, 1999). However, there does not appear to be any difference in the pharmacodynamics of alprazolam (McAuley & Friedman, 1999) or triazolam (Rukstalis & de Wit, 1999) in relation to the fluctuations of endogenous progesterone across the menstrual cycle, implying that a dose adjustment on the basis of menstrual timing is not required.

Antidepressants with sedating properties are often used in the management of in-somnia. Tricyclic antidepressants and (to a greater extent) monoamine oxidase inhibitors suppress REM sleep, and their discontinuation is associated with rebound REM that is frequently accompanied by nightmares and intense dreams (Minot et al., 1993; Sharpley & Cowen, 1995). Many, but not all, of the new-generation antidepressants produce in-creased physiological arousal during sleep, reduce delta activity, and suppress REM (Armitage et al., 1995b). Serotonin receptor modulators, such as trazodone and nefazo-done, increase sleep continuity and do not reduce SWS (Sharpley & Cowen, 1995), but their overall sedative effect is not limited to the night.

Nonprescription substances that facilitate sleep include camomile tea, valerian root, tryptophan, and melatonin. None of these substances has been shown to be helpful for persistent insomnia. It should also be emphasized that the consumer cannot be assured of purity because these substances are not regulated by the U.S. Food and Drug Administra-tion. Although there are promising results on the sleep-inducing effects of melatonin (e.g.,

Zhdanova et al., 1995), important questions about dose and long-term effects have yet to be answered.

Nonpharmacological Approaches

Two meta-analyses concluded that nonpharmacological interventions for insomnia produce reliable and durable clinical benefits (Morin et al., 1994; Murtagh & Greenwood, 1995). As a group, patients with sleep onset difficulties fell asleep faster after treatment than 81% of untreated controls, and patients with sleep maintenance problems had less disrupted sleep after treatment than 74% of untreated controls (Morin et al., 1994).

Behavioral Components

Teaching a patient to self-administer relaxation exercises (rather than listening to taped instructions) can promote sleep by reducing overall arousal. Patients who tend to worry a lot, either about sleep or about other topics, often benefit from postponing worries that emerge throughout the day to a scheduled daily period of "worry time." This technique has been effective in reducing symptoms of generalized anxiety disorder, but its effects on sleep have not been systematically investigated (Borkovec et al., 1983).

Stimulus control (Bootzin et al., 1991) is a central behavioral component for most successful interventions. The instructions are designed to strengthen the bed as a cue for sleep and to weaken it as a cue for activities that are not consistent with sleep. Stimulus control instructions are also designed to strengthen internal cues for sleep and to stabilize the sleep–wake rhythm. These are achieved by instructing patients to adhere to the following five rules: (1) to go to bed only when sleepy; (2) not to use the bedroom for any activity other than sleep (with the exception of sex); (3) to leave the bed and bedroom when unable to fall asleep; (4) to wake up at a regular time regardless of how well or how long the patients slept at night; and (5) to avoid taking naps unless these naps are short and taken regularly. Adherence and efficacy of the procedure are increased when the rationale for each instruction is explained as it is presented, and when a patient's progress and difficulties are carefully monitored in daily sleep logs and addressed in subsequent follow-up sessions.

The goal of the first rule is to help patients become more sensitive to internal cues of sleepiness, and to increase the likelihood that they will fall asleep quickly. The second rule is designed to remove from the bedroom activities that are associated with arousal. This rule is designed to help break maladaptive bedtime routines and replace them by routines that are less likely to interfere with sleep. The third rule is intended to disassociate the bed from frustration about not being able to fall asleep. Keeping a consistent wake times serves two purposes. In the short run, it is likely to produce some sleep deprivation that will facilitate sleep onset the following night, thus strengthening the association between the bed and sleep. In the long run, consistent wake times affect the biological clock regulating sleep and wakefulness, and help develop a more stable sleep rhythm. The goal of the last rule is to prevent irregular napping that might destabilize the sleep rhythm. A short nap (less than 1 hour) that takes place daily at about the same time is permissible.

Research has shown that the stimulus control procedure is effective both for sleep onset insomnia and for sleep maintenance insomnia. Improvements usually begin after a week or two of following the instructions. Compliance issues need to be carefully examined and addressed for this method to be successful.

Older adults with poor sleep often benefit from the addition of sleep restriction (Spielman et al., 1987). Patients are instructed to restrict the time in bed to their estimated total sleep time, leading to partial sleep deprivation. This initial sleep deprivation helps consolidate sleep and increase sleep efficiency. Patients are then instructed to gradually increase time spent in bed as long as sleep efficiency remains high. With time, the increased sense of control and self-efficacy will lead to longer and more efficient sleep.

Cognitive Components

Cognitive components of treatment typically target a patient's expectations and attribution styles and are designed to increase a sense of self-efficacy. They are usually used in combination with one or more of the behavioral interventions reviewed above. The basic elements of cognitive treatments for insomnia include setting realistic expectations, decatastrophizing the consequences of a bad night, highlighting small gains, examining and changing maladaptive coping styles, and shifting a patient away from attributions that are inconsistent with good sleep. Patients who experience premenstrual insomnia can benefit from the same behavioral strategies and cognitive components. In particular, understanding the time-limited nature of premenstrual exacerbation can prevent the use of maladaptive coping strategies that tend to prolong the duration of insomnia.

Light Exposure

Bright light significantly affects the circadian sleep–wake rhythm. The combination of bright light during wake and total darkness during sleep is a particularly strong entraining influence and can facilitate adjustment to changes in sleep schedules (Czeisler et al., 1989). The direction of the shift depends on the timing of the exposure to light. A phase advance is achieved by light exposure in the morning and can be used in the treatment of insomnia when evidence of delayed sleep tendencies is present. Morning light exposure has been found to reduce sleep onset latency in sleep onset insomnia (Lack, 1995; Guilleminault et al., 1995a). Evening light has been found to delay wake-up time, increase total sleep (Lack & Wright, 1993), and increase sleep efficiency (Campbell et al., 1993) in those with sleep maintenance insomnia. The timing and dose of light exposure is important, and a consultation with a sleep specialist is recommended. Possible side effects of light therapy include eye irritation and headache. Light therapy should not be used in patients with retinopathies.

PARASOMNIAS

The parasomnias include unusual sleep-related behaviors such as sleepwalking, night terrors, sleep talking, teeth grinding, bedwetting, REM behavior disorders, and nightmares. Some parasomnias, such as sleepwalking, night terrors, and sleep talking, are disorders of partial arousal from SWS (deep sleep) and are most common during childhood, with no significant gender differences (Ohayon et al., 1997). Other parasomnias, such as REM behavior disorders and nightmares, occur during REM sleep and emerge during adulthood. REM behavior disorder is most common in men (ASDA, 1997), whereas night-mares and sleep-related eating are twice as common in women (Ohayon et al., 1997; Schenck & Mahowald, 1994). There have been a few reports of premenstrual exacerba-tion of sleepwalking (Schenck & Mahowald, 1995). The parasomnias require careful dif-ferential diagnoses but remain beyond the scope of this chapter.

Prescription of benzodiazepines is the most common treatment for both REM and NREM parasomnias (e.g., Keefauver & Guilleminault, 1994). It is indicated when dan-gerous behaviors are involved and when there is a change in the sleep environment so that the parasomnia might be more dangerous or embarrassing. To minimize injuries re-lated to odd sleep behaviors, steps need to be taken to make the sleep environment safe (e.g., covering glass windows, locking doors and windows, and placing an alarm on the bedroom door). Parasomnias often worsen during periods of stress or sleep deprivation, and even when sleep is fragmented as a result of high caffeine intake (Lee et al., 1999). The frequency of parasomnia is often reduced with relaxation, stress management tech-niques, and the prevention of sleep deprivation and sleep fragmentation. Hypnosis has been reported efficacious for night terrors and sleepwalking (Reid et al., 1981). Chronic nightmares, considered a parasomnia in the sleep disorders nosology, can be treated with a cognitive-behavioral technique called "imagery rehearsal" (Krakow et al., 1995). The patient is instructed to recall the nightmare in detail, change its content so it is no longer frightening, and visualize the new set of images.

COMORBID PSYCHIATRIC DISORDERS

The high prevalence of psychiatric comorbidity in those with insomnia poses a therapeu-tic challenge. Should one treat the psychopathology first and then treat residual sleep symptoms, or should one target the sleep difficulties without waiting to see whether treat-ment of the comorbid psychiatric condition resolves the sleep problem? A report on the patterns of symptomatic recovery in psychotherapy indicates that sleep complaints do not change as a result of general psychotherapy (Kopta et al., 1994) and implies that sleep complaints need to be specifically targeted if they are to be changed. Components from the nonpharmacological interventions for sleep can be integrated into the treatment of the presenting problem, and the impact of any pharmacological agent on sleep symptoms needs to be considered. The following is a review of the most salient sleep symptoms and sleep abnormalities in mood and anxiety disorders.

Mood Disorders

Patients with major depression experience difficulties with sleep onset, sleep mainte-nance, and/or early morning awakenings. The main alterations in sleep architecture of depressed patients include a decrease in the latency to the first REM episode; an in-crease in the amount of REM sleep in the beginning of the night (e.g., Kupfer & Reynolds, 1992); and a reduction in the amount of SWS, which is more pronounced in men than in women (Reynolds et al., 1990). Although these alterations in EEG sleep parameters are not unique to mood disorders (Gillin et al., 1990; Mendelson et al., 1987), they appear to predict therapeutic efficacy (e.g., Vogel, 1975). Another gender difference in sleep abnormality associated with depression is a greater amount of fast-frequency EEG activity during sleep in depressed women than in depressed men (Armitage et al., 1995a). Daytime sleepiness may also be an associated feature of depression. Individuals with major depression tend to spend a greater amount of time in bed—a fact that may contribute to reports of daytime somnolence more than any actual increase in the amount of time spent sleeping. Sleepiness per se is more commonly reported with cyclothymia or bipolar depression.

Sleep abnormalities of patients with bipolar disorder during a depressive episode are similar to those found in patients with major depression. A manic episode is typically associated with short sleep durations, long sleep latencies, and decreased SWS (ASDA, 1997). In contrast, the sleep of patients with dysthymia is comparable to that of normal controls (Arriaga et al., 1990).

Anxiety Disorders

Although individuals with insomnia frequently (50%) have high scores on anxiety scales (Mellinger et al., 1985), the proportion of those with self-reported insomnia meeting DSM-III diagnostic criteria for anxiety disorders in one study was only about 15% (Tan et al., 1984). On the other hand, patients with generalized anxiety disorder and patients with obsessive–compulsive disorder frequently complain about difficulties initiating or maintaining sleep (Insel et al., 1982; Reynolds et al., 1983). Sleep onset difficulties of patients with obsessive–compulsive disorder are often related to obsessive or compulsive behaviors that focus on sleep, such as checking rituals at bedtime (Insel et al., 1982). About a third of patients with panic disorder report repeated nocturnal panic episodes, the majority of which commonly arise out of NREM sleep (Mellman & Uhde, 1989). Sleep abnormalities associated with posttraumatic stress disorder include recurrent disturbing nightmares; a greater number of arousals and awakenings, particularly from REM sleep; and extended time awake after sleep onset compared with controls (e.g., Mellman et al., 1995).

SUMMARY AND CONCLUSIONS

In the past decade, sleep researchers have begun to pay attention to factors that are specific to women's sleep. There is an accumulation of evidence that gonadal hormones affect sleep and circadian rhythms, but the clinical significance of these findings is not clear. Attention to factors such as menstrual cycle phase and hormonal status will improve the diagnosis and treatment of sleep disorders in women. Treatment of women's sleep disturbances can be further improved by research into the impact of endogenous and exogenous hormones on sleep. If, as suggested by Manber and Armitage (1999), disruptions in sleep continuity are caused by an abnormally sharp premenstrual drop in progesterone then clinical trials with different regimens of hormonal therapy could lead to improvement in the treatment of insomnia in women. Similarly, if we understand the impact of repeated monthly fluctuations in the amplitude of the temperature rhythm, we may be able to improve women's ability to adapt to shift work and the impact of shift work on the reproductive system. The increased attention to the effects of gonadal hormones on sleep has clearly indicated that the issues are complex, and that many questions remain unanswered.

REFERENCES

American Psychiatric Association. (1994). *Diagnostic and statistical manual of mental disorders* (4th ed.). Washington, DC: Author.

American Sleep Disorders Association (ASDA). (1997). *The International Classification of Sleep Disorders: Diagnostic and coding manual*. Rochester, MN: Author.

American Sleep Disorders Association (ASDA), Atlas Task Force. (1993). Recording and scoring leg movements. *Sleep, 16*, 748–759.

Armitage, R., Hudson, A., Trivedi, M., et al. (1995a). Sex differences in the distribution of EEG frequencies during sleep: Unipolar depressed outpatients. *Journal of Affective Disorders, 34*, 121–129.

Armitage, R., Trivedi, M., Rush, A. J., et al. (1995b). The effects of fluoxetine on period-analyzed sleep EEG in depression. *Sleep Research, 24*, 381.

Arriaga, F., Rosasdo, P., & Paiva, T. (1990). The sleep of dysthymic patients: A comparison with normal controls. *Biological Psychiatry, 27*, 649–656.

Asplund, R., & Aberg, H. (1995). Body mass index and sleep in women aged 40 to 64 years. *Maturitas, 22*, 1–8.

Ballenger, C. (1976). Subjective sleep disturbance at the menopause. *Journal of Psychosomatic Research, 20*, 509–513.

Barrett, J., Lack, L., & Morris, M. (1993). The sleep-evoked decrease of body temperature. *Sleep, 16*(2), 93–99.

Berry, R. (1995). Sleep related breathing disorders. In R. George, R. Light, M. Matthay, & R. Matthay (Eds.), *Chest medicine: Essentials of pulmonary and critical care medicine* (2nd ed., pp. 125–140). Baltimore: Williams & Wilkins.

Berthon-Jones, M., & Sullivan, C. (1984). Ventilation and arousal responses to hypercapnia in normal sleeping humans. *Journal of Applied Physiology, 57*(1), 59–67.

Bixler, E. O., Kales, A., Vela-Bueno, A., et al. (1982). Nocturnal myoclonus and nocturnal myoclonic activity in a normal population. *Research Communications in Chemical Pathology and Pharmacology, 36*, 129–140.

Bliwise, D. (1994). Normal aging. In M. Kryger, T. Roth, & W. Dement (Eds.), *Principles and practices of sleep medicine* (pp. 26–39). Philadelphia: W.B. Saunders.

Bonnet, M., & Arand, D. (1992). Caffeine use as a model of chronic and acute insomnia. *Sleep, 15*, 526–536.

Bonnet, M., & Arand, D. (1995). Twenty-four hour metabolic rate in insomniacs and matched normal sleepers. *Sleep, 18*, 581–588.

Bonnet, M., & Arand, D. (1997). Heart rate variability: Sleep stage, time of night, and arousal influences. *Electroencephalography and Clinical Neurophysiology, 102*(5), 390–396.

Bootzin, R., Epstein, D., & Wood, J. (1991). Stimulus control instructions. In P. Hauri (Ed.), *Case studies in insomnia* (pp. 19–28). New York: Plenum Press.

Borkovec, T. D., Wilkinson, L., Folensbee, R., et al. (1983). Stimulus control applications to the treatment of worry. *Behaviour Research and Therapy, 21*(3), 247–251.

Brown, S. L., Salive, M. E., Pahor, M., et al. (1995). Occult caffeine as a source of sleep problems in an older population. *Journal of the American Geriatrics Society, 43*, 860–864.

Brownell, L., West, P., & Kryger, M. (1986). Breathing during sleep in normal pregnant women. *American Review of Respiratory Disease, 133*, 38–41.

Burgess, H. J., Trinder, J., & Kim, Y. (1996). Cardiac parasympathetic nervous system activity does not increase in anticipation of sleep. *Journal of Sleep Research, 5*, 83–89.

Burgess, H. J., Trinder, J., Kim, Y., et al. (1997). Sleep and circadian influences on cardiac autonomic nervous system activity. *American Journal of Physiology, 273*(4, Pt 2), 1761–1768.

Campbell, S., Dawson, D., & Anderson, M. (1993). Alleviation of sleep maintenance insomnia with time exposure to bright light. *Journal of the American Geriatrics Society, 41*, 829–836.

Campbell, S., Gillin, J., & Kripke, D. (1989). Gender differences in the circadian temperature rhythms of healthy elderly subjects: Relationships to sleep quality. *Sleep, 12*(6), 529–536.

Carter, A., & Soliman, M. R. (1998). Estradiol and progesterone alter ethanol-induced effects on mu-opioid receptors in specific brain regions of ovariectomized rats. *Life Sciences, 62*(2), 93–101.

Coble, P. A., Reynolds, C. F., III, Houck, P., et al. (1994). Childbearing in women with and without a history of affective disorder: I. Psychiatric symptomatology. *Comprehensive Psychiatry, 35*, 205–214.

Collado-Seidel, V., Kazenwadel, J., Wetter, T. C., et al. (1999). A controlled study of additional sr-L-dopa in L-dopa-responsive restless legs syndrome with late-night symptoms. *Neurology, 52*(2), 285–290.

Colrain, I. M., Trinder, J., & Fraser, G. (1990). Ventilation during sleep onset in normal females. *Sleep, 13*(6), 491–501.

Colrain, I. M., Trinder, J., Fraser, G., et al. (1987). Ventilation during sleep onset. *Journal of Applied Physiology, 63*(5), 2067–2074.

Czeisler, C., Kronauer, R., Allen, J., et al. (1989). Bright light induction of strong (type 0) resetting of the human circadian pacemaker. *Science, 244*, 1328–1333.

Czeisler, C., Weitzman, E., & Moore-Ede, M. (1980). Human sleep: Its duration and organization depend on its circadian phase. *Science, 210*, 1264–1267.

Douglas, N., White, D., Weil, J., et al. (1982). Hypercapnic ventilatory response in sleeping adults. *American Review of Respiratory Disease, 126*, 758–762.

Driver, H., Dijk, D., Werth, E., et al. (1996). Sleep and the sleep electroencephalogram across the menstrual cycle in young healthy women. *Journal of Clinical Endocrinology and Metabolism, 81*, 728–735.

Ferini-Strambi, L., Zucconi, M., Castronovo, V., et al. (1999). Snoring and sleep apnea: A population study in Italian women. *Sleep, 22*(7), 859–864.

Friess, E., Tagaya, H., Trachsel, L., et al. (1997). Progesterone-induced changes in sleep in male subjects. *American Journal of Physiology, 272*(5, Pt. 1), E885–E891.

Gee, K., Bolger, M., Brinton, R., et al. (1988). Steroid modulation of the chloride ionophore in rat brain: Structure–activity requirements, regional dependence, and mechanism of action. *Journal of Pharmacology and Experimental Therapeutics, 246*(2), 803–812.

Gillberg, M., & Akerstedt, T. (1982). Body temperature and sleep at different times of day. *Sleep, 5*(4), 378–388.

Gillin, J. C. (1994). Sleep and psychoactive drugs of abuse and dependence. In M. Kryger, T. Roth, & W. Dement (Eds.), *Principles and practices of sleep medicine* (2nd ed., pp. 934–942). Philadelphia: W.B. Saunders.

Gillin, J. C., Smith, T. L., Irwin, M., et al. (1990). Short REM latency in primary alcoholic patients with secondary depression. *American Journal of Psychiatry, 147*, 106–109.

Glotzbach, S., & Heller, H. (1994). Temperature regulation. In M. Kryger, T. Roth, & W. Dement (Eds.), *Principles and practice of sleep medicine* (2nd ed., pp. 201–275). Philadelphia: W.B. Saunders.

Goodman, D., Brodie, C., & Ayida, G. (1988). Restless leg syndrome in pregnancy. *British Medical Journal, 297*, 1101–1102.

Gora, J., Colrain, I., & Trinder, J. (1999). Respiratory-related evoked potentials at the transition from wake- to sleep-type activity in the EEG. *Journal of Sleep Research, 8*(2), 123–134.

Greenblatt, D. J. (1992). Pharmacology of benzodiazepine hypnotics. *Journal of Clinical Psychiatry, 53*(6, Suppl.), 7–13.

Guilleminault, C., Clerk, A., Black, J., et al. (1995a). Nondrug treatment trials in psychophysiological insomnia. *Archives of Internal Medicine, 155*, 838–844.

Guilleminault, C., Stoohs, R., Clerk, A., et al. (1993). A cause of excessive daytime sleepiness: The upper airway resistance syndrome. *Chest, 104*(3), 781–787.

Guilleminault, C., Stoohs, R., Clerk, A., et al. (1992). From obstructive sleep apnea syndrome to upper airway resistance syndrome: Consistency of daytime sleepiness. *Sleep, 15*(6, Suppl.), S13–S16.

Guilleminault, C., Stoohs, R., Kim, Y., et al. (1995b). Upper airway sleep-disordered breathing in women. *Annals of Internal Medicine, 122,* 493–501.

Hening, W., Allen, R., Earley, C., et al. (1999). The treatment of restless legs syndrome and periodic limb movement disorder: An American Academy of Sleep Medicine review. *Sleep, 22*(7), 970–999.

Henke, K., Dempsey, J., Kowitz, J., et al. (1990). Effects of sleep-induced increases in upper airway resistance on ventilation. *Journal of Applied Physiology, 69,* 617–624.

Hertz, G., Fast, A., Feinsilver, S., et al. (1992). Sleep in normal late pregnancy. *Sleep, 15*(3), 246–251.

Humphreys, J., Lee, K., Neylan, T., et al. (1999). Sleep patterns of sheltered battered women. *Journal of Nursing Scholarship, 31*(2), 139–143.

Insel, T., Gillin, C., Moore, A., et al. (1982). The sleep of patients with obsessive–compulsive disorder. *Archives of General Psychiatry, 39,* 1372–1377.

Ishizuka, Y., Pollak, C., Shirakawa, S., et al. (1992). Sleep spindle frequency changes during the menstrual cycle. *Journal of Sleep Research, 3,* 26–29.

Kamimori, G., Joubert, A., Otterstetter, R., et al. (1999). The effect of the menstrual cycle on the pharmacokinetics of caffeine in normal, healthy eumenorrheic females. *European Journal of Clinical Pharmacology, 55,* 445–449.

Keefauver, S., & Guilleminault, C. (1994). Sleep terrors and sleep walking. In M. Kryger, T. Roth, & W. Dement (Eds.), *Principles and practices of sleep medicine* (2nd ed., pp. 5567–5573). Philadelphia: W.B. Saunders.

Kirmil-Gray, K., Eagleston, J., Thorensen, C., et al. (1985). Brief consultation and stress management treatment for drug-dependent insomnia: Effects on sleep quality, self-efficacy, and daytime stress. *Journal of Behavioral Medicine, 8,* 79–99.

Kopta, S., Howard, K., Lowry, J., et al. (1994). Patterns of symptomatic recovery in psychotherapy. *Journal of Consulting and Clinical Psychology, 62,* 1009–1016.

Krakow, B., Kellner, R., Pathak, D., et al. (1995). Imagery rehearsal treatment for chronic nightmares. *Behaviour Research and Therapy, 33,* 837–843.

Kryger, M., Roth, T., & Dement, W. (Eds.). (2000). *Principles and practices of sleep medicine* (3rd ed.). Philadelphia: W.B. Saunders.

Kupfer, D., & Reynolds, C. I. (1992). Sleep and affective disorders. In E. Paykel (Ed.), *Handbook of affective disorders* (2nd ed., pp. 311–323). Edinburgh: Churchill Livingstone.

Lack, L., & Wright, H. (1993). The effect of evening bright light in delaying the circadian rhythms and lengthening the sleep of early morning awakening insomniacs. *Sleep, 16,* 436–443.

Lack, L., Wright, H., & Paynter, D. (1995). The treatment of sleep onset insomnia with morning bright light. *Sleep Research, 24A,* 338.

Lane, J., Steege, J., Rupp, S., et al. (1992). Menstrual cycle effects on caffeine elimination in the human female. *European Journal of Clinical Pharmacology, 43,* 543–546.

Lee, K. A. (1988). Circadian temperature rhythms in relation to menstrual cycle phase. *Journal of Biological Rhythms, 3,* 255–263.

Lee, K. A. (1998). Alterations in sleep during pregnancy and postpartum: A review of 30 years of research. *Sleep Medicine Reviews, 2,* 231–242.

Lee, K. A., McEnary, G., & Weekes, D. (1999). Gender differences in sleep patterns for early adolescents. *Journal of Adolescent Health, 24*(1), 16–20.

Lee, K. A., McEnary, G., & Weekes, D. (2000a). REM sleep and mood state in childbearing women: Sleepy or weepy? *Sleep, 23*(7), 877–885.

Lee, K. A., Shaver, J. F., Giblin, E. C., et al. (1990). Sleep patterns related to menstrual cycle phase and premenstrual affective symptoms. *Sleep, 13,* 403–409.

Lee, K. A., Zaffke, M. E., & Baratte-Beebe. (in press). Restless legs syndrome and sleep disturbances during pregnancy: The role of folate and iron. *Journal of Women's Health and Gender-
Based Medicine.*

Lee, K. A., Zaffke, M. E., & McEnary, G. (2000b). Parity and sleep patterns during and after pregnancy. *Obstetrics and Gynecology, 95*(1), 14–18.

Lugaresi, E., Cirignotta, F., & Zucconi, M. (1983). Good and poor sleepers: An epidemiological
survey of San Marino population. In C. Guilleminault & E. Lugaresi (Eds.), *Sleep/wake disorders: Natural history, epidemiology, and longterm evolution* (pp. 1–12). New York: Raven
Press.

Manber, R., & Armitage, R. (1999). Sex, steroids, and sleep: A review. *Sleep, 22*(5), 540–555.

Manber, R., & Bootzin, R. (1997). Sleep and the menstrual cycle. *Health Psychology, 16*, 1–6.

Manber, R., Bootzin, R., & Bradley, K. (1997). Menstrual cycle effects on sleep of female insomniacs. *Sleep Research, 26*, 248.

Matthews, K., Wing, R., Kuller, L., et al. (1990). Influence of natural menopause on psychological
characteristics and symptoms of middle-aged healthy women. *Journal of Consulting and Clinical Psychology, 58*, 345–351.

McAuley, J., & Friedman, C. (1999). Influence of endogenous progesterone on alprazolam
pharmacodynamics. *Journal of Clinical Psychopharmacology, 19*, 233–239.

McClusky, H., Milby, J., Switzer, P., et al. (1991). Efficacy of behavioral versus triazolam treatment
in persistent sleep-onset insomnia. *American Journal of Psychiatry, 148*, 121–126.

Mellinger, G., Balter, M., & Uhlenhuth, E. (1985). Insomnia and its treatment: Prevalence and correlates. *Archives of General Psychiatry, 42*, 225–232.

Mellman, T., Kulick-Bell, R., Ashlock, L., et al. (1995). Sleep events among veterans with combat-
related posttraumatic stress disorder. *American Journal of Psychiatry, 152*(1), 110–115.

Mellman, T., & Uhde, T. (1989). Sleep panic attacks: New clinical findings and theoretical implications. *Amercian Journal of Psychiatry, 146*(9), 1204–1207.

Mendelson, W. B., Sack, D. A., James, S. P., et al. (1987). Frequency analysis of the sleep EEG in
depression. *Psychiatry Research, 21*, 89–94.

Minot, R., Luthringer, R., & Macher, J. (1993). Effects of miclobemide on the psychophysiology of
sleep/wake cycle: A neuroelectrophysiological study of depressed paients administered with
miclobemide. *International Clinical Psychopharmaology, 7*, 181–189.

Montplaisir, J., Godbout, R., Pelletier, G., et al. (1994). Restless legs syndrome and periodic limb
movements during sleep. In M. Kryger, T. Roth, & W. Dement (Eds.), *Principles and practices
of sleep medicine* (pp. 589–597). Philadelphia: W.B. Saunders.

Morin, C., Colecchi, C., Stone, J., et al. (1999). Behavioral and pharmacological therapies for late-
life insomnia: A randomized controlled trial. *Journal of the American Medical Association,
281*, 991–999.

Morin, C., Culbert, J., & Schwartz, S. (1994). Nonpharmacological interventions for insomnia: A
meta-analysis of treatment efficacy. *American Journal of Psychiatry, 151*, 1172–1180.

Mumenthaler, M., Taylor, J., O'Hara, R., et al. (1999). Effects of menstrual cycle and female sex
steroids on ethanol pharmacokinetics. *Alcoholism: Clinical and Experimental Research, 23*,
250–255.

Murtagh, D., & Greenwood, K. (1995). Identifying effective psychological treatments for insomnia: A meta-analysis. *Journal of Consulting and Clinical Psychology, 63*, 79–89.

Nicholson, A. (1994). Hypnotics: Clinical pharmacology and therapeutics. In M. Kryger, T. Roth,
& W. Dement (Eds.), *Principles and practice of sleep medicine* (2nd ed., pp. 355–363). Philadelphia: W.B. Saunders.

Ohayon, M., Morselli, P., & Guilleminault, C. (1997). Prevalence of nightmares and their relationship to psychopathology and daytime functioning in insomnia subjects. *Sleep, 20*, 340–348.

Owens, J. F., & Mathews, K. A. (1998). Sleep disturbance in healthy middle aged women.
Maturitas, 30, 41–50.

Parry, B., Berga, S., Mostofi, N., et al. (1997). Plasma melatonin circadian rhythms during the menstrual cycle and after light therapy in premenstrual dysphoric disorder and normal control subjects. *Journal of Biological Rhythms, 12,* 47–64.

Parry, B., Mendelson, W., Duncan, W., et al. (1989). Longitudinal sleep EEG, temperature, and activity measurements across the menstrual cycle in patients with premenstrual depression and age matched controls. *Psychiatry Research, 30,* 285–303.

Phillipson, E., & Bowes, G. (1986). Control of breathing during sleep. In N. Cherniack & J. Widdicombe (Eds.), *Handbook of physiology: Control of breathing* (Section 3, Vol. 2, pp. 649–690). Bethesda, MD: American Physiological Society.

Pickett, C., Regensteiner, J., Woodward, W., et al. (1989). Progestin and estrogen reduce sleep-disordered breathing in postmenopausal women. *Journal of Applied Physiology, 66,* 1656–1661.

Polo-Kantola, P., Erkkola, R., Helenium, H., et al. (1998). When does estrogen replacement therapy improve sleep quality? *American Journal of Obstetrics and Gynecology, 178*(5), 1002–1009.

Popovic, R. M., & White, D. P. (1995). Influence of gender on waking genioglossal electromyogram and upper airway resistance. *American Journal of Respiratory and Critical Care Medicine, 152,* 725–773.

Popovic, R. M., & White, D. P. (1998). Upper airway muscle activity in normal women: influence of hormonal status. *Journal of Applied Physiology, 84*(3), 1055–1062.

Purdie, D., Empson, J., Crichton, C., et al. (1995). Hormone replacement therapy, sleep quality and psychological well-being. *British Journal of Obstetrics and Gynaecology, 102,* 735–739.

Rechtschaffen, A., & Kales, A. (Eds.). (1968). *A manual of standardized terminology, techniques and scoring system for sleep stages of human subjects.* Los Angeles: UCLA Brain Information Service/Brain Research institute.

Reid, W., Ahmed, I., & Levie, C. (1981). Treatment of sleep walking: A controlled study. *American Journal of Psychotherapy, 35,* 27–37.

Reynolds, C. F., III, Kupfer, D., Thase, M., et al. (1990). Sleep, gender, and depression: An analysis of gender effects on the electroencephalographic sleep of 302 depressed outpatients. *Biological Psychiatry, 28,* 673–684.

Reynolds, C. F., III, Shaw, D., Newton, T., et al. (1983). EEG sleep in outpatients with generalized anxiety. *Psychiatry Research, 8,* 81–89.

Roehrs, T., Zorick, F., Sicklesteel, J., et al. (1983). Age related sleep–wake disorders at a sleep disorders clinic. *Journal of the American Geriatrics Society, 31,* 364–370.

Rukstalis, M., & de Wit, H. (1999). Effects of triazolam at three phases of the menstrual cycle. *Journal of Clinical Psychopharmacology, 19,* 450–458.

Salih, A. M., Gray, R. E., Mills, K. R., et al. (1994). A clinical, serological and neurophysiological study of restless legs syndrome in rheumatoid arthritis. *British Journal of Rheumatology, 33*(1), 60–63.

Sanchez, R., & Bootzin, R. (1985). A comparison of white noise and music: Effects of predictable and unpredictable sounds on sleep. *Sleep Research, 14,* 121.

Satinoff, E. (1988). Thermal influences on REM sleep. In R. Lydic & J. Biebuyck (Eds.), *Clinical physiology of sleep* (pp. 135–144). New York: Oxford University Press.

Saunders, D. G. (1994). Posttraumatic stress symptom profiles of battered women: A comparison of survivors in two settings. *Violence and Victims, 9,* 31–44.

Scharf, M., McDonnald, M., Stover, R., et al. (1997). Effects of estrogen replacement therapy on rates of cyclic alternating patterns and hot-flash events during sleep in postmenopausal women: A pilot study. *Clinical Therapeutics, 19,* 304–311.

Schenck, C., & Mahowald, M. (1994). Review of nocturnal sleep-related eating disorders. *International Journal of Eating Disorders, 15*(4), 343–356.

Schenck, C., & Mahowald, M. (1995). Two cases of premenstrual sleep terrors and injurious sleepwalking. *Journal of Psychosomatic Obstetrics and Gynaecology, 16,* 79–84.

Schiff, I., Regestein, Q., Tulchinsky, D., et al. (1979). Effects of estrogen on sleep and psychological state of hypogonadal women. *Journal of the American Medical Association, 242*, 2405–2407.

Schoene, R. B., Robertson, T., Pierson, D. J., et al. (1981). Respiratory drives and exercise in menstrual cycles of athletic and non athletic women. *Journal of Applied Physiology, 50*, 1300–1305.

Schutte, S., Del Conte, A., Doghramji, K., et al. (1994). Snoring during pregnancy and its impact on fetal outcome. *Sleep Research, 23*, 325.

Selye, H. (1941). Acquired adaptation to the anesthetic effect of steroid hormones. *Journal of Immunology, 41*, 259–268.

Severino, S., Wagner, M., Hurt, S., et al. (1991). High nocturnal temperature in premenstrual syndrome and late luteal phase dysphoric disorder. *American Journal of Psychiatry, 148*, 1329–1335.

Sharpley, A., & Cowen, P. (1995). Effect of pharmacologic treatments on the sleep of depressed patients. *Biological Psychiatry, 37*(2), 85–98.

Skomro, R., & Kryger, M. (1999). Clinical presentations of obstructive sleep apnea syndrome. *Progress in Cardiovascular Disease, 41*(5), 331–340.

Somers, V., Dyken, M., Mark, A., et al. (1993). Sympathetic-nerve activity during sleep in normal subjects. *New England Journal of Medicine, 328*, 303–307.

Spielman, A., Saskin, P., & Thorpy, M. (1987). Treatment of chronic insomnia by restriction of time in bed. *Sleep, 10*, 45–56.

Stepanski, E., Zorick, F., Roehrs, T., et al. (1988). Daytime alertness in patients with chronic insomnia compared with asymptomatic control subjects. *Sleep, 11*, 54–60.

Tan, T., Kales, J., Kales, A., et al. (1984). Biopsychobehavioral correlates of insomnia: IV. Diagnoses based on DSM-III. *American Journal of Psychiatry, 141*, 356–362.

Vogel, G. (1975). A review of REM sleep deprivation. *Archives of General Psychiatry, 32*, 749–761.

Voordouw, B. C., Euser, R., Verdonk, R. E., et al. (1992). Melatonin and the melatonin–progestin combinations alter pituitary–ovarian function in women and can inhibit ovulation. *Journal of Clinical Endocrinology and Metabolism, 74*, 108–117.

Waterhouse, J., Minors, D., & Waterhouse, M. (1990). *Your body clock: How to live with it, not against it*. New York: Oxford University Press.

White, D. (1986). Occlusion pressure and ventilation during sleep in normal humans. *Journal of Applied Physiology, 61*(4), 1279–1287.

Whittle, A. T., Marshall, I., Mortimore, I. L., et al. (1999). Neck soft tissue and fat distribution: Comparison between normal men and women by magnetic resonance imaging. *Thorax, 4*(4), 323–328.

Woodward, S., & Freedman, R. (1994). The thermoregulatory effects of menopause hot flashes on sleep. *Sleep, 17*, 497–501.

Young, T., Palta, M., Dempsey, J., et al. (1993). The occurrence of sleep-disordered breathing among middle-aged adults. *New England Journal of Medicine, 328*, 1230–1235.

Zhdanova, I., Wurtman, R., Lynch, H., et al. (1995). Sleep inducing effects of low melatonin doses. *Sleep Research, 24*, 66.

16

Body Dysmorphic Disorder

KATHARINE A. PHILLIPS

Body dysmorphic disorder (BDD), also known as dysmorphophobia, is an intriguing, underrecognized, and sometimes difficult-to-treat condition that is relatively common in women. BDD was first described more than a century ago (Morselli, 1891), and since then has been reported around the world (Phillips, 1991). Although the disorder's symptoms may sound trivial, they can cause severe distress, notably impaired functioning and suicide (Phillips et al., 1993).

Classified as a somatoform disorder in the *Diagnostic and Statistical Manual of Mental Disorders*, fourth edition (DSM-IV), BDD consists of a distressing and/or impairing preoccupation with a nonexistent or slight defect in appearance (American Psychiatric Association, 1994). In addition, the appearance preoccupations must not be better accounted for by another psychiatric disorder, such as anorexia nervosa. BDD's delusional variant is classified in DSM-IV as delusional disorder, somatic type. Delusional BDD can be double-coded as both delusional disorder and BDD (that is, delusional patients may receive both diagnoses), reflecting the likelihood that the disorder's delusional and nondelusional variants are the same disorder spanning a spectrum of insight, rather than two distinct disorders (Phillips et al., 1994).

Despite BDD's long historical tradition, systematic research on it has only recently begun. Currently, little is known about gender-related aspects of BDD, although research on these and other aspects of BDD is rapidly increasing. This chapter provides a clinically focused overview of BDD, including its prevalence, clinical features, diagnosis, and treatment, as well as what is known about gender-related aspects of this disorder.

EPIDEMIOLOGY/PREVALENCE

The prevalence of BDD in the community is unclear. One community survey ($n = 673$) in Florence, Italy, reported a 1-year prevalence figure of 0.7%; in this study, all individuals with BDD were women (Faravelli et al., 1997). Community studies from the United States have reported rates of 2.3% (in adolescents; Mayville et al., 1999) and 1.1% (Bienvenu et al., 2000). In contrast, a study of 102 undergraduate students, the majority of whom were women, found a much higher rate of 13% (Biby, 1998). A limitation of these studies is that they do not appear to have used a reliable and valid instrument for diagnosing BDD. BDD has been reported in 12% of dermatology patients (Phillips et al., 2000) and 6–15% of patients seeking cosmetic surgery (Ishigooka et al., 1998; Sarwer et al., 1998a, 1998b). Reported rates of BDD in psychiatric settings range from 8–37% in patients with obsessive–compulsive disorder (OCD) (Brawman-Mintzer et al., 1995; Hollander et al., 1993; Simeon et al., 1995), 11–13% in patients with social phobia (Brawman-Mintzer et al., 1995; Wilhelm et al., 1997), 26% in patients with trichotillomania (Soriano et al., 1996), to 0–42% in patients with major depression (Brawman-Mintzer et al., 1995; Nierenberg et al., in press; Perugi et al., 1998; Phillips et al., 1996).

CLINICAL FEATURES

Demographic Characteristics

The reported sex ratio of BDD has varied in different studies. In the largest published series of patients with DSM-IV BDD ($n = 188$), 49% were women (Phillips & Diaz, 1997). Some clinical series have contained more men than women (59% in Perugi et al., 1997a, and 60% in Hollander et al., 1993), whereas another had more women than men (76% in Veale et al., 1996a). In the only published series of children and adolescents with BDD, nearly all (91%) of the subjects were female (Albertini & Phillips, 1999); because BDD's age of onset appears similar for women and men, the large percentage of females in this study probably reflects their greater willingness to seek evaluation and treatment.

Most studies have found that a majority of patients with BDD have never been married (Phillips et al., 1994). Two studies that assessed gender differences in BDD found that 17% (Perugi et al., 1997a) and 22% (Phillips & Diaz, 1997) of women were married, with the latter study finding that women were more likely to be married than were men.

Bodily Preoccupations

Individuals with BDD are preoccupied with the thought that some aspect of their appearance is unattractive, ugly, deformed, or "not right" in some way. A study from the United States found that women with BDD are most often preoccupied with their skin (71%), hair (52%), or nose (40%) (Phillips & Diaz, 1997), whereas a study from Italy found that they are most often preoccupied with their face (38%) and legs (25%) (Perugi et al., 1997a). However, the appearance concerns can involve any body area and may involve overall appearance. The U.S. study found that women were more likely than men to focus on their hips and weight, whereas men were more likely to focus on their genitals and body build; women were more likely to view themselves as too large or fat, whereas men were more likely to consider themselves too small and inadequately muscular (Phillips & Diaz, 1997). Although hair concerns were equally common in men and women, men were more likely to worry about thinning hair. In the study from Italy, women were more likely to focus on their breasts and legs, and men were more likely to focus on their genitals, height, and excessive body hair (Perugi, 1997a).

BDD preoccupations are distressing, time-consuming, and usually difficult to resist or control. The preoccupations are typically associated with low self-esteem (Biby, 1998; Rosen & Ramirez, 1998), rejection sensitivity (Phillips et al., 1996), and feelings of shame, embarrassment, and unworthiness (Phillips, 1996). Insight in BDD is usually poor or absent. One study ($n = 100$) found that more than half of subjects had beliefs about their perceived defects that were delusional (Phillips et al., 1994). A majority also have prominent ideas or delusions of reference, believing that others take special notice of the supposed defects—for example, talk about them, stare at them, or mock them (Phillips et al., 1994). For example, one woman with BDD thought that other people laughed at her and stared at her minor skin blemishes through binoculars whenever she left her house.

BDD-Related Behaviors

Although BDD's definition does not mention or require the presence of BDD-related behaviors, nearly all patients perform one or more of them. The usual intent of these behaviors is to examine, improve, or hide the perceived defects. Common behaviors include excessive mirror checking; excessive grooming (e.g., applying makeup, hair styling, or hair cutting); camouflaging (e.g., with clothes or makeup); seeking reassurance; comparing with others; skin picking; dieting; excessive exercising; and seeking surgical, dermatological, and other nonpsychiatric medical treatment (Hollander et al., 1993; Phillips & Diaz, 1997). However, the behaviors patients may engage in to improve their appearance are virtually unlimited (e.g., excessive showering to get one's hair "right"). Such behaviors typically consume many hours a day. A study from the United States found that women are more likely than men to pick their skin and camouflage with makeup, whereas men are more likely to camouflage with a hat (Phillips & Diaz, 1997). The study from Italy found that women are more likely than men to check mirrors and use camouflaging behaviors (Perugi et al., 1997a).

Although the usual intent of these behaviors is to decrease anxiety, anxiety often increases (Phillips, 1996a). Patients often, for example, feel more anxious after checking the mirror and being distressed by what they perceive. Although women who pick their skin may feel less anxious while picking, they usually feel more anxious and depressed later when they realize the damage they have caused. Occasionally, skin picking can be life-threatening, as in the case of a woman who picked at a pimple on her neck with tweezers to the point where she exposed her carotid artery and required emergency surgery (O'Sullivan et al., 1999).

Complications

Although level of functioning varies in BDD, most studies have reported significantly impaired functioning in individuals with this disorder (Perugi et al., 1997b; Phillips et al., 1993; Veale et al., 1996a). For example, in the largest published series of women with BDD ($n = 93$), 99% experienced social impairment and 78% academic/occupational impairment because of their BDD symptoms (Phillips & Diaz, 1997). Many women with

BDD have few friends, avoid dating and other social interactions, or get divorced because of their symptoms. They often avoid specific situations, such as restaurants, beaches, or shopping, in which they feel particularly self-conscious about their appearance. Women with BDD may also perform their school work or job below their capacity, or may not work at all, because of their symptoms. Their symptoms may also interfere with caring for their children. In the previously mentioned series, 48% of women had a history of psychiatric hospitalization, 29% had been completely housebound for at least 1 week because of their BDD symptoms, and 27% had attempted suicide (Phillips & Diaz, 1997). In the previously noted series of child/adolescent patients, most of whom were female, 39% had been psychiatrically hospitalized and 21% had attempted suicide (Albertini & Phillips, 1999). A recent study of dermatology patients who committed suicide reported that most had either acne or BDD; all of the patients with BDD were women (Cotterill & Cunliffe, 1997).

Patients with BDD also experience unusually high levels of perceived stress (DeMarco et al., 1998) and have markedly poor quality of life. In the only study that has assessed quality of life in BDD, mental-health-related quality of life was markedly worse than that of the general population, as well as worse than normative data for patients with depression, diabetes, or a recent myocardial infarction (Phillips, 2000b). Their mental-health-related quality of life was also poorer than has been reported for patients with OCD or schizophrenia.

Comorbidity

In clinical series, major depression is the disorder most often comorbid with BDD, with lifetime rates of 31% to 82% reported (Phillips, 1999). Social phobia, substance-related disorders, and OCD also commonly co-occur with BDD (Hollander et al., 1993; Perugi et al., 1997b; Phillips & Diaz, 1997), although a study from England found fairly low rates of Axis I comorbidity (Veale et al., 1996a). One study found that women with BDD were more likely than men to have comorbid bulimia nervosa and less likely to have alcohol abuse or dependence (Phillips & Diaz, 1997). Another study found that women were more likely to have bulimia nervosa, panic disorder, and generalized anxiety disorder, whereas men were more likely to have bipolar disorder (Perugi et al., 1997a). Reported rates of a comorbid personality disorder range from 57% to 100% (Neziroglu et al., 1996; Phillips & McElroy, 2000; Veale et al., 1996a), with avoidant personality disorder the most common in several studies.

Course of Illness

Virtually all studies that have assessed age of BDD onset have found that the disorder usually begins during adolescence and not infrequently begins in childhood (Albertini & Phillips, 1999). Available retrospective data suggest that BDD is usually chronic, with the largest study reporting a mean duration of illness in women of approximately 16 years (Phillips & Diaz, 1997).

In contrast, the only follow-up study of BDD found that treated patients generally had a fairly good outcome. This chart review study of 82 outpatients treated in a specialty BDD program found that over a follow-up period of 6 months to 7 years, a majority of patients improved; however, BDD symptoms often remitted only partially, and only a minority of patients achieved and maintained full remission (Phillips et al., 1999). Prospective longitudinal studies are needed to confirm these findings.

Additional Gender-Related Aspects of the Clinical Presentation

Virtually nothing is known about psychiatric aspects of the menstrual cycle, pregnancy, postpartum period, and menopause in women with BDD. Anecdotal evidence suggests that many women experience increased BDD symptoms premenstrually, although no data are available to confirm or disconfirm this impression. It appears that relatively few women with BDD have children, although no published data are available on this issue; as noted previously, a relatively low percentage of women with BDD are married. It is also worth noting that although I have consulted on and treated an estimated 300 women with BDD, only two of these women were pregnant, and their BDD symptoms continued during their pregnancy. From an anecdotal perspective, many women report feeling too self-conscious and ashamed of their appearance to be in a relationship, and many avoid sexual relationships. Some women report not wanting to have children because they worry that their children will suffer from BDD. One published case of "BDD by proxy" described a woman who terminated three pregnancies because she worried that her children would be unattractive (Laugharne et al., 1997).

DIAGNOSIS AND DIFFERENTIAL DIAGNOSIS

BDD is underrecognized and usually goes undiagnosed in clinical settings. One study found that of 17 inpatients subsequently diagnosed with BDD, BDD symptoms had been noted in only 5 charts and no patient received the diagnosis, although it was a significant problem in all cases and in some cases was the major reason for hospitalization (Phillips et al., 1993). In studies of depressed patients and general outpatients, BDD was missed by the clinician in every case (Phillips et al., 1996; Zimmerman & Mattia, 1998).

BDD can be difficult to diagnose because patients often keep their symptoms secret due to embarrassment and shame (Phillips, 1996). They may volunteer only depression, anxiety, or discomfort in social situations. Thus BDD may be misdiagnosed as depression, social phobia, agoraphobia, or avoidant personality disorder (due to secondary social anxiety and isolation). It may also be misdiagnosed as OCD (due to obsessional preoccupations and compulsive behaviors), panic disorder (because situational panic attacks may occur—e.g., when a patient is out in public or looking in the mirror), or trichotillomania (in patients who cut or pluck their hair to improve their appearance). Delusional patients are sometimes misdiagnosed with schizophrenia or psychotic depression.

To diagnose BDD, the symptoms typically need to be asked about directly, using questions such as the following:

- Have you ever been very worried about your appearance in any way? (If yes:) What was your concern?
- Did this concern preoccupy you? Did you think about it a lot and wish you could worry about it less?
- What effect has this preoccupation with your appearance had on your life? Has it

caused you a lot of distress or significantly interfered with your social life, school work, job, or other activities? Has it affected your family or friends?

Clues to the diagnosis include the BDD-related behaviors noted above, ideas or delusions of reference; social anxiety and self-consciousness; being housebound; depression, anxiety, or suicidal ideation; or unnecessary surgical or dermatological treatment (Phillips, 1996).

TREATMENT

Surgical, Dermatological, and Other Nonpsychiatric Medical Treatment

Most women with BDD seek nonpsychiatric treatment, which is often costly. In a series of 131 women with BDD, 78% sought and 70% received such treatment (Phillips et al., in press-a). Dermatological treatment and surgery were most commonly sought and received. Conversely, it has been reported that 7% of women seeking cosmetic surgery have BDD (Sawrer et al., 1998a). Other types of medical or dental treatment may also be received. Many women finally receive the requested treatment after being refused treatment by numerous physicians, and some have multiple procedures. One study found that although men and women were equally likely to seek and receive nonpsychiatric treatment for BDD, women received a greater number of treatments than men (Phillips et al., in press-a). Most women with BDD are dissatisfied with such treatment; many dislike their appearance even more or develop new appearance preoccupations (Fukuda, 1977; Phillips et al., in press-a). Occasionally, dissatisfied patients sue their physicians or even become violent toward them (Phillips, 1996a).

Pharmacotherapy and Other Somatic Treatments

Although BDD has been said to be "extremely difficult" to treat (Munro & Chmara, 1982), available data suggest that serotonin reuptake inhibitors (SRIs) are often, and perhaps preferentially, effective for this disorder. In a series of 130 patients (who received a total of 316 medications) for whom response was assessed retrospectively, 42% of 65 SRI trials resulted in "much" or "very much" improvement, compared to 30% of 23 trials with monoamine oxidase inhibitors (MAOIs), 15% of 48 trials with non-SRI tricyclics, 3% of trials with neuroleptics, 6% with a variety of other medications (e.g., mood stabilizers), and 0% of trials with electroconvulsive therapy (ECT) (Phillips, 2000a). In a retrospective study of 50 patients, 35 SRI trials resulted in much improvement, whereas 18 trials of non-SRI tricyclics led to no overall improvement in BDD symptoms (Hollander et al., 1994). In a study of 45 patients openly treated in a clinical practice, 70% of SRI trials (43 of 61) resulted in much or very much improvement (Phillips, 2000a).

Two systematic open-label pharmacotherapy studies, both with fluvoxamine, have been published. A 16-week trial (n = 30) reported an intent-to-treat response rate of 63%, with a mean fluvoxamine dose of 238.3 ± 85.8 mg/day; the mean time to response was 6.1 ± 3.7 weeks (range = 1–16 weeks) (Phillips et al., 1998). In another open-label fluvoxamine trial (n = 15), 10 subjects responded (Perugi et al., 1996). In the only published controlled pharmacotherapy study, a double-blind crossover trial, clomipramine was more effective than desipramine (Hollander et al., 1999). In the first placebo-controlled treatment study (N = 74), fluoxetine was more effective than placebo

(Phillips et al., in press-b). Of interest, available data indicate that delusional patients often respond to SRIs without antipsychotics, and that insight and referential thinking may improve with SRI treatment (Hollander et al., 2000; Phillips et al., 1998). The one study that examined gender differences in treatment outcome (assessments were retrospective) found no gender differences in response to SRIs or other medications (Phillips & Diaz, 1997).

Augmentation of an SRI with buspirone (mean dose of 56.5± 15.2 mg/day) was effective in 33% of the trials (Phillips et al., in press-a). Augmentation of an SRI with a neuroleptic, or combining a selective SRI with clomipramine (and monitoring clomipramine levels), may be another promising strategy when an SRI is not adequately effective, although published data on the efficacy of these approaches is limited (Phillips et al., in press-a). Some patients, especially those who are severely depressed, may improve with stimulant or lithium augmentation of an SRI (Phillips et al., in press-a). Patients who do not respond to one adequate SRI trial may respond to another SRI or venlafaxine (Phillips et al., in press-a). If none of these strategies are effective, an MAOI may be considered. All of these strategies, though promising, require further research.

Other medications used as single agents have not been well studied, although the previously noted retrospective studies and the clomipramine/desipramine study found that non-SRIs were often not effective. An intriguing preliminary finding is that antipsychotics alone are generally ineffective for delusional BDD, whereas SRIs are often effective (Phillips et al., 2000a). Antipsychotics deserve further study in BDD as both single and augmenting agents. Because pimozide has been reported (Munro & Chmara, 1982) to be particularly effective for monosymptomatic hypochondriacal psychosis (the previous term for delusional disorder, somatic type), this medication in particular deserves further investigation.

Medication discontinuation studies have not been done, but in one of the previously noted fluvoxamine studies, six responders discontinued fluvoxamine after completing the study, all of whom relapsed, with BDD symptoms significantly improving in all four patients who restarted an SRI (Phillips et al., 1998). In a chart-review study, discontinuation of an effective SRI resulted in relapse of BDD in 83% (n = 31) of cases (Phillips et al., 2001). Many patients require and maintain improvement with long-term treatment.

ECT was ineffective in six published case reports (Phillips, 1991) and effective in two (Carroll, 1994; Hay, 1970). In a subsequent series of 130 cases, none of eight ECT trials were successful, although the data were largely retrospective (Phillips, 2000a). Regarding psychosurgery, one case report noted improvement in BDD symptoms with a modified leucotomy (Hay, 1970) and another with a bilateral anterior cingulotomy and subcaudate tractotomy (E. Cassem, personal communication). In one case a capsulotomy was effective (P. Mindus, personal communication), but in two other cases an anterior internal capsulotomy was ineffective (S. A. Rasmussen, personal communication, 2000).

Cognitive-Behavioral Therapy

Preliminary data suggest that cognitive-behavioral therapy (CBT) may be effective for BDD. Several investigators have reported that strategies such as cognitive restructuring, exposure (e.g., exposing the defect in social situations and preventing avoidance behaviors), and response prevention (avoiding compulsive behaviors, such as mirror checking and reassurance seeking) are effective for a majority of patients. In one report, four of five patients improved with such approaches in 90-minute sessions 1 day or 5 days per week, with the total number of sessions ranging from 12 to 48 (Neziroglu & Yaryura-Tobias, 1993). Techniques included having patients cover or remove mirrors, limit grooming time, and stop using makeup. Exposure techniques were used after developing an anxiety hierarchy that included having patients go to avoided restaurants or stores, sit in crowded waiting rooms, and mess up their hair before interacting with other people.

In a pilot study of 19 patients (primarily women) who were randomly assigned to a CBT group or a no-treatment waiting-list control group, the CBT group improved more than the control group (Veale et al., 1996b). Seven of nine patients who received CBT no longer met criteria for BDD at the end of the study. Another study reported that group therapy utilizing exposure and response prevention plus cognitive techniques was effective in 77% of 27 women (Rosen et al., 1995). This study used similar techniques (e.g., exposure to social situations and avoiding camouflage, resisting body-checking behaviors, and changing negative self-statements about appearance). Subjects in the treatment group improved more than those in a no-treatment waiting-list control group. The subjects in this study appeared to have relatively mild BDD, and many seemed to be in a "diagnostic gray zone" between BDD and eating disorders. An open case series of 13 patients treated in small CBT-focused groups that met for 12 weekly 90-minute sessions found that BDD significantly improved (Wilhelm et al., 1999). The only longer-term (i.e., maintenance) study of CBT found that response was maintained in 10 patients after 6 months (McKay et al., 1997).

As is the case for pharmacotherapy, well-controlled studies are needed to confirm CBT's effectiveness (only waiting-list controls have been used). One unanswered question pertains to the length and number of sessions needed: If patients have access to only a few sessions (as is often the case), is the treatment effective and worth doing? Another unanswered question is this: How effective is CBT for delusional or severely depressed patients?

No studies have been done on the effectiveness of combining CBT and pharmacotherapy, although clinical experience suggests that some patients benefit from this approach, and that it should be considered when patients do not respond to CBT or medication alone.

Other Treatments

Available data, although limited, suggest that BDD is unlikely to improve significantly with supportive or insight-oriented psychotherapy alone (Phillips et al., 1993). Severely ill and delusional patients appear particularly unlikely to respond to this treatment. Nonetheless, some patients benefit from and need psychotherapy in addition to CBT or medication. Insight-oriented or supportive therapy may be effective for other disorders or problems the patients may have, and may help patients in coping with their illness.

Treating Women with BDD

Because available data, while limited, indicate that SRIs and CBT are often effective for BDD and are more effective than other treatments, one of these approaches should be tried. My practice is to recommend CBT for mildly ill patients without significant comorbidity (if qualified CBT therapists are available). For more moderately to severely ill patients, and for those with comorbidity requiring medication, treatment with an SRI is warranted. An SRI is always indicated for suicidal patients. More severely ill patients often refuse or are unable to engage in CBT; others are unable to tolerate the temporary anxiety this approach can cause. In such cases, partial response to an SRI may enable patients to participate in CBT.

Based on available data, an SRI should be tried for at least 12 weeks, and the highest dose recommended by the manufacturer should be tried if lower doses are ineffective. Clinical experience suggests that a successful SRI should be continued for a minimum of 1 year. If an SRI is ineffective, another SRI or an augmentation or combination strategy should be tried. If CBT is ineffective, more frequent sessions should be considered. Patients who receive CBT should be monitored for relapse.

Educating the patient about BDD is an important aspect of treatment (Phillips, 1996). Educating family members and significant others, when clinically appropriate, can also facilitate treatment. Family members should be advised to avoid assisting with BDD rituals (e.g., they should be asked to avoid holding mirrors or lights for the patient, providing reassurance, or participating in grooming rituals). Family members should not allow their lives to be severely disrupted by the patient's illness, and they should encourage the patient to function at as high a level as possible, while recognizing her limitations.

Virtually nothing is known about treating pregnant women with BDD. CBT would seem preferable to medication, although more severely ill or very depressed patients may require an SRI, and treatment decisions must be tailored to the individual patient. One pregnant woman with BDD whom I treated had had an excellent response to 60 mg/day paroxetine prior to her pregnancy. When she became pregnant, she wished to continue an SRI, and paroxetine was changed to fluoxetine because at the time more data were available on the use of fluoxetine during pregnancy. On fluoxetine (40 mg/day), the patient was more symptomatic than on paroxetine, but the dose was not increased because she wished to keep it as low as possible while pregnant. However, the patient then experienced increased BDD and depressive symptoms; as a result, she stopped eating and had suicidal ideation. Fluoxetine was gradually increased to 80 mg/day (during the second trimester), resulting in remission of all symptoms. The patient subsequently gave birth to a healthy baby and has continued in remission postpartum on fluoxetine.

It is sometimes difficult to get patients (especially those who are delusional) to accept psychiatric treatment. Some refuse treatment because they are convinced that surgical, dermatological, or other medical treatment is needed; others refuse because they are convinced that their views of their defects are accurate and that psychiatric treatment will not be helpful. Psychoeducation that emphasizes the potential benefits of treatment is essential in such cases. It is usually unproductive to try to talk delusional patients out of their beliefs; a more useful approach is to focus on the potential for treatment to decrease their preoccupation, suffering, and functional impairment.

Psychiatrists may need to confer with dermatologists, plastic surgeons, and other nonpsychiatric physicians from whom patients request or receive treatment. Although no one can predict how an individual patient will respond to such treatment, available data indicate that patients usually do not improve and may get worse. Occasionally, such treatment precipitates psychosis, suicidal behavior, or violence. For these reasons, it seems wise to advise patients to try psychiatric treatment before obtaining surgery, and to avoid more aggressive dermatological treatment such as dermabrasion or isotretinoin. Patients who damage their skin by picking often require and benefit from a combination of dermatological and psychiatric treatment, in which case it is important and beneficial for the psychiatrist and dermatologist to collaborate.

CONCLUSIONS AND FUTURE DIRECTIONS

BDD can cause severe impairment in functioning and is associated with notably poor quality of life. SRIs and CBT are promising treatment approaches. Research on BDD is still in its early stages, and much more investigation is needed. In particular, research on aspects of BDD that are relevant to women is currently lacking and greatly needed. For example, how common is premenstrual worsening of symptoms, and what happens to BDD symptoms during pregnancy? Is the postpartum period a time of increased risk for the onset of or worsening of BDD symptoms? How should BDD be treated during pregnancy?

In the meantime, it is important for clinicians to be aware that BDD appears to be relatively common but usually undiagnosed in women. Clinicians should be aware of the clues to BDD and should screen women for this disorder. Although much remains to be learned about treatment, the approaches discussed in this chapter are very promising for women who suffer from this distressing and often disabling disorder.

REFERENCES

Albertini, R. S., & Phillips, K. A. (1999). 33 cases of body dysmorphic disorder in children and adolescents. *Journal of the American Academy of Child and Adolescent Psychiatry, 38,* 453–459.

American Psychiatric Association. (1994). *Diagnostic and statistical manual of mental disorders* (4th ed.). Washington, DC: Author.

Biby, E. L. (1998). The relationship between body dysmorphic disorder and depression, self-esteem, somatization, and obsessive–compulsive disorder. *Journal of Clinical Psychology, 54,* 489–499.

Bienvenu, O. J., Samuels, J. F., Riddle, M. A., et al. (2000). The relationship of obsessive–compulsive disorder to possible spectrum disorders: Results from a family study. *Biological Psychiatry, 48,* 287–293.

Brawman-Mintzer, O., Lydiard, R. B., Phillips, K. A., et al. (1995). Body dysmorphic disorder in patients with anxiety disorders and major depression: A comorbidity study. *American Journal of Psychiatry, 152,* 1665–1667.

Carroll, B. J. (1994). Response of major depression with psychosis and body dysmorphic disorder to ECT [Letter to the editor]. *American Journal of Psychiatry, 151,* 288–289.

Cotterill, J. A., & Cunliffe, W. J. (1997). Suicide in dermatological patients. *British Journal of Dermatology, 137,* 246–250.

DeMarco, L. M., Li, L. C., Phillips, K. A., et al. (1998). Perceived stress in body dysmorphic disorder. *Journal of Nervous and Mental Disease, 186,* 724–726.

Faravelli, C., Salvatori, S., Galassi, F., et al. (1997). Epidemiology of somatoform disorders: A community survey in Florence. *Social Psychiatry and Psychiatric Epidemiology, 32,* 24–29.

Fukuda, O. (1977). Statistical analysis of dysmorphophobia in out-patient clinic. *Japanese Journal of Plastic and Reconstructive Surgery, 20,* 569–577.

Hay, G. G. (1970). Dysmorphophobia. *British Journal of Psychiatry, 116,* 399–406.

Hollander, E., Allen, A., Kwon, J., et al. (1999). Clomipramine vs. desipramine crossover trial in body dysmorphic disorder: Selective efficacy of a serotonin reuptake inhibitor in imagined ugliness. *Archives of General Psychiatry, 56,* 1033–1039.

Hollander, E., Cohen, L. J., & Simeon, D. (1993). Body dysmorphic disorder. *Psychiatric Annals, 23,* 359–364.

Hollander, E., Cohen, L. J., Simeon, D., et al. (1994). Fluvoxamine treatment of body dysmorphic disorder [Letter to the editor]. *Journal of Clinical Psychopharmacology, 14,* 75–77.

Ishigooka, J., Iwao, M., Suzuki, M., et al. (1998). Demographic features of patients seeking cosmetic surgery. *Psychiatry and Clinical Neuroscience, 52,* 283–287.

Laugharne, R., Upex, T., & Palazidou, E. (1997). Dysmorphophobia by proxy. *Journal of the Royal Society of Medicine, 91,* 266.

Mayville, S., Katz, R. C., Gipson, M. T., et al. (1999). Assessing the prevalence of body dysmorphic disorder in an ethically diverse group of adolescents. *Journal of Child and Family Studies, 8,* 357–362.

McKay, D., Todaro, J., Neziroglu, F., et al. (1997). Body dysmorphic disorder: A preliminary evaluation of treatment and maintenance using exposure with response prevention. *Behaviour Research and Therapy, 35,* 67–79.

Morselli, E. (1891). Sulla dismorfofobia e sulla tafefobia. *Bolletinno della Accademia di Genova, 6,* 110–119.

Munro, A., & Chmara, J. (1982). Monosymptomatic hypochondriacal psychosis: A diagnostic checklist based on 50 cases of the disorder. *Canadian Journal of Psychiatry, 27,* 374–376.

Neziroglu, F. A., McKay, D., Todaro, J., et al. (1996). Effect of cognitive behavior therapy on persons with body dysmorphic disorder and comorbid Axis II diagnoses. *Behavior Therapy, 27,* 67–77.

Neziroglu, F. A., & Yaryura-Tobias, J. A. (1993). Exposure, response prevention, and cognitive therapy in the treatment of body dysmorphic disorder. *Behavior Therapy, 24,* 431–438.

Nierenberg, A. A., Phillips, K. A., Petersen, T. J., et al. (in press). Body dysmorphic disorder in outpatients with major depression. *Journal of Affective Disorders.*

O'Sullivan, R. L., Phillips, K. A., Keuthen, N. J., et al. (1999). Near fatal skin picking from delusional body dysmorphic disorder responsive to fluvoxamine. *Psychosomatics, 40,* 79–81.

Perugi, G., Akiskal, H. S., Giannotti, D., et al. (1997a). Gender-related differences in body dysmorphic disorder (dysmorphophobia). *Journal of Nervous and Mental Disease, 185,* 578–582.

Perugi, G., Akiskal, H. S., Lattanzi, L., et al. (1998). The high prevalence of "soft" bipolar (II) features in atypical depression. *Comprehensive Psychiatry, 39,* 63–71.

Perugi, G., Giannotti, D., Di Vaio, S., et al. (1996). Fluvoxamine in the treatment of body dysmorphic disorder (dysmorphophobia). *International Clinical Psychopharmacology, 11,* 247–254.

Perugi, G., Giannotti, D., Frare, F., et al. (1997b). Prevalence, phenomenology and comorbidity of body dysmorphic disorder (dysmorphophobia) in a clinical population. *International Journal of Psychiatry in Clinical Practice, 1,* 77–82.

Phillips, K. A. (1991). Body dysmorphic disorder: The distress of imagined ugliness. *American Journal of Psychiatry, 148,* 1138–1149.

Phillips, K. A. (1996). *The broken mirror: Understanding and treating body dysmorphic disorder.* New York: Oxford University Press.

Phillips, K. A. (1999). Body dysmorphic disorder and depression: Theoretical considerations and treatment strategies. *Psychiatric Quarterly, 70,* 313–331.

Phillips, K. A. (2000a). Pharmacologic treatment of body dysmorphic disorder: A review of empirical data and a proposed treatment algorithm. *Psychiatric Clinics in North America, 7,* 59–82.

Phillips, K. A. (2000b). Quality of life for patients with body dysmorphic disorder. *Journal of Nervous and Mental Disease, 188,* 170–175.

Phillips, K. A., Albertini, R. S., & Rasmussen, S. A. (in press-b). A randomized placebo-controlled trial of fluoxetine in body dysmorphic disorder. *Archives of General Psychiatry.*

Phillips, K. A., Albertini, R. S., Siniscalchi, J., et al. (2001). Effectiveness of pharmacotherapy for body dysmorphic disorder: A chart-review study. *Journal of Clinical Psychiatry, 62,* 721–727.

Phillips, K. A., & Diaz, S. (1997). Gender differences in body dysmorphic disorder. *Journal of Nervous and Mental Disease, 185,* 570–577.

Phillips, K. A., Dufresne, R., Wilkel, C., et al. (2000). Prevalence of body dysmorphic disorder in dermatology patients. *Journal of the American Academy of Dermatology, 42,* 436–441.

Phillips, K. A., Dwight, M. M., & McElroy, S. L. (1998). Efficacy and safety of fluvoxamine in body dysmorphic disorder. *Journal of Clinical Psychiatry, 59,* 165–171.

Phillips, K. A., Grant, J., Albertini, R. S., Stout, R., et al. (1999). Retrospective follow-up study of body dysmorphic disorder. *New Research Program and Abstracts, American Psychiatric Association 152nd Annual Meeting.* Washington, DC: American Psychiatric Association, 151.

Phillips, K. A., Grant, J. D., Siniscalchi, J., et al. (in press-a). Surgical and nonpsychiatric medical treatment of patients with body dysmorphic disorder. *Psychosomatics.*

Phillips, K. A., & McElroy, S. L. (2000). Personality disorders and traits in patients with body dysmorphic disorder. *Comprehensive Psychiatry, 41,* 229–236.

Phillips, K. A., McElroy, S. L., Keck, P. E., Jr., et al. (1993). Body dysmorphic disorder: 30 cases of imagined ugliness. *American Journal of Psychiatry, 150,* 302–308.

Phillips, K. A., McElroy, S. L., Keck, P. E., Jr., et al. (1994). A comparison of delusional and nondelusional body dysmorphic disorder in 100 cases. *Psychopharmacology Bulletin, 30,* 179–186.

Phillips, K. A., Nierenberg, A. A., Brendel, G., et al. (1996). Prevalence and clinical features of body dysmorphic disorder in atypical major depression. *Journal of Nervous and Mental Disease, 184,* 125–129.

Rosen, J. C., & Ramirez, E. (1998). A comparison of eating disorders and body dysmorphic disorder on body image and psychological adjustment. *Journal of Psychosomatic Research, 44,* 441–449.

Rosen, J. C., Reiter, J., & Orosan, P. (1995). Cognitive-behavioral body image therapy for body dysmorphic disorder. *Journal of Consulting and Clinical Psychology, 63,* 263–269.

Sarwer, D. B., Wadden, T. A., Pertschuk, M. J., et al. (1998a). Body image dissatisfaction and body dysmorphic disorder in 100 cosmetic surgery patients. *Plastic and Reconstructive Surgery, 101,* 1644–1649.

Sarwer, D. B., Whitaker, L. A., Pertschuk, M. J., et al. (1998b). Body image concerns of reconstructive surgery patients: An underrecognized problem. *Annals of Plastic Surgery, 40,* 403–407.

Simeon, D., Hollander, E., Stein, D. J., et al. (1995). Body dysmorphic disorder in the DSM-IV field trial for obsessive compulsive disorder. *American Journal of Psychiatry, 152,* 1207–1209.

Soriano, J. L., O'Sullivan, R. L., Baer, L., et al. (1996). Trichotillomania and self-esteem: A survey of 62 female hair pullers. *Journal of Clinical Psychiatry, 57,* 77–82.

Veale, D., Boocock, A., Gournay, K., et al. (1996a). Body dysmorphic disorder: A survey of fifty cases. *British Journal of Psychiatry, 169,* 196–201.

Veale, D., Gournay, K., Dryden, W., et al. (1996b). Body dysmorphic disorder: A cognitive behavioural model and pilot randomized controlled trial. *Behaviour Research and Therapy, 34,* 717–729.

Wilhelm, S., Otto, M. W., Lohr, B., et al. (1999). Cognitive behavior group therapy for body dysmorphic disorder: A case series. *Behaviour Research and Therapy, 37,* 71–75.

Wilhelm, S., Otto, M. W., Zucker, B. G., et al. (1997). Prevalence of body dysmorphic disorder in patients with anxiety disorders. *Journal of Anxiety Disorders, 11,* 499–502.

Zimmerman, M., & Mattia, J. I. (1998). Body dysmorphic disorder in psychiatric outpatients: Recognition, prevalence, comorbidity, demographic, and clinical correlates. *Comprehensive Psychiatry, 39,* 265–270.

17

Somatoform Disorders

ONDRIA C. GLEASON
WILLIAM R. YATES

Somatoform disorders are characterized by physical complaints that are not fully accounted for by physical findings, by substance use, or by another psychiatric disorder, and that are not under voluntary control. Although medically unexplained physical symptoms are common in the general population, treatment seeking for these symptoms is not as common. A patient with a somatoform disorder may become a very high utilizer of care, presenting to multiple physicians with the same or similar complaints. Multiple evaluations are sought because negative findings and reassurance do not reduce the patient's concern that a medical disorder is present. This high rate of health care utilization places the patient at risk for iatrogenic complications, increases health care costs, and often leads to frustration for both the patient and physicians. The somatoform disorders include the following diagnostic categories: somatization disorder, conversion disorder, undifferentiated somatoform disorder, pain disorder, hypochondriasis, body dysmorphic disorder, and somatoform disorder not otherwise specified. Table 17.1 outlines the diagnostic criteria for somatization disorder, conversion disorder, hypochondriasis, and pain disorder from the *Diagnostic and Statistical Manual of Mental Disorders*, fourth edition (DSM-IV-TR, American Psychiatric Association, 2000). This chapter focuses on the epidemiology, presentation, course, comorbidity, and treatment of somatoform disorders, as well as the few data available concerning effects of reproductive cycle events on the course of somatoform presentations. Body dysmorphic disorder is discussed extensively by Phillips in Chapter 16 of this volume, and thus receives less attention here than the other disorders.

EPIDEMIOLOGY

Few population-based studies have examined the epidemiology of somatoform disorders. Most of the information comes from clinical populations, and is focused on somatization

TABLE 17.1. DSM-IV-TR Diagnostic Criteria for Selected Somatoform Disorders

Somatization Disorder

A. A history of many physical complaints beginning before age 30 years that occur over a period of several years and result in treatment being sought or significant impairment in social, occupational, or other important areas of functioning.

B. Each of the following criteria must have been met, with individual symptoms occurring at any time during the course of the disturbance:

(1) *four pain symptoms*: a history of pain related to at least four different sites or functions . . .

(2) *two gastrointestinal symptoms*: a history of at least two gastrointestinal symptoms other than pain . . .

(3) *one sexual symptom*: a history of at least one sexual or reproductive symptom other than pain . . .

(4) *one pseudoneurological symptom*: a history of at least one symptom or deficit suggesting a neurological condition not limited to pain . . .

C. Either (1) or (2):

(1) after appropriate investigation, each of the symptoms in Criterion B cannot be fully explained by a known general medical condition or the direct effects of a substance (e.g., a drug of abuse, a medication)

(2) when there is a related general medical condition, the physical complaints or resulting social or occupational impairment are in excess of what would be expected from the history, physical examination, or laboratory findings

D. The symptoms are not intentionally produced or feigned (as in Factitious Disorder or Malingering).

Conversion Disorder

A. One or more symptoms or deficits affecting voluntary motor or sensory function that suggest a neurological or other general medical condition.

B. Psychological factors are judged to be associated with the symptom or deficit because the initiation or exacerbation of the symptom or deficit is preceded by conflicts or other stressors.

C. The symptom or deficit is not intentionally produced or feigned (as in Factitious Disorder or Malingering).

D. The symptom or deficit cannot, after appropriate investigation, be fully explained by a general medical condition, or by the direct effects of a substance, or as a culturally sanctioned behavior or experience.

E. The symptom or deficit causes clinically significant distress or impairment in social, occupational, or other important areas of functioning or warrants medical evaluation.

F. The symptom or deficit is not limited to pain or sexual dysfunction, does not occur exclusively during the course of Somatization Disorder, and is not better accounted for by another mental disorder.

Hypochondriasis

A. Preoccupation with fears of having, or the idea that one has, a serious disease based on the person's misinterpretation of bodily symptoms.

B. The preoccupation persists despite appropriate medical evaluation and reassurance.

C. The belief in Criterion A is not of delusional intensity (as in Delusional Disorder, Somatic Type) and is not restricted to a circumscribed concern about appearance (as in Body Dysmorphic Disorder).

D. The preoccupation causes clinically significant distress or impairment in social, occupational, or other important areas of functioning.

E. The duration of the disturbance is at least 6 months.

TABLE 17.1. (*continued*)

F. The preoccupation is not better accounted for by Generalized Anxiety Disorder, Obsessive–Compulsive Disorder, Panic Disorder, a Major Depressive Episode, Separation Anxiety, or another Somatoform Disorder.

Pain Disorder

A. Pain in one or more anatomical sites is the predominant focus of the clinical presentation and is of sufficient severity to warrant clinical attention.

B. The pain causes clinically significant distress or impairment in social, occupational, or other important areas of functioning.

C. Psychological factors are judged to have an important role in the onset, severity, exacerbation, or maintenance of the pain.

D. The symptom or deficit is not intentionally produced or feigned (as in Factitious Disorder or Malingering).

E. The pain is not better accounted for by a Mood, Anxiety, or Psychotic Disorder and does not meet criteria for Dyspareunia.

Note. Reprinted with permission from the Diagnostic and Statistical Manual of Mental Disorders, Fourth Edition, Text Revision. Copyright 2000 American Psychiatric Association.

disorder and conversion disorder. The Epidemiologic Catchment Area (ECA) survey was a multisite study of prevalence rates of psychiatric illness (defined according to DSM-III criteria) in the general population, undertaken in collaboration with the National Institute of Mental Health in the early 1980s in the United States. The ECA survey found the lifetime prevalence for somatization disorder to be 0.13% (Myers et al., 1984; Swartz et al., 1986). These low prevalence estimates stem from the relatively high symptom count (a total of eight pain symptoms) for somatization disorder criteria in DSM-III. Escobar et al. (1989) proposed a "somatization syndrome" that required only four somatization symptoms for men and six somatization symptoms for women, to determine whether lesser symptom counts would also indicate significant problems. When these lesser criteria were used, somatization syndrome was 30–150 times more prevalent than somatization disorder, with 11.6% of the U.S. population meeting criteria for somatization syndrome at some time in their lives.

The differences in the prevalence of somatization disorder in men and women are notable. Figure 17.1 illustrates the gender distribution of various somatoform disorders, including somatization disorder, seen by a consultation service in an academic setting over a 2-year period (Yates, 1999). The predominance of female patients is striking. The ECA study found an estimated lifetime prevalence of somatization disorder in men of 0.02%, compared to an estimated rate of 0.23% in women; lifetime prevalence rates for the broader-based somatization syndrome were 8.68% for men and 14.30% for women (Swartz et al., 1991). Female gender stands out as the most important risk factor for somatization disorder. Kroenke and Spitzer (1998) studied gender differences in the reporting of 13 common physical symptoms in 1,000 patients evaluated with the Primary Care Evaluation of Mental Disorders interview. They found that 10 of the 13 symptoms were reported more often in women, and concluded that women report most physical symptoms at least 50% more often than men. In this study, gender was identified as the most important demographic factor, associated with the reporting of physical symptoms, fol-

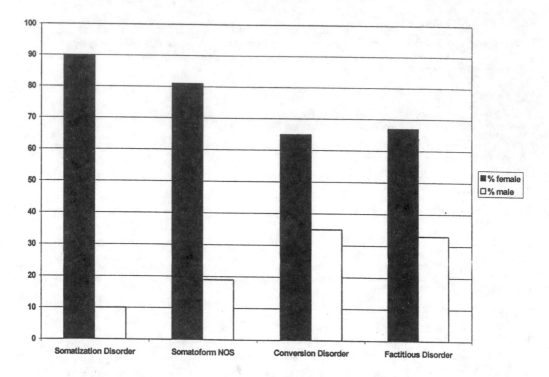

FIGURE 17.1. Gender distributions for somatoform disorders in a psychiatry consultation series.

lowed by low educational level. Other risk factors for somatization disorder included genetic and family factors, younger age, and nonwhite race.

Wool and Barsky (1994) reviewed the evidence that women tend to somatize more than men. This review included studies of both the general population and groups seen in the medical care setting. In general, women demonstrated more somatic symptoms and more somatoform disorders than men. Wool and Barsky proposed five possible mechanisms for higher rates of somatization in women: (1) Somatic symptoms may be more culturally approved in women than in men, making it less likely for men to report somatic symptoms when they do occur; (2) women may be more ready to seek medical attention when symptoms develop; (3) psychiatric disorders associated with somatization, such as mood disorders and anxiety disorders, are found more commonly in women; (4) women have higher rates of childhood physical and sexual trauma (factors suggested as important etiological events; and (5) women may have an innate sensitivity to bodily sensations, which may produce higher rates of endorsement of somatic symptoms.

The rate estimates for hypochondriasis are variable. Escobar et al. (1998) found a 3% prevalence rate among primary care patients. Gureje et al. (1997) found a prevalence rate of 0.8% for hypochondriasis as defined by the *International Classification of Diseases*, 10th revision, and 2.2% for a less restrictive definition of the disorder, in a Nigerian ambulatory setting. It has been suggested that hypochondriasis may not be an independent disorder, but rather a feature of other psychiatric disorders, including somatization disorder. Noyes et al. (1997) proposed this idea after finding increased rates of somatization disorder among first-degree relatives of patients with hypochondriasis.

The rate estimates for conversion disorder in the general population have ranged from 11 per 100,000 to 500 per 100,000 (American Psychiatric Association, 2000). Like somatization disorder, conversion disorder is more common in females than in males (Boffeli & Guze, 1992). Tomasson et al. (1991) reviewed the medical records of 65 patients with somatization disorder and 51 patients with conversion disorder. They found that 95% of the former patients and 78% of the latter patients were female. Folks et al. (1984) found similar results in a sample of 62 patients discharged from a general hospital carrying a diagnosis of conversion disorder. Eighty-five percent of these patients were female.

Faravelli et al. (1997) studied the prevalence rates of DSM-III-R somatoform disorders in Florence, Italy. They found 1-year prevalence rates as follows: hypochondriasis, 4.5%; undifferentiated somatoform disorder, 13.8%; somatization disorder, 0.7%; body dysmorphic disorder, 0.7%; and somatoform pain disorder, 0.6%.

PRESENTATION

Somatoform disorders present in a variety of settings to a variety of medical and mental health professionals. Many contacts occur in the primary care setting. Patients may present in settings related to their primary symptoms. For example, conversion disorder commonly presents with pseudoseizures, sudden motor paralysis, or loss of bodily sensation—symptoms that would routinely be managed by a neurologist. Pain is a common somatization symptom and is commonly evaluated in settings where treatment for pain can occur (hospitals, surgical clinics, pain clinics). Since abdominal pain is common in somatization disorder, gastroenterology clinics are often sites of evaluation for these patients.

The primary concern for the initial symptom evaluation must be the potential for a medical disorder. Patients with somatization disorder do not have increased risk for medical illness or death; however, this does not mean that medical illnesses cannot be present. Therefore, some evaluation of potential medical causes must be done. However, the extent and intensity of this evaluation are best minimized to prevent potential iatrogenic complications. Following the ruling out of medical causes, potential psychological factors can be pursued.

Patients with somatoform disorders often present to multiple physicians for evaluation of the same complaint and may not acknowledge all of the medical contact that they have experienced. This lack of important information can complicate the presentation and evaluation. Withholding of medical history stems from several factors. Patients may feel that a new physician may be biased by the negative findings from another physician. They do not agree with the previous findings and often hope that another physician will be able to make a medical diagnosis to explain what is causing their symptoms. In addition, patients may feel embarrassed about all the evaluation that they have completed.

There are few differences in the clinical presentation of women and men with somatization disorder. Golding et al. (1991) recruited 12 men and 68 women (by mass media advertisement and by primary care physician referral) who met DSM-III criteria for somatization disorder. There were no statistically significant differences demographically.

Men and women had equal numbers of symptoms. The only symptom more common in women was dizziness. They did find that men were more likely than women to be work-disabled (defined as "unemployment due to health problems"). Interestingly, men in this study were more likely to have been recruited through the mass media (50% of men vs. 13% of women) and women were more likely to be referred by their primary care physicians (55% of women vs. 8% of men), despite there being no differences between the genders in the numbers of physician visits 6 months prior to the study. The authors concluded that physicians are less likely to suspect somatization disorder in men than in women.

The psychiatric differential diagnosis for presentations common in somatoform disorders can be quite complex. Clinicians should be diligent in searching for evidence of primary mood and anxiety disorders. Understanding a patient's presentation is facilitated when additional information from a collateral source can be obtained. A thorough review of all medical records can often clear up a complex presentation and confirm a diagnosis of somatization disorder.

COURSE

Somatoform disorders tend to be chronic and marked by high utilization of health care. Despite no evidence of significant medical problems, patients with somatization disorder display disability consistent with severe medical illness. These patients are often functionally disabled and rate themselves as suffering from severe medical illness. Fatigue is a common somatic symptom. In the ECA data set, subjects endorsing current fatigue had higher lifetime rates of somatization disorder than those without fatigue and had increased rates of medical care utilization (Walker et al., 1993). Bass et al. (1999) also found complaints of fatigue to be associated with increased visits in a gastroenterology clinic. Eighty percent of these "frequent attenders" reported fatigue as a significant complaint, and somatoform disorders were the most prevalent psychiatric disorders found in this group.

The ECA study also found that 95% of persons with somatization disorder were seen in a general health outpatient setting in the 6 months prior to the survey. This is significantly higher than the 57% rate of contact by those without somatization disorder. More remarkable is the increase in hospitalization: 45% of persons with somatization disorder were hospitalized for medical reasons in the prior 6 months, compared to only 13% of the rest of the ECA sample (Swartz et al., 1991).

Barsky et al. (1998) prospectively studied patients with hypochondriasis over 4–5 years. At follow-up, the group displayed less somatization; however, 63% still met diagnostic criteria for hypochondriasis. This study showed that there can be a decline in symptoms; however, in general, hypochondriasis (like other somatoform disorders) is a chronic condition marked by morbidity, functional impairment, and personal distress.

Spertus et al. (1999) studied gender differences in adjustment to chronic pain, related to prior trauma history. They concluded that a history of significant trauma associated with emotional distress may adversely affect one's ability to manage pain effectively, particularly among men.

The patient with a somatoform disorder is at risk for iatrogenic complications related to frequent and often extensive medical evaluations. One potential iatrogenic problem in somatoform disorders is the development of dependence on prescription drugs used for the treatment of medical and psychiatric symptoms/disorders co-occurring with the somatoform disorder (Singh, 1998). Since pain is a frequent physical symptom in somatization, physicians often get trapped into prescribing increasingly potent analgesics. Patients with somatoform disorder patients then become physiologically dependent on the narcotic analgesics and develop withdrawal symptoms and medication-seeking behavior. This drug dependence then becomes a comorbid diagnosis complicating the management of the somatoform disorder. Such problems can be avoided by accurately diagnosing somatoform disorders and recognizing the futility of symptom resolution as a treatment goal.

There has been little study of the effects of reproductive cycle events on the course of somatoform disorders. Stewart et al. (1992) found increased rates of psychological distress, including somatization, during the perimenopausal years. However, Ballinger (1976) found hypochondriacal preoccupation to be more common following menopause.

COMORBIDITY

Axis I Comorbidity

Somatization disorder frequently occurs with comorbid Axis I disorders. In the ECA study, all of the other Axis I diagnoses studied were more prevalent in subjects with somatization disorder compared to subjects without somatization disorder (Swartz et al., 1991). One hundred percent of the ECA sample with somatization disorder had another psychiatric diagnosis, compared to 34% of the sample without somatization disorder. Somatization disorder increases the risk of comorbid panic disorder more than any other disorder, with a prevalence ratio of nearly 25. Somatization disorder also increases the risk of comorbid major depression, obsessive–compulsive disorder, manic episode, and schizophrenia, with prevalence ratios all exceeding 10. Clinical sample studies of Axis I comorbidity in somatization disorder have also been published. Brown et al. (1990) found the highest risk ratios were for panic disorder (16.25), major depression (9.41), schizophrenia (7.77) and obsessive compulsive disorder (7.04).

Noyes et al. (1994) examined psychiatric comorbidity in a series of subjects with hypochondriasis. These subjects were compared to a control group of medical outpatients who scored low on measures of hypochondriasis. The subjects with hypochondriasis were more likely to have a comorbid psychiatric diagnosis than were those without hypochondriasis were (62% vs. 30%). Panic disorder and major depression were the most common diagnoses. Major depression often occurred after the diagnosis of hypochondriasis, whereas panic disorder often preceded the diagnosis of hypochondriasis. It has been suggested that hypochondriasis be classified with the anxiety disorders (Noyes, 1999). Hypochondriasis appears to be most closely related to phobic disorders—specific phobia of illness, in particular.

Conversion disorder is also associated with significant psychiatric comorbidity. Binzer et al. (1997) studied psychiatric comorbidity among 30 patients with conversion disorder and found that 33% met criteria for other Axis I disorders.

The timing of the onset of two psychiatric disorders is particularly important in studying the relationship between the disorders. Rief et al. (1992) studied the relationship between somatoform disorders and mood disorders in a series of subjects with somatoform disorders. Eighty seven percent of the patients with somatoform disorders had a lifetime comorbid mood disorder. In the majority of patients with mood disorder comorbidity (73%), the somatoform disorder preceded the onset of the mood disorder. The length of time from the onset of the somatoform disorder to the onset of the mood disorder was at least 1 year. Patients with both disorders tended to have separate courses for the individual disorders. The somatoform disorder tended to be of long duration with chronic symptoms. The mood disorder tended to be episodic with periods of remission.

The most difficult timing-of-onset relationship to untangle is that of somatization disorder and panic disorder. Here, 35% of the comorbid cases had a first symptom of somatization disorder, 41% had a panic disorder symptom occurring first, and 24% of cases could not be classified, suggesting nearly simultaneous emergence of symptoms. Swartz et al. (1991) conclude that for the majority of instances of comorbidity, somatization disorder appears to be a distinct disorder not dependent on a preexisting primary condition. They also conclude that somatization disorder appears to have a life of its own, distinct from other major psychiatric disorders.

Like the somatic symptoms associated with somatization disorder, the psychiatric symptoms tend to be chronic and many times unresponsive to standard psychopharmacological approaches. It is often best to treat the psychiatric symptoms associated with somatization disorder like the medical symptoms—not seeking symptom elimination as a goal, but pursuing symptom management with a goal of reduction in morbidity associated with medical treatment or intervention.

Axis II Comorbidity

Personality disorders are more common in patients with somatization disorder then the general population. Rost et al. (1992) studied a series of patients with somatization disorder for concurrent Axis II diagnoses. All patients received the Structured Clinical Interview for DSM-III-R, Axis II Personality Disorders (Spitzer, 1990). Sixty-one percent demonstrated at least one personality disorder, with 37% having two or more personality disorders. The most frequent personality disorder diagnoses were avoidant (26.7%), paranoid (21.3%), self-defeating (19.1%), and obsessive–compulsive (17.1%). Histrionic personality disorder and antisocial personality disorder were found in 12.8% and 7.4% of the patients with somatization disorder, respectively. The Axis II disorders in the group with somatization disorder were then compared to those in a control group of general medical patients. This study found individual personality disorders to be 2.5 to 24.8 times more likely in the former group than in the latter group. The risk ratios were highest for schizotypal (24.8), avoidant (11.6), paranoid (9.3), and dependent (5.0) personality disorders.

In another study of personality disorder among patients with somatization disorder in a medical population, Stern et al. (1993) compared 25 such patients to matched controls with either a mood or an anxiety disorder. Despite this control selection, the rate of personality disorders in the patients with somatization disorder remained twice that in the control group (72% vs. 36%). Personality traits found to be increased in somatization disorder included histrionic, passive–dependent, and sensitive–dependent. In the Binzer et al. (1997) study discussed earlier, elevated rates of coexisting personality disorders were found in patients with conversion disorder. Fifty percent of patients with conversion disorder in this study had an associated personality disorder, compared to 17% in the control group.

Few studies have targeted the personality disorder comorbidity in hypochondriasis. Barsky et al. (1992) studied a series of 76 outpatients with DSM-III-R hypochondriasis, recruited from a medical clinic. According to the Personality Diagnostic Questionnaire impairment/distress subscale, 63% of the case group met criteria for a personality disorder—three times higher than that for a control group of medical outpatients recruited from the same clinic.

Studies of patients with chronic pain have demonstrated high rates of personality disorder comorbidity. Fishbain et al. (1986) found that 59% of patients admitted to a pain unit met criteria for a personality disorder. The most frequent diagnoses were dependent, passive–aggressive, and histrionic personality disorders. Compulsive and dependent traits were found in both the men and women participating in the study.

Comorbidity may have several clinical implications. First, symptoms of more than one illness can produce diagnostic confusion. In addition, once one psychiatric diagnosis is made, there is often a tendency to stop the diagnostic interview process and forget that an additional diagnosis may be present. Comorbidity is frequently associated with a more severe form of mental illness. Severity of illness may be displayed in higher severity of target symptoms, poorer response to treatment, or more impairment or disability in an area of functioning such as work or social activities. Knowledge of comorbidity alerts the clinician to the increased likelihood of more severe disorder that is less likely to be simply managed. This information can allow the clinician to revise expectations and provide for a multidisciplinary strategy for treatment.

TREATMENT RESPONSE

Somatization Disorder

The treatment of somatization disorder begins with a paradigm shift in the physician's role in treatment. Physicians who continue to pursue symptom resolution as the goal of treatment are likely to become quickly frustrated by patients with somatization disorder. The goal of treatment needs to be shifted from symptom resolution to reduction of impairment and minimization of unnecessary health care utilization. This approach also recognizes the need to reduce the risk of iatrogenic complications related to medically unnecessary tests and operations. Symptoms become not something to relieve, but something to interpret and to manage in the context of a patient's functioning and lifestyle.

The physician needs to begin by acknowledging the patient's symptoms. A brief physical exam targeted to the site of the patient's complaint reinforces the physician's concern about potential medical sources for the complaint. Following this exam, the physician may state that there is no evidence that the patient's symptoms are the result of a life-threatening or potentially disabling medical condition. The physician can then validate the symptom by stating that he or she will want to continue monitoring the symptom over time and to schedule a follow-up visit for reevaluation. Reduction of impairment begins by acknowledging the presence of symptoms but encouraging the patient to maintain normal daily activities as much as possible.

Psychiatrists can become involved in the management of somatization disorder, although there is no evidence that specialist treatment is more effective than that provided by primary care physicians. Patients often resist referral to a psychiatrist and see it as a rejection of their medical problems by the referring physician. For a patient resisting psychiatric management, the psychiatrist can provide direction to the primary care physician. Referring physicians may benefit by the suggestion of a one-time psychiatric consultation to help in assessment, while scheduling the patient back for primary management. Some patients with somatization disorder endorse psychiatric as well as medical symptoms. For these patients, psychiatric referral and management may be accepted for the psychiatric component of their complaints.

McLeod and Budd (1997) have described a 6-week structured group intervention that holds promise for the management of patients with somatization. One hundred seventy-one participants at Harvard Pilgrim Health Care completed the study. The 6-week Personal Health Improvement Program included classroom videos, exercises and home study assignments. One year after the course, participants reported decreases in emotional and physical distress, increases in functional status, and high levels of satisfaction. Medical records also revealed decreased use of medical resources.

A three-step approach to the psychological management of somatization was outlined by Luff and Garrod (1935). The three steps include (1) establishment of a strong physician–patient relationship; (2) education of the patient in the nature of his or her symptoms and the concept of somatization; and (3) provision of support, reassurance, and availability for follow-up and monitoring of the patient's condition.

The establishment of a strong psychiatrist–patient relationship will require many of the components described earlier: acknowledgment of the patient's symptom, concern for the need for medical evaluation, and monitoring of the symptoms over time. Education about somatization and somatization disorder can be helpful. The psychiatrist can inform the patient that this is a valid condition, and that a great deal has been learned about this problem from the study of others with it. The psychiatrist can reassure the patient that the problem will be monitored. Over time, the role of stress and environmental issues in contributing to the physical symptoms can be discussed. The focus on medical symptoms can often be shifted to concerns the patient may have about relationships and other life issues. Praise for continuing high levels of functioning provides the patient with motivation for continued limitation of the impairment related to the symptom.

Few studies of specific psychotherapy treatments for somatization disorder exist. Speckens et al. (1995) conducted a randomized controlled trial of cognitive-behavioral therapy in a series of patients with medically unexplained physical symptoms. From 6 to 16 sessions of cognitive-behavioral therapy were administered to the case group. The control group continued to be managed by the primary care providers. The intervention targeted the identification and modification of dysfunctional automatic thoughts as the key procedure. Follow-up measures were completed at 6 and 12 months. In general, the treated group improved on measures of somatic symptoms, physical distress, sickness impact, functional impairment, and hypochrondriacal beliefs.

No effective pharmacological interventions for somatization disorder have been reported. However, very few systematic controlled trials of medication approaches for the management of somatization disorder exist. This lack of study is probably due in part to the clinical experience that few patients with somatization disorder benefit from psychotropic management. In addition, these patients tend to be particularly sensitive to medication side effects.

Hypochondriasis

For a patient with hypochondriasis, one must first determine whether the hypochondriasis is primary or secondary to another psychiatric disorder. If the patient has a primary mood or anxiety disorder with secondary hypochondriasis, successful treatment of the patient's primary disorder often results in reduction of secondary somatic symptoms. The pharmacological treatment of primary hypochondriasis is even less clear than that of somatization disorder.

Cognitive-behavioral therapy holds promise for hypochondriasis, because the core feature is the cognitive misperception of a symptom as indication of a serious disease. All people experience physical symptoms on a daily basis, and most are able to correctly interpret these symptoms as normal and not indicative of a serious illness; however, patients with hypochondriasis interprets these normal symptoms as indication of a possible serious illness. This interpretation leads to rumination, heightened arousal, increased surveillance for additional symptoms, and a tendency to focus on the most serious of medical illnesses as the cause for their symptoms. The tendency to misinterpret physical symptoms can be explained as an indication of an underlying dysfunctional assumption about health and illness.

Warwick (1995) completed a trial of cognitive-behavioral treatment for 32 patients with DSM-III-R hypochondriasis. Half of the patients received weekly cognitive-behavioral therapy for 4 months; the other half remained on a waiting list. The active treatment group demonstrated a highly significant decrease in global severity of hypochondriasis, as well as a highly significant decrease in depression and anxiety ratings.

Warwick described the principles of cognitive-behavioral therapy used in this study. The first principle is to explore each patient's symptom pattern and explain that these symptoms can be addressed through the cognitive model. Patients may often express relief with this approach, as many medical practitioners have probably spent a great deal of time telling them what their symptoms are not, but not what they are. The second principle is to have patients begin self-monitoring their physical symptoms, anxiety about their health, negative thoughts, and behavior related to their belief that they are ill. Attention to somatic triggers, the degree of anxiety, associated negative thoughts, and the resultant behavior form the core of monitoring.

A third step is the active reattribution of a patient's negative thoughts. Dysfunctional assumptions can be the basis for hypochondriacal fears and need to be challenged. An example of a dysfunctional assumption is a perception that one will develop cancer because a relative had cancer. Such dysfunctional assumptions can be attacked in a rational fashion. The therapist can provide family members with a realistic plan to dealing with requests for reassurance. Therapists can encourage patients to challenge their beliefs about themselves. Patients can also be encouraged to begin a medically appropriate exercise program.

Next, the therapist must stop the cycle of hypochondriacal behavior through the use of exposure with response prevention. Responses triggered by hypochrondriacal anxiety can include visiting physicians or repetitively seeking reassurance from friends or family members. The therapist can induce the symptoms by simulating cues and then block the patient's usual response to the symptoms. Family members can become involved to assist in the blocking of repeated reassurance seeking.

Group therapy approaches to hypochondriasis also show promise. Stern and

Fernandez (1991) used a cognitive-behavioral approach to the treatment of hypo-chondriasis in a group of six hospitalized patients. The mean duration of the patients' hypochondriasis was 12 years. The treatment intervention included nine sessions. Sessions focussed on a variety of topics, including general education, the attention focus of hypochondriasis, relaxation exercises, use of symptom diaries, family factors, and depression. Following group treatment, participants reported less medical utilization and lowered preoccupation with illness.

Conversion Disorder

There are essentially no controlled studies documenting specific efficacy for the treatment of conversion disorder. One reason for this lack of research is the relatively rare prevalence rate for this disorder, making it difficult to plan and carry out such studies. Despite the lack of controlled research, reports of single cases and small case series provide some direction for the management of conversion disorder symptoms. Various strategies for management of conversion disorder have been described, including hypnosis, amobarbital-assisted interviews, behavior therapy, pharmacological management, electroconvulsive therapy, physical therapy, and biofeedback. Treatment efficacy for acute conversion disorder is generally better than for chronic conversion disorder.

Patients with conversion disorder appear to have above-average susceptibility to hypnosis (VanDyck & Hoogduin, 1989). The use of hypnosis has been described for conversion disorder since the 19th century. Patients are placed under hypnosis, and after satisfactory induction, additional historical information about the potential precipitating events can be elicited. The suggestion that hypnosis can be curative is provided before, during, and after hypnosis. Hypnosis may be more appropriate for loss of motor function than for pseudoseizures, which occur intermittently and may be less treatable by hypnotic suggestion.

Amobarbital interviews can help provide information for assessment, as well as a treatment modality for acute conversion disorder. A general procedure for completing an amobarbital interview has been described by Perry et al. (1997). Although generally safe, amobarbital has been associated with laryngospasm, so it should be done in a setting where resuscitation can be accomplished if necessary. Patients can be told that many people experience great benefit from such interviews and that improvement can be expected. During an interview, a patient is asked about the life stressors that may have contributed to his or her current condition. The amobarbital may reduce defenses and allow the patient to discuss important precipitants. If a motor deficit is the presenting condition, the patient can be instructed to move the affected area under amobarbital; this technique can help diagnostically and provide support for the suggestion that the interview will help and the patient will be improved afterward.

Behavior therapy appears to hold promise in the treatment of conversion disorder (Donohue et al., 1997; Gooch et al., 1997; Silver, 1996; Speed, 1996). An inpatient behavioral modification program can be developed that is targeted to the patient's presenting symptom. A contract can be drawn up that outlines the steps of the behavioral treatment program. Patients are praised and provided positive reinforcement for doing well (e.g., going a day without a pseudoseizure). Positive reinforcement needs to be customized to the individual patient. When targeted behaviors worsen, the behaviors are not reinforced but ignored. Behavior therapy can be often used in conjunction with physical therapy or speech therapy for aphonia. The behavioral modification program works best when tied to a program at home at the time of discharge. In addition, the stresses related to the precipitating event need to be identified and modified prior to a patient's discharge from the hospital.

As in hypochondriasis, pharmacotherapy can play a key role in the management of conversion disorder in the treatment of underlying depression or anxiety disorders. For significant anxiety associated with a severe stressor, short-term benzodiazepine treatment can be used in conjunction with behavioral therapy.

Pain Disorder with Psychological Features

Barkin et al. (1996) have summarized the psychological principles of pain management. Psychological approaches can be utilized for all patients with pain, but appear particularly important in those with significant psychological features to their pain problem. Three primary approaches can be utilized: cognitive-behavioral treatment (including relaxation training and relapse prevention), operant learning, and biofeedback. Comparative studies suggest that each approach appears to be effective in improving pain complaints and functional status. Combining approaches does not appear to provide additional benefit. Because space prohibits a discussion of all three of these approaches here, we concentrate on cognitive-behavioral treatment.

Cognitive-behavioral treatment begins with educating a patient about his or her pain disorder. Patients may have significant misinformation about their condition that reduces their level of functioning. For example, a patient with chronic back pain may feel that any activity increases the risk of causing permanent injury. When informed that prudent exercise and activity are associated with minimum risk of permanent injury, the patient may be more likely to engage in therapeutic activities. The therapist must be aware of the patient's perception of his or her illness and future expectations for pain. Cognitive distortions like catastrophizing can contribute to increased pain and disability. A primary cognitive intervention is to get the patient to see him- or herself as capable of increased functioning, with the potential for remission of the pain condition. Coping skills training and activity-pacing skills appear to also provide benefit as part of the cognitive-behavioral treatment of chronic pain.

Relaxation training can provide reduction in pain related to psychologically induced muscle tension. Relaxation training can include progressive muscle relaxation, stretch-based relaxation, and breathing exercises. Individual training in relaxation can be augmented by audiotapes that patients can use at home during the acute and maintenance phases of therapy. Imagery training can provide additional assistance in relaxation or can be targeted to specific pain management techniques.

Consideration needs to be given to the prevention of relapse. Patients need to be placed in a maintenance program with specific strategies for dealing with pain recurrence. Returning to work should be encouraged, with a gradual increase in activities at the work site. Family members and employers should be educated about the maintenance-phase plan of treatment.

Psychotropic drugs, particularly antidepressants, can also be useful in the management of chronic pain. Phillip and Fickenger (1993) reviewed studies of the use of psychotropic drugs in the management of chronic pain syndromes. Most individual studies found that 50–70% of subjects improved with antidepressant treatment, compared to

30–40% of subjects receiving a placebo. Despite the limited study, doses for pain control generally range from 50% to 75% of the dosages commonly recommended in the treatment of depression.

One important issue in chronic pain management is the potential for the development of prescription drug misuse (abuse or dependence). Clinicians must carefully weigh the risks and benefits in the prescription of narcotic pain medications. Although aggressive use of narcotics carries the risk of abuse or dependence, hesitancy in narcotic use runs the risk of inadequate control of pain in patients with legitimate clinical indications for narcotic use.

Fishbain et al. (1992) reviewed studies of drug abuse, dependence, and addiction in patients with chronic pain. Within these studies, the prevalence of drug abuse, dependence and addiction was in the range of 3.2–18.9%. Patients at risk for prescription drug misuse include those with antisocial personality disorder, prior alcohol abuse or dependence, prior drug abuse or dependence, or significant family history of alcohol or drug problems. It is best to carefully consider non-narcotic analgesic use for patients with one of these risk factors. For those without one of these risk factors the potential for drug abuse or dependence appears small. Despite this, it is felt that narcotic analgesics are not effective for chronic pain management, and chronic use should be avoided. Psychological factors may play in key role in problems weaning patients away from chronic narcotic use.

CONCLUSION

Individuals with somatoform disorders make high use of medical services, and often present to physicians other than psychiatrists. Comorbid psychiatric disorders, especially mood disorders, are common and often develop after the onset of a somatoform disorder. Patients with somatoform disorders can be challenging to manage medically. Physicians must modify the primary goal of treatment; rather than symptom resolution, they must think in terms of symptom reduction and minimization of unnecessary health care utilization. This includes the establishment of a strong patient–physician relationship, acknowledgment of the patient's symptoms, support, reassurance, and availability. Further studies of treatment efficacy in the somatoform disorders should be done, in light of the considerable psychological distress and cost associated with these disorders.

REFERENCES

American Psychiatric Association. (2000). *Diagnostic and statistical manual of mental disorders, Fourth Edition, Text Revision*. Washington, DC: Author.

Ballinger, C. B. (1976). Psychiatric morbidity and the menopause: Clinical features. *British Medical Journal, i*(6019), 1183–1185.

Barkin, R. L., Lubenow, T. R., Bruehl, S., et al. (1996). Management of chronic pain: Part II. *Disease-A-Month, 42*, 457–507.

Barsky, A. J., Fama, J. M., Bailey, E. D., et al. (1998). A prospective 4-to 5-year study of DSM-III-R hypochondriasis. *Archives of General Psychiatry, 55*(8), 737–744.

Barsky, A. J., Wyshak, G., & Klerman, G. L. (1992). Psychiatric comorbidity in DSM-III-R hypochondriasis. *Archives of General Psychiatry, 49*, 101–108.

Bass, C., Bond, A., Gill, D., et al. (1999). Frequent attenders without organic disease in a gastroenterology clinic: Patient characteristics and health care use. *General Hospital Psychiatry, 21*(1), 30–38.

Binzer, M., Andersen, P. M., & Kullgren, G. (1997). Clinical characteristics of patients with motor disability due to conversion disorder: A prospective control group study. *Journal of Neurology, Neurosurgery and Psychiatry, 63*(1), 83–88.

Brown, F. W., Golding, J. M., & Smith, G. R., Jr. (1990). Psychiatric comorbidity in primary care somatization disorder. *Psychosomatic Medicine, 52*(4), 445–451.

Boffeli, T. J., & Guze, S. B. (1992). The simulation of neurologic disease. *Psychiatric Clinics of North America, 15*(2), 301–310.

Donohue, B., Thevenin, D. M., & Runyon, M. K. (1997). Behavioral treatment of conversion disorder in adolescence: A case example of globus hystericus. *Behavioral Modification, 21*(2), 231–251.

Escobar, J. I., Gara, M., Waitzkin, H., et al. (1998). DSM-IV hypochondriasis in primary care. *General Hospital Psychiatry, 20*(3), 155–159.

Escobar, J. I., Rubio-Stipec, M., Canino, G., et al. (1989). Somatic symptom index (SSI): A new and abridged somatization construct. Prevalence and epidemiologic correlates in two large community samples. *Journal of Nervous and Mental Disease, 177*, 140–146.

Faravelli, C., Salvatori, S., Galassi, F., et al. (1997). Epidemiology of somatoform disorders: A community survey in Florence. *Social Psychiatry and Psychiatric Epidemiology, 32*(1), 24–29.

Fishbain, D. A., Goldberg, M., & Meagher, B. R. (1986). Male and female chronic pain patients categorized by DSM-III psychiatric diagnostic criteria. *Pain, 26*, 181–197.

Fishbain, D. A., Rosomoff, H. L., & Rosomoff, R. S. (1992). Drug abuse, dependence, and addiction in chronic pain patients. *Clinical Journal of Pain, 8*, 77–85.

Folks, D. G., Ford, C. V., & Regan, W. M. (1984). Conversion symptoms in a general hospital. *Psychosomatics, 25*, 285–295.

Golding, J. M., Smith, G. R., Jr., & Kashner, T. M. (1991). Does somatization disorder occur in men?: Clinical characteristics of women and men with multiple unexplained somatic symptoms. *Archives of General Psychiatry, 48*(3), 231–235.

Gooch, J. L., Wolcott, R., & Speed, J. (1997). Behavioral management of conversion disorder in children. *Archives of Physical Medicine and Rehabilitation, 78*(3), 264–268.

Gureje, O., Ustun, T. B., & Simon, G. E. (1997). The syndrome of hypochondriasis: A cross-national study in primary care. *Psychological Medicine, 27*(5), 1001–1010.

Kroenke, K., & Spitzer, R. L. (1998). Gender differences in the reporting of physical and somatoform symptoms. *Psychosomatic Medicine, 60*(2), 150–155.

Luff, M. C., & Garrod, M. (1935). The after-results of psychotherapy in 500 adult cases. *British Medical Journal, ii*, 54–59.

McLeod, C. C., & Budd, M. A. (1997). Treatment of somatization in primary care: Evaluation of the Personal Health Improvement Program. *HMO Practice, 11*(2), 88–94.

Myers, J. K., Weissman, M. M., Tischler, G. I., et al. (1984). Six month prevalence of psychiatric disorders in three communities. *Archives of General Psychiatry, 41*, 959–967.

Noyes, R., Jr. (1999). The relationship of hypochondriasis to anxiety disorders. *General Hospital Psychiatry, 21*(1), 8–17.

Noyes, R., Jr., Holt, C. S., Happel, R. L., et al. (1997). A family study of hypochondriasis. *Journal of Nervous and Mental Disease, 185*(4), 223–232.

Noyes, R., Jr., Kathol, R. G., Fisher, M. M., et al. (1994). Psychiatric comorbidity among patients with hypochondriasis. *General Hospital Psychiatry, 16*(2), 78–87.

Perry, P. J., Alexander, B., & Liskow, B. I. (1997). *Psychotropic drug handbook* (7th ed.). Washington, DC: American Psychiatric Press.

Phillip, M., & Fickinger, M. (1993). Psychotropic drugs in the management of chronic pain syndromes. *Pharmacopsychiatry, 26*, 221–234.

Rief, W., Schaefer, S., Hiller, W., et al. (1992). Lifetime diagnoses in patients with somatoform disorders: Which came first? *European Archives of Psychiatry and Clinical Neuroscience, 241*(4), 236–240.

Rost, K. M., Akins, R. N., Brown, F. W., et al. (1992). The comorbidity of DSM-III-R personality disorders in somatization disorder. *General Hospital Psychiatry, 14*(5), 322–326.

Silver, F. W. (1996). Management of conversion disorder. *American Journal of Physical Medicine and Rehabilitation, 75*(2), 134–140.

Speckens, A. E., van Hemert, A. M., Spinhoven, P., et al. (1995). Cognitive behavioral therapy for medically unexplained physical symptoms: A randomized controlled trial. *British Medical Journal, 311*, 1328–1332.

Speed, J. (1996). Behavioral management of conversion disorder: Retrospective study. *Archives of Physical Medicine and Rehabilitation, 77*(2), 147–154.

Spertus, I. L., Burns, J., Glenn, B., et al. (1999). Gender differences in associations between trauma history and adjustment among chronic pain patients. *Pain, 82*(1), 97–102.

Spitzer, R. (1990). *Structured Clinical Interview for DSM-III-R Personality Disorders SCID-II (Version 1.0).* Washington, DC: American Psychiatric Press.

Stern, J., Murphy, M., & Bass, C. (1993). Personality disorders in patients with somatization disorder. A controlled study. *British Journal of Psychiatry, 163*, 785–789.

Stern, R., & Fernandez, M. (1991). Group cognitive and behavioral treatment for hypochondriasis. *British Medical Journal, 303*, 1229–1331.

Stewart, D. E., Boydell, K., Derzko, C., et al. (1992). Psychological distress during the menopausal years in women attending a menopause clinic. *International Journal of Psychiatry in Medicine, 22*(3), 213–220.

Swartz, M. S., Blazer, D. G., Woodbury M. M., et al. (1986). Somatization disorder in a community population. *American Journal of Psychiatry, 143*, 1403–1408.

Swartz, M., Landerman, R., George, L. K., et al. (1991). Somatization disorder. In L. N. Robins & D. A. Regier (Eds.), *Psychiatric disorders in America: The Epidemiologic Catchment Area study* (pp. 220–257). New York: Free Press.

Tomasson, K., Kent, D., & Coryell, W. (1991). Somatization and conversion disorders: Comorbidity and demographics at presentation. *Acta Psychiatrica Scandinavica, 84*(3), 288–293.

VanDyck, R., & Hoogduin, K. (1989). Hypnosis and conversion disorders. *American Journal of Psychotherapy, 43*(4), 480–493.

Walker, E. A., Katon, W. J., & Jemelka, R. P. (1993). Psychiatric disorders and medical care utilization among people in the general population who report fatigue. *Journal of General Internal Medicine, 8*, 426–440.

Warwick, H. M. C. (1995). Treatment of hypochondriasis. In R. Mayou, C. Bass, & M. Sharpe (Eds.), *Treatment of functional somatic symptoms* (pp. 163–174). Oxford: Oxford University Press.

Wool, C. A., & Barsky, A. J. (1994). Do women somatize more than men?: Gender differences in somatization. *Psychosomatics, 35*, 445–452.

Yates, W. R. (1999). Epidemiology of psychiatric disorders in the medically ill. In R. G. Robinson & W. R. Yates (Eds.), *Psychiatric treatment of the medically ill* (pp. 41–64). New York: Marcel Dekker.

18

Personality Disorders

PAULA L. HENSLEY
H. GEORGE NURNBERG

DEFINITIONS

According to the fourth edition of the *Diagnostic and Statistical Manual of Mental Disorders* (DSM-IV; American Psychiatric Association, 1994) a personality disorder (PD) is a stable, durable pattern of behavior and internal experience that differs sharply from cultural expectations, is rigid and pervasive, begins in adolescence or early adulthood, and results in impairment or distress. DSM-IV classifies 10 specific PDs (aside from the "not otherwise specified" category) into three clusters.

Cluster A, the "odd" cluster, includes paranoid, schizoid, and schizotypal PDs. Paranoid PD, according to DSM-IV, is characterized by a pattern of suspicion and distrust of others, and an interpretation of their motives as malign. Patients with schizoid PD demonstrate a consistent pattern of aloofness from social relationships and restricted emotional expressiveness in interpersonal environments. Schizotypal PD (STPD) is characterized by strong discomfort with, and little capacity for, close relationships, as well as by distorted cognitions or perceptions and eccentric behaviors. According to DSM-IV, all of the Cluster A disorders are slightly more common in males.

Cluster B, the "dramatic" cluster, includes antisocial, borderline, histrionic, and narcissistic PDs. Antisocial PD (ASPD) has as its essential feature a consistent pattern of disregarding and violating others' rights; this pattern develops in childhood or early adolescence and endures in adulthood. DSM-IV identifies ASPD as more frequently diagnosed in men, with overall prevalence in community samples of 3% in men and 1% in women. Borderline PD (BPD) is characterized by a durable pattern of unstable relationships, self-concept, and affects, as well as strong impulsivity, that begins by young adulthood and is manifested in various contexts. According to DSM-IV, BPD is a clinical diagnosis predominantly made in women (approximately 75% of cases). Individuals with histrionic PD show excessive and all-encompassing emotionality and seek attention constantly. Histrionic PD is clinically diagnosed more frequently in women; however, the sex ratio is not significantly different from the sex ratio of women within the clinical settings in which the diagnoses are made. Narcissistic PD has as its essential feature an enduring pattern of grandiosity, craving for admiration, and absence of empathy that begins by young adulthood and is seen in various contexts. DSM-IV notes that 50–75% of people diagnosed with narcissistic PD are men.

In Cluster C, the "anxious" cluster, are avoidant, dependent, and obsessive–compulsive PDs. Individuals with avoidant PD are socially inhibited, feel inadequate, and are hypersensitive to negative evaluation. According to DSM-IV, avoidant PD occurs with equal frequency in males and females. Dependent PD is characterized by an overpowering need to be taken care of that leads to submission, clinging, and separation fears. Dependent PD is diagnosed predominantly in women; however, as is the case with histrionic PD, the sex ratio is not significantly different from that within the clinical settings in which the diagnoses are made. Obsessive–compulsive PD has as its essential feature an excessive concern with being orderly, perfect, and in mental and interpersonal control, to the detriment of being open, flexible, and efficient. DSM-IV notes that this PD is diagnosed about twice as often in males as in females.

Appendix B of DSM-IV, which lists criteria sets provided for further study, includes two additional PDs—depressive and passive–aggressive (also called negativistic). Depressive PD has as its essential feature a widespread and enduring pattern of depressive behaviors and cognitions that begins by young adulthood and occurs in various contexts, but that does not occur only during episodes of major depression and is not better explained by dysthymia. Passive–aggressive PD was part of the PD grouping in DSM-III-R, but was removed for excess comorbidity and questions regarding its suitability as an independent diagnostic entity. It is characterized by negative attitudes and passive resistance to performance demands in occupational and social contexts.

Finally, DSM-IV recognizes the potential contributions of a dimensional nosology as an alternative to its current categorical approach. That is, it acknowledges the possibility (1) that PDs may be maladaptive forms of personality traits that merge gradually into normality and into each other, or (2) that the three PD clusters may be viewed as dimensions of personality dysfunction on a continuum with Axis I disorders. Possible dimensional approaches are discussed further below.

EPIDEMIOLOGY

Although DSM-IV acknowledges that social stereotypes about gender roles and behaviors influence the diagnosis of PDs, and cautions against overdiagnosing and underdiagnosing certain PDs in particular genders, clinical practice suggests otherwise.

Some authors have suggested that gender differences in PD diagnoses exist due to differences in personality characteristics, such as a tendency for females to internalize and males to externalize their responses to pain and suffering (Widom, 1999). Such a contrast can be due to one or multiple factors, which can be split along the lines of nature versus nurture. Perhaps females have a hard-wired predisposition to internalize emotions, due to structural brain differences, hormonal differences, or an interaction of the two. Cyranowski et al. (2000) offer a model for understanding the adolescent onset of the gender difference in rates of depression. These authors argue that females have social relationships marked by a stronger affiliative style than do men; they hypothesize that this tendency is probably the result of biological and social factors evolving from different reproductive challenges presented to females and males. On the nurture side of the argument, social norms and parental expectations may contribute to an inclination for females to internalize. For example, a study of adults (mothers) who were misled about an infant's gender showed a tendency for these mothers to smile more at an infant thought to be female and a tendency to offer an infant dressed as a male a more action-oriented toy—a toy train rather than a doll (Will & Self, 1976). This study suggests that the power of parental and social expectations, starting at a very young age, is quite strong.

Studies examining the prevalence of PDs by gender present a confusing array of findings. Alnaes and Torgersen (1988) examined outpatients with different Axis I diagnoses and found that men were more likely to have STPD and obsessive–compulsive, passive–aggressive, paranoid, and narcissistic PDs than were women. They found that women had fewer PDs and did not predominate in any of the PDs.

Weissman (1993) reviewed work by Neugebauer et al. (1980) and concluded:

> Based on an unequal sex ratio, the specific types of personality disorders tend to cancel each other out, and the sex ratio for total rates of personality disorder is almost equal. These rates seem to be, from the Neugebauer et al. review, fairly consistent across age groups, with a slight decrease in the older age groups, and with higher rates in the urban rather than rural areas, and higher rates in the lower socioeconomic groups than in the upper classes. (p. 50)

Reich (1987) studied the sex distribution of outpatients with a DSM-III diagnosis of a PD; he found that histrionic PD was more commonly diagnosed in women, and that paranoid and compulsive PDs and ASPD were more commonly diagnosed in men. The Epidemiologic Catchment Area (ECA) study found a higher rate of ASPD in men (Robins et al., 1984); however, that was the only PD considered for assessment. (Other PDs were excluded for lack of construct validity.) Secondary analysis (Samuels et al., 1994) of the ECA data from eastern Baltimore showed a higher, but not statistically significant, prevalence of PDs in men (12.3% vs. 6.8% in women). In psychiatric inpatients studied by Jackson et al. (1991), ASPD was the only DSM-III or DSM-III-R PD with a clear gender difference (i.e., greater frequency in males). A common limitation of these studies was a failure to control for Axis I comorbidity by examining a group of patients with the same or similar Axis I pathology.

Two more recent studies examined gender differences in PDs in a depressed population. Golomb et al. (1995) examined a group of patients with a primary DSM-III-R diagnosis of major depression and found that men were significantly more likely than women to meet DSM-III-R criteria for ASPD and for narcissistic and obsessive–compulsive PDs as measured by the Personality Diagnostic Questionnaire—Revised, and for narcissistic and obsessive–compulsive PDs as measured by the Structured Clinical Interview for DSM-III-R, Axis II (SCID-II). Neither the SCID-II nor the Personality Diagnostic Questionnaire—Revised, which have poor concurrent validity between them, revealed a higher prevalence of any PD in women. This study supports earlier studies that challenge the methodology in findings of more frequent diagnoses of BPD and of histrionic and dependent PDs in women.

A second study that partially replicates and extends the findings of Golomb et al. (1995) is the work of Carter et al. (1999). Subjects in this second study were recruited from outpatients with major depression (DSM-III-R criteria) and were assessed with a Structured Clinical Interview for DSM-III-R, Personality Questionnaire (SCID-PQ) and SCID-II. The authors gathered data on both PD diagnoses and symptoms. Females did not predominate in any PD symptomatology or diagnosis, although men were more likely to meet full criteria for ASPD, BPD, STPD, and paranoid, narcissistic, and obsessive–compulsive PDs. Men, more than women, tended to have symptoms of (but not necessarily to meet full criteria for) STPD, ASPD, and schizoid, narcissistic, and obsessive–compulsive PDs.

Although these studies attempted to control for Axis I disorders, a limitation to generalizability is that both were restricted to outpatients seeking care for depression. Carter et al. (1999) suggest that the higher proportion of PDs found in depressed men may reflect a higher threshold of psychopathology needed for men to seek treatment. The more salient confound is that the base rate of major depressive disorder is twofold higher in women.

The gender distribution of PD characteristics has been hypothesized to be similar to that of the actual PDs. Zimmerman and Coryell (1990) examined the DSM-III PDs from a dimensional perspective and found that men scored higher on the paranoid, schizoid, compulsive, antisocial, and narcissistic dimensions. In contrast, women scored higher on histrionic, dependent, and avoidant dimensions.

In summary, gender comparisons of PD prevalences are confounded by multiple determinants: (1) gender-specific base rates of comorbid Axis I disorders (e.g., major depressive disorder, panic and other anxiety disorders; (2) differential environmental exposures and impact as risk factors (e.g., females are more likely to be sexually assaulted (Stein & Barrett-Connor, 2000), whereas males are more likely to be physically assaulted); (3) social role training; (4) biologically influenced adaptive styles (e.g., different cognitive processing); (5) differential treatment response; (6) diagnostic biases by clinicians; and (7) differential threshold for treatment seeking.

NOSOLOGICAL MODELS

As noted earlier, a possible alternative to the categorical approach to diagnosis used in DSM-IV and previous editions of the DSM is a dimensional perspective. Lensenweger (1999) examined a nonclinical university population and found considerable evidence for the stability of PD features over time. Loranger et al. (1991) demonstrated that although dimensional features changed to some degree, categorical diagnoses showed consistency over time and with change in Axis I. The dimensional approach may be more sensitive to state (Axis I) factors; for example, patients with remitted depression may show improvement in PD criteria. A follow-up study of adolescents with a DSM-III-R diagnosis of BPD found that the diagnosis was stable over the 2-year follow-up period for only 33% of the study group (Garnet et al., 1994). It may be difficult to draw conclusions from the Garnet et al. (1994) study, because significant changes typically occur in concurrent diagnoses during adolescence (e.g., heavy drinking in adolescence), affecting Axis II diagnoses.

Many authors have examined personality characteristics and cite the considerable overlap of criteria sets among the different categories. Despite the finding that 50% or more of patients with PDs, when systematically assessed, have two or more coexisting PD diagnoses (Oldham et al., 1992; Pfohl et al., 1986; Nurnberg et al., 1991; Fryer et al.,

1988; Morey, 1988), clinicians in practice rarely make multiple PD diagnoses. Nurnberg et al. (1999) applied a form of latent trait modeling—the application of grade-of-membership (GoM) analysis—to DSM-III-R PDs and identified four personality groupings. One type, a core PD group, represents a naturally occurring, perhaps qualitatively distinct type, characterized by marked PD pathology. This type is egocentric, entitled, envious, exploiting, externalizing, and emotionally volatile in the context of disturbed interpersonal relationships. Impulsivity, angry outbursts, affective instability, hypersensitivity to criticism, excessive need for approval, and suspiciousness are further indicators of behavioral deficits. The moral code is selective, self-serving, and even dishonest. In DSM-III-R nosology, this type is characterized by criteria defining the ASPD, BPD, and paranoid, narcissistic, histrionic, and passive–aggressive PD categories. These individuals are extremely maladaptive and alloplastic. No significant gender differences were found in the rate of diagnosing this personality type.

A second latent type is socially anxious and detached, with predominantly compulsive and avoidant adaptational features. Individuals in this personality trait domain are emotionally distant, solitary, moralistic, perfectionistic, pessimistic, indecisive, and overly conscientious. Avoidant, schizoid, obsessive–compulsive, and self-defeating PD criteria in DSM-III-R characterize them. They seem to be characterized primarily by exaggerated traits, which may be more or less maladaptive. Males predominate in this group.

A third personality type is characterized by quantitative dependent and self-defeating traits. These individuals are sociable, need relationships, and undervalue themselves. A person in this group is sensitive to criticism, self-sacrificing, and emotionally expressive. The mode of function is relatively more adaptive and autoplastic; females predominate in this group.

A fourth personality type is essentially asymptomatic and characterized by the absence of items that define PDs. This type is autonomous, self-assured, decisive, feels appreciated, accepts criticism, and has a stable sense of identity or self. Individuals assigned to this group rarely meet criteria for PD diagnoses; neither gender predominates. The GoM analysis failed to confirm the natural occurrence of any single specific Axis II PD or cluster in this group. Interestingly, gender-specific distinctions could be made with males predominanting in Group 2, female predominance in Group 3, and equal gender distribution in Groups 1 and 4. GoM, a fuzzy degree of membership modeling, provides a more parsimonious handling of the PD criteria than does the categorical approach of the DSM.

Support for a dimensional approach comes from the work done in behavioral genetics. Behavioral genetic studies have consistently found evidence for the variable heritability of personality traits. Such genetic studies are used to support proponents of a dimensional model of PD classification. Livesley et al. (1993) examined 18 dimensions of personality in volunteer twin pairs from the general population to determine estimates of genetic and environmental influences. Of the 18 dimensions, 12 had heritabilities in the 40–60% range. These 12 were affective lability, anxiousness, callousness, cognitive distortion, identity problems, narcissism, oppostitionality, rejection, restricted expression, social avoidance, stimulus seeking, and suspiciousness. The dimensions with less than 40% heritability were compulsivity, conduct problems, insecure attachment, intimacy problems, self-harm, and submissiveness. The authors suggest that the similarity between these results and those results reported for normal personality support the hypothesis that "personality disorders involve extremes of normal variation and hence a dimensional classification" (Livesley et al., 1993, p. 1830). Later work by Livesley et al. (1998) examined phenotypic and genetic structures underlying personality traits, and revealed four phenotypic components (Emotional Dysregulation, Dissocial Behavior, Inhibitedness, and Compulsivity) that were similar across three samples: patients with PDs, general population subjects, and volunteer twin pairs. These four phenotypic components were similar to four genetic and environmental factors that multivariate genetic analysis yielded. The authors write, "Our data clearly show that the phenotypic structure of personality disorder traits closely reflects the underlying genetic architecture" (Livesley et al., 1998, p. 945). Thus these results support a dimensional representation of personality traits in classifying PDs. However, which dimensions are core and essential remains to be determined.

Evidence from earlier family studies indicated that STPD is genetically linked to schizophrenia and that BPD is not (Kety et al., 1975; Kendler et al., 1981; Baron et al., 1985; Gunderson et al., 1983). This supported the DSM-III division of the broad borderline concept into schizotypal and borderline categories, and permitted two genetic propositions: (1) Mentally ill biological relatives of persons with chronic schizophrenia have STPD and not BPD; (2) the mentally ill relatives of those with BPD preponderantly have BPD themselves (Tarnopolsky, 1992). Seven further studies (Pope et al., 1983; Loranger et al., 1982; Akiskal, 1981; Stone et al., 1981; Andrulonis et al., 1981; Soloff & Millward, 1983; Schulz et al., 1989) found no link to schizophrenia among relatives of patients with BPD. Loranger et al. (1982) found BPD to occur 10 times more often in relatives of female patients with BPD than in relatives of female patients with schizophrenia. Although Soloff and Millward (1983) found higher than predicted rates of schizophrenia among patients with a mixed BPD-STPD pattern, other reports (Baron et al., 1985; Schulz et al., 1989) showed a preponderance of DSM-III affective disorder and schizophrenia in relatives of depressed and nondepressed probands with mixed BPD-STPD. Twin studies extend the independent status of these PDs, finding monozygotic twins of patients with STPD to have genetically determined STPD and not BPD (Torgersen, 1984). In addition, BPD transmission demonstrates a greater environmental than genetic mode of inheritance. The relationship of STPD as a *forme fruste* of schizophrenia would further support a categorical conceptualization of PDs. In the *International Statistical Classification of Diseases and Related Health Problems*, 10th revision (ICD-10), STPD is incorporated into the schizophrenia grouping (World Health Organization, 1992).

Initial reports (Pope et al., 1983; Akiskal, 1981; Stone et al., 1981; Andrulonis et al., 1981; Soloff & Millward, 1983; Schulz et al., 1989; Gunderson & Elliott, 1985) documenting higher than expected prevalences of DSM-III affective disorder in relatives of patients with BPD served to link the conditions. However, DSM-III influenced this finding by separating out the schizophrenia-psychosis-related schizotypal subgroup and using four criteria (i.e., 3, 4, 5, and 7) from the affective domain for diagnosing BPD. Pope et al. (1983), Zanarini et al. (1988), Silverman et al. (1993), and Andrulonis and Vogel (1984) determined that the higher frequency of affective disorder in relatives was accounted for by concurrent affective disorder in the probands with BPD. Torgersen (1984) found cotwins with an affective disorder to be cotwins of patients with BPD and affective disorder. Relatives with STPD and BPD have equal prevalences of depression among their relatives (Soloff & Millward, 1983; Schulz et al., 1989). The first study (Coryell & Zimmerman, 1989) to examine all PDs in relatives of depressed patients did not find BPD to be more prevalent than other PDs among them. Probands with BPD also show familial aggregation of other types of psychopathology, such as substance abuse, antisocial behavior, eating disorders, and DSM-III attention deficit disorder (Akiskal et al., 1985;

Loranger et al., 1982; Andrulonis et al., 1981; Schulz et al., 1989; Zanarini et al., 1988; Links et al., 1988; Loranger & Tulis, 1985). Therefore, the evidence does not support a biogenetic linkage between BPD and affective disorder (Gunderson & Phillips, 1991).

A familial aggregation of BPD, borderline traits, and PDs with related traits (e.g., histrionic PD and ASPD) is consistent with strong evidence for a genetic heritability (35–50%) to individual differences in personality (Schulz et al., 1989; Silverman et al., 1991; McGuffin & Thapar, 1992). It is apparent that the PD constructs are not discrete, but rather polymorphic phenotypes. These entities can be regarded as variants along multiple-component dimensions with complex modes of transmission (e.g., oligogenic) at different quantitative trait loci. Therefore, PD transmission may be better understood by a dimensional approach in which several relatively distinct related temperaments aggregate in families, instead of a categorical model that conceptualizes the PD constructs as entities with discrete boundaries. Consistent with this hypothesis, Silverman et al. (1991) found an increased risk for affective and impulsive personality traits operating as independent factors in relatives of probands with BPD, without a relationship to affective disorders. This does not rule out the possibility that a phenotype may be dimensional and the genotype categorical, or the reverse.

ETIOLOGY

Data from a community-based longitudinal study indicates that people with a history of childhood abuse or neglect are more likely to have PDs and elevated PD symptoms during early adulthood (Johnson et al., 1999). These authors found that people with documented childhood abuse or neglect were more than four times as likely as those not abused or neglected to be diagnosed with PDs during early adulthood. The findings suggest that childhood physical abuse, sexual abuse, and neglect play an important role in the onset of some PDs. The authors examined the different forms of abuse to determine whether certain forms were associated with specific PDs. They found that documented physical abuse was associated with elevated ASPD and depressive PD symptoms; sexual abuse was associated with elevated BPD symptoms; and neglect was associated with elevated symptoms of ASPD, BPD, and avoidant, narcissistic, and passive–aggressive PDs. Johnson et al. (1999) cite several possible mechanisms for these associations:

> Childhood maltreatment may independently increase the risk for PDs; maladaptive parenting, rather than childhood maltreatment, may increase the risk for PDs; childhood maltreatment may increase the risk for PDs among persons with biological diatheses for psychiatric disorders; and/or childhood maltreatment may be an indicator of preexisting PDs. Childhood abuse and neglect may increase the risk for PDs independent of childhood and parental psychiatric disorders. (p. 604)

Many authors cite ASPD as an example of a diagnosis more common in men. It is not surprising, then, that the majority of research done on ASPD has focused on male subjects. One study of outpatients in an addiction treatment center found similar prevalence rates for men (10%) and women (22%) (Galen et al., 2000). Studies of female subjects with ASPD may be particularly revealing of explanations for this gender difference. Examination of data on adult outcomes of adolescent girls with antisocial behavior by

Pajer (1998) demonstrates the difficulty of studying the multiple factors that may lead to perceived gender differences in PDs. Pajer questions the accuracy of criminal statistics, because the justice system itself tends to underreport rates of female juvenile delinquency—in part due to a reluctance to arrest girls with antisocial behavior and a trend to refer them for psychiatric treatment. Biases also exist in clinicians' beliefs about how an adolescent girl demonstrates antisocial behavior. A common belief is that such behavior is predominantly sexual in nature, manifesting itself as precocious sexual activity. Alternatively, prostitution tends to be associated with histrionic PD, BPD, trauma spectrum, and females; and prostitutes tend to be adolescent female runaways with a high prevalence of sexual abuse. Another common belief is that women are less violent than men. Although the most common pathological outcome for boys with antisocial behavior has been shown to be adult criminality, the adult course for girls has been assumed to be more benign. However, Pajer (1998) concludes that women with a history of adolescent antisocial behavior have higher mortality rates, a 10- to 40-fold increase in criminal behavior, a variety of psychiatric problems, dysfunctional and sometimes violent relationships, poor educational achievement, less stable work histories, and higher rates of service utilization. Evidence is also presented that the rate of violent crime among females is increasing.

One study examining adult women is a notable exception to the predominance of research focusing on male subjects. Rutherford et al. (1999) have examined the lifetime prevalence of ASPD and explored the relationship between ASPD and psychopathology. The authors compared five classification systems for the diagnosis of ASPD (DSM-III, DSM-III-R, DSM-IV, the Feighner criteria, and the Research Diagnostic Criteria) by using them to diagnose ASPD in women with cocaine dependence who sought substance use treatment. The five classification systems are similar but not interchangeable, as demonstrated by the wide range of rates of diagnosis of ASPD. Rates of subjects meeting diagnostic criteria ranged from 11% (Research Diagnostic Criteria) to 61% (DSM-III). In all five systems, the authors found a weak relationship between the childhood and adult antisocial behaviors seen in women. Work by Caspi et al. (1993) indicates that precursors of antisocial behavior in women may be more closely related to the early taking on of adult roles and norm-breaking behaviors as a way of obtaining adult possessions (e.g., money, clothes, drugs).

The influence of childhood abuse and neglect on the development of ASPD has yielded findings similar to those in other PDs. Luntz and Widom (1994) examined to what extent childhood abuse and neglect increased the risk of an adult diagnosis of ASPD. They hypothesized that (1) childhood victims of abuse and/or neglect would be more likely to meet criteria for ASPD as young adults and to have a greater number of antisocial symptoms than control subjects without a history of abuse and/or neglect, and (2) the hypothesized relationship would persist even when criminal history was controlled for. The authors interviewed a group of young adults (227 men and 189 women) with documented histories of childhood abuse and/or neglect; the National Institute of Mental Health Diagnostic Interview Schedule, which makes the diagnosis of ASPD with DSM-III-R criteria, was used. Comparison subjects who were not abused or neglected were interviewed with the same instrument. The findings supported the first hypothesis— 13.5% of subjects abused or neglected as children, versus 7.1% of comparison subjects, met criteria for ASPD. Males had a greater rate of ASPD than females in both groups of subjects. Of the survivors of childhood abuse and/or neglect, 20.3% of men and 5.3% of women met criteria for ASPD. Of the comparison subjects, 10.1% of men and 2.6 % of women were diagnosed with ASPD. Statistical analysis of these data implies that child-hood maltreatment is a risk factor for adult ASPD in males but not in females, because the results for females did not reach statistical significance. The authors attempted an analysis of the influence of the type of maltreatment; the data suggest that the type of maltreatment makes little difference in the extent of risk for ASPD, but the small numbers for some types of maltreatment prevent definitive conclusions.

Attempts to understand the etiology of ASPD have yielded several models. These de-velopmental models suggest that antisocial behavior that emerges early and occurs across diverse settings is prognostic of persistence (Myers et al., 1998). Myers et al. (1998) also state that "Antisocial behavior is predictive of adolescent and adult involvement in sub-stance abuse" (p. 499). The authors examined adolescents with a history of inpatient sub-stance use treatment to evaluate the persistence of antisocial behavior in the context of substance abuse. They found that "of the variables included in the logistic regression, early onset of conduct disorder behavior (at age 10 or earlier), greater diversity of con-duct disorder behavior occurring independent of substance involvement, and greater re-cent use of drugs were significant predictors of the antisocial personality disorder diagno-sis in late adolescence/early adulthood" (Myers et al., 1998, p. 483). Of an original sample in which 40% were female, male subjects were more likely to be diagnosed with ASPD at 4 years after treatment (71% vs. 29%).

BPD is commonly assumed to be more prevalent in women; many argue that child-hood sexual abuse is often the cause of BPD. Examining the origins of BPD may shed some light onto differences in how PDs arise. Goldman et al. (1992) examined a group of outpatient children with BPD to determine whether they were more likely to have a his-tory of physical or sexual abuse. The authors found that the group with BPD had a greater prevalence of physical and combined physical–sexual abuse. Zanarini et al. (1997) also found a high rate of abuse and neglect in a sample of inpatients with BPD. Compared to inpatients diagnosed with other PDs, the group with BPD was more likely to report emotional and physical abuse by caretakers and sexual abuse by noncaretakers. The authors assert that the childhood sexual abuse reported by patients with BPD may represent a marker of the severity of family dysfunction, in addition to being traumatic in itself. Also, the patients with BPD were more likely to report caretakers' emotional with-drawal, inconsistent treatment, denial of the patients' thoughts and feelings, placement of the patients in a parental role, and failure to provide protection. The authors identified four significant predictors of a BPD diagnosis: female gender, sexual abuse by a male noncaretaker, emotional denial by a male caretaker, and inconsistent treatment by a fe-male caretaker (Zanarini et al., 1997).

Laporte and Guttman (1996) studied a group of women with a diagnosis of a PD to determine whether trauma in childhood was unique to BPD or present in other PDs as well. The women with BPD in their sample experienced more losses and separations in childhood (except for death of a parent and placement in foster homes) than women with other PDs. The authors also demonstrated that women with a diagnosis of BPD experi-enced more overall verbal (46% vs. 23%), physical (52% vs. 28%), and sexual (49% vs. 22%) abuse, and witnessed more violence (39% vs. 25%), than women with other PDs (Laporte & Guttman, 1996).

The etiology of BPD continues to intrigue researchers. An interesting approach to the question is presented by another study from Goldman et al. (1993) in which they exam-ined psychopathology in families of children and adolescents with BPD. The gender ratio of the group with BPD was approximately 2.6 boys to 1.0 girls. The authors found a higher rate of psychopathology in the families of children with BPD. These children also had a significantly greater likelihood of having both parents with psychopathology. Over-all, substance abuse, depression, and antisocial behavior were more common in the fami-lies of the children with BPD. Finding greater rates of familial psychopathology in chil-dren with BPD implies that both biological and environmental risk factors are operative. Although the authors are careful to warn against inferring causality, they suggest that abuse and parental psychopathology, mediated both biologically and environmentally, are likely contributors to the etiology of BPD (Goldman et al., 1993).

Somatization disorder is an Axis I disorder with important relationships to histrionic PD, BPD, and ASPD. DSM-IV reports that the lifetime prevalence rates of somatization disorder are greater in women—0.2% to 2% in women, and less than 0.2% in men. Guze et al. (1986) found an association between somatization disorder and ASPD in male and female relatives. Male relatives of females with somatization disorder show an increased rate of ASPD and alcoholism (Cloninger et al., 1975; Woerner & Guze, 1968). Several authors have examined patients with somatization disorder to determine which, if any, PDs may be present. BPD and somatization disorder were found by both Hudziak et al. (1996) and Cloninger et al. (1997) to share features. Cloninger et al. (1975) observed, "Hysteria (Briquet's Syndrome) and sociopathy cluster in the same families instead of seg-regating as independent traits" (p. 29). They examined population and family data about both men and women with sociopathy, and women with hysteria. ("Sociopathy" in this context is roughly equivalent to ASPD, and "hysteria" corresponds to somatization dis-order.) The authors' findings supported their hypothesis that the same process may cause sociopathy and hysteria in women. Their data also supported a familial association of sociopathy and hysteria (Cloninger et al., 1975).

Paris (1997) has reviewed the phenomenology, behavioral symptoms, epidemiologi-cal studies, risk factors, outcome, and treatment of BPD and ASPD. The author summa-rizes the main differences between the two disorders and states that these differences re-flect a distinction between aggressiveness and victimization. Paris (1997) concludes that "similar traits in men and women can have different behavioral expression. . . . [I]mpul-sivity in men is more likely to be expressed through exploitation of others, whereas impulsivity in women is more likely to be expressed in self-destructive behaviors" (p. 240). Perhaps BPD and ASPD represent the same entity, according to gender.

COMORBIDITY

Studies of the comorbidity of Axis I and Axis II indicate that the presence of an Axis II disorder severely affects the response of the Axis I disorder to treatment. The influence of BPD on the treatment outcome of anxiety disorders was the subject of work by Nurnberg et al. (1989). Estimates of the prevalence of anxiety disorders in patients with BPD range from 3% to 10% (Akiskal et al., 1980; Carroll et al., 1981; Kroll et al., 1981; Pope et al., 1983). Conversely, estimates of the prevalence of BPD in patients with anxiety disorders are 6–16% in patients with panic disorder (Reich et al., 1987), 4–20% in patients with obsessive–compulsive disorder (Hermesh et al., 1987; Rasmussen & Tsuang, 1987), and 70% in patients with chronic posttraumatic stress disorder (Lindy et al., 1984). The prev-alence of PDs in patients with anxiety disorders in general is estimated to range from

35% to 65%. Nurnberg et al. (1989) reported that patients with BPD (with and without comborbid anxiety disorders) had significantly worse outcomes than patients with other PDs or no PD, but that the patients with comorbid anxiety disorders and BPD had the worst outcome. Gender as an independent variable showed no significant interaction with PD or anxiety disorder group. A more recent study that examined gender differences in a patient sample diagnosed with panic disorder found that males were more likely to meet criteria for schizoid PD and BPD (Barzega et al., 2001). Women, in contrast, were more likely to be diagnosed with diagnosed with histrionic and cluster PDs (Barzega et al., 2001).

Nurnberg and Raskin (1997) examined groups of outpatients with and without panic disorder (hereafter referred to as the PAD and NPAD groups, respectively) to determine whether the PAD group had greater rates of childhood physical or sexual abuse, childhood psychiatric disorder, and/or current PDs. Using the Inventory for Childhood Disturbance, 11 (35%) of the 31 patients in the PAD group and 2 (18%) of the 11 patients in the NPAD group reported abuse in general. The types and rates of abuse in the two groups were as follows: (1) physical abuse (typically involving repeated beatings that led to some degree of physical injury in the child), 35% PAD and 9% NPAD; (2) sexual abuse, 10% PAD and 18% NPAD; (3) emotional mistreatment (repeated ridicule or humiliation), 55% PAD and 27% NPAD; (4) witnessing parental violence, 29% PAD and 18% NPAD; and (5) neglect (including medical neglect and lack of response to childhood truancy), 23% PAD and 18% NPAD. Overall, 80% of the individuals in the PAD group rated positive for at least one measure of gross childhood disturbance or had at least one other disturbance present.

Thirty-four subjects—87% of the PAD group and 64% of the NPAD group—had mild to moderate symptoms of anxiety in childhood, but none had been treated for anxiety as children. Thirty-one of the 42 patients (74%)—27 of 31 (87%) in the PAD group and 4 of 11 (36%) in the NPAD group—received a diagnosis of PD; most had multiple diagnoses. In the PAD group's total of 61 PD diagnoses, 37 diagnoses were in the anxious cluster (including 5 self-defeating), 13 in the dramatic cluster, and 6 in the odd cluster. Significant intercorrelations between physical and emotional abuse, childhood anxiety, and adult PD were obtained at the $p < .01$ level of significance (Nurnberg & Raskin, 1997).

Patients in the PAD group who had PD and trauma histories proved to be more resistant to standard treatment combining psychotherapy and medication, which is generally quite successful for the treatment of less complicated panic disorder. Those patients with associated BPD had the poorest outcome. The results of the study suggest that for at least a subgroup of patients with panic disorder, a biological diathesis—interacting in a complex way within a matrix of abusive toxic childhood developmental environmental events—is longitudinally expressed over a continuum of childhood anxiety disorder, PD (primarily of the anxious cluster), and panic disorder in the adults. Sexual abuse was not found to be a significant distinguishing factor when compared with the apparently stronger contribution by psychological and physical abuse, except when in combination with other forms of abuse. Multiple forms of abuse seem to be the rule in this patient population.

Pepper et al. (1995) investigated the comorbidity of PDs with dysthymia and major depression by gathering data from direct interviews with patients and from interviews with knowledgeable informants. They found that the patients with dysthymia were more likely than the patients with episodic major depression to meet criteria for at least one PD. Of their study population, 60% of patients with early-onset dysthymia met criteria for at least one PD. Pepper et al. (1995) noted that "dysthymic patients exhibited significantly higher rates of borderline, histrionic, avoidant, and self-defeating personality disorder than patients with episodic major depression" (p. 242). Of the patients with episodic major depression, only 18% were diagnosed with a PD. The study population included a group of patients with "double depression" (dysthymia and major depression). According to Pepper et al. (1995), "patients with double depression exhibited significantly higher rates of any personality disorder, any cluster B and C disorder, and borderline, histrionic, and self-defeating personality disorders than patients with episodic major depression" (p. 245). Patients with pure dysthymia showed higher rates of any PD, any PD in cluster B, BPD, and histrionic PD.

TREATMENT

Treatment studies of PDs have primarily focused on borderline PD. Prior to the introduction of the selective serotonin reuptake inhibitors (SSRIs), monoamine oxidase inhibitors (MAOIs) were found to treat "hysteroid dysphoria," a syndrome characterized by a particular pattern of affective symptoms found in many patients considered to have BPD. According to Liebowitz and Klein (1981),

> Hysteroid dysphoria is defined as a chronic nonpsychotic disturbance involving repeated episodes of abruptly depressed mood in response to feeling rejected. Individuals with this disorder, who are usually but not exclusively women, characteristically spend much of their time seeking approval, applause, attention and praise, especially in the context of a romantic interrelationship, to which they respond with elevation of mood and energy. (pp. 69–70)

Data from Liebowitz and Klein (1981) suggest that most of their patients with hysteroid dysphoria seeking outpatient psychiatric treatment met DSM-III criteria for BPD prior to treatment. Treatment with MAOIs and psychotherapy proved effective for feelings of chronic emptiness and boredom, difficulty tolerating being alone, impulsivity, angry outbursts, unstable relationships, and self-damaging physical acts. Affective lability and identity disturbance (including problems of gender identity and long-term goal setting) showed little response to treatment with MAOIs and psychotherapy.

Psychopharmacological approaches to patients with BPD have involved virtually every class of agents, and provide further testimony to the various hypotheses on the affiliation of the disorder and its heterogeneity. Several earlier studies reported efficacy for low-dose, high-potency neuroleptics in BPD for cognitive dysfunction, transient psychosis, hostility, behavioral dyscontrol, anger, depression, and overall social functioning (Brinkley et al., 1979; Serban & Siegel, 1984; Goldberg et al., 1986). Although many reports on neuroleptics are favorable, patients are often noncompliant with neuroleptic regimens because of subjectively dysphoric effects. Clinicians have also been reluctant to use traditional neuroleptics out of concern for tardive dyskinesia. With the advent of the atypical antipsychotics and their reported improved side effect profile, possibly including a lower risk of tardive dyskinesia, interest in this class of agents can be expected to be renewed. Report of beneficial effects of clozapine in open trials with treatment-refractory patients who have BPD supports this direction of further inquiry (Benedetti et al., 1998).

The generally unsatisfactory experience with tricyclic antidepressant medication for depression and BPD is consistent with a boundary distinction with mood disorder. In the one double-blind study (Soloff et al., 1986a, 1986b) comparing amitriptyline, haloperidol, and placebo in patients with BPD (some with concurrent major depression), (1) haloperidol was superior even for depressive symptoms; (2) major depression did not predict response; and (3) a number of patients with BPD showed paradoxical clinical worsening in impulsivity, aggression, and suicidal behaviors on amitriptyline. In terms of antidepressant class, MAOIs seem to be more efficacious in BPD—particularly for depressive symptoms related to reactivity, such as hypersomnia, craving for sweets, and weight gain (Hedberg et al., 1971; Liebowitz et al., 1988; Cowdry & Gardner, 1988). Soloff et al. (1993) did not replicate the earlier finding of overall efficacy for haloperidol. This subsequent study compared phenelzine, haloperidol, and placebo; phenelzine was superior for anger and hostility, and not effective for atypical depressive symptoms (Soloff et al., 1993). Even when modestly effective acutely, neither phenelzine nor haloperidol has shown persistent efficacy in continuation therapy (Cornelius et al., 1993). The emergent finding from studies of antidepressant drug treatment of depression in subjects with coexisting BPD is that the traditional somatic treatments—heterocyclics (Black et al., 1988; Pfohl et al., 1984), MAOIs (Tyrer, 1988), and electroconvulsive therapy (Zimmerman et al., 1986)—are substantially less effective (15–25%) than in patients with depression without co-occurring BPD.

Because of BPD's seemingly biological heterogeneity, investigation into pharmacological treatment has shifted focus to various dimensions of temperamental pathology (e.g., affective dysregulation, impulsivity, and aggressive dyscontrol behaviors). Cowdry and Gardner (1988) compared alprazolam (a short-acting benzodiazepine), carbamazepine (an anticonvulsant used in treating bipolar disorder and impulsive aggression), trifluoperazine (a typical antipsychotic), tranylcypromine (an MAOI), and placebo. The medications were studied in a double-blind crossover design of patients with BPD and without concurrent major depression. The authors found no evidence for predictors of specific drug response. Tranylcypromine improved physician and patient ratings of mood and impulsivity. Physicians rated patients taking carbamazepine to have improved mood, but patients rated themselves as not improved by this medication. However, actual behavioral dyscontrol was dramatically reduced in frequency and severity. Trifluoperazine, if tolerated to completion of the trial, improved physician ratings of anxiety and suicidality; for patients, ratings of depression, anxiety, and rejection sensitivity improved significantly during the trial. Alprazolam seemed to disinhibit the patients in this study, as demonstrated by an increase in suicidality and frequency of behavioral dyscontrol. Some patients reported a paradoxical improvement in mood and increase in behavioral dyscontrol. This combination received positive ratings from patients and negative ratings from physicians. No predictors for response to alprazolam were found in the data analysis (Cowdry & Gardner, 1988).

More limited studies have suggested that other agents may have beneficial effects for certain BPD subgroups: lithium for emotional instability (Rifkin et al., 1972) and aggressive behavior (Sheard, 1971); psychostimulants for impulsive adults with a history of childhood DSM-III attention deficit disorder with hyperactivity (Wender et al., 1981); and naltrexone for self-injurious behavior (Winchel & Stanley, 1991). With the exception of patients with intermittent explosive disorder related to temporal lobe epilepsy, caution is indicated for the use of benzodiazepines, which can disinhibit and induce angry or aggressive reactions in patients with BPD (Stein, 1992).

The shift from a molar to a more molecular approach toward treatment of BPD symptomatology shows greater promise, particularly hypothesized serotonergic dysregulation and irritable impulsive aggression. Preliminary open-label trials of SSRIs (Cornelius et al., 1990; Norden, 1989; Markovitz et al., 1991) suggested beneficial effects on poor impulse control (independent of concurrent depression) by acting on primary serotonin-mediated behavior rather than on mood. Two more recent placebo control studies (Coccaro & Kavoussi, 1997; Salzman et al., 1995) validate the impulsivity/aggression reducing effect of SSRIs in individuals with BPD and other PDs. Coccaro and Kavoussi (1997) showed a sustained drug effect, independent of a relationship to depression, anxiety, or alcohol use, from the end of 2 through 3 months of SSRI treatment. Whether the antiaggressive action persists with continuation treatment remains to be determined. Parallel observations of potential significant implications from animal studies and now human subjects show that SSRI drug action can modulate indices of hostility and affiliative behavior, even in the absence of baseline clinical depression or other psychopathology (Knutson et al., 1998). Some data suggest that the newer generation of antidepressants which are combined-action agents may offer additional treatment options (Schatzberg, 2000).

Although post-DSM-III treatment studies have focused heavily on pharmacological approaches, the psychosocial treatment literature has also made important contributions. A recent review of the psychotherapeutic treatment of PDs suggests that psychotherapy is effective in the treatment of PDs but no approach has clear superiority (Bateman & Fonagy, 2000). The Menninger Clinic project (Kernberg et al., 1972) initially compared supportive, modified analytically oriented, and traditional psychoanalytic therapies as treatment for patients with BPD and found that the best response occurred with the modified technique. Wallerstein's (1986) follow-up study showed that the treatment outcomes of the first two groups converged over time, further supporting the finding that patients with BPD do more poorly with traditional psychoanalytic therapy. High dropout rates (60%) in the first 6 months of individual psychotherapy treatment distinguish patients with BPD from those with other PDs (Stein, 1992). Intense transference reactions, regression in therapy, primitive defenses, and exacerbation of suicidal behaviors seem to characterize the individual psychodynamically oriented treatment failures of patients with BPD (Higgitt & Fonagy, 1992).

Dialectical behavior therapy (DBT), designed for chronically suicidal patients with BPD, represents a promising advance in psychosocial treatment modalities (Linehan et al., 1991; Bohus et al., 2000). This manualized cognitive-behavioral treatment has demonstrated persistent anger reduction, decreased parasuicidal behaviors, improved social functioning, and reduction in therapy attrition compared to standard treatment (psychotherapy). At present, in the absence of a definitive unimodal treatment for BPD, combined forms of individual, group, behavior, family, cognitive, and drug therapies are used (Higgitt & Fonagy, 1992; Waldinger, 1987; Linehan et al., 1991). A new generation of studies on the potential synergy of combined treatments is now possible and needs to be developed (e.g., studies on DBT plus SSRIs).

SUMMARY

The empirical literature indicates that a number of PDs have achieved levels of diagnostic validity comparable to or exceeding those of other well-accepted diagnoses. However, further improvement is needed to reduce extensive overuse and overlap with other PDs. The recent findings linking serotonergic systems with impulsive aggression also imply that specific biological substrates may correlate better with component traits than with specific diagnostic categories. Further diagnostic changes can no longer rely on expert consensus; instead, they should be based on extensive empirical testing of how alterations in criteria and algorithms that are considered descriptively parsimonious improve or diminish predictive power in conjunction with external factors, independent of the defining phenomena.

The current DSM-IV PDs are unlikely to achieve construct validity as mutually exclusive diagnoses with unique causal pathways. The features that characterize individuals with PDs are all etiologically heterogeneous and phenomenologically quantitative (Rutter, 1987). A PD can be conceptualized as a maladaptive response to disturbances in regulation along a spectrum of pathologies (e.g., affective, impulsive, anxious, cognitive), manifested in an interpersonal context by signs and symptoms, and expressed as a characterological variant. Given the orthogonal dimensional nature of personality structure, a better understanding of the constructs may be obtained through a paradigm shift away from discrete nosological categories to alternative models, which reject a priori assumptions of unitary syndromes, recognize that character pathology can cross conceptual borders of nosological categories, and endorse concepts of complexly regulated component behavioral clusters common to multiple diagnostic categories (Nurnberg et al., 1991).

The search for more parsimonious and correct approaches to classifying inherently complex and multiple overlapping maladaptive personality traits has intensified the debate on whether a dimensional or a categorical system should be used (Widiger et al., 1987). As evidence that mental disorders are continuous variations, dimensional proponents cite the following: There has been a persistent failure to find discontinuities between symptoms and outcome (Kendall, 1982); PD criteria reflect extreme variants of normal traits (Cloninger, 1987); a dimensional approach allows multiple diagnoses to exist more appropriately in several grades of severity (Widiger et al., 1987); and multidimensional scaling can order the DSM-III PD subtypes more efficiently (Cloninger, 1987). Although he supports the categorical approach, Rutter (1987) sees little justification to retaining the current quantitative-trait-defined disorders. In his view, they are useful descriptors, but they are without clear boundaries and better placed in one overall category.

Meehl (1992) has shown empirically that a PD can be a qualitatively discrete phenotypic expression of a genetically transmitted latent taxon on a spectrum of pathology leading to an Axis I condition (e.g., schizogene → schizotaxic defect → STPD → clinical schizophrenia). Because either a categorical or a dimensional variable can appear phenotypically discrete or continuous as a result of its interactions with other variables, advanced taxometric techniques have to be used distinguish these otherwise difficult-to-distinguish illness concepts, and provide a more interpretable and meaningful structure for the hypothetical constructs (Grayson, 1987).

The current DSM-IV system of PD classification is actually an opportunistic admixture of both qualitative-typal and quantitative-trait-defined constructs. Recognizing that these system constructs are not mutually exclusive but need to be classified differently, we propose a synthetic approach. Conjectured categorical constructs (e.g., schizotypal, paranoid, schizoid, avoidant) could be classified within corresponding Axis I groupings, whereas dimensional trait-defined constructs (e.g., narcissistic, histrionic, dependent, compulsive, passive–aggressive) could be placed within a general PD category, perhaps as defined within a broad BPD concept (Rutter, 1987). Research could then proceed more appropriately according to type of category. For example, with dimensional constructs, more accurate identification of common biological or clinical covariates is provided by examining a patient's position on a particular continuum, rather than by assignment to a specific arbitrary category (Fleiss, 1972). Distinguishing these conjectured constructs should be a priority for developing an improved nosology for PDs (Grove & Tellegen, 1991).

REFERENCES

Akiskal, H. S. (1981). Subaffective disorders: Dysthymic, cyclothymic and bipolar II disorders in the "borderline" realm. *Psychiatric Clinics of North America, 4*, 25–46.

Akiskal, H. S., Chen, E. S., Davis, G. C., et al. (1985). Borderline: An adjective in search of a noun. *Journal of Clinical Psychiatry, 46*, 41–48.

Akiskal, H. S., Rosenthal, T. L., Haykal, R. F., et al. (1980). Characterologic depressions: Clinical and sleep EEG findings separating 'subaffective dysthymia' from 'character spectrum disorders.' *Archives of General Psychiatry, 37*, 777–783.

Alnaes, R., & Torgersen, S. (1988). DSM-III symptom disorders (Axis I) and personality disorders (Axis II) in an outpatient population. *Acta Psychiatrica Scandinavica, 78*, 348–355.

American Psychiatric Association. (1994). *Diagnostic and statistical manual of mental disorders* (4th ed.). Washington, DC: Author.

Andrulonis, P. A., Glueck, B. C., Stroebel, C. F., et al. (1981). Organic brain dysfunction and the borderline syndrome. *Psychiatric Clinics of North America, 4*(1), 47–66.

Andrulonis, P. A., & Vogel, N. G. (1984). Comparison of borderline personality subcategories to schizophrenic and affective disorders. *British Journal of Psychiatry, 144*, 358–363.

Barzega, G., Maina, G., Venturello, A., et al. (2001). Gender-related distribution of personality disorders in a sample of patients with panic disorder. *European Psychiatry, 16*, 173–179.

Baron, M., Gruen, R., Asnis, L., et al. (1985). Familial transmission of schizotypal and borderline personality disorders. *American Journal of Psychiatry, 142*(8), 927–934.

Bateman, A. W., & Fonagy, P. (2000). Effectiveness of psychotherapeutic treatment of personality disorder. *British Journal of Psychiatry, 177*, 138–143.

Benedetti, F., Sforzini, L., Colombo, C., et al. (1998). Low-dose clozapine in acute and continuation treatment of severe borderline personality disorder. *Journal of Clinical Psychiatry, 59*(3), 103–107.

Black, D. W., Bell, S., Hulbert, J., et al. (1988). The importance of Axis II in patients with major depression: A controlled study. *Journal of Affective Disorders, 14*, 115–122.

Bohus, M., Haaf, B., Stiglmayr, C., et al. (2000). Evaluation of inpatient dialectical–behavioral therapy for borderline personality disorder—a prospective study. *Behavioral Research Therapy, 38*, 875–887.

Brinkley, J. R., Beitman, B. D., & Friedel, R. O. (1979). Low-dose neuroleptic regimens in the treatment of borderline patients. *Archives of General Psychiatry, 36*, 319–326.

Carroll, B. J., Greden, J. T., Feinberg, M., et al. (1981) Neuroendocrine evaluation of depression in borderline patients. *Psychiatric Clinics of North America, 4*(1), 89–99.

Carter, J. D., Joyce, P. R., Mulder, R. T., et al. (1999). Gender differences in the frequency of personality disorders in depressed outpatients. *Journal of Personality Disorders, 13*(1), 67–74.

Caspi, A., Lynam, D., Moffitt, T. E., et al. (1993). Unraveling girls' delinquency: Biological, disposition, and contextual contributions to adolescent misbehavior. *Developmental Psychology, 29*, 19–30.

Cloninger, C. R. (1987). A systematic method for clinical description and classification of personality variants. *Archives of General Psychiatry, 44,* 573–588.

Cloninger, C. R., Bayon, C., & Przybeck, T. R. (1997). Epidemiology and axis I comorbidity of antisocial personality. In D. M. Stoff, J. Breiling, & J. D. Master (Eds.), *Handbook of antisocial behavior.* New York: Wiley.

Cloninger, C. R., Reich, T., & Guze, S. B. (1975). The multifactorial model of disease transmission: III. Familial relationship between sociopathy and hysteria (Briquet's syndrome). *British Journal of Psychiatry, 127,* 23–32.

Coccaro, E. F., & Kavoussi, R. J. (1997). Fluoxetine and impulsive aggressive behavior in personality-disordered subjects. *Archives of General Psychiatry, 54,* 1081–1088.

Cornelius, J. R., Soloff, P. H., Perel, J. M., et al. (1990). Fluoxetine trial in borderline personality disorder. *Psychopharmacology Bulletin, 26*(1), 151–154.

Cornelius, J. R., Soloff, P. H., Perel, J. M., et al. (1993). Continuation pharmacotherapy of borderline personality disorder with haloperidol and phenelzine. *American Journal of Psychiatry, 150*(12), 1843–1848.

Coryell, W. H., & Zimmerman, M. (1989). Personality disorder in the families of depressed, schizophrenic, and never-ill probands. *American Journal of Psychiatry, 146,* 496–502.

Cowdry, R. W., & Gardner, D. L. (1988). Pharmacotherapy of borderline personality disorder. *Archives of General Psychiatry, 45,* 111–119.

Cyranowski, J. M., Frank, E., Young, E., et al. (2000). Adolescent onset of the gender difference in lifetime rates of major depression: A theoretical model. *Archives of General Psychiatry, 57,* 21–27.

Fleiss, J. L. (1972). Classification of the depressive disorders by numerical typology. *Journal of Psychiatric Research, 9,* 141–153.

Fryer, M. R., Frances, A. J., Sullivan, T., et al. (1988). Comorbidity of borderline personality disorder. *Archives of General Psychiatry, 45,* 348–352.

Galen, I. W., Brower, K. J., Gillespie, B. W., et al. (2000). Sociopathy, gender, and treatment outcome among outpatient substance abusers. *Drug Alcohol Dependence, 61,* 23–33.

Garnet, K. E., Levy, K. N., Mattanah, J. J. F., et al. (1994). Borderline personality disorder in adolescents: Ubiquitous or specific? *American Journal of Psychiatry, 151*(9), 1380–1382.

Goldberg, S. C., Schulz, S. C., Schulz, P. M., et al. (1986). Borderline and schizotypal personality disorders treated with low-dose thiothixene vs. placebo. *Archives of General Psychiatry, 43,* 680–686.

Goldman, S. J., D'Angelo, E. J., & DeMaso, D. R. (1993). Psychopathology in the families of children and adolescents with borderline personality disorder. *American Journal of Psychiatry, 150*(12), 1831–1835.

Goldman, S. J., D'Angelo, E. J., DeMaso, D. R., et al. (1992). Physical and sexual abuse histories among children with borderline personality disorder. *American Journal of Psychiatry, 149*(12), 1723–1726.

Golomb, M., Fava, M., Abraham, M., et al. (1995). Gender differences in personality disorders. *American Journal of Psychiatry, 152*(4), 579–582.

Grayson, D. A. (1987). Can categorical and dimensional views of psychiatric illness be distinguished? *British Journal of Psychiatry, 151,* 355–361.

Grove, W. M., & Tellegen, A. (1991). Problems in the classification of personality disorders. *Journal of Personality Disorders, 5,* 31–41.

Gunderson, J. G., & Elliott, G. R. (1985). The interface between borderline personality disorder and affective disorder. *American Journal of Psychiatry, 142*(3), 277–288.

Gunderson, J. G., & Phillips, K. A. (1991). A current view of the interface between borderline personality disorder and depression. *American Journal of Psychiatry, 148*(8), 967–975.

Gunderson, J. G., Siever, L. J., & Spaulding, E. (1983). The search for the schizotype: Crossing the border again. *Archives of General Psychiatry, 40,* 15–22.

Guze, S. B., Cloninger, C. R., Martin, R. L., et al. (1986). A follow-up and family study of Briquet's syndrome. *British Journal of Psychiatry, 149,* 17–23.

Hedberg, D. L., Hauch, J. H., & Gleuch, B. C., Jr. (1971). Tranylcypromine–trifluoperazine combination in the treatment of schizophrenia. *American Journal of Psychiatry, 127*(9), 1141–1146.

Hermesh, H., Shahar, A., & Munitz, H. (1987). Obsessive–compulsive disorder and borderline personality disorder. *American Journal of Psychiatry 144*(1), 120–121.

Higgitt, A., & Fonagy, P. (1992). Psychotherapy in borderline and narcissistic personality disorder. *British Journal of Psychiatry, 161,* 23–43.

Hudziak, J. J., Boffeli, T. J., Kriesman, J. J., et al. (1996). Clinical study of the relation of borderline personality disorder to Briquet's syndrome (hysteria), somatization disorder, antisocial personality disorder, and substance abuse disorders. *American Journal of Psychiatry, 153*(12), 1598–1606.

Jackson, H. J., Whiteside, H. L., Bates, G. W., et al. (1991). Diagnosing personality disorders in psychiatric inpatients. *Acta Psychiatrica Scandinavica, 83,* 206–213.

Johnson, J. G., Cohen, P., Brown, J., et al. (1999). Childhood maltreatment increases risk for personality disorders during early adulthood. *Archives of General Psychiatry, 56,* 600–606.

Kendall, R. E. (1982). The choice of diagnostic criteria for biological research. *Archives of General Psychiatry, 39,* 1334–1339.

Kendler, K. S., Gruenberg, A. M., & Strauss, J. S. (1981). An independent analysis of the Copenhagen sample of the Danish adoption study of schizophrenia: II. The relationship between schizotypal personality disorder and schizophrenia. *Archives of General Psychiatry, 38,* 982–984.

Kernberg, O. F., Burstein, E. D., Coyne, L., et al. (1972). Psychotherapy and psychoanalysis: Final report of the Menninger Foundation's Psychotherapy Research Project. *Bulletin of the Menninger Clinic, 36,* 1–277.

Kety, S. S., Rosenthal, D., Wender, P. H., et al. (1975). Mental illness in the biological and adoptive families of adopted individuals who have become schizophrenic: A preliminary report based on psychiatric interview. In R. Fieve, D. Rosenthal, & H. Brill (Eds.), *Genetic research in psychiatry.* Baltimore: John Hopkins University Press.

Knutson, B., Wolkowitz, O. W., Cole, S. W., et al. (1998). Selective alteration of personality and social behavior by serotonergic intervention. *American Journal of Psychiatry, 155*(3), 373–379.

Kroll, J., Sines, L., Martin, K., et al. (1981). Borderline personality disorder: Construct validity of the concept. *Archives of General Psychiatry, 38,* 1021–1026.

Laporte, L., & Guttman, H. (1996). Traumatic childhood experiences as risk factors for borderline and other personality disorders. *Journal of Personality Disorders, 10*(3), 247–259.

Lensenweger, M. F. (1999). Stability and change in personality disorder features: The longitudinal study of personality disorders. *Archives of General Psychiatry, 56,* 1009–1015.

Liebowitz, M. R., & Klein, D. F. (1981). Interrelationship of hysteroid dysphoria and borderline personality disorder. *Psychiatric Clinics of North America, 4*(1), 67–87.

Liebowitz, M. R., Quitkin, F. M., Stewart, J. W., et al. (1988). Antidepressant specificity in atypical depression. *Archives of General Psychiatry, 45,* 129–137.

Lindy, J. D., Grace, M. C., & Green, B. L. (1984). Building a conceptual bridge between civilian trauma and war trauma: Preliminary psychological findings from a clinical sample of Vietnam veterans. In B. A. van der Kolk (Ed.), *Post-traumatic stress disorder: Psychological and biological sequelae.* Washington, DC: American Psychiatric Press.

Linehan, M. M., Armstrong, H. E., Suarez, A., et al. (1991). Cognitive-behavioral treatment of chronically parasuicidal borderline patients. *Archives of General Psychiatry, 48,* 1060–1064.

Links, P. S., Steiner, M., & Huxley, G. (1988). The occurrence of borderline personality disorder in the families of borderline patients. *Journal of Personality Disorders, 2,* 14–20.

Livesley, W. J., Jang, K. L., Jackson, D. N., et al. (1993). Genetic and environmental contributions to dimensions of personality disorder. *American Journal of Psychiatry, 150*(12), 1826–1831.

Livesley, W. J., Jang, K. L., & Vernon, P. A. (1998). Phenotypic and genetic structure of traits delineating personality disorder. *Archives of General Psychiatry, 55*, 941–948.

Loranger, A. W., Oldham, J. M., & Tullis, E. H. (1982). Familial transmission of DSM-III borderline personality disorder. *Archives of General Psychiatry, 39, 795–799*.

Loranger, A. W., Lenzenweger, M. F., Gartner, A. F., et al. (1991). Trait–state artifacts and the diagnosis of personality disorders. *Archives of General Psychiatry, 48, 720–728*.

Loranger, A. W., & Tulis, E .H. (1985). Family history of alcoholism in borderline personality disorder. *Archives of General Psychiatry, 42, 153–157*.

Luntz, B. K., & Widom, C. S. (1994). Antisocial personality disorder in abused and neglected children grown up. *American Journal of Psychiatry, 151(5), 670–674*.

Markovitz, P. J., Calabrese, J. R., Schulz, S. C., et al. (1991). Fluoxetine in the treatment of borderline and schizotypal personality disorders. *American Journal of Psychiatry, 148(8), 1064–1067*.

McGuffin, P., & Thapar, A. (1992). The genetics of personality disorder. *British Journal of Psychiatry, 160, 12–23*.

Meehl, P. E. (1992). Factors and taxa, traits and types, differences of degree and differences in kind. *Journal of Personality, 60, 117–177*.

Morey, L. C. (1988). Personality disorders in DSM-III-R: Convergence, coverage, and internal consistency. *American Journal of Psychiatry, 145, 573–577*.

Myers, M. G., Stewart, D. G., & Brown, S. A. (1998). Progression from conduct disorder to antisocial personality disorder following treatment for adolescent substance abuse. *American Journal of Psychiatry, 155(4), 479–485*.

Neugebauer, R., Dohrenwend, B. P., & Dohrenwend, B. S. (1980). Formulation of hypotheses about the true prevalence of functional psychiatric disorders among adults in the U.S. In B. P. Dohrenwend, B. S. Dohrenwend, M. S. Gould, et al. (Eds.), *Mental illness in the United States: Epidemiological estimates*. New York: Praeger.

Norden, M. J. (1989). Fluoxetine in borderline personality disorder. *Progress in Neuropsychopharmacology and Biological Psychiatry, 13, 885–893*.

Nurnberg, H. G., Raskin, M., Levine, P. E., et al. (1989). Borderline personality disorder as a negative prognostic factor in anxiety disorders. *Journal of Personality Disorders, 3(3), 205–216*.

Nurnberg, H. G., Raskin, M., Levine, P. E., et al. (1991). The comorbidity of borderline personality disorder and other DSM-III-R Axis II personality disorders. *American Journal of Psychiatry, 148, 1371–1377*.

Nurnberg, H. G., & Raskin, M. (1997). Childhood abuse experiences in adult panic disorder. *Medscape Mental Health, 2(3)*.

Nurnberg, H. G., Woodbury, M. A., & Bogenschutz, M. P. (1999). A mathematical typology analysis of DSM-III-R personality disorder classification: Grade of membership technique. *Comprehensive Psychiatry, 40(1), 61–71*.

Oldham, J. M., Skodol, A. E., Kellman, H. D., et al. (1992). Diagnosis of DSM-III-R personality disorders by two structured interviews: Patterns of comorbidity. *American Journal of Psychiatry, 149, 213–220*.

Pajer, K. A. (1998). What happens to "bad" girls?: A review of the adult outcomes of antisocial adolescent girls. *American Journal of Psychiatry, 155(7), 862–870*.

Paris, J. (1997). Antisocial and borderline personality disorders: Two separate diagnoses or two aspects of the same psychopathology? *Comprehensive Psychiatry, 38(4), 237–242*.

Pepper, C. M., Klein, D. N., Anderson, R. L., et al. (1995). DSM-III-R Axis II comorbidity in dysthymia and major depression. *American Journal of Psychiatry, 152(2), 239–247*.

Pfohl, B., Coryell, W., Zimmerman, M., et al. (1986). DSM-III personality disorders: Diagnostic overlap and internal consistency of individual DSM-III criteria. *Comprehensive Psychiatry, 27, 21–34*.

Pfohl, B., Staugh, D., & Zimmerman, M. (1984). The implications of DSM-III personality disorders for patients with major depression. *Journal of Affective Disorders, 7, 309–318*.

Pope, H. G., Jr., Jonas, J. M., Hudson, J. I., et al. (1983). The validity of DSM-III borderline personality disorder: A phenomenologic, family history, treatment response, and long-term follow-up study. *Archives of General Psychiatry, 40,* 23–30.

Rasmussen, S. A., & Tsuang, M. T. (1987). Drs. Rasmussen and Tsuang reply [Letter to the editor]. *American Journal of Psychiatry, 144*(1), 121–122.

Reich, J. (1987). Sex distribution of DSM-III personality disorders in psychiatric outpatients. *American Journal of Psychiatry, 144*(4), 485–488.

Reich, J., Noyes, R., Jr., & Troughton, E. (1987). Dependent personality disorder associated with phobic avoidance in patients with panic disorder. *American Journal of Psychiatry, 144*(3), 323–326.

Rifkin, A., Quitkin, F., Carrillo, C., et al. (1972). Lithium carbonate in emotionally unstable character disorders. *Archives of General Psychiatry, 27,* 519–523.

Robins, L. N., Helzer, J. E., Weissman, M. M., et al. (1984). Lifetime prevalence of specific psychiatric disorders in three sites. *Archives of General Psychiatry, 41,* 949–958.

Rutherford, M. J., Cacciola, J. S., & Alterman, A. I. (1999). Antisocial personality disorder and psychopathy in cocaine-dependent women. *American Journal of Psychiatry, 156*(6), 849–856.

Rutter, M. (1987). Temperament, personality and personality disorder. *British Journal of Psychiatry, 150,* 443–458.

Salzman, C., Wolfson, A. N., Schatzberg, A., et al. (1995). Effect of fluoxetine on anger in symptomatic volunteers with borderline personality disorder. *Journal of Clinical Psychopharmacology, 15,* 23–29.

Samuels, J. F., Nestadt, G., Romanoski, A. J., et al. (1994). DSM-III personality disorders in the community. *American Journal of Psychiatry, 151*(7), 1055–1062.

Schatzberg, A. F. (2000). New indications for antidepressants. *Journal of Clinical Psychiatry, 61,* 9–17.

Schulz, P. M., Soloff, P. H., Kelly, T., et al. (1989). A family history study of borderline subtypes. *Journal of Personality Disorders, 3,* 217–229.

Serban, G., & Siegel, S. (1984). Response of borderline and schizotypal patients to small doses of thiothixene and haloperidol. *American Journal of Psychiatry, 141*(1), 1455–1458.

Sheard, M. H. (1971). Effect of lithium on human aggression. *Nature, 230,* 113–114.

Silverman, J. M., Pinkham, L., Horvath, T. B., et al. (1991). Affective and impulsive personality disorder traits in the relatives of patients with borderline personality disorder. *American Journal of Psychiatry, 148*(10), 1378–1385.

Silverman, J. M., Siever, L. J., Horvath, T. B., et al. (1993). Schizophrenia-related and affective personality disorder traits in relatives of probands with schizophrenia and personality disorders. *American Journal of Psychiatry, 150*(3), 435–442.

Soloff, P. H., Cornelius, J., George, A., et al. (1993). Efficacy of phenelzine and haloperidol in borderline personality disorder. *Archives of General Psychiatry, 50,* 377–385.

Soloff, P. H., George, A., Nathan, R. S., et al. (1986a). Paradoxical effects of amitriptyline on borderline patients. *American Journal of Psychiatry, 143*(12), 1603–1605.

Soloff, P. H., George, A., Nathan, R. S., et al. (1986b). Progress in pharmacotherapy of borderline disorders. *Archives of General Psychiatry, 43,* 691–697.

Soloff, P. H., & Millward, J. W. (1983). Psychiatric disorders in the families of borderline patients. *Archives of General Psychiatry, 40,* 37–44.

Stein, G. (1992). Drug treatment of the personality disorders. *British Journal of Psychiatry, 161,* 167–184.

Stein, M. B., & Barrett-Connor, E. (2000). Sexual assault and physical health: Findings from a population-based study of older adults. *Psychosomatic Medicine, 62,* 838–843.

Stone, M. H., Kahn, E., & Flye, B. (1981). Psychiatrically ill relatives of borderline patients: A family study. *Psychiatric Quarterly, 53,* 71–84.

Tarnopolsky, A. (1992). The validity of the borderline personality disorder. In D. M. Silver (Ed.), *Handbook of borderline disorders*. Madison, CT: International Universities Press.

Torgersen, S. (1984). Genetic and nosological aspects of schizotypal and borderline personality disorders: A twin study. *Archives of General Psychiatry, 41, 546–554*.

Tyrer, P. (1988). The management of personality disorder. In P. Tyrer (Ed.), *Personality disorders*. London: Wright.

Waldinger, R. J. (1987). Intensive psychodynamic therapy with borderline patients: An overview. *American Journal of Psychiatry, 144*(3), 267–274.

Wallerstein, R. (1986). *Forty-two lives in treatment*. New York: Guilford Press.

Weissman, M. M. (1993). The epidemiology of personality disorders: A 1990 update. *Journal of Personality Disorders, 7*(Suppl.), 44–62.

Wender, P. H., Reimherr, F. W., & Wood, D. R. (1981). Attention deficit disorder ('minimal brain dysfunction') in adults: A replication study of diagnosis and drug treatment. *Archives of General Psychiatry, 38*, 449–456.

Widiger, T. A., Trull, T. T., Hurt, S. W., et al. (1987). A multi-dimensional scaling of the DSM-III personality disorders. *Archives of General Psychiatry, 44, 557–563*.

Widom, C. S. (1999). Childhood victimization and the development of personality disorders: Unanswered questions remain. *Archives of General Psychiatry, 56, 607–608*.

Will, J. A., & Self, P. A. (1976). Maternal behavior and perceived sex of infant. *American Journal of Orthopsychiatry, 46*(1), 135–139.

Winchel, R. M., & Stanley, M. (1991). Self-injurious behavior: A review of the behavior and biology of self-mutilation. *American Journal of Psychiatry, 148*(3), 306–317.

Woerner, P. I., & Guze, S. B. (1968). A family and marital study of hysteria. *British Journal of Psychiatry, 114, 161–168*.

World Health Organization. (1992). *International statistical classification of diseases and related health problems* (10th rev.). Geneva: World Health Organization.

Zanarini, M. C., Gunderson, J. G., & Marino, M. F. (1988). DSM-III disorders in the families of borderline outpatients. *Journal of Personality Disorders, 2*(4), 292–302.

Zanarini, M. C., Williams, A. A., Lewis, R. E., et al. (1997) . Reported pathological childhood experiences associated with the development of borderline personality disorder. *American Journal of Psychiatry, 154*(8), 1101–1106.

Zimmerman, M., & Coryell, W. H. (1990). DSM-III personality disorder dimensions. *Journal of Nervous and Mental Disease, 78*(11), 686–692.

Zimmerman, M., Coryell, W., Pfohl, B., et al. (1986). ECT response in depressed patients with and without a DSM-III personality disorder. *American Journal of Psychiatry, 143*(8), 1030–1032.

19

Complementary and Alternative Medicine

DANIEL A. MONTI
MARIE STONER

"Complementary and alternative medicine" (CAM), also referred to in the literature as "unconventional," "unorthodox," or "nontraditional medicine," caught the attention of the medical community in 1993 when an article appearing in the *New England Journal of Medicine* reported the results of a national survey on the prevalence, costs, and patterns of use of unconventional medical treatments (Eisenberg et al., 1993). To the surprise of many, this study found that one in three respondents had used an unconventional or CAM treatment in the past year. The majority did so for chronic, as opposed to life-threatening, medical conditions; most (89%) did so without referrals from their physicians; and almost three-quarters (72%) did not tell their physicians about their use of an unconventional therapy. Extrapolation of the data to the U.S. population suggested that in 1990 Americans made an estimated 425 million visits to CAM providers, which exceeded the number of visits to all U.S. primary care physicians (388 million). An estimated $10.3 billion was paid out of pocket for CAM treatments, which was comparable to the total annual out-of-pocket expenditures for all hospitalizations in the United States.

Several studies since have suggested that the use of CAM in the United States is substantial and increasing, and that disclosure rates to physicians remains low (Elder et al., 1997; Eisenberg et al., 1998). Given these trends, health care providers should have some understanding of CAM treatments. The available demographic data on CAM users suggests that health care providers especially needing a knowledge base in CAM are those who specialize in mental health, women's health, and the treatment of chronic illnesses.

BACKGROUND AND SIGNIFICANCE

The term "complementary and alternative medicine" refers to the broad range of health systems, modalities, and practices that are not part of the conventional and politically dominant health system (O'Connor et al., 1997). Functionally defined, CAM refers to those interventions that are neither taught widely in medical schools nor generally available in U.S. hospitals (Eisenberg et al., 1993). Several practices that are considered CAM in the United States include complex traditional health care systems from other cultures, such as traditional Chinese medicine, as well as components of these systems that are practiced as distinct entities, such as acupuncture (Eskinazi, 1998). Although there are many different CAM practices, three fundamental principles are common to many of the CAM health systems:

1. *Holism*—the theory that living nature is correctly seen in terms of interacting wholes (as of living organisms) that are more than the mere sum of elementary particles. In the realm of health this translates to all aspects of the person (including, physical, emotional, mental, diet, and lifestyle) as being interrelated and important to treatment, not just the specific disease or specific body part that is affected (Dossey & Swyers, 1992).

2. *Vitalism*—the doctrine that the functions of a living organism are due to a vital principle distinct from physiochemical forces. This vital principal has different names and elaboration among the CAM systems. For example, in traditional Chinese medicine, it is referred to as *qi* (or *ch'i*); in traditional Indian medicine it is known as *prana*; and in Western traditions such as homeopathy and chiropractic, it is called "vital force" or "life force" (Eskinazi, 1998).

3. *Energy*—a term that refers to the vitalistic force necessary to achieve balance or harmony in the system. In traditional Chinese medicine, for example, the energetic imbalance of a particular organ is described in terms of *yin* and *yang*. When there is an imbalance in either direction, it is thought to disrupt the harmony of the entire system, with ramifications beyond the organ itself.

In the United States, many of the CAM practices that have recently come into vogue were commonly used prior to the start of the 20th century. During the 1800s two important scientific observations both shaped the course of, and established a stronghold for, what is now considered conventional Western medicine: (1) Pathogens such as bacteria cause disease states; and (2) certain substances can help an individual ward off the effects of these pathogens (Dossey & Swyers, 1992). With this knowledge, scientists began to conquer infectious diseases and improve surgical procedures. This eventually led to a mindset that all physical and mental afflictions should be treatable with the appropriate vaccine, antibiotic, or chemical compound (Gordon, 1980). Hence biomedicine developed around the philosophical construct of "materialism", whereby biological entities are considered as equal to the sum of their anatomical parts, and disease is understood in terms of molecular, physiological, and pathological mechanisms believed to form the basis of biological processes (Eskinazi, 1998). The position of biomedicine in the United States during the early 1900s was further strengthened by growing political support (King, 1984).

It should be noted that not all practices considered within the realm of CAM are derived from a traditional health system or a paradigm of holism. For example, a physician who practices chelation therapy for atherosclerosis may believe that ethylenediamine-tetraacetic acid (EDTA) affects blood vessel calcium in a manner that *mechanistically* differs from the manner posited by current mainstream medical thinking. Such a practitioner may or may not have a holistic or otherwise alternative orientation.

CAM DEMOGRAPHICS

Demographic data on CAM users in the U.S. population suggests that women use CAM therapies significantly more than men (Eisenberg et al., 1993). CAM therapies are most commonly used for chronic conditions, such as back problems, anxiety, depression, and headaches (Eisenberg et al., 1998; Astin, 1998; Davidson et al., 1998; Unutzer et al., 2000). Other common features of CAM users are (1) an age range of 35–49 years (2) some college education, and (3) annual incomes higher than $50,000. Similar socioeconomic features of CAM users were found in a Canadian study by Kelner and Wellman (1997), who studied a group of 300 patients receiving care from either a family practitioner or one of five different types of alternative health care providers. They also found distinctions among the different alternative groups, suggesting that users of CAM should not be regarded as a homogeneous population. Also, those who used CAM generally did not do so to the exclusion of conventional medicine. Rather, people tended to choose different treatments for different problems.

CAM PRACTICES

Table 19.1 provides an overview of the U.S. National Institutes of Health (NIH) categorization of CAM practices. The remainder of this chapter is devoted to a focussed discussion of a few CAM health systems. The CAM practices discussed have been preferentially chosen based upon actual supportive data and relevance to the topic of women's health, especially mental health. In addition to illnesses such as depression, anxiety, and substance-related disorders, there is mention of problems thought to be influenced by stress and psychological issues, as well as problems that are unique to women such as reproductive medicine.

HERBAL MEDICINE

"Herbal medicine," also known as "phytotherapy," "herbalism," and "botanical medicine," is the treatment of illness with plants or plant extracts. The use of herbal medicine dates back to antiquity, and it remains the mainstay of medical treatment in many developing countries (Akerele, 1985; Barrett et al., 1999). Herbal remedies have also played a significant role in the medical histories of those areas of the world considered to be more "developed." In fact, substances first isolated from plants account for 25% of Western pharmaceutical products, with another 25% derived from modification of chemicals first found in plants (Farnsworth & Soajarto, 1993).

In the United States, the Food and Drug Administration (FDA) regards botanicals and their extracts as nutritional supplements; they can only be packaged as such, and

TABLE 19.1. Classification Of Alternative Medicine Practices with Examples

---

Mind-Body Interventions

Behavioral, psychological, social, and spiritual approaches to health.

Hypnosis	Imagery
Meditation	Biofeedback
Yoga	Prayer and Mental Healing

Alternative Medical Systems

Complete systems of theory and practice that have been developed outside of the Western biomedical model.

Traditional Oriental Medicine	Naturopathic Medicine
Acupuncture	Homeopathic Medicine
Ayurvedic Medicine	Environmental Medicine

Pharmacological and Biological Treatments

Drugs and vaccines not accepted by mainstream medicine.

Cartilage Products	Neural Therapy
EDTA Chelation Therapy	Apitherapy
Ozone	Aromatherapy

Herbal Medicine

Plant-derived preparations used for therapeutic and preventive purposes.

Ginkgo biloba extract	Valarian
Hypericum	Ginseng

Manual Healing Methods

Systems that are based on manipulation and/or movement of the body.

Chiropractic	Postural Reeducation Therapies
Massage Therapy	Bioenergetical Systems
Pressure Point Therapies	Biofield Therapies

Bioelectromagnetics

The unconventional use of electromagnetic fields for medical purposes

---

Source. Adapted from *Alternative Medicine: Expanding Medical HorizonsI*, A Report to the National Institutes of Health on Alternative Medical Systems and Practices in the United States. NIH pub #94-066.* Washington, D.C.: U.S. Government Printing Office, 1994.

may be sold over the counter. Since herbs cannot be patented, it has been cost-prohibitive for manufacturers to pay for the kind of rigorous studies required by the FDA for approval as medicinal treatments. Although most untested herbal remedies are probably harmless, the contents of herbal products do not always correspond to their labels, and there have been reports of tainted products (Angell & Kassirer, 1998). Even though these problems may make it difficult for health care providers and patients to objectively evaluate the use of herbal preparations, the U.S. botanical market is booming and was purported to approach $4 billion in retail in 1999 (Brevoort, 1998).

Numerous herbal products have been claimed to be effective for a variety of mental health problems. There are several herbs in popular use, three of which have some significant supportive data.

Hypericum perforatum, commonly known as St. John's wort, has become increasingly popular as an alternative treatment for depression. There are numerous clinical research reports, mostly from Europe, and four literature reviews of controlled studies on this herbal treatment (Harrer & Schulz, 1995; Ernst, 1995; Linde et al., 1996; Volz, 1997). The review by Linde et al. (1996) included a meta-analysis of pooled results of 1,757 patients treated in 23 studies. Overall, it appears that St. John's wort may be useful in treating mild to moderate depression (Field et al., 2000). However, a randomized controlled trial by Shelton et al. (2001) did not find St. John's wort effective for the treatment of severe major depression.

It remains unclear which of St. John's wort's active components account for the antidepressant effect. There are several potential side effects, which include gastrointestinal disturbances, photosensitivity, and altered metabolism of certain drugs (e.g., digoxin) (Greeson et al., 2001). It should also be noted that preparations of the herb are not standardized or regulated in the United States as they are in Europe, which makes dosing a problem. There is currently a 3-year, multicenter NIH drug trial underway to investigate this intriguing herbal remedy (Bender, 2001). Completion of this study is expected in the near future.

Gingko biloba, commonly known as ginkgo, is gaining increasing popularity as a treatment for improving memory and cognition, especially in elderly persons and in patients with dementia. The extract of *Gingko biloba* referred to as EGb 761 is an approved treatment for dementia in Germany, where more than 5 million prescriptions are written for it each year. Kleijnin and Knipschild (1992) reviewed 40 clinical trials, 8 of which were considered "well-performed," and noted benefits on all reported outcomes. Barrett et al. (1999) reviewed four subsequent placebo-controlled, double-blind, randomized clinical trials (Rai et al., 1992; Hofferberth, 1994; Kanowski et al., 1997; Maurer et al., 1997), again finding promising outcomes. A fifth study by Le Bars et al. (1997) was noted to have a high dropout rate, although the intention to treat analysis did show significant improvement. Recently, Le Bars (2000) completed another placebo-controlled, double-blind trial if EGb 761, finding mild improvement in cognitive functioning, daily living, and social behavior.

Valeriana officinalis, commonly known as valerian, is most often used as an antispasmodic, sedative, and sleep aid (Hobbs, 1993). Animal studies on valerian lend support to the suggestion of sedative and hypnotic effects (Houghton, 1988), and the adverse effects profile appears favorable (Bos et al., 1997). Barrett et al. (1999) reviewed the five blinded clinical trials that have been reported. Three reported improved sleep quality and decreased sleep latency in valerian-treated patients; one reported positive polysomnographic changes in valerian-treated participants; and one reported decreased anxiety with a combination of valerian and St. John's wort as compared to diazepam. The available data suggest that valerian is a potentially useful treatment that warrants further investigation.

HOMEOPATHY

German physician Samuel Hahnemann founded "homeopathy" in the late 18th century. In this system of health, illness is viewed as a vital force disturbance that manifests itself in a unique pattern of physical, mental, and emotional responses. The disturbance is treated with remedies of highly diluted (often untraceable) amounts of a substance (plant, mineral, animal product, or chemical) that is chosen for it's ability to produce the pathological symptoms when taken in larger doses. Homeopathic practitioners maintain that the remedies become more effective as they are diluted (potentization by dilution). It is thought that the electromagnetic energy of the substance remains as a "memory" in the remedy (Cassileth, 1998).

Linde et al. (1997) performed a meta-analysis of homeopathic research to test the hypothesis that the clinical effects of homeopathy were entirely placebo effects. The authors found 89 studies that met the inclusion criteria of placebo control and randomized assignment or double-blind conditions. These studies were drawn from 13 countries, had a mean sample size of 118 patients, and looked at 24 different clinical categories (including migraine, menopause, and premenstrual syndrome). The overall odds ratio for the 89 studies was 2:45 in favor of homeopathy; the odds ratio for the 26 high-quality studies was 1:66 in the same direction. The authors concluded that despite its implausibility, homeopathy warrants serious research, particularly trials testing the effectiveness of remedies on single clinical conditions.

Homeopathy is more widely used and researched in Europe than in the United States. In England, it has been part of the National Health Service since 1948. Women in particular are attracted to homeopathic remedies for treatment of life cycle issues. There are reports that suggest that homeopathy may be efficacious for pregnancy-related symptoms such as nausea (Katz, 1995), and for changes associated with menopause (Warenik-Szymankiewicz et al., 1997).

ACUPUNCTURE

"Acupuncture" is a form of treatment based in traditional Chinese philosophy which regards health as a relative balance between the individual and the surrounding environment (Beal, 1999). It is thought that human life is empowered by a basic vital force referred to as *qi* (or *ch'i*). *Qi* is described as flowing through the body in a network of pathways called "meridians," and it is particularly accessible at specific locations along the meridians called "acupuncture points." The qualitative difference of *qi* along the meridians is described in terms of *yin* and *yang*. *Yin* and *yang* harmony can be described in terms of active and passive, masculine and feminine, heat and cold, and stimulating and calming. It is thought that everything in the universe has a *yin* and *yang* aspect, and that *yin* and *yang* balance each other in a homeostatic manner. The goal of acupuncture treatment is to achieve *yin* and *yang* balance of the meridians by affecting the flow of *qi*. This is accomplished by systematically placing tiny needles through the skin at designated acupuncture points.

Compelling data suggest that acupuncture may be efficacious in the treatment of several types of pain (Patel et al., 1989; Dickens & Lewith, 1989). Particularly pertinent to woman, there have been positive outcomes in the treatment of pain associated with migraine headache (Vincent, 1990) and menstruation (Helms, 1987). Moreover, numerous studies have assessed the efficacy of acupuncture in drug addictions. Most but not all reported positive results (Bullock et al., 1989, 1999; Lipton et al., 1990; Margolin et al., 1993; Konefal et al., 1994; Wells et al., 1995).

There have been several interesting reports regarding the use of acupuncture in women's reproductive health care. It should be noted that most of these studies are small and require replication. Beal (1999) reviewed 12 placebo-controlled trials for the treatment of morning sickness, finding positive results for acupuncture in 11 of them. Budd (1995) reviewed the mostly British literature on the use of acupuncture for the induction of labor, concluding that it was generally safe, but required lengthier treatment times than standard techniques. Some studies have reported that acupuncture can reduce the duration of labor (Zeisler et al., 1998), presumably by affecting maternal serum biochemistry (Tempfer et al., 1998).

CHIROPRACTIC

Traditional chiropractic medicine, founded by D. D. Palmer in 1895, focuses on the achievement of optimal health through manual manipulation of supposed slippages in the spine called "subluxations." Chiropractic philosophy places particular emphasis on the concept that the human body has an innate self-healing ability and seeks to achieve homeostasis. Original chiropractic doctrine suggested subluxation as the cause of all disease; this philosophical approach is referred to as "straight chiropractic." Alternative chiropractic programs were developed soon after the beginning of the 20th century. They incorporated other disease models and therapies, and are referred to as "mixers." There are now various subspecialties and a wide range of techniques within the chiropractic profession. There is a large body of research on the use of chiropractic treatments. Although there are some discrepancies among the available clinical trials, the data overall suggest that chiropractic may be useful for the treatment of musculoskeletal disorders, especially low-back problems (Haldeman et al., 1992).

The "NeuroEmotional Technique" (NET) is a treatment intervention that specifically addresses emotions, cognition, and behavior. Developed by chiropractor Scott Walker (1992), NET is based upon the concept that emotional trauma can cause an aberrant neurological pattern in the body, which does not resolve on its own. The NET treatment protocol is complex in that it integrates chiropractic philosophy with acupuncture reflex points and psychological principles. It also incorporates a manual muscle test to assess the congruency of mental images and verbal statements; that is, a muscle tests stronger in a congruent condition than an incongruent one (Monti et al., 1999). NET is used to treat a variety of cognitive, emotional, and physical problems (Hall, 1999), and is practiced by a wide array of healthcare providers. There is one randomized, controlled, double-blind clinical trial that demonstrates the effectiveness of NET in reducing phobic symptoms (Peterson, 1997). Additional studies are needed.

MIND–BODY MEDICINE

"Mind–body medicine" refers to a collection of treatments that recognize the bidirectional nature of psyche and soma. Hypnosis and biofeedback are two mind–body therapies that have been well documented in the literature.

"Hypnosis" refers to a state of focused attention in which a willing participant is responsive to suggestions. This state, also referred to as "trance," is characterized by a modified sensorium, an altered psychological state and characteristically minimal motor functioning. In addition to achieving deep relaxation, the hypnotic treatment may include direct suggestions for specific changes in physiology and cognition (Spiegel & Spiegel, 1978). Guided imagery is often an integral part of hypnotic technique.

Although the American Medical Association has recognized hypnosis since 1958, its classification as CAM is based upon its use in complex mind–body problems such as immune enhancement (Goldberg, 1985) and accelerated healing of bone fractures (Ginandes & Rosenthal, 1999). There are data suggesting that hypnosis may be efficacious for a variety of mental health problems such as anxiety disorders (Marks et al., 1968; Stanton, 1993), nicotine addiction (Crasilneck & Hall, 1985), and methadone addiction (Manganiello, 1984). The use of hypnosis is also indicated in the treatment of physical disorders that are exacerbated by stress, such as psoriasis and gastrointestinal disorders (Brown & Fromm, 1987; Galovski & Blanchard, 1998). A NIH Technology Assessment Panel (1996) found strong evidence for the use of hypnosis in alleviating chronic pain conditions, including pain associated with cancer, irritable bowel syndrome, temporomandibular joint syndrome, and tension headaches.

"Biofeedback" is a treatment program designed to develop one's ability to control autonomic nervous system functions, such as heart rate, blood pressure, skin temperature, and muscle contractions. These functions are monitored on electronic equipment attached to a patient while modulation techniques are being learned. Biofeedback has become commonplace in clinical settings as a complementary treatment for a number of somatic disorders, including myofacial pain (Flor & Birbaumer, 1993), incontinence (Susset et al., 1990), and Raynaud's syndrome (Freedman et al., 1981; Yocum et al., 1985). There is also some data on its use in premenstrual syndrome (Van Zak, 1994). Numerous reports suggest its clinical efficacy in the treatment of anxiety disorders (Clark & Hirschman, 1990; Rice et al., 1993; Altocchi et al., 1994). Electroencephalogram biofeedback for the treatment of mood disorders has shown promising results in a preliminary study by Rosenfeld (in press). This application is based upon previous observations that hypoactivation of the left frontal cortex can be a state and trait marker for depression (Davidson, 1995).

YOGA

"Yoga" is an ancient Eastern Indian system of health that prescribes a multiphasic approach to healthy living, including proper diet, behavior, physical exercise, and adequate sleep. Modern practice in the United States, however, consists mainly of yogic postures (*asanas*), breathing (*pranayama*), and meditation techniques; these are typically used to relax and strengthen the body, and to promote mental clarity and proper flow of energy (*prana*).

In experimental studies, yogic techniques have been shown to attenuate autonomic activation, as well as to decrease adrenocortical activity (Sudsang et al., 1991). Clinically, the practice of yoga has been correlated with a reduction in cardiovascular risk factors (Schmidt et al., 1997) and with improvement in medical disorders such as asthma, non-insulin-dependent diabetes, musculoskeletal disorders, arthritis, and carpal tunnel syndrome (Janssen, 1989; Jain et al., 1993; Garfinkel et al., 1998).

Wood (1993) investigated the effect of yoga versus visualization or relaxation techniques, on mood, physical energy, and mental alertness. The findings showed higher improvements in the yoga group. Yoga was also an important component of stress reduction programs that were shown to improve mood disturbances, anxiety, and pain levels (Ornish, 1996; Kabat-Zin et al., 1985). Shannahoff-Khalsa et al. (1999) recently demonstrated improvement of obsessive–compulsive disorder symptoms in patients who employed a 12-month yoga protocol.

FUTURE DIRECTIONS

Although CAM has become quite popular in the United States, there is an overall dearth of acceptable research on the validity, efficacy, and safety of these treatments. CAM therapies have been at a disadvantage in this regard, because until recently, investigators at recognized research institutions were often discouraged from studying anything in the realm of CAM. These problems are compounded by the inherent difficulty in studying many of the CAM systems with the "gold standard" of placebo-controlled, double-blind clinical trials (Margolin et al., 1998).

Recently the political and academic climate has become more favorable toward CAM. In 1991, the U.S. Congress instructed the NIH to create an Office of Unconventional Medical Practices, later renamed the Office of Alternative Medicine. In late 1998, that office was upgraded and renamed the National Center for Complementary and Alternative Medicine (NCCAM). In 1999, the NCCAM was given an annual operating budget of $56 million to pursue scientific investigation of CAM (*NCCAM Newsletter,* 1998). The study of CAM practices has now become much more attractive, acceptable and legitimate to researchers. In addition, a recent survey of U.S. medical schools suggests that more than 60% of them include CAM in some part of the curriculum (Wetzel et al., 1998). All of these factors have contributed to the growing trend for physicians to integrate some aspect of CAM into their clinical practices; hence the emerging term "integrative medicine." However, the degree to which conventional medicine will embrace specific CAM therapies ultimately depends upon the results of large, multisite clinical trials. Some of the CAM therapies already have begun building a foundation of supportive research, and several sophisticated studies are currently underway. Now more than ever there are opportunities to explore innovative approaches to studying these intriguing health alternatives.

REFERENCES

Akerele, O. (1985). The WHO Traditional Medicine Programme: Policy and implementation. *International Traditional Health Newsletter, 1,* 1.

Altocchi, J., Dasta, R., & Danton, W. (1994). Nondrug treatment of anxiety. *American Family Physician, 10,* 161–166.

Angell, M., & Kassirer, J. (1998). Alternative medicine—The risks of untested and unregulated remedies. *New England Journal of Medicine, 339,* 839–841.

Astin, J. A. (1998). Why patients use alternative medicine: Results of a national study. *Journal of the American Medical Association, 279,* 1548–1553.

Barrett, B., Kiefer, D., & Rabago, D. (1999). Assessing the risks and benefits of herbal medicine: An overview of scientific evidence. *Alternative Therapies, 5*(4), 19–40.

Beal, M. (1998). Women's use of complementary and alternative therapies in reproductive health care. *Journal of Nurse-Midwifery, 43*(3), 224–234.

Beal, M. (1999). Acupuncture and acupressure: Applications to women's reproductive health care. *Journal of Nurse Midwifery, 44*(3), 217–230.

Bender, J. (2001). *Duke University 3-year study on the effects of St. John's wort.* Unpublished research, Duke University, Durham, NC.

Brevoort, P. (1998). The booming US botanical market: A new overview. *HerbalGram, 44,* 33–46.

Brown, D. P., & Fromm, E. (1987). *Hypnosis and behavioral medicine.* Hillsdale, NJ: Erlbaum.

Budd, S. (1995). Acupuncture. In D. Tiran & S. Mack (Eds.), *Complementary therapies for pregnancy and childbirth* (pp. 43–58). London: Baillière Tindall.

Bullock, M. L., Culliton, P., & Olander, R. (1989). Controlled trial of acupuncture for severe recidivist alcoholism. *Lancet, i*(8659), 1435–1439.

Bullock, M. L., Kiresuk, T. J., Pheley, A. M., et al. (1999). Auricular acupuncture in the treatment of cocaine abuse: A study of efficacy and dosing. *Journal of Substance Abuse Treatment, 16*(1), 31–38.

Cassileth, B. (1998). *The alternative medicine handbook.* New York: Norton.

Clark, M. E., & Hirschman, R. (1990). Effects of paced respiration on anxiety reduction in a clinical population. *Biofeedback and Self-Regulation, 15*(3), 273–284.

"Complementary Alternative Medicine" (1998, Fall). *NCCAM Newsletter, 5*(3), 1–3.

Crasilneck, H., & Hall, J. (1985). *Clinical hypnosis: Principles and applications.* Orlando, FL: Grune & Stratton.

Davidson, J. R. T., Rampes, H., Eisen, M., et al. (1998). Psychiatric disorders in primary care patients receiving complementary medical treatments. *Comprehensive Psychiatry, 39*(1), 16–20.

Davidson, R. J. (1995). Cerebral asymmetry, emotion and affective style. In R. J. Davidson & K. Hugdahl (Eds.), *Brain asymmetry* (pp. 361–387). Cambridge, MA: MIT Press.

Dickens, E., & Lewith, G. (1989). A single-blind controlled and randomized clinical trial to evaluate the effect of acupuncture in the treatment of trapezio-metacarpal osteoarthritis. *Complementary Medical Research, 3,* 5–8.

Dossey, L., & Swyers, J. P. (1994). Introduction. In *Alternative medicine: Expanding medical horizons* (pp. 37–48). A report to the National Institutes of Health on alternative medical systems and practices in the United States (NIH Publication No. 94-066). Washington, DC: U.S. Government Printing Office.

Eisenberg, D. M., Davis, R. B., Ettner, S. L., et al. (1998). Trends in alternative medicine use in the United States, 1990–1997: Results of a follow-up national survey. *Journal of the American Medical Association, 280*(18), 1569–1575.

Eisenberg, D. M., Kessler, R. C., Foster, C., et al. (1993). Unconventional medicine in the United States: Prevalence, costs, and patterns of use. *New England Journal of Medicine, 328*(4), 246–252.

Elder, N., Gillcrist, A., & Minz, R. (1997). Use of alternative health care by family practice patients. *Archives of Family Medicine, 6,* 181–184.

Ernst, E. (1995). St. John's wort, an anti-depressant?: A systematic, criteria-based review. *Phytomedicine, 2,* 67–71.

Eskinazi, D. (1998). Policy perspectives: Factors that shape alternative medicine. *Journal of the American Medical Association, 280*(18), 1621–1623.

Farnsworth, N., & Soejarto, D. (1991). Global importance of medicinal plants. In O. Akerele (Ed.), *Conservation of medicinal plants* (pp. 16–52). Cambridge, England: Cambridge University Press.

Field, H. L., Monti, D. A., Greeson, J. M., et al. (2000). St. John's wort. *International Journal of Psychiatry in Medicine, 30*(3), 203–219.

Flor, H., & Birbaumer, N. (1993). Comparisons of electromyographic biofeedback, cognitive-behavioral therapy, and conservative medical interventions in the treatment of chronic musculoskeletal pain. *Journal of Consulting and Clinical Psychology, 61,* 653–658.

Freedman, R. R., Lynn, S. J., Ianni, P., et al. (1981). Biofeedback treatment of Raynaud's disease and phenomenon. *Biofeedback and Self-Regulation, 6*(3), 355–365.

Galovski, T., & Blanchard, E. (1998). The treatment of irritable bowel syndrome with hypnotherapy. *Applied Psychophysiology and Biofeedback, 23*(4), 219–232.

Garfinkel, M., Singhal, A., Katz, W. A., et al. (1998). Yoga-based intervention for carpal tunnel syndrome. *Journal of the American Medical Association, 280,* 1601–1603.

Ginandes, C., & Rosenthal, D. (1999). Using hypnosis to accelerate the healing of bone fractures: A randomized controlled pilot study. *Alternative Therapies,, 3*(2), 67–75.

Goldberg, B. (1985). Hypnosis and the immune response. *International Journal of Psychosomatics, 32*(3), 34–36.

Gordon, J. S. (1980). The paradigm of holistic medicine. In A. Hastings (Ed.), *Health for the whole person* (pp. 14–45). Boulder, CO: Westview Press.

Greeson, J. M., Sanford, B., & Monti, D. A. (2001). St. John's wort: A review of the current pharmacological, toxicological, and clinical literature. *Psychopharmacology, 153*(1), 402–414.

Haldeman, S., Chapman-Smith, D., & Peterson, D. M. (1992). *Guidelines for chiropractic quality assurance and practice parameters.* Gaithersburg, MD: Aspen.

Hall, L. D. (1999). *Good news for people who hurt.* Amarillo, TX: Agape Associates.

Harrer, G., & Schulz, V. (1994). Clinical investigation of the antidepressant effectiveness of hypericum. *Journal of Geriatriatric Psychiatry and Neurology, 7*(Suppl. 1), S6–S8.

Hobbs, C. (1993). *Valerian, the relaxing and sleep herb* (M. Miovic & B. Baugh, Eds.). San Francisco, CA: Botanica Press.

Hofferberth, B. (1994). The efficacy of Egb 761 in patients with senile dementia of the Alzheimer type: A double-blind, placebo-controlled study on different levels of investigation. *Human Psychopharmacology, 9,* 215–222.

Houghton, P. (1988). The biological activity of valerian and related plants. *Journal of Pharmacology, 22,* 121–142.

Jain, S. C., Uppal, A., Bhatnagar, S. O. D., et al. (1993). A study of response pattern of non-insulin-dependent diabetics to yoga therapy. *Diabetes Research and Clinical Practice, 19,* 69–74.

Janssen, G. W. H. M. (1989). The application of Maharishi Ayur-Veda in the treatment of ten chronic diseases: A pilot study. *Nederlands Tijdschrift Voor Integrale Geneeskunde, 5,* 586–594.

Kabat-Zinn, J., Lipworth, L., & Burney, R. (1985). The clinical use of mindfulness meditation for the self-regulation of chronic pain. *Journal of Behavioral Medicine, 8*(2), 163–190.

Kanowski, S., Hermann, W. M., Stephan, K., et al. (1997). Proof of efficacy of the *Ginkgo biloba* special extract Egb 761 in outpatients suffering from mild to moderate primary dementia of the Alzheimer type or multi-infarct dementia. *Phytomedicine, 4,* 3–13.

Katz, T. (1995). The management of pregnancy and labour with homeopathy. *Complementary Therapies in Nursing and Midwifery, 1*(6), 159–164.

Kelner, M., & Wellman, B. (1997). Who seeks alternative health care?: A profile of the users of five modes of treatment. *Journal of Alternative and Complementary Medicine, 3*(2), 127–140.

King, L. S. (1984). The Flexner report of 1910. *Journal of the American Medical Association, 251*(8), 1079–1086.

Kleijnen, J., & Knipschild, P. (1992). *Ginkgo biloba* for cerebral insufficiency. *British Journal of Clincal Pharmacology, 34,* 352–358.

Konefal, J., Duncan, R., & Clemence, C. (1994). The impact of the addition of an acupuncture treatment program to an existing Metro–Dade County outpatient substance abuse treatment facility. *Journal of Addictive Disorders, 13,* 71–99.

Le Bars, P. L., Katz, M. M., & Berman, N. (1997). A placebo-controlled, double-blind, randomized trial of an extract of Ginkgo biloba for dementia. North America EGb Study Group. *Journal of the American Medical Association, 278*(16), 1327–1332.

Le Bars, P. L., Kieser, M., & Itil, K. Z. (2000). A 26-week analysis of a double-blind, placebo-controlled trial of the ginkgo biloba extract EGb 761 in dementia. *Dementia and Geriatric Cognitive Disorders, 11*(4), 230–237.

Linde, K., Ramirez, G., Mulrow, C. D., et al. (1996). St. John's wort for depression: An overview and meta-analysis of randomized clinical trials. *British Medical Journal, 313*, 253–258.

Linde, L., Clausius, N., Ramirez, G., et al. (1997). Are the clinical effects of homeopathy placebo effects?: A meta-analysis of placebo-controlled trials. *Lancet, 350*, 834–843.

Lipton, D., Brewington, V., & Smith, M. (1990, August). *Acupuncture and crack addicts: A single-blind placebo test of efficacy.* Paper presented at Advances in Cocaine Treatment, a NIDA Technical Review Meeting, Washington, DC.

Manganiello, A. (1984). A comparative study of hypnotherapy and psychotherapy in the treatment of methodone addicts. *American Journal of Clinical Hypnosis, 26*(4), 273–279.

Margolin, A., Avants, S. K., Chang, P., et al. (1993). Acupuncture for the treatment of cocaine dependence in methadone-maintained patients. *American Journal of Addiction, 2*, 194–201.

Margolin, A., Avants, S. K., & Kleber, H. D. (1998). Investigating alternative medicine therapies in randomized controlled trials. *Journal of the American Medical Association, 280*(18), 1626–1628.

Marks, I. M., Gelder, M. G., & Edwards, G. (1968). Hypnosis and desensitization for phobics: A controlled prospective trial. *British Journal of Psychiatry, 114*, 1263–1274.

Maurer, K., Ihl, R., Dierks, T., et al. (1997). Clinical efficacy of ginkgo biloba special extract Egb 761 in dementia of the Alzheimer type. *Journal of Psychiatric Research, 31*, 645–655.

Monti, D. A., Sinnott, J., Marchese, M., et al. (1999). Muscle test comparisons of congruent and incongruent self-referential statements. *Perceptual and Motor Skills, 88*, 1019–1028.

National Institutes of Health (NIH). (1994). *Alternative medicine: Expanding medical horizons.* A report to the National Institutes of Health on alternative medical systems and practices in the United States (NIH Publication No. 94-066). Washington, DC: U.S. Government Printing Office. Bethesda, MD: U.S. Department of Health and Human Services, Public Health Service, NIH, Office of Medical Applications of Research.

National Institutes of Health (NIH), Technology Assessment Panel on Integration of Behavioral and Relaxation Approaches into the Treatment of Chronic Pain and Insomnia. (1996). *Special communication.*

O'Connor, B. B., & Lazar, J. S. (1997). Talking with patients about their use of alternative therapies. *Primary Care: Clinics in Office Practice, 24*(4), 699–714.

Ornish, D. (1996). *Dr. Dean Ornish's program for reversing heart disease: The only system scientifically proven to reverse heart disease without drugs or surgery.* New York: Ivy Books.

Panel on Definition and Description, CAM Research Methodology Conference, April, 1995. (1997). Defining and describing complementary and alternative medicine. *Alternative Therapies, 3*(2), 49–51.

Patel, M., Gutzwiller, F., Paccaud, F., et al. (1989). A meta-analysis of acupuncture for chronic pain. *International Journal of Epidemiology, 18*, 900–906.

Peterson, K. B. (1997). The effects of spinal manipulation on the intensity of emotional arousal in phobic subjects exposed to threat stimulus: A randomized, controlled, double-blind clinical trial. *Journal of Manipulative and Physiological Therapeutics, 20*, 602–606.

Rai, G. S., Shovelin, C., & Wesnes, K. A. (1992). A double blind, placebo-controlled study of *Ginkgo biloba* extract in elderly outpatients with mild to moderate memory impairment. *Current Medical Research and Opinion, 12*, 350–355.

Rice, K. M., Blanchard, E. B., & Purcell, M. (1993). Biofeedback treatments of generalized anxiety disorder—Preliminary results. *Biofeedback and Self-Regulation, 18*(2), 93–106.

Rosenfeld, J. P. (2000). An EEG biofeedback protocol for affective disorders. *Clinical Electroencephalography, 31*, 7–12.

Schmidt, T., Wijga, A., Von Zur Muhlen, A., et al. (1997). Changes in cardiovascular risk factors and hormones during a comprehensive residential three month kriya yoga training and vegetarian nutrition. *Acta Physiologica Scandinavica, 640,* 158–162.

Shannahoff-Khalsa, D., Ray, L. E., Levine, S., et al. (1999). Randomized controlled trial of yogic mediation techniques for patients with obsessive–compulsive disorder. *CNS Spectrums, 4*(12), 34–47.

Shelton, R. C., Keller, M. B., Gelenberg, A., et al. (2001). Effectiveness of St. John's wort in major depression. *Journal of the American Medical Association, 285*(15), 1978–1986.

Spiegel, H., & Spiegel, D. (1978). *Trance and treatment: Clinical uses of hypnosis.* New York: Basic Books.

Stanton, H. E. (1993). Using hypnotherapy to overcome examination anxiety. *American Journal of Clinical Hypnosis, 35*(3), 198–204.

Sudsang, R., Chentanez, V., & Veluvan, K. (1991). Effect of Buddhist meditation on serum cortisol and total protein levels, blood pressure, pulse rate, lung volume and reaction time. *Physiology and Behavior, 50*(3), 543–548.

Susset, J., Galea, G., & Read, L. (1990). Biofeedback therapy for female incontinence due to low urethral resistance. *Journal of Urology, 124,* 1205–1208.

Tempfer, C., Zeisler, H., Heinzl, H., et al. (1998). Influence of acupuncture on maternal serum levels of interleukin-8, prostaglandin F_{2alpha}, and beta-endorphin: A matched pair study. *Obstetrics and Gynecology, 92*(2), 245–248.

Unützer, J., Klap, R., Sturm, R., et al. (2000). Mental disorders and the use of alternative medicine: Results from a national survey. *American Journal of Psychiatry, 157*(11), 1851–1857.

Van Zak, D. B. (1994). Biofeedback treatments for premenstrual and premenstrual affective syndromes. *International Journal of Psychosomatics, 41,* 53–60.

Vincent, C. (1990). A controlled trial in the treatment of migraine by acupuncture. *Clinical Journal of Pain, 5,* 305–312.

Volz, H. P. (1997). Controlled clinical trials of hypericum extracts in depressed patients—An overview. *Pharmacopsychiatry, 30*(Suppl.), S72–S76.

Walker, S. (1992). Ivan Pavlov, his dog and chiropractic. *Digest of Chiropractic Economics, 34,* 36–46.

Warenik-Szymankiewicz, A., Meczekalski, B., & Obrebowska, A. (1997). Feminon N in the treatment of menopausal symptoms. *Ginekologia Polska, 68*(2), 89–93.

Wells, E. A., Jackson, R., Diaz, R. O., et al. (1995). Acupuncture as an adjunct to methadone treatment services. *American Journal of Addiction, 4,* 198–214.

Wetzel, M. S., Eisenberg, D. M., & Kaptchuk, T. J. (1998). Courses involving complementary and alternative medicine at U.S. medical schools. *Journal of the American Medical Association, 280,* 784–787.

Wood, C. (1993). Mood changes and perceptions of vitality: A comparison of the effects of relaxation, visualization and yoga. *Journal of the Royal Society of Medicine, 86,* 251–258.

Yocum, D. E., Hodes, R., Sundstrom, W. R., et al. (1985). Use of biofeedback training in treatment of Raynaud's disease and phenomenon. *Journal of Rheumatology, 12*(1), 90–93.

Zeisler, H., Tempfer, C., Mayerhofer, et al. (1998). Influence of acupuncture on duration of labor. *Gynecologic and Obstetric Investigations, 46,* 22–25.

Part III

Psychiatric Consultation in Women

20

Gynecology

DIANA L. DELL

Over the past two decades, the interface between psychiatry and gynecology has evolved into a very narrow subspecialty for a few medical practitioners. But almost every practicing obstetrician–gynecologist and every practicing psychiatrist encounter this interface on a daily basis when dealing with patients and their families. Several areas of interface related to reproductive function have been covered in greater detail in earlier chapters of this volume: psychiatric aspects of the menstrual cycle (Steiner & Born, Chapter 3), psychiatric issues in pregnancy (Nonacs et al., Chapter 4), postpartum and breastfeeding issues (Arnold et al., Chapter 5), psychiatric aspects of hormonal contraception (Warnock & Blake, Chapter 6), and psychiatric aspects of menopause (Ayubi-Moak & Parry, Chapter 7). This chapter explores two other areas where psychiatrists are often consulted for assistance in optimizing patient management: bereavement reactions related to reproductive events, and chronic pelvic pain (CPP).

BEREAVEMENT REACTIONS RELATED TO REPRODUCTIVE EVENTS

After many years in clinical practice, one begins to see an almost inevitable connection between reproduction and grieving—whether it is the loss of innocence that accompanies an unintended pregnancy, the loss of "feeling normal" that accompanies infertility, the loss of "self" that can accompany even the most sought-after pregnancy, or the profound sorrow that accompanies fetal anomaly or fetal death. Grieving may be transient and supportive of emotional growth when it accompanies the shifting roles from individual to partner to parent. It may be devastating and all-consuming when it is related to the loss of one's fertility or the loss of a child.

Infertility and Mood Symptoms

It is estimated that at least 14% of couples of reproductive age who desire pregnancy are unable to conceive within 1 year. Infertility is experienced by most couples as a life crisis in which they feel isolated and powerless. Feelings of frustration, anger, depression, guilt, grief, anxiety, and marital dissatisfaction are common (Lukse & Vacc, 1999). There appear to be significant gender differences in the way men and women experience both the global stress related to infertility and specific stressors (Newton et al., 1999). Psychotherapeutic interventions that address those reactions in gender-specific ways can improve the quality of life for infertile women, and may even improve conception rates (Beutel et al., 1999).

Most studies over the last two decades that have addressed mood symptoms among infertile women have shown rates of distress and depression far exceeding those found in fertile women. The literature less clearly indicates whether higher rates of depression cause infertility or result from failure to conceive or carry a pregnancy.

Assisted Reproductive Technology

The process of conceiving is a complex and expensive maze for infertile couples to navigate. Assisted reproductive technology usually begins with pituitary down-regulation via Gn-RH analogues, followed by high-dose gonadotropin stimulation in an effort to create numerous oocytes (Hammond & Stillman, 1999). During down-regulation, women experience menopausal symptoms (hot flushes, mood changes, headaches, and sleep disturbances); with gonadotropin stimulation, they experience depressive symptoms, restlessness, agitation, and increasing pelvic pain/pressure secondary to bilateral development of large ovarian follicles.

If *in vitro* fertilization (IVF) or gamete intrafallopian transfer (GIFT) is planned, monitoring of follicular development requires serial transvaginal ultrasound examinations, which may become increasingly uncomfortable as the follicles mature. Egg retrieval is commonly performed by transvaginal needle aspiration under ultrasound guidance (Hammond & Stillman, 1999). Many infertile women are reluctant to express their discomfort during these procedures, but may describe their distress and discomfort in great detail in the wake of failed conception.

Following retrieval, oocytes are combined with male gametes and cultured in the laboratory, using increasingly sophisticated technology. With IVF, the goal is uterine pre-embryo replacement at the four- to eight-cell stage, which is usually 48–72 hours in culture. Intrauterine placement is done transvaginally. With GIFT techniques, less rigorous laboratory conditions are needed since the fallopian tube will serve as its own incubator, but placement of the gametes into the fallopian tube requires laparoscopic surgery and general anesthesia (Hammond & Stillman, 1999).

Women undergoing infertility treatments initiate each treatment cycle with high expectations and a high level of hope that conception will finally take place. But the high expectations and hope that are necessary to enable women to cope with expensive and often uncomfortable treatment regimens can also create an emotional setup for disappointment if they do not conceive (Lukse & Vacc, 1999). Failure to conceive is marked by the onset of menstruation—an event that becomes associated with anger, grief, and a sense of devastation, all of which have been well documented in both research and clinical settings.

Women with comorbid eating disorders may have secondary infertility related to their eating pattern. The eating disorders are often underrecognized by health care providers and/or denied by these patients during their fertility workups (Brkovich & Fisher, 1999).

Pregnancy Loss

Parents begin forming attachments to a pregnancy very early in the process. In a planned pregnancy or in a case where the partners have impaired fertility, this attachment begins well before conception. Unfortunately, 45–50% of all pregnancies probably end in spontaneous miscarriage; many such pregnancies go unrecognized, because miscarriage occurs before the next expected menstrual period. Approximately 20% of recognized pregnancies are spontaneously lost in the first trimester or early second trimester. In addition, there are 1.5 million induced abortions per year in the United States (McElroy & Moore, 1997). (Induced abortions are discussed more fully later.)

Elevated degrees of emotional distress following miscarriage will be seen in women under the following conditions (Brier, 1999):

- The pregnancy was planned and desired.
- It took a long time or took intensive infertility management to conceive (heightening fear that future pregnancy might not occur).
- A woman has a history of elective abortions and residual guilt (miscarriage may be perceived as punishment).
- There were no warning signs of miscarriage (and thus little time to prepare coping strategies).
- The loss occurs later in pregnancy.
- A woman has a history of pregnancy loss (the current loss may well trigger earlier grief).
- A couple has no living children.
- A woman experiences feelings of isolation due to absence of social support and/or strain between her and her partners.
- A woman has a history of poor coping, especially depression (which tends to be associated with self-blame and guilt).

Grieving is more difficult with miscarriage or stillbirth, since societal norms often do not validate the experience in a way that facilitates healing of the loss. Parents may grieve for the spontaneous loss of a 6-week fetus or a stillborn infant as intensely as for any other loss in their lives. For many young parents, it may be the first significant loss that they have experienced.

Stages of Perinatal Grief

When told of fetal death or a major fetal anomaly, many parents experience shock and emotional numbing. They may express an unrealistic sense that "this is not really happening" and respond with denial and disbelief (American College of Obstetricians and Gynecologists [ACOG], 1985). They often feel empty and lonely. If the obstetrical condition is not emergent, allowing time for parents to make an initial accommodation to the loss at this stage can be very important. Parents should be encouraged to make as many choices about the proposed obstetrical intervention as are feasible. This tactic restores some sense of control in a situation in which they feel completely out of control. They should be encouraged to see the products of conception after evacuation of the uterus or to hold their stillborn infant after delivery; this is the only time they will ever have with their infant. Seeing and holding also facilitate appropriate grieving by allowing the parents to claim the infant and establish the reality of the loss. Photographs should be taken and offered to the parents. If they do not wish to have them, the photos should be held in a file where parents will have access to them in the future. Patients commonly request these materials as their grief lessens.

As the experience becomes more "real," a searching stage emerges as the parents look for a reason for the loss (ACOG, 1985). The searching may take many forms: blaming themselves, blaming the caretakers or hospital, or blaming God. They may experience vivid dreams about the baby or the birth process. Pseudohallucinations of hearing an infant crying are not uncommon. The parents may openly or unconsciously blame each other, which inhibits the grieving process and their ability to comfort each other. They may experience hostility toward other pregnant women and jealousy toward those women's live-born infants. They need assurance to understand that these feelings are normal and will lessen over time.

With increasing acceptance of the loss comes disorientation (ACOG, 1985). This occurs over a variable period of time after the death of the fetus/neonate. Grieving parents may be socially isolated by virtue of their sadness and despair. Support groups of other patients and partners who have experienced perinatal loss are especially helpful at this stage. Depressive symptoms are also common, and supportive psychotherapy may be helpful. If occupational or academic dysfunction is severe or ongoing, antidepressants may be indicated.

As time passes, an ongoing reorganization takes place (ACOG, 1985). The parents begin to integrate the loss and return to normal activities. The pain is never completely gone, but it no longer immobilizes them. During the first 6 months after pregnancy loss, women have higher rates of depression, anxiety, and somatization than women who have given birth to live infants. After 1 year, most women have returned to baseline (Janssen et al., 1996). Support groups have been widely utilized and appear to be one of the most helpful modalities in assisting patients and their partners during this stressful life event.

The process of bereavement may take up to 2 years to resolve. Individuals with difficult bereavement experiences may have difficulty in four different areas: delayed onset of grieving, unusually intense grief symptoms, prolonged grief symptoms, or "getting stuck" in one of the bereavement stages.

Bereavement is more difficult when death is unexpected, as is commonly the case during childbearing. It is also more difficult when the pregnancy itself was surrounded by marked ambivalence or when there are unresolved issues related to the events surrounding the pregnancy loss.

Unplanned Pregnancy and Abortion

Every year in America, more than 6 million women become pregnant—roughly 11% of all reproductive-age women. It is estimated that 50–60% of those pregnancies are unintended or mistimed, and that about half of them will be electively aborted. Two-thirds of the women in America will have at least one unintended pregnancy by the time they reach menopause. More than half of all couples seeking abortion were using a contraceptive method during the month they conceived. The psychological stress associated with detection of an unwanted or mistimed pregnancy may precipitate emotional crisis for the mother. Debilitating ambivalence, disturbances of sleep and appetite, and suicidal ideation are common (Brown & Eisenberg, 1995).

Numerous studies show that women who carry unintended or mistimed pregnancies begin prenatal care later in pregnancy and receive less adequate prenatal care than women with wanted pregnancies. Their ability to proceed normally through the emotional stages of adjustment to pregnancy is often impaired. Such a woman is also at greater risk for depression, and for physical abuse, and the relationship with her partner is at greater risk of dissolution. Both parents may suffer economic hardship and may fail to achieve their educational and career potentials. The fetus is more likely to be exposed to harmful substances (e.g., tobacco and alcohol). The child produced by an unwanted pregnancy, as distinguished from a mistimed one, is at greater risk of being born at low birthweight, of dying within its first year of life, of being abused, and of not receiving sufficient resources for healthy development (Brown & Eisenberg, 1995).

Postabortion Syndrome

Before abortion was legalized, there was an accumulation of case reports about psychological impairment secondary to the abortion events (extreme pain, fear of dying, or rape by the abortion provider). Since abortion was legalized in the United States in 1971, more than 250 studies have looked at the psychological effects secondary to induced abortion. In 1989, U.S. Surgeon General C. Everett Koop, himself opposed to abortion, concluded that the data were "insufficient . . . to support the premise that abortion does or does not produce a post-abortion syndrome" (quoted in Brown & Eisenberg, 1995, p. 54).

All studies agree that the negative emotional effects of abortion are nearly always transient, and that most women who choose abortion feel increasingly relieved and comfortable over time (Minden & Notman, 1991; Stotland, 1993). Patients are at higher risk for psychiatric illness following induced abortion if they were pressured or coerced into abortion, if they had marked ambivalence about their decision, if they have limited social support, and if they have had prior psychiatric illness (Blumenthal, 1991; Brown & Eisenberg, 1995).

There is clinical evidence that postpartum depression may occur following either spontaneous or induced abortion. Clinically, early intervention with psychotherapy and/or antidepressants shortens dysfunction and should improve outcome. In the rare instances when patients experience profound impairment after induced abortion, early intervention directed toward resolution of the trauma is mandated; whatever therapeutic modality seems most appropriate for a particular patient should be employed.

CHRONIC PELVIC PAIN

Most patients with CPP are initially seen by their gynecologists or other primary care physicians. In the early stages of their pain experience, the patients' pain complaints are treated symptomatically with medical interventions that have been proven effective for managing acute pain. If the pain does not respond, there is a progressive escalation of diagnostic and treatment modalities. If a patient is seeing a general practitioner, she will often be referred to a gynecologist. If a patient is seeing a gynecologist, she will often be prepared for diagnostic surgery. CPP is the reason cited for up to 10% of outpatient gynecological referrals; it is the indication for up to 35% of diagnostic laparoscopies and up to 12% of the hysterectomies performed in the United States (Reiter, 1990).

In current gynecological practice, those women referred for psychiatric evaluation or treatment of CPP have almost always had a diagnostic or operative laparoscopy that has "ruled out" significant gynecological pathology (Stegge & Stout, 1993). The referral often reflects increasing physician frustration after weeks or months of unsuccessful treatment attempts with different modalities.

From a patient's perspective, she has endured numerous painful physical examinations, diagnostic tests, medication trials, and surgeries without significant diminution of her pain. Her pain experience has begun to affect other areas of her life. She has begun to experience increasing physical and mental fatigue, periods of depression, episodes of crying, and difficulty sleeping. Her sense of herself and her self-confidence have often been eroded. As one participant in an ethnographic study stated "I pray that they will find out what's wrong so I can show the doctors I am not crazy" (quoted in Zadinsky & Boyle, 1996, p. 228).

In general, the experience of pain involves four basic domains: nociception, pain, suffering, and pain behavior (ACOG, 1996).

"Nociception" is the initiation of a neurological signal based on a noxious event. A limited number of stimuli can initiate these signals: thermal events, mechanical events (including stretch, distension, or muscle contraction), and chemical events (including liberation of histamines, prostaglandins, and other noxious substances).

"Pain" is the recognition of the neural signal as noxious. In the event of a noxious thermal stimulus, for example, previous experience compels one to rapidly locate the source of the noxious stimulus and to remove one's hand from the hot object. Pain in the abdomen or pelvis is much more complex. Parietal sensation travels via fast pain fibers, which generate a sensation that is sharp and easily localized. Visceral sensation, however, is transmitted via slow pain fibers, which result in pain characterized as burning or aching in nature and difficult to localize. Neither slow nor fast fibers adapt to a stimulus, so they continue to generate the pain signal for as long as the stimulus is present. In addition, visceral and parietal pain fibers take different routes to the central nervous system, which may further alter the perceived location of pain. Unfortunately, as both surgeons and patients have discovered, direct palpation or movement of an internal organ that reproduces the pain does *not* necessarily signify that removal of that organ will get rid of the pain (ACOG, 1996).

"Suffering" is the affective response generated by the pain event. The extent of affective response will vary greatly with prior pain experiences, duration of pain experiences, previous life events, and many other factors. Patients with prior pain experience may have a broad range of reactions—from regression and dependency to learned helplessness, anger directed toward the caregiver, and detachment. Over time, many women express increasing frustration about continued symptoms in the face of negative diagnostic tests. If the first discussion about the psychological impact of chronic pain or a referral for mental health evaluation takes place during this period of frustration, it can markedly disrupt the therapeutic alliance. It is at this point that many patients seek out another medical opinion. For a woman who seeks mental health evaluation for CPP, the most common presenting complaint is that others believe her pain is "all in her head."

"Pain behavior" reflects the adaptive changes made because of the pain experience. The extent to which pain behavior is functional or dysfunctional also depends on prior pain experiences, duration of the pain experience, and previous life events.

Pain is generally classified as "acute" when it lasts less than 3 months, "subacute" when it lasts 3–6 months, and "chronic" when it has been present for 6 months or more. CPP was first described in 1952 (Duncan & Taylor, 1952). In current usage, a diagnosis of CPP implies a syndrome with persistent or recurrent lower abdominal, pelvic, or back pain. It is often associated with fatigue, headache, gastrointestinal disorders, and sexual dysfunction (Heim et al., 1998).

Early studies implied that CPP was psychogenic in origin. Studies from the 1950s described women with this disorder as having dysfunctional families of origin, in which maternal warmth was lacking. They characterized this group as having a high prevalence of female identity problems, conflicts about adult sexuality/intimacy, and histories of incest/abuse. Over the next 30 years, researchers continued to identify family dysfunction and early traumatic sexual experiences in women with CPP in ways implying causation. More recent work, however, with better control groups and comparisons to subpopulations with other chronic pain conditions, appears to negate a unique relationship between sexual abuse and CPP (Rapkin et al., 1990; Savidge & Slade, 1997).

It now seems more obvious that abusive experiences of any kind can increase a person's vulnerability to various painful conditions, many of which are chronic (Savidge & Slade, 1997). For example, as many as one-third of women with irritable bowel syndrome also have a history of CPP. In one recent study (Walker et al., 1996), women with both disorders were significantly more likely to have current/lifetime psychiatric disorders, to have experienced childhood sexual abuse, and to have had a hysterectomy. Those psychiatric conditions identified as most likely to occur were dysthymia, panic, and somatization. The study also suggests that the number of medically unexplained physical symptoms may be a proxy for the level of psychiatric distress (Walker et al., 1996).

Historically, the most commonly reported psychiatric disturbances among patients with CPP have been depression, anxiety, and anger/hostility. Current research provides evidence that these symptoms are not the cause of the CPP, but are more likely secondary to the psychological experience of living with a chronic pain condition (Savidge & Slade, 1997).

Both men and women have predictable behavioral, cognitive, and physiological responses to chronic pain. At a behavioral level, they reduce their activity level, narrow their range of activities, relinquish home and work responsibilities, increase dependence on family members, and markedly increase their dependence on medications. Cognitively, they develop passive or inflexible coping styles, become preoccupied with their pain, and tend toward catastrophizing and negative pain-related thinking. Physically, patients develop muscle tension and spasm in adjacent areas. Over time, they become physically deconditioned secondary to lack of activity (Keefe & Goli, 1996).

Treatment regimens for women with CPP often require multidisciplinary services (Hammer & Valentino-Hammer, 1996). It is extremely important to treat the underlying disorder whenever possible, since hyperalgesia may occur with chronic stimulation of pain receptors. Treatment of coexisting mood, anxiety, and sleep disorders is also essential.

Both liaison psychiatrists and primary care providers must emphasize that mood, anxiety, and sleep disorders typically coexist with CPP and can make the pain experience worse. Direct acknowledgment that both a woman's pain and her suffering are real may help to allay her concerns that doctors believe her pain is "all in her head" (Zadinsky & Boyle, 1996).

Modern medicine stigmatizes illnesses that have strong psychosomatic components. Patients with CPP and other types of chronic pain who feel health care providers' empathy and respect will come to realize that they are not culpable for their conditions and will begin to regain control of their own lives (Elks, 1997). Individual psychotherapy and group therapy can provide places where patients with chronic pain can process changes in their lives and plan for their future.

Pharmacological treatment of pain symptoms should be initiated promptly and continued on a regular basis. Analgesics should be taken on a time schedule instead of taken "as needed" for pain. Similarly, follow-up visits with both the gynecologist and the psychiatrist should be scheduled at regular intervals rather than in response to periods of distress. Medication should be chosen carefully, with attention to side effects and half-lives being especially important. Narcotics and benzodiazepines should be used with caution because of their potential for habituation. On the other hand, those medications should not be withheld if other therapies are not effective. If such agents are used, their use should be targeted toward objectives such as increasing activity level, not just pain relief. Placebos should never be used to assess pain response. Practitioners should avoid drug combinations that increase sedation without enhancing analgesia (ACOG, 1996).

A significant portion of treatment planning must be directed toward reversing changes in behavior that have occurred secondary to pain. Scheduling activity–rest cycles will be necessary to help patients with long-standing pain return to a normal level of activity. A structured program of physical exercise will increase strength and endurance, which may also enhance a patient's overall sense of well-being. As the patient increases her capabilities, finding ways to increase the range of activities available to her is essential (Keefe & Goli, 1996).

Cognitive techniques that decrease catastrophizing and negative pain-related thinking should be emphasized. Cognitive coping strategies such as imagery and distraction methods will give patients a renewed sense of control and decrease their dependence on medications for pain relief. Relaxation training and biofeedback can also assist in this process. Family members can help by learning to reinforce "well" behaviors and to limit attention to pain behaviors (Keefe & Goli, 1996).

CONCLUSIONS AND FUTURE DIRECTIONS

In the evolving interface between psychiatry and gynecology, increased clinical and research attention must be focused on comorbid gynecological and psychiatric disorders. Failure to recognize that comorbidity will result in unnecessary human suffering and unnecessary expenditure of health care dollars. This comorbidity is especially poignant in cases where unresolved grief associated with reproductive events results in significant somatization, and in cases involving CPP. New educational strategies are needed for both psychiatrists and obstetrician–gynecologists that emphasize understanding of the emotional reactions to all reproductive and pain-related issues.

REFERENCES

American College of Obstetricians and Gynecologists (ACOG). (1985). *Grief related to perinatal death* (ACOG Technical Bulletin No. 86). Washington, DC: Author.

American College of Obstetricians and Gynecologists (ACOG). (1996). *Chronic pelvic pain* (ACOG Technical Bulletin No. 223). Washington, DC: Author.

Beutel, M., Kupfer, J., Kirchmeyer, P., et al. (1999). Treatment-related stresses and depression in couples undergoing assisted reproductive treatment by IVF or ICSI. *Andrologia, 31*(1), 27–35.

Blumenthal, S. J. (1991). Psychiatric consequences of abortion: Overview of research findings. In N. L. Stotland (Ed.), *Psychiatric aspects of abortion* (pp. 17–37). Washington, DC: American Psychiatric Press.

Brier, N. (1999). Understanding and managing the emotional reactions to miscarriage. *Obstetrics and Gynecology, 93*, 151–155.

Brkovich, A. M., & Fisher, W. A. (1998). Psychological distress and infertility: Forty years of research. *Journal of Psychosomatic Obstetrics and Gynecology, 19*(4), 218–228.

Brown, S. S., & Eisenberg, L. (1995). *The best intentions: Unintended pregnancy and the well-being of children and families* (pp. 1–20). Washington, DC: National Academy Press.

Duncan, C. H., & Taylor, II. C. (1952). A psychosomatic study of pelvic congestion. *American Journal of Obstetrics and Gynecology, 64*, 1–12.

Elks, M. L. (1997). 'I'm OK; you're not': Medical socialization and psychosomatic illness. *Medical Hypotheses, 48*, 33–36.

Hammer, M., & Valentino-Hammer, V. (1996). Managing chronic pain: A multidisciplinary approach. *Resident and Staff Physician, 42*(2), 12–18.

Hammond, C. B., & Stillman, R. J. (1999). Infertility and assisted reproduction. In R. J. Scott, P. J. DiSaia, C. B. Hammond, & W. N. Spellacy (Eds.), *Danforth's obstetrics and gynecology* (pp. 649–667). Philadelphia: Lippincott Williams & Wilkins.

Heim, C., Ehlert, U., Hanker, J. P., et al. (1998). Abuse-related posttraumatic stress disorder and alterations of the hypothalamic–pituitary–adrenal axis in women in chronic pelvic pain. *Psychosomatic Medicine, 60*, 309–318.

Janssen, H. J. E. M., Cuisinier, M. C. J., Hoogduin, K. A. L., et al. (1996). Controlled prospective study on the mental health of women following pregnancy loss. *American Journal of Psychiatry, 153*(2), 226–230.

Keefe, F. J., & Goli, V. (1996). A practical guide to behavioral assessment and treatment of chronic pain. *Journal of Practical Psychiatry and Behavioral Health, 3*, 151–161.

Lukse, M. P., & Vacc, N. A. (1999). Grief, depression, and coping in women undergoing infertility treatment. *Obstetrics and Gynecology, 93*(2), 245–251.

McElroy, S. W., & Moore, K. A. (1997). Trends over time in teenage pregnancy: The critical changes. In R. A. Maynard (Ed.), *Kids having kids* (pp. 23–53). Washington, DC: Urban Institute Press.

Minden, S. L., & Notman, M. T. (1991). Psychotherapeutic issues related to abortion. In N. L. Stotland (Ed.), *Psychiatric aspects of abortion* (pp. 119–133). Washington, DC: American Psychiatric Press.

Newton, C. R., Sherrard, W., & Glavac, I. (1999). The Fertility Problem Inventory: Measuring perceived infertility-related stress. *Fertility and Sterility, 72*(1), 54–62.

Rapkin, A. J., Kames, L. D., Darke, L. L., et al. (1990). History of physical and sexual abuse in women with chronic pelvic pain. *Obstetrics and Gynecology, 76*, 92–96.

Reiter, R. C. (1990). A profile of women with chronic pelvic pain. *Clinical Obstetrics and Gynecology, 33*, 130–136.

Savidge, C. J., & Slade, P. (1997). Psychological aspects of chronic pelvic pain. *Journal of Psychosomatic Research, 42*(5), 433–444.

Stegge, J. F., & Stout, A. L. (1993). Chronic gynecologic pain. In D. E. Stewart & N. L. Stotland

(Eds.), *Psychological aspects of women's health care* (pp. 249–266). Washington, DC: American Psychiatric Press.

Stotland, N. L. (1993). Induced abortion. In D. E. Stewart & N. L. Stotland (Eds.), *Psychological aspects of women's health care* (pp. 207–225). Washington, DC: American Psychiatric Press.

Walker, E. A., Gelfand, A. N., Gelfand, M. D., et al. (1996). Chronic pelvic pain and gynecological symptoms in women with irritable bowel syndrome. *Journal of Psychosomatic Obstetrics and Gynecology, 17,* 39–46.

Zadinsky, J. K., & Boyle, J. S. (1996). Experiences of women with chronic pelvic pain. *Health Care for Women International, 17,* 223–232.

21

Oncology

Women with Breast, Gynecologic, or Lung Cancer

EMMIE I. CHEN
ELISABETH J. S. KUNKEL

In this chapter, we discuss the medical and psychological aspects of some of the common malignancies faced by women: breast, gynecologic, and lung cancer. Breast and gynecologic malignancies pose specific challenges for women related not only to the impact of the cancer and its treatments, but also to changes in sexuality, femininity, gender, and maternal issues. Lung cancer has become the leading cause of cancer-related death in women in the United States; as a result, one must include it in any discussion of women's mental health. The woman with cancer must abdicate some or all of her responsibilities for child care, housekeeping, and/or work while simultaneously adjusting to changes in her appearance and relationships. There needs to be a reliable, integrated system of mental health screening and services in order to assess patients throughout the course of illness and to intervene when appropriate.

BREAST CANCER

Breast cancer is the most common form of cancer and the second leading cause of cancer death among North American women. In 2001, the American Cancer Society estimated that 192,000 new invasive cases of breast cancer among women in the United States and 40,200 deaths would occur (American Cancer Society, 2001). The risk of breast cancer increases with advanced age, but it is not a lethal disease for the majority of women (Phillips et al., 1999; American Cancer Society, 2001). Rapid advances in early detection, resulting from screening mammography and the use of adjuvant chemotherapy for early-stage disease, have led to increased disease-free survival and improved quality of life among diagnosed women (Phillips et al., 1999; Farrow et al., 1992; Kunkel, 1994; Parker et al., 1996). Therapeutic interventions are toxic and intensive, resulting in increased physical and emotional demands to cope with the cancer and treatment sequelae (Rowland & Massie, 1998). Although there is great variability in women's responses to dealing with cancer, and although psychologically healthy women usually respond well, breast cancer has a uniquely complex impact that raises concerns related to femininity, sexuality, body image, self-esteem, and mortality.

Psychosocial factors in prevention, early detection, treatment, and prognosis play a key role in breast cancer care (Rowland & Massie, 1998; Glanz & Lerman, 1992). Controversy remains regarding who should and who should not be screened. Increased availability and acceptance of surgical options (e.g., lumpectomy with radiation, mastectomy with or without breast reconstruction) and higher patient consumerism have increased women's participation in the decision-making process. Patient adherence to treatment and communication among patient, doctor, and family have become more crucial in the face of aggressive, multimodal treatment regimens. Moreover, genetic testing and chemo-prevention have brought attention to the psychological effects on unaffected women who are at increased risk for breast cancer, sometimes referred to as the "worried well" (Rowland & Massie, 1998; Lerman et al., 1991). Recent progress in identifying genetic susceptibility—for example, the presence of breast cancer 1 and 2 (BRCA1 and/or BRCA2) mutations—has intensified the need to define the benefits and risks of early detection, genetic testing, and preventative measures (e.g., prophylactic bilateral mastectomy, prophylactic oophorectomy). Pre- and posttesting counseling for women undergoing genetic testing, as well as attention to their psychological problems, is critical. These care-related changes have developed amidst a greater demand by patients for involvement in their own care, consumer activism, attention to ethical and informed consent issues, use of quality-of-life assessment in treatment outcomes, managed care, and the emphasis on cost-effective care. There is a growing demand for medical professionals to understand, recognize, and address the psychosocial impact of breast cancer throughout the course of care (Rowland & Massie, 1998).

Early Detection and Decision Making

Mammography, followed by ultrasound examination of suspicious lesions, is the standard approach for early detection. Mammography is used in conjunction with monthly breast self-examination (BSE) and yearly physician breast examination. Women under 35 years old who have a symptomatic mass, and/or a strong family history, are referred for a baseline mammogram. Regardless of their risk status, all women should have a baseline mammogram at or before age 35. Women from 40 to 49 years old should repeat a mammogram every 1 to 2 years, and women after 50 should have yearly mammograms (Kunkel, 1994; Early Breast Cancer Trialists' Collaborative Group, 1990).

Although monthly BSE is useful for detecting new masses, a woman who is particularly anxious about getting breast cancer may start doing daily BSE as a means of reassurance. Alternatively, a woman who is extremely fearful of finding cancer may not examine herself at all. Recommending a physician who can do periodic, frequent breast examinations is particularly helpful for the anxious woman who will not examine herself. The primary care physician serves as the first line of intervention and reassurance for women who need guidance and recommendations in reaching a decision concerning early detection. False-positive results from screening tests may produce unnecessary anxiety and complications (Sox, 1998).

The Biopsychosocial Impact of Breast Cancer

Sociocultural, psychosocial, and medical factors all contribute to women's psychological response to, and the ways they cope with, breast cancer. Comprehensive care should address problems across the illness trajectory in all three areas. Within the sociocultural realm, the growing attention to the patient's role in medical decision making, increased demand for and greater public involvement in the assessment of research in the prevention and treatment of breast cancer, and more federal support for research on the psychosocial and behavioral aspects of cancer affect the public's view of breast cancer (Rowland & Massie, 1998). Women who play a more active role with their physicians in decision making now shoulder an increased burden of responsibility for making the right choices. Many women report that the decision-making process is highly stressful; however, women who are given a choice about treatment fare better than those who are not (Ashcroft et al., 1985; Morris & Royle, 1988; Glynn et al., 1987; Fallowfield et al., 1990). Occasionally, a woman will find herself emotionally paralyzed by the decision-making process; in such a case, referral for psychiatric consultation is often beneficial.

According to Meyerowitz (1980), psychological and psychosocial factors affect women diagnosed with breast cancer in three ways: (1) psychological discomfort (anxiety, depression, and anger); (2) changes in life patterns (consequent to physical discomfort, marital or sexual disruption, and/or altered activity levels); and (3) fears and concerns (about mastectomy/loss of breast, cancer recurrence, and death). The life stage at which the cancer occurs, previous emotional stability, and the presence of interpersonal supports are also key factors in psychosocial adaptation to illness (Rowland & Massie, 1998; Spiegel et al., 1989). Studies suggest that patients with breast cancer who use an active problem-solving approach to the stresses of illness and exhibit flexibility in their coping efforts are less distressed and adapt better (Penman, 1979; Taylor et al., 1985; Hilton, 1989). However, the relative efficacy of coping styles may be situation-specific (Suls & Fletcher, 1985). For example, use of denial and avoidant coping strategies during active chemotherapy or radiation (as opposed to information-seeking and problem-solving skills during treatment planning) may be more helpful in reducing treatment side effects (Glanz & Lerman, 1992). The lay belief that women can cause their own illnesses by being poor copers has added another psychological burden for many women with breast cancer (e.g., not having a "fighting spirit" or not laughing enough). Prolonged anxiety or depression is not expected as an emotional reaction to a cancer diagnosis.

Psychiatric consultation is normally requested for women who are at high genetic risk for breast cancer and request prophylactic mastectomy; for those who fear cancer and are considering prophylactic mastectomy (despite their lack of high risk factors); for those unable to make a decision about treatment; and for those with a current or past psychiatric history of anxiety, depression, substance abuse/dependence, or other mental disorders. Patients who present as management problems for the physician and staff and/or those who are unable to comply with hospital rules also tend to receive psychiatric attention. Moreover, if suicidal thinking is expressed, a formal psychiatric evaluation should always be requested (Rowland & Massie, 1998).

Medical factors that may have an impact upon coping include disease stage, treatment(s), responses to treatment, and clinical course, including rehabilitation. A sensitive, supportive surgeon, radiation oncologist, or oncologist can communicate clearly and can monitor emotional as well as physical well-being. Hair loss, control of nausea and vomiting, and body image are frequent areas of concern. Women who are psychologically healthy tend to present with earlier-stage disease. They can be taught to screen themselves for new masses, swelling, dimpling, nipple retraction, discharge, color changes, sores, and asymmetry. With more advanced disease, the focus of treatment shifts from survival and cure to palliative care. If psychological health is poor, women tend to cope less well with their disease.

The National Comprehensive Cancer Network (NCCN) Psychosocial Distress Practice Guidelines Panel (1999) has proposed the establishment of standards of care for the management of distress, as well as treatment guidelines. The panel has proposed an evaluation and treatment model, including a primary oncology team, a multidisciplinary committee, professional educational programs, and outcome research studies. The goal is to routinely and rapidly assess patients in medical and surgical clinics for distress (psychological/psychiatric, social, or spiritual/religious), so that no distressed patient goes unrecognized and/or untreated (NCCN Psychosocial Distress Practice Guidelines Panel, 1999). Patients with mild distress are referred to the primary oncology team. Patients with moderate to severe distress are referred for mental health, social work, and/or pastoral services.

Mastectomy

Although mastectomy was the standard breast cancer treatment for a long time, recent surgical practice has been to offer more conservative surgical approaches (General Accounting Office, 1994), partly in the hope that sparing breast tissue will reduce the psychosocial morbidity associated with surgery. The loss of one or both breasts evokes feelings of mutilation and altered body image; diminished self-worth; loss of a sense of femininity; decrease in sexual attractiveness and function; anxiety, depression, and hopelessness; guilt and shame; and fears of recurrence, abandonment, and/or death (Meyerowitz, 1980; Lewis & Bloom, 1978–1979). The removal of a breast should be understood as an amputation of a body part—a part that symbolizes sexuality, femininity, gender and maternal issues. Women may complain of phantom breast sensations or phantom breast pain, and must adapt to alterations in body image. The more invested the woman is in her body image for her sense of self-esteem, the harder it may be for her to deal with the cancer (Kunkel, 1994).

Mourning the loss of a cherished body part and the threat to life are universal, but there seems to be variability in the extent to which other events are experienced (Rowland & Massie, 1998). At 1 year, women whose disease was discovered at an early stage and who were well adjusted before they had a mastectomy can expect to have a quality of life equal to that of unaffected peers. Predictors of poor psychological adaptation include more advanced disease, concurrent physical or emotional illness, stress, expectation of poor support from others, and a tendency to perceive life events as less under one's own control (Psychological Aspects of Breast Cancer Study Group, 1987; Hughson et al., 1988). More recent studies suggest that while most women report improvement in emotional and physical well-being over time, for a significant minority (20–25%), problems persist beyond 2 years after treatment (Irvine et al., 1991).

Lumpectomy and Radiation Therapy

Women who choose mastectomy have as good a prognosis as those who pick lumpectomy and radiation therapy. Early on, women receiving lumpectomy and radiation adapt better than those receiving mastectomy. In the long term, however, women choosing lumpectomy fare no differently from (or may do even worse than) those who choose mastectomy (Maunsell et al., 1989; Omne-Ponten et al., 1994; Levy et al., 1992). Specifically, women undergoing radiation therapy are at higher risk of depressive symptoms at the end of radiation treatments (Lasry et al., 1987; Monroe et al., 1989), presumably related to loss of support and fears of recurrence with diminished surveillance.

Currently, American women can choose between lumpectomy and mastectomy. However, legislation regarding informed consent on treatment options is mandated in fewer than half the states (Rowland & Massie, 1998). Medical decision making also includes making choices regarding the nature of the care (e.g., high-quality radiation therapy) and the site of care delivery (e.g., academic medical centers) (Farrow et al., 1992; Nattinger et al., 1992; Hynes, 1994). Physician recommendations continue to exert the most significant influence on treatment choices for the majority of women (Ashcroft et al., 1985; Margolis et al., 1989).

Adjuvant Chemotherapy

The need for adjuvant chemotherapy demands psychological adjustment to another treatment modality. Chemotherapy is administered over a lengthy treatment period; serves as a reminder of the threat to life implicit in the need for systemic therapy; and results in nausea, vomiting, and hair loss. When used for disease recurrence, it may reactivate concerns about death and dying, contributing to fear that the cancer is spreading. In addition to drug-induced nausea and vomiting, anticipatory nausea and vomiting, a conditioned reflex, can occur without the emetic agent. Although antiemetic medications can be used for women with anticipatory nausea and vomiting, this reflex is exacerbated by anxiety and responds well to behavioral interventions (e.g., relaxation, distraction). Many of the antiemetic agents are neuroleptics (e.g., prochlorperazine, metoclopramide), which may produce akathisia. Patients are frequently unprepared for this side effect and feel as if they are "going crazy" (Farrow et al., 1992; Kunkel, 1994). Newer antiemetic agents (e.g., ondansetron, granesitron) are more costly, but do not produce akathisia.

Alopecia, a very common side effect of chemotherapy, is very anxiety-provoking in some women because of the role hair plays in appearance, femininity, and sexuality. Some women fear their partners will reject them if they turn bald. Weight gain, problems with concentration, and premature menopause in younger women are other troublesome side effects. Despite fear of experiencing such side effects, few women refuse to start treatment, and most comply with their treatment regimens (Taylor et al., 1984). Planning for emotional reactions to ending treatment is important, as fears of recurrence peak at this time. Women experience more severe reactive anxiety and depression during treatment completion than they do earlier in treatment (Rowland & Massie, 1998).

Hormonal Therapy

Tamoxifen is the most commonly prescribed adjuvant therapy. It significantly reduces re-currence and mortality rates in all age groups of women with breast cancer (National Al-liance of Breast Cancer Organizations [NABCO], 1998; Hortobagyi, 1998). For women with a high risk of recurrent disease, the combination of tamoxifen (or ovarian ablation for premenopausal women) and chemotherapy is recommended (Hortobagyi, 1998). However, antiestrogens like tamoxifen may cause distressing hot flashes in premeno-pausal women. Premature menopause, depression, and weight gain also occur with the use of tamoxifen. Patients with breast cancer whose treatment leads to menopausal symp-toms may be at higher risk for depression, and thus, should be targets for psychiatric screening (Duffy et al., 1999).

In 1998, the Breast Cancer Prevention Trial (BCPT) revealed that tamoxifen for high-risk women is highly effective in preventing breast cancer. Other reports suggest that tamoxifen is particularly effective in elderly women. In the fall of 1998, the National Surgical Adjuvant Breast and Bowel Project (NSABP) began its "STAR" breast cancer prevention trial comparing tamoxifen with raloxifene over a 5-year period in 22,000 high-risk women (NABCO, 1998).

Bone Marrow Transplantation

Although there has not been focused research on the psychological effects of bone mar-row transplantation for breast cancer, it is clear that this intensive therapy often takes a high toll on the quality of life. Ensuring that psychological support is provided across the course of transplantation and follow-up is crucial, so that optimal survival and quality of life are achieved (Cassileth et al., 1980). Efforts are underway to measure the long-term effectiveness of bone marrow transplantation in women with breast cancer. Recent stud-ies suggest that bone marrow transplantation may not offer benefits over conventional treatment (Memorial Sloan Kettering Cancer Center, 1999).

Advanced Disease

Care for women with advanced breast cancer is aimed at palliative care, providing comfort and symptom control. The most common sites of metastatic disease are skin, lymph nodes, bone, lung parenchyma, pleura, and liver. The keys to successful supportive care are conti-nuity of care with physicians and staff, and support from friends and family. Attention to pain control is crucial. Spiegel and Bloom (1983) found that for women with metastatic breast cancer, beliefs about the meaning of the pain in relation to the illness predicted the pain level better than the metastatic site did. Psychiatric consultation should be considered when emotional distress is not responsive to the usual supportive measures. Evaluation of new-onset cognitive disorders (e.g., delirium, dementia) should include at the least com-puted tomography or magnetic resonance imaging of the head; liver function tests; calcium; a workup for infection; a complete blood count and differential; vitamin B_{12}; folate; rapid plasma reagin (RPR); and thyroid-stimulating hormone levels. All unnecessary medications should be discontinued (Patkar & Kunkel, 1997). The newest treatments for metastatic breast cancer include using monoclonal antibodies (e.g., trastuzumab) for women with tu-mors that produce the HER2 protein (Memorial Sloan Kettering Cancer Center, 1999).

Psychosocial Interventions

Today there are many different psychosocial interventions for women with breast cancer, varying in type (individual or group), orientation (behavioral, cognitive, or supportive), duration (time-limited or open-ended), timing (pre- or posttreatment or during treatment), and target population (early vs. advanced, under 40 vs. older, high-risk, etc.). The central purpose of psychosocial and psychoeducational interventions is to provide each woman with the skills or resources needed to cope with her illness and to improve the quality of her life (Rowland & Massie, 1998). Group interventions help patients through their illness and may increase survival. One of the most important factors for increasing survival may be permission to express anger in the group (Spiegel & Kato, 1996). Support from other women who have been through the same illness and procedures is often extremely helpful. Many women view cancer as a transitional event, and a shared group experience can help minimize the negative impact of illness on recovery and well-being (Rowland & Massie, 1998). Studies suggest that psychological parameters may also have a significant impact on immune cell subsets (Tjemsland et al., 1997; Cohen et al., 1998). Treatment of depression may improve quality of life, immune function, and possibly also survival time (Spiegel, 1996).

Role and Care of the Family

A positive relationship between social support and health or illness outcome is a consistent finding (Wallston et al., 1983). For most patients, family members provide the primary support. Today there are greater demands on the family members in the decision-making process, in the provision of emotional support, and as care providers. Absence of social support, or loss of a significant person who withdraws during the illness, adds stress that may be more emotionally painful than the illness itself (Dunkel-Schetter & Wortman, 1982). The impact of cancer can be as devastating to a family member as to the patient herself. Involvement of the spouse or partner in the decision-making process, early hospital visitation, and early viewing of scars are important for facilitating psychological adjustment. Early resumption of sexual relations reduces the likelihood of uncomfortable emotional and physical distance. Despite increased provider sensitivity to sexual issues, staff avoidance contributes to wide variations in the use of effective sexual interventions. Furthermore, women may worry about their children's risks of breast cancer. Adolescent daughters may be particularly vulnerable during the course of illness, possibly due to fears of developing the disease and/or increased responsibilities.

Although most women who are referred for psychiatric consultation have already been diagnosed with breast cancer, there are also women who have had benign biopsies of lumps in their breasts and are concerned about getting the disease, often because of extensive family histories of breast cancer. Others have premorbid psychiatric diagnoses, making coping with the stress of breast cancer more difficult. The focus of psychiatric treatment may shift rapidly among individual outpatient work, crisis intervention, family treatment, and supportive treatment while a patient is admitted to the medical unit. Researchers are continuing to develop new models of intervention that will help reduce distress, increase compliance, and foster adaptive coping in women with breast cancer. Today many different health care practitioners are helping to provide individual psychotherapy, pharmacotherapy, family therapy, and pain management for these patients (Kunkel, 1994).

GYNECOLOGIC CANCER

In 2001, the American Cancer Society estimated that gynecologic cancer would be diagnosed in approximately 80,300 women and would result in an estimated 26,300 deaths (American Cancer Society, 2001). It is most common in older women and includes cancers of the ovaries, fallopian tubes, uterine corpus, cervix, vagina, and vulva. Screening is only available for cervical cancer. Gynecologic cancers tend to present late. Women typically experience mild, vague, or somewhat familiar symptoms, and, therefore, are reluctant to seek care. Because treatment frequently begins with the diagnosis of an advanced-stage cancer, the psychological and medical issues are by necessity more complicated (Auchincloss & McCartney, 1998).

Women experience cumulative side effects from surgery, chemotherapy, and/or radiation therapy. Coping with gynecologic cancer is enormously physically and psychologically challenging for the patient and those around her. Commonly, the cancer and its treatments change the patient's hormonal, sexual, reproductive, and bowel and bladder function. During the course of illness, patients struggle with altered self-perception, fear of dying, treatment-related menopause, impaired or lost fertility, sexual dysfunction, and relationship problems (Auchincloss, 1995).

Approximately 20–25% of hospitalized patients with gynecologic cancer have major depressive disorders (Cain et al., 1983; Evans et al., 1986). Women at highest risk for depression have a history of a mood disorder, are in advanced stages of cancer, and/or have poorly controlled pain (Cain et al., 1983; Bukberg et al., 1984; Massie & Holland, 1990). Certain chemotherapeutic agents (e.g., vincristine, vinblastine) are potentially life-saving but may have depressive side effects (Massie & Holland, 1990). Psychiatrists can assist patients in coping with their unpleasant side effects (McCartney, 1993). The understanding and support of the oncology team are crucial for a patient's recovery. Various formats (support groups, newsletters, videotapes, Internet sites) have begun to develop in order to link women with gynecologic cancer to each other and to their care providers, through treatment information, support, and referral services (Auchincloss & McCartney, 1998).

Issues across All Sites

Stigma and Loneliness

Gynecologic cancer carries a stigma related to its historically poor prognosis and its location at the site of female sexual response and reproduction. For the general population, gynecologic cancer is often equated with a death sentence. Due to a lack of public understanding and difficulty finding local support, women often feel isolated and socially estranged. Women with gynecologic cancer may refrain from open discussion about their disease and may have irrational feelings of shame, embarrassment, and guilt for years. The special challenge for the gynecologic oncology team is that these tumors not only are keenly distressing because of their malignant nature; they also present difficult prognostic situations, involving complex and still-evolving treatment protocols, fertility loss, damaged sexual responses, and the acute onset of menopause. The power of stigma, avoidance, the rarity of some tumors, the accompanying sense of isolation, and the extensive ripple effects on a patient's emotional ties to others can be both overwhelming and stressful (Auchincloss & McCartney, 1998).

Physical Changes

Gynecologic cancer treatment often involves loss of ovarian function, and for pre-menopausal women this leads to treatment-related menopause. The onset of hot flushes, vaginal dryness, hair and skin changes, and mood disturbance—all related to lack of estrogen—may augment the sense of premature aging. Thus careful medical attention and support, including discussion and management of menopausal symptoms, are very help-ful, especially when the transition to menopause is abrupt and untimely (Auchincloss & McCartney, 1998).

Women spend much time and emotional energy in the first 2 years of survival accom-modating to other treatment-related changes and learning to live with them. These changes include fatigue; surgical scars; pain; sadness over lost body integrity or lost youthfulness; al-teration of gastrointestinal, bladder, and sexual function; skin changes (from radiation); and changes in hair thickness or texture after chemotherapy. These physical changes alter a woman's sense of identity, femininity, and sexuality, and may alter the way others perceive her. The oncology team must remain sensitive to the fact that even a small physical change may require a significant process of adaptation by the patient.

A referral to a mental health professional who is particularly skilled in counseling women with cancer can be invaluable for women dealing with more extensive body changes (e.g., ostomies) or changes due to radiation or surgery. Psychiatric evaluation and treatment can gradually restore a sense of body acceptance and comfort—common concerns after cancer treatment. A support group may provide insight into various ways that others have accepted their changed bodies after cancer and may foster individual emotional expression. For women who undergo radical surgical procedures (e.g., pelvic exenteration or vulvectomy), discussing feelings about their bodies, as well as changes in both sexuality and elimination, can help women to arrive at a sense of themselves as vig-orous, whole, and worthwhile (Auchincloss & McCartney, 1998).

Sexuality, Sexual Dysfunction, and Infertility

Although most women find satisfaction in their lives and relationships after gynecologic cancer treatment, a high proportion experience persistent problems with sexual function-ing (Schover et al., 1989). Women are particularly vulnerable to these problems, as the cancer arises at the site of pelvic sexual response. Treatment modalities may adversely af-fect sexual function as well. Furthermore, emotional, relationship, and fertility concerns are closely linked to sexual expression for these women. With hysterectomy or with infer-tility due to chemotherapy, the inability to conceive children can be catastrophic. In addi-tion, loss of sexual desire and dyspareunia (painful intercourse) can result in decreased sexual frequency or even sexual abstinence. Good medical management is essential to im-proving impaired sexual function and to reestablishing the possibility of comfortable sex. Decreased sexual activity is not solely linked to the degree of physical damage; psycho-logical and social variables may play a primary role in the development of posttreatment sexual problems (Schover et al., 1987; Schover, 1991). Psychosocial variables may be more critical than physical variables for sexual rehabilitation (Weijmar Schultz et al., 1990; Weijmar Schultz & van de Wiel, 1992). Addressing psychosocial and sexual out-comes following cancer treatment and emphasizing partner involvement in sexual reha-bilitation are keys to providing optimal therapeutic interventions.

Site-Specific Issues

Cervical Cancer

In 2001, the American Cancer Society estimated that 12,900 diagnoses of invasive cervical cancer and approximately 4,400 deaths would occur (American Cancer Society, 2001). The prevalence of Pap screening has made carcinoma *in situ* of the cervix much more frequent than invasive cancer (American Cancer Society, 2001). Factors contributing to increased risk include exposure to sexually transmitted diseases; exposure to the human papillomavirus (due to early, frequent, unprotected sexual contacts); smoking; substance abuse or dependence; and immunosuppression. For example, immunosuppressed women with HIV have a 15- to 20-fold increase in risk of cervical cancer (Auchincloss & McCartney, 1998). The Pap test should be performed annually, along with an internal pelvic exam, in women, who are or have been, sexually active or who have reached age 18. Signs and symptoms of cervical cancer include abnormal vaginal bleeding or spotting, abnormal vaginal discharge, and (with more advanced disease) pain and systemic complaints.

With behavioral modifications or early detection, cervical cancer is preventable. Cervical dysplasia progresses to carcinoma over a period of months to years. When detected early, invasive cervical cancer is one of the most successfully treatable cancers, with a 5-year survival rate of 91% for localized cancers (American Cancer Society, 2001). Knowledge that the sexually transmitted human papillomavirus is a major etiological factor causes many women to blame themselves for having had unprotected intercourse or, alternatively, to fear that others will assume that they have been promiscuous (Auchincloss & McCartney, 1998).

Persistent vaginal changes may compromise sexual activity, resulting in significant emotional distress (Bergmark et al., 1999). Although sexual dysfunction is worse when surgery is combined with radiation than when surgery alone is performed, Schover et al. (1989) found that marital stability and happiness were not affected by treatment modality. Information, support, and education can minimize the impact of radiation. For example, every woman who receives pelvic radiation could be provided with a vaginal dilator. Educational counseling and follow-up are crucial. Women feel better when given specific instructions for how to maintain a healthy vagina. Sexual experiences related to gynecologic dysfunction (e.g., pain) can be addressed as a separate issue. This approach helps women to regain a sense of control over their sexual function, allowing them to handle sexual situations with a more relaxed attitude (Auchincloss & McCartney, 1998).

Counseling prior to discharge or in outpatient support groups may be helpful in assisting women who are facing difficult treatment sequelae, such as fistulae, bladder and gastrointestinal obstruction, and/or inflammation (e.g., cystitis, proctitis). Hospital-based and community supports are now more widespread for women with ostomies. Patients may feel angry about treatment-related morbidity, and may question their physicians and treatments out of a sense of frustration. Patients who undergo pelvic exenteration for widespread disease require special counseling to recover psychologically, manage their ostomy care, and regain sexual comfort (Lamont et al., 1978). Recent studies advocate combinations of radiation therapy and chemotherapy for females with cervical cancer (Rose et al., 1999).

Uterine/Endometrial Cancer

In 2001, the American Cancer Society estimated that there would be 38,300 new diagnoses of cancer of the uterine corpus (usually of the endometrium) and 6,600 associated deaths, primarily in postmenopausal women. Signs and symptoms of uterine cancer include abnormal vaginal bleeding or spotting, with pain and systemic symptoms presenting as later manifestations. Estrogen-related exposure is the major risk factor for endometrial cancer: hormone replacement therapy with unopposed estrogen (estrogen replacement therapy); tamoxifen (weakly estrogenic in the uterine lining); early menarche; late menopause; nulliparity; polycystic ovarian disease; and/or chronic anovulation. Hormone replacement therapy (progesterone plus estrogen replacement therapy) is thought to largely offset the increased risk related to unopposed estrogen replacement therapy. Other factors that increase one's risk include infertility, obesity, gall bladder disease, diabetes, and hypertension. Pregnancy and the use of oral contraceptives appear to reduce the risk of endometrial cancer. Women aged 40 and over should have an annual pelvic exam, and endometrial biopsy is recommended at menopause and periodically thereafter for women at high risk of developing endometrial cancer* (American Cancer Society, 2001; Benedet & Miller, 1999).

Surgical staging is the favored initial treatment approach. Further treatment (radiation, hormones, and/or chemotherapy) is determined based upon surgical staging. Effective chemotherapeutic agents have yet to be established, and adjunctive therapy usually includes radiation. Currently endometrial cancer treatment has a favorable prognosis; the 1-year relative survival rate is 92% (American Cancer Society, 2001). Surgical treatment alone has less of an impact on sexual response and comfort than either radiation or chemotherapy does.

Younger women are often aware of the rareness of endometrial cancer in their age range and may feel particularly lonely. For example, Auchincloss and McCartney (1998) note an example in which one young woman in a gynecologic cancer support group went around the room checking the type of gynecologic cancer each of the other women had, and when each had answered and all had cervical or ovarian cancer, she sat back and said quietly, "I'm the only one." When a younger woman cannot retain her ovaries to avoid treatment-related menopause or cannot use her own ova for reproduction, she faces both menopause and loss of fertility.

Ovarian Cancer

In 2001, the American Cancer Society estimated that 23,400 cases of ovarian cancer would be diagnosed, accounting for 4% of all cancers among women. An estimated 13,900 deaths were expected from ovarian cancer—more than from any other cancer of the female reproductive system (American Cancer Society, 2001). Factors associated with increased risk of ovarian cancer are increased age, a personal history of breast cancer, and/or a family history of ovarian cancer. Continued surveillance is necessary for women with a strong family or personal history of breast cancer; in general, ovarian cancer appears later than breast cancer (Hartmann et al., 1999). Pregnancy and oral contraceptive use are associated with decreased risk.

Ovarian cancer is often diagnosed at an advanced stage because of the silent onset of the disease and the lack of early, accurate detection methods. Primary stages of the disease may present with few or mild symptoms, such as mild abdominal fullness, bloating, and unexplained, vague digestive disturbances. Occasionally, women experience anger as-

---

*Women with hereditary non-polyposis colon cancer (or at risk for it) should be screened annually with endometrial biopsies for cancer.

sociated with delay in diagnosis due to both physician-related and patient-related factors. Initial treatment includes surgical staging and debulking; tumor debulking is thought to improve the chemotherapy outcome (American Cancer Society, 2001).

Ovarian cancer presents with a range of psychological symptoms during diagnosis, treatment, and survival. Women at risk, especially young women with poor social support, are vulnerable to high levels of depression and anxiety. Various physiological stressors, including surgical menopause, steroid therapy, and pain during active treatment, are risk factors for depression and anxiety. Although improved surgical and chemotherapeutic regimens for ovarian cancer have resulted in a better prognosis, the general public still perceives this cancer as lethal and incurable. Loneliness is common among women with ovarian cancer. Such patients face the risk of recurrence, the need for second-look surgery, and retreatment (possibly over years) (Auchincloss & McCartney, 1998).

Chemotherapeutic agents inflict both acute and long-term toxicity. Symptoms of anxiety and depression are common immediately after chemotherapy and during palliative care. Palliative care includes management of pain, fatigue, nausea, and depression. Women in psychological distress may benefit from psychological counseling and/or brief group or individual supportive psychotherapies. When possible, a psychiatric consultant knowledgeable in psycho-oncology should pharmacologically address pain, discomfort, and severe mood symptoms (Hamilton, 1999).

Other Gynecologic Cancers

Rarer tumor types include vulvar, vaginal, and fallopian tube cancers, which were expected to be diagnosed in an estimated 5,700 women and to result in approximately 1,400 deaths in 2001 (American Cancer Society, 2001). Vulvar cancer accounts for more than half of these deaths and is usually diagnosed in postmenopausal women. The possibility of surgical cure is the hallmark of treatment. However, the standard treatment of radical vulvectomy is now being reconsidered due to its physically mutilating procedure, associated with bilateral lymphedema and a high incidence of sexual dysfunction. Women who undergo radical vulvectomy are often dismayed and depressed. Research on the psychosocial and sexual response to vulvectomy suggests that psychological and social variables are more crucial for rehabilitation than physical variables. Counseling may be integral to restoring the patient's self-esteem as a woman and as a potential sexual partner.

Corney et al. (1992a, 1992b, 1993) described a group of 105 patients who had undergone radical pelvic surgery for carcinoma of the cervix or vulva; they found that many were still anxious and depressed, and reported chronic sexual problems up to 5 years following surgery. Of the 75 previously sexually active women, 57 (76%) experienced postoperative sexual difficulties (Corney et al., 1993). Loss of desire was the most commonly reported sexual dysfunction. Many of the patients wanted more information, and a large group of the younger patients preferred that their partners be involved.

LUNG CANCER

Lung and bronchial cancer are the leading cause of cancer-related death in women in the United States; an estimated 78,800 new diagnoses and 67,300 deaths were projected in

2001 for women alone (American Cancer Society, 2001). Cigarette smoking is the primary risk factor. Other risk factors include exposure to certain industrial substances; certain organic chemicals; radon and asbestos, particularly for those who smoke; radiation exposure from occupational, medical, and environmental sources; air pollution; tuberculosis; and secondhand tobacco smoke in nonsmokers. The 5-year relative survival rate for all stages combined is only 14%. Although 49% of patients will survive if the disease is localized, only 15% of lung cancers are found when the disease is still localized (American Cancer Society, 2001). The high mortality is largely due to problems with early detection and the lack of effective screening procedures. Signs and symptoms (persistent cough, sputum streaked with blood, chest pain, and recurring pneumonia or bronchitis) often do not appear until the disease is advanced. As a result, most lung carcinomas are discovered only at an advanced stage, and palliative treatment (i.e., symptom management) is the only option for care.

Treatment

Treatment depends on the type and stage of the cancer and includes surgery, radiation therapy, and chemotherapy. Initially, small-cell lung cancers are responsive to chemotherapy and radiation therapy. Chemotherapy is used systemically, but central nervous system (CNS) irradiation may be added to reduce CNS involvement, usually requiring 6 to 12 months of intensive outpatient treatment. The more common non-small-cell lung cancers are usually diagnosed at an advanced stage, where palliation is usually the focus of treatment. In these cases, the cancer is widespread, usually involving CNS and bony metastases (Sarna, 1998). Poor prognosis may be associated with apathy and treatment nihilism in both patients and clinicians (Sarna, 1998; McVie, 1996).

Before treatment begins, informing patients with cancer of the potential psychological effects of the chemotherapeutic agents in their treatment regimen can be of significant value. In one study, patients with localized small-cell lung carcinoma were treated with either of two combination chemotherapy regimens; one regimen caused less depression and fatigue than the other, despite lack of differences in tumor response (Silberfarb et al., 1983). Physicians should be aware of the effects of chemotherapy on mental functioning and choose, among equally efficacious regimens, the one that causes less psychological morbidity.

Emotional and Symptom Distress

In their classic study, Weisman and Worden (1976–1977) noted that patients with lung cancer were found to experience greater emotional distress than those with other advanced cancers. Emotional distress peaks with diagnosis, falls off during treatment, and then increases again with disease progression and elevated symptom distress (Sarna, 1998). Anxiety and depression can intensify suffering and somatization. Younger age and lower socioeconomic status are associated with increased distress (Ryan, 1996). Although studies indicate that the prevalence of psychiatric disorders (e.g., anxiety and depression) is low, women with lung cancer have a high prevalence of subsyndromal psychological symptoms (Anonymous, 1989; Bleehan et al., 1993). The first indication of lung cancer for some patients may be the occurrence of personality changes (or other psychiatric symptoms or diagnoses) secondary to brain metastases. Particularly in small-cell lung cancer, assessment and treatment of psychological distress may be particularly difficult due to cognitive impairment resulting from brain metastases, paraneoplastic syndromes, or treatment side effects. Traditional measures of depression may not be valid for patients with lung cancer, as disease- and treatment-related symptoms such as fatigue, anorexia, and sleep disturbances may confound depression scores. Anxiety can arise as a manifestation of the disease, a reaction to treatment, or an exacerbation of a preexisting anxiety disorder. Anxiety is frequently triggered by poorly controlled pain, unanticipated events, the discovery of a new tumor, and frightening or painful procedures (Ryan, 1996).

Sarna and Brecht (1997) reported that fatigue, disillusionment, frequent pain, and difficulties in sleeping were the most distressing, prevalent concerns raised by women with advanced lung cancer. Other symptoms secondary to advanced lung cancer and to side effects of palliative treatment include functional decline, weight loss, difficulties in concentration, cough, dyspnea, bowel disruption, CNS effects, and paresthesias. Dyspnea is often linked to severe fatigue, impaired cognitive function, and poor appetite, all of which can promote a patient's social withdrawal (Brown et al., 1986; Ryan, 1987). Patients with lung cancer commonly fear suffocation, shortness of breath, choking, intense pain, loss, and death (Ryan, 1996). Compared to short-term symptoms related to treatment (nausea, vomiting), disease-related symptoms (pain, fatigue, dyspnea, functional decline, anorexia, and alterations in sleep) seem to have a greater effect on emotional well-being (Moinpour, 1994). Chemotherapy-induced changes in appetite and nausea may persist long after emetic agents have been discontinued (Sarna & Brecht, 1997). Psychological distress is often the result of uncontrolled physical symptoms, and effective symptom management may be the key to alleviating distress for many patients (Sarna, 1998). Such distress may predict survival, even after functional status, age, and personality traits are controlled for (Kukull et al., 1986)

Distressing symptoms also affect the emotional well-being of family members and caregivers (Sarna & McCorkle, 1996). Spouses or partners commonly suffer profound emotional distress (Wellisch et al., 1983), and the family burden may be greatly increased by the need for family members to assume the woman's traditional housekeeping and caretaking roles. In addition to the cost of treatment, the financial and emotional burden on the family may escalate as health care moves increasingly to the home (Sarna, 1998).

Tools such as the Lung Cancer Symptom Scale (Hollen et al., 1993; Hollen & Gralla, 1996) and the Functional Assessment of Cancer Therapy—Lung scale (Cella et al., 1995), now provide reliable and valid methods to screen for disruptions in quality of life and for the need for further psychiatric assessment and/or intervention. In a comprehensive review of literature from 1970 to 1995 on the quality of life in patients with lung cancer, Montazeri et al. (1998) found that the European Organization for Research and Treatment of Cancer's Quality of Life Lung Cancer Questionnaire—(QLQ-LC13), in conjunction with this organization's core cancer questionnaire (QLQ-C30), was the best-developed instrument. Bernhard and Ganz (1991) suggest that prior to the initiation of a treatment protocol, brief neuropsychiatric testing should be performed in order to obtain a cognitive baseline, as cognitive changes due to chemotherapeutic agents can be subtle and easily missed.

Relaxation, meditation, imagery, and cognitive therapies may reduce both emotional and physical distress. Such behavioral interventions have been shown to reduce the nausea and vomiting associated with chemotherapy, to decrease suffering from pain, and to reduce anxiety related to dyspnea. Individual, family, and group interventions can help participants to learn new coping skills and develop a sense of competence, control, and support that enhances hope and quality of life (Ryan, 1996). The course of treatment should include routine, systematic screening for anxiety, depression, symptom distress, impaired functional status, and emotional distress, in order to detect patients who require a more detailed assessment and possibly more intensive psycho-oncology interventions. Effective psychological treatment may require an interdisciplinary approach with the aim of reducing emotional distress and managing physical symptoms (NCCN Psychosocial Distress Practice Guidelines Panel, 1999; Sarna, 1998). Montazeri et al. (1998) argue that improvement in quality of life for a patient with lung cancer involves palliation of symptoms, psychosocial interventions, and understanding patients' feelings and concerns.

Tobacco Use

Tobacco-related diseases will become the leading cause of preventable death throughout the world in the 21st century. Although the rate of increase in the incidence of lung cancer among women began to slow in the 1990s, decreasing smoking patterns among women still lag behind those of men (American Cancer Society, 2001). Patients often misunderstand the 20- to 40-year lag time between smoking initiation and a diagnosis of lung cancer (Peto et al., 1994), as well as the length of time after cessation before risk reduction occurs. This can lead to frustration in patients diagnosed with lung cancer, especially for those who quit smoking before the diagnosis. Surprisingly, most patients do not even acknowledge the relationship between their smoking behavior and their lung cancer (Mumma & McCorkle, 1982; Lebovits et al., 1981). On the other hand, patients without a smoking history (almost 25% of women with lung cancer; Zang & Winder, 1996), who may have been exposed to secondhand smoke at work or at home, may exhibit anger and resentment (Sarna, 1998). Psychological support, skills training, nicotine replacement, and/or slow-releasse bupropion may be necessary for both patients and family members who smoke. Sarna (1995) found that although most women stopped smoking soon after being diagnosed with lung cancer, many relatives continued to smoke. Relatives who blame patients with lung cancer for having smoked or for continuing to smoke after diagnosis may complicate the patients' adjustment to the lung cancer (Sarna, 1998).

Long-Term Survivors and Emotional Well-Being

Among the few studies that address cancer survivorship, one (Schag et al., 1994) suggested that disease-free survivors of lung cancer (n = 57, 44% female) had more problems than did survivors of colon cancer (n = 117, 34% female) and prostate cancer (n = 104). The survivors of lung cancer experienced severe, persistent problems in work, daily activities, and pain. Anxiety, depression, sleep disturbances, and cognitive problems in concentration and memory were also worse among survivors of lung cancer than colon and prostate cancer. The survivors of lung cancer also expressed difficulties with sexual functioning (e.g., decrease in intercourse and difficulties with arousal), which may have been due to the impact of reduced lung capacity on sexual performance. Among the survivors, 58% were worried that the cancer was progressing. In this study, the length of survival was not a critical factor in quality-of-life ratings for survivors of lung cancer, and the Karnofsky Performance Status, a standard measure of functional status, was most predictive of quality of life for all three groups of survivors

(Schag et al., 1994). In another study, worry about cancer progression significantly impaired quality of life (Sarna, 1993).

CONCLUSIONS/FUTURE DIRECTIONS

Psychological issues for patients with cancer have been the subject of increasing research in the past few years. Studies are helping to refine screening instruments and to elucidate effective interventions across the course of illness, from screening and diagnosis to palliative treatment or survivorship. There is increasing emphasis on the need to integrate screening for psychosocial distress into the routine medical care of all patients with cancer (NCCN Psychosocial Distress Practice Guidelines Panel, 1999). Women continue to grapple with decisions regarding early detection, treatment, and treatment side effects.

Improvements in early detection and in cancer treatment of have resulted in encouraging statistics regarding cancer survival. Refinements in Pap screening have introduced increased choices for physicians (e.g., traditional Pap vs. ThinPrep Pap vs. others), and informed patients may wish to have a say in how screening proceeds. The newest advances in smoking cessation include the use of new medications that minimize nicotine cravings, along with behavioral therapies aimed at long-term cessation and prevention of relapse.

These advances also create new issues in medical decision making for both women and their treatment teams. As genetic testing advances, issues for women who are at increased risk for cancer will become increasingly complex. Legal, ethical, and social issues already complicate the emotional, psychological, and medical aspects of screening and testing for cancer predisposition genes. For example, will insurance companies and disability carriers label women who are BRCA1- or BRCA2-positive as having a "preexisting condition"? Cancer risk assessment programs should involve professionals specialized in genetics, oncology, psychiatry/psychology, social work, and pastoral care. Women should be informed of the potential risks and benefits associated with presymptomatic genetic testing. At the other end of the treatment continuum, potentially curative treatments may result in long-term sequelae that are manifested as chronic or late effects appearing months to years later (Loescher et al., 1989). Health care providers must realize the possibility that long-term and/or late effects may cause physiological or psychosocial disability in survivors (Memorial Sloan Kettering Cancer Center, 1999). The survivor population is exploding, and such patients must deal with a variety of issues related to reintegration, long-term effects of cancer treatment, employment, disability, sexuality, family, and social networks. Screening for distress related to psychological, spiritual/religious, and/or social concerns can provide guidance for service delivery to those in need (NCCN Psychosocial Distress Practice Guidelines Panel, 1999).

ACKNOWLEDGMENTS

We wish to acknowledge the thoughtful writings of Rowland and Massie (1998), Auchincloss and McCartney (1998), and Sarna (1998) which contributed to the organization and content expressed in this chapter. We also acknowledge the technical assistance of Dr. Philip Lartey in the preparation of this chapter.

REFERENCES

American Cancer Society. (2001). *Cancer facts and figures–2001*. Atlanta, GA: Author.

Anonymous. (1989). Survival, adverse reactions and quality of life during combination chemotherapy compared with selective palliative treatment for small-cell lung cancer. Report to the Medical Research Council by its Lung Cancer Working Party. *Respiratory Medicine, 83,* 51–58.

Ashcroft, J. J., Leinster, S. J., & Slade, P. A. (1985). Breast cancer—Patient choice of treatment: Preliminary communication. *Journal of the Royal Society of Medicine, 78,* 43–46.

Auchincloss, S. S. (1995). After treatment—Psychological issues in gynecologic cancer survivorship. *Cancer, 76*(Suppl.), 2117–2124.

Auchincloss, S. S., & McCartney, C. F. (1998). Gynecologic cancer. In J. C. Holland, W. Breitbart, P. B. Jacobsen, et al. (Eds.), *Psycho-oncology* (pp. 359–370). New York: Oxford University Press.

Benedet, J. L., & Miller, D. M. (1999). Gynecologic cancer. In R. E. Pollack (Ed.), *UICC International Union against Cancer manual of clinical oncology* (7th ed., pp. 537–562). New York: Wiley-Liss.

Bergmark, K., Avall-Lundqvist, E., Dickman, P. W., et al. (1999). Vaginal changes and sexuality in women with a history of cervical cancer. *New England Journal of Medicine, 340,* 1383–1389.

Bernhard, J., & Ganz, P. A. (1991). Psychosocial issues in lung cancer patients (Part 2). *Chest, 99,* 480–485.

Bleehen, N. M., Girling, D. J., Machin, D., et al. (1993). A randomised trial of three or six courses of etoposide cyclophosphamide methotrexate and vencristine or six courses of etoposide and ifosfamide in small cell lung cancer (SCLC): II. Quality of life. *British Journal of Cancer, 68,* 1157–1166.

Brown, M. L., Carrieri, V., Janson-Bjerklic, S., et al. (1986). Lung cancer and dyspnea: The patient's perception. *Oncology Nursing Forum, 13,* 19–23.

Bukberg, J., Penman, D., & Holland, J. C. (1984). Depression in hospitalized cancer patients. *Psychosomatic Medicine, 46,* 199–212.

Cain, E. N., Kohorn, E. I., Quinlan, D. M., et al. (1983). Psychosocial reactions to the diagnosis of gynecologic cancer. *Obstetrics and Gynecology, 62,* 635–641.

Cassileth, B. R., Zupkis, R. V., Sutton-Smith, K., et al. (1999). Information and participation preferences among cancer patients. *Annals of Internal Medicine, 92,* 832–836.

Cella, D. F., Bonomi, A. E., Lloyd, S. R., et al. (1995). Reliability and validity of the Functional Assessment of Cancer Therapy—Lung (FACT-L) quality of life instrument. *Lung Cancer, 12,* 199–220.

Cohen, M. J., Kunkel, E. J. S., & Levenson, H. (1998). Associations between psychosocial stress and malignancy. In J. R. Hubbard & E. A. Workman (Eds.), *Handbook of stress medicine: An organ system approach* (pp. 205–228). Boca Raton, FL: CRC Press.

Corney, R. H., Crowther, M. E., & Howells, A. (1993). Psychosexual dysfunction in women with gynaecologic cancer following radical pelvic surgery. *British Journal of Obstetrics and Gynaecology, 100,* 73–78.

Corney, R. H., Everett, H., Howells, A., et al. (1992a). Psychosocial adjustment following major gynaecological surgery for carcinoma of the cervix and vulva. *Journal of Psychosomatic Research, 36,* 561–568.

Corney, R. H., Everett, H., Howells, A., et al. (1992b). The care of patients undergoing surgery for gynaecological cancer: The need for information, emotional support and counselling. *Journal of Advanced Nursing, 17,* 667–671.

Duffy, L. S., Greenberg, D. B., Younger, J., et al. (1999). Iatrogenic acute estrogen deficiency and psychiatric syndromes in breast cancer patients. *Psychosomatics, 40,* 304–308.

Dunkel-Schetter, C., & Wortman, C. (1982). The interpersonal dynamics of cancer: Problems in social relationships and their impact on the patients. In J. S. Friedman & R. M. DiMatteo (Eds.), *Interpersonal issues in health care*. New York: Academic Press.

Early Breast Cancer Trialists' Collaborative Group. (1990). *Treatment of early breast cancer: Vol. 1. Worldwide evidence 1985–1990*. Oxford: Oxford University Press.

Evans, D. L., McCartney, C. F., Nemeroff, C. B., et al. (1986). Depression in women treated for gynecological cancer: Clinical and neuroendocrine assessment. *American Journal of Psychiatry, 143*, 447–452.

Fallowfield, L. J., Hall, A., Maguire, G. P., et al. (1990). Psychological outcomes of different treatment policies in women with early breast cancer outside a clinical trial. *British Medical Journal, 301*, 575–580.

Farrow, D. C., Hunt, W. C., & Samet, J. M. (1992). Geographic variation in the treatment of localized breast cancer. *New England Journal of Medicine, 326*, 1097–1101.

General Accounting Office. (1994, November 15). *Breast conservation versus mastectomy: Patient survival in day-to-day medical practice and in randomized studies*. Washington, DC: U.S. Government Printing Office.

Glanz, K., & Lerman, C. (1992). Psychosocial impact of breast cancer: A critical review. *Annals of Behavioral Medicine, 14*, 204–212.

Glynn, O. R., Ashcroft, J. J., Leinster, S. J., et al. (1987). Informal decision analysis with breast cancer patients: An aid to psychological preparation for surgery. *Journal of Psychosocial Oncology, 5*(2), 23–33.

Hamilton, A. B. (1999). Psychological aspects of ovarian cancer. *Cancer Investigation, 17*, 335–341.

Hartmann, L. C., Schaid, D. J., Woods, J. E., et al. (1999). Efficacy of bilateral prophylactic mastectomy in women with a family history of breast cancer. *New England Journal of Medicine, 340*, 77–84.

Hilton, B. A. (1989). The relationship of uncertainty, control, commitment, and threat of recurrence to coping strategies used by women diagnosed with breast cancer. *Journal of Behavioral Medicine, 12*, 39–54.

Hollen, P. J., & Gralla, R. J. (1996). Comparison of instruments for measuring quality of life in patients with lung cancer. *Seminars in Oncology, 23*, 31–40.

Hollen, P. J., Gralla, R. J., Kris, M. G., et al. (1993). Quality of life assessment in individuals with lung cancer—testing the Lung Cancer Symptom Scale (LCSS). *European Journal of Cancer, 29A*, S51–S58.

Hortobagyi, G. N. (1998). Treatment of breast cancer. *New England Journal of Medicine, 339*, 974–984.

Hughson, A. V., Cooper, A. F., McArdle, C. S., et al. (1988). Psychosocial consequences of mastectomy: Levels of morbidity and associated factors. *Journal of Psychosomatic Medicine, 32*, 383–391.

Hynes, D. M. (1994). The quality of breast cancer care in local communities: Implications for health care reform. *Medical Care, 32*, 328–340.

Irvine, D., Brown, B., Crooks, D., et al. (1991). Psychosocial adjustment in women with breast cancer. *Cancer, 67*, 1097–1117.

Kukull, W. A., McCorkle, R., & Driever, M. (1986). Symptom distress, psychosocial variables and lung cancer survival. *Journal of Psychosocial Oncology, 4*, 91–104.

Kunkel, E. J. (1994, February). Patients with breast cancer: The role of psychological factors. *Carrier Foundation Medical Education Letter, 185*, 1–7.

Lamont, J. A., DePetrillo, A. D., & Sargent, E. S. (1978). Psychosexual rehabilitation and exenterative surgery. *Gynecologic Oncology, 6*, 236–242.

Lasry, J.-C. M., Margolese, R. G., Poisson, R., et al. (1987). Depression and body image following mastectomy and lumpectomy. *Journal of Chronic Disease, 40*, 529–534.

Lebovits, A. H., Chahinian, A. P., & Gorzynski, J. G. (1981). Psychological aspects of asbestos-related mesothelioma and knowledge of high risk for cancer. *Cancer Detection and Prevention, 4,* 181–184.

Lerman, C., Rimer, B. K., & Engstrom, P. F. (1991). Cancer risk notification: Psychosocial and ethical implications. *Journal of Clinical Oncology, 9,* 1275–1282.

Levy, S. M., Haynes, L. T., Herberman, R. B., et al. (1992). Mastectomy versus breast conservation surgery: Mental health effects at long-term follow-up. *Health Psychology, 11,* 349–354.

Lewis, F. M., & Bloom, J. R. (1978–1979). Psychosocial adjustment to breast cancer: A review of selected literature. *International Journal of Psychiatry in Medicine, 9,* 1–17.

Loescher, L. J., Wech-McCaffrey, D., Leigh, S. A., et al. (1989). Surviving adult cancers: Part I. Physiologic effects. *Annals of Internal Medicine, 11,* 411–432.

Margolis, G. J., Goodman, R. L., Rubin, A., et al. (1989). Psychological factors in the choice of treatment for breast cancer. *Psychosomatics, 30,* 192–197.

Massie, M. J., & Holland, J. C. (1990). Depression and the cancer patient. *Journal of Clinical Psychiatry, 51*(Suppl.), 12–19.

Maunsell, E., Brisson, J., & Deschenes, L. (1989). Psychological distress after initial treatment for breast cancer: A comparison of partial and total mastectomy. *Journal of Clinical Epidemiology, 42,* 765–771.

McCartney, C. F. (1993). Gynecologic oncology. In D. E. Stewart & N. L. Stotland (Eds.), *Psychological aspects of women's health care* (pp. 291–312). Washington, DC: American Psychiatric Press.

McVie, J. C. (1996). Non-small lung cancer—Meta-analysis of efficacy of chemotherapy. *Seminars in Oncology, 23,* 12–16.

Memorial Sloan Kettering Cancer Center. (1999, August). MSK fine-tunes treatment for breast cancer. *Center News,* pp. 1, 4.

Meyerowitz, B. E. (1980). Psychosocial correlates of breast cancer and its treatment. *Psychological Bulletin, 87,* 108–131.

Moinpour, C. M. (1994). Measuring quality of life—An emerging science. *Seminars in Oncology, 21*(Suppl.), 48–63.

Monroe, A. J., Biruls, R., Griffin, A. V., et al. (1989). Distress associated with radiotherapy for malignant disease: A quantitative analysis based on patients' perceptions. *British Journal of Cancer, 60,* 370–374.

Montazeri, A., Gillis, C. R., & McEwen, J. (1998). Quality of life in patients with lung cancer: A review of literature from 1970 to 1995. *Chest, 113,* 467–491.

Morris, J., & Royle, G. T. (1988). Offering patients a choice of surgery for early breast cancer: A reduction in anxiety and depression in patients and their husbands. *Social Science and Medicine, 26,* 583–585.

Mumma, C., & McCorkle, R. (1982). Causal attribution and life-threatening disease. *International Journal of Psychiatry in Medicine, 12,* 311–319.

National Alliance of Breast Cancer Organizations (NABCO). (1998, July). *NABCO News,* pp. 1, 5.

National Comprehensive Cancer Network (NCCN) Psychosocial Distress Practice Guidelines Panel. (1999). NCCN practice guidelines for the management of psychosocial distress. *NCCN Proceedings: Oncology, 13,* 113–147.

Nattinger, A. B., Gottlieb, M. S., Veum, J., et al. (1992). Geographic variation in the use of breast-conserving treatment for breast cancer. *New England Journal of Medicine, 326,* 1102–1107.

Omne-Ponten, M., Homberg, L., & Sjoden, P.-O. (1994). Psychosocial adjustment among women with breast cancer stages I and II: Six-year follow-up of consecutive patients. *Journal of Clinical Oncology, 12,* 1778–1782.

Parker, S. L., Tong, T., Bolden, F., et al. (1996). Cancer statistics, 1996. *CA: A Cancer Journal for Clinicians, 46,* 5–27.

Patkar, A. A., & Kunkel, E. J. (1997). Treating delirium among elderly patients. *Psychiatric Services, 48,* 46–48.

Penman, D. T. (1979). *Coping strategies in adaptation to mastectomy.* Unpublished doctoral dissertation, Yeshiva University.

Peto, R., Lopez, A. D., Boreham, J., et al. (1994). *Mortality in relation to smoking in developed countries, 1950–2000: Indirect estimates from national vital statistics, 1994.* New York: Oxford University Press.

Phillips, K., Glendon, G., & Knight, J. A. (1999). Putting the risk of breast cancer in perspective. *New England Journal of Medicine, 340,* 141–144.

Psychological Aspects of Breast Cancer Study Group. (1987). Psychological response to mastectomy: A prospective comparison study. *Cancer, 59,* 189–196.

Rose, P. G., Bundy, B. N., Watkins, E. B., et al. (1999). Concurrent cisplatin based radiotherapy and chemotherapy for locally advanced cervical cancer. *New England Journal of Medicine, 340,* 1144–1153.

Rowland, J. H., & Massie, J. M. (1998). Breast cancer. In J. C. Holland, W. Breitbart, P. B. Jacobsen, et al. (Eds.), *Psycho-oncology* (pp. 380–401). New York: Oxford University Press.

Ryan, L. S. (1987). Lung cancer: Psychosocial implications. *Seminars in Oncology Nursing, 3,* 222–227.

Ryan, L. S. (1996). Psychosocial issues and lung cancer: A behavioral approach. *Seminars in Oncology Nursing, 12,* 318–323.

Sarna, L. (1993). Women with lung cancer: Impact on quality of life. *Quality of Life Research, 2,* 13–22.

Sarna, L. (1995). Smoking behaviors of women after diagnosis with lung cancer. *Image, 27,* 35–41.

Sarna, L. (1998). Lung cancer. In J. C. Holland, W. Breitbart, P. B. Jacobsen, et al. (Eds.), *Psycho-oncology* (pp. 340–348). New York: Oxford University Press.

Sarna, L., & Brecht, M. (1997). Dimensions of symptom distress in women with advanced lung cancer: A factor analysis. *Heart and Lung, 26,* 23–30.

Sarna, L., & McCorkle, R. (1996). Burden of care and lung cancer. *Cancer Practice, 4,* 245–251.

Schag, C. A., Ganz, P. A., Wing, D. S., et al. (1994). Quality of life in adult survivors of lung, colon, and prostate cancer. *Quality of Life Research, 3,* 127–141.

Schover, L. R. (1991). The impact of breast cancer on sexuality, body image, and intimate relationships. *CA: A Cancer Journal for Clinicians, 4,* 112–120.

Schover, L. R., Evans, R. B., & von Eschenbach, A. C. (1987). Sexual rehabilitation in a cancer center: Diagnosis and outcome in 384 consultations. *Archives of Sexual Behavior, 16,* 445–461.

Schover, L. R., Fife, M., & Gershenson, D. (1989). Sexual dysfunction and treatment for early stage cervical cancer. *Cancer, 63,* 204–212.

Silberfarb, P. M., Holland, J. C., Anbar, D., et al. (1983). Psychological response of patients receiving two drugs regimens for lung carcinoma. *American Journal of Psychiatry, 140,* 110–111.

Sox, H. C. (1998). Benefit and harm associated with screening for breast cancer. *New England Journal of Medicine, 338,* 1145–1146.

Spiegel, D. (1996). Cancer and depression. *British Journal of Psychiatry, 168,* 109–113.

Spiegel, D., & Bloom, J. R. (1983). Group therapy and hypnosis reduce metastatic breast carcinoma pain. *Psychosomatic Medicine, 4,* 333–339.

Spiegel, D., Bloom, J. R., Kraemer, H. C., et al. (1989). Effect of psychosocial treatment on survival of patients with metastatic breast cancer. *Lancet, ii,* 888–891.

Spiegel, D., & Kato, P. M. (1996). Psychosocial influences on cancer incidence and progression. *Harvard Review of Psychiatry, 4,* 10–26.

Suls, J., & Fletcher, B. (1985). The relative efficacy of avoidant and non-avoidant coping strategies: A meta-analysis. *Health Psychology, 4,* 249–288.

Taylor, S. E., Lichtman, R. R., & Wood, J. V. (1984). Compliance with chemotherapy among breast cancer patients. *Health Psychology, 3,* 553–562.

Taylor, S. E., Lichtman, R. R., Wood, J. V., et al. (1985). Illness-related and treatment-related factors in psychological adjustment to breast cancer. *Cancer, 55,* 2506–2513.

Tjemsland, L., Søreide, J. A., Matre, R., et al. (1997). Preoperative psychological variables predict immunological status in patients with operable breast cancer. *Psycho-oncology, 6,* 311–320.

Wallston, B. S., Alagna, S. W., DeVellis, B. M., et al. (1983). Social support and physical health. *Health Psychology, 2,* 367–391.

Weijmar Schultz, W. C. M., & van de Wiel, H. B. M. (1992). Sexual rehabilitation after gynecologic cancer treatment. *Journal of Sexual Education and Therapy, 18,* 286–293.

Weijmar Schultz, W. C. M., van de Wiel, H. B. M., Bouma, J., et al. (1990). Psychosexual functioning after the treatment of cancer of the vulva: A longitudinal study. *Cancer, 66,* 402–407.

Weisman, A. D., & Worden, J. W. (1976–1977). The existential plight in cancer: Significance of the first 100 days. *International Journal of Psychiatry in Medicine, 7,* 1–15.

Wellisch, D., Fawzy, F., Landsverk, J., et al. (1983). Evaluation of psychosocial problems of the home-bound cancer patient: The relationship of disease and the sociodemographic variables of patients to family problems. *Journal of Psychosocial Oncology, 1,* 1–15.

Zang, E. A., & Winder, E. L. (1996). Differences in lung cancer risk between men and women—examination of the evidence. *Journal of the National Cancer Institute, 88,* 183–192.

22

Rheumatological Diseases

CATHERINE A. STAROPOLI
CHRISTINE SKOTZKO

Rheumatological diseases are more common in women than in men (Table 22.1). These illnesses also appear to be affected by hormonal changes associated with menstruation and pregnancy, which may influence the development and course of the illnesses. Diagnosis is based on the presence or absence of symptoms and ancillary data that define these syndromes. This chapter briefly describes the history, diagnostic features, purported mechanism of disease, and treatment factors associated with the more commonly seen rheumatological disorders, including chronic fatigue syndrome (CFS), fibromyalgia (FM), systemic lupus erythematosus (SLE), and rheumatoid arthritis (RA).

As a group, these disorders appear to exhibit some phenomenological and genetic relationships to major depression. It is therefore not surprising that concurrent psychiatric disorders are common. It is important to remember that these are clinical syndromes rather than disease entities, and as such may present with differential psychological impact. Mood symptoms can be conceptualized as being akin to treatment-resistant depressive disorders. Somatoform and anxiety disorders are also frequent comorbid disorders and similarly difficult to treat.

Rheumatological disorders may present insidiously or with a dramatic alteration in psychological and/or physical functioning. SLE is a good example, as it may be associated with purely central nervous system (CNS) involvement. Hypomania is a common presentation, but psychosis, cognitive disturbance, and/or coma can also occur.

CHRONIC FATIGUE SYNDROME

CFS is associated with debilitating fatigue and a combination of symptoms that predominantly feature self-reported impairments in concentration, short-term memory, and sleep, as well as musculoskeletal pain. Various terms have been used to describe this illness over

TABLE 22.1. Ratio of Men to Women with Selected Autoimmune Diseases

Selected autoimmune diseases	M:F ratio
Systemic lupus erythematosus	1:9
Rheumatoid arthritis	1:4
Sjogren's syndrome	1:9
Myasthenia gravis	1:2
Autoimmune adrenal disease	1:3
Multiple sclerosis	1:5

Note. Adapted from Lahita (1996). Copyright 1996 by MSP International, Inc. Adapted by permission.

the past century, including "myalgic encephalomyelitis," "chronic fatigue," "immune dysfunction syndrome," and "postviral fatigue syndrome."

Price et al. (1992) reported that 24% of a general U.S. adult population had fatigue lasting longer than 2 weeks, with 59–64% of these people reporting no medical cause for their fatigue. Manu et al. (1993) reported that a psychiatric diagnosis explaining chronic complaints of fatigue was present in 74% of individuals, and that physical disorders were diagnosed in 7% of patients. The relative risk of women's developing fatigue is 1.7 as compared to men's risk (David et al., 1990; Cathebras et al., 1992)

In 1988, researchers from the Centers for Disease Control established criteria for the diagnosis of CFS to facilitate comparison of research efforts in the area of chronic fatigue. These were later further revised (Fukuda et al., 1994) and are presented below. This definition does not clearly describe a homogeneous group of individuals with a discrete disorder, but rather a syndrome with a heterogeneous group of triggering mechanisms that may share a common pathway, leading to the complex of symptoms seen (Komaroff, 1997).

CFS is severe disabling fatigue lasting for at least 6 months, of new and definite onset, not alleviated by rest, and associated with at least 4 of the following symptoms: impaired memory or concentration, sore throat, tender lymphadenopathy, myalgias, arthralgias, new headache, unrefreshing sleep, and postexertion malaise. A CFS diagnosis can only be made after alternative tests for medical and psychiatric causes of chronic fatiguing illness have been ruled out. (Fukuda et al., 1994, 1994, pp. 953–959)

Presently, 1 in 1,000 U.S. adults meet these criteria for CFS (Buchwald et al., 1995), whereas in primary care practice the prevalence is 1 in 100 (Bates et al., 1993). Bates et al. (1993) also noted that patients with CFS have a high prevalence of concurrent psychiatric disorders in general (78%) and somatoform disorders in particular (28%).

The cause of CFS is unknown. McCluskey (1993) hypothesized that CFS is a primary disorder of sleep regulation. Research has attempted to determine various objective biological abnormalities that can be found in patients with CFS. Komaroff (1997) suggests that there is evidence of an underlying CNS process. Magnetic resonance imaging (MRI) and single-photon emission computed tomography (SPECT) abnormalities have been reported to occur more often in patients with CFS than in healthy controls (Natelson et al., 1993; Tirelli et al., 1998), but Greco et al. (1997) did not discern a pattern of white matter abnormalities particular to CFS. Neuroendocrine abnormalities have been reported, with evidence of hypofunctioning of corticotropin-releasing hormone neurons in the hypothalamus (Demitrack et al., 1991), and lower evening salivary cortisol in nondepressed patients with CFS than in depressed individuals and controls (Strickland et al., 1998). Tilt table testing also revealed more hypotension in patients with CFS than in controls, suggesting a neurally mediated etiology (Rowe & Calkins, 1998). Chronic immune activation has been demonstrated (Whiteside & Friberg, 1998). A postinfective association has been shown with mononucleosis, upper respiratory tract infections, Epstein–Barr virus, and other infectious agents as well (White et al., 1995; Salit, 1997). Stress is commonly noted prior to the onset of CFS (Salit, 1996). Recent work has found an excess prevalence of both infectious events and negative life events during the 3 months preceding the onset of CFS (Theorell et al., 1999).

A diagnosis of CFS can only be made after excluding medical and psychiatric causes of chronic fatiguing illness (Fukuda et al., 1994). When CFS is suspected, evaluation should include a thorough physical examination, as well as a medical and psychological history, including particular attention to descriptions of episodes of medically unexplained symptoms; substance use history; and use of over-the-counter medications, herbal products, and vitamin supplements. A mental status exam should be done to identify abnormalities in mood, cognition, and personality.

A minimum battery of screening tests to exclude other diagnoses includes a complete blood count with leukocyte differential; a test of erythrocyte sedimentation rate (ESR); serum levels of alanine aminotransferase, total protein, albumin, globulin, alkaline phosphatase, calcium, phosphorus, glucose, blood urea nitrogen, electrolytes, creatinine, and thyroid-stimulating hormone; and a urinalysis (Fukuda et al., 1994). Presently there is no single laboratory test with adequate sensitivity or specificity to diagnose CFS.

Little is known about the prognosis of patients with CFS. Only a minority of patients show significant deterioration over time. Komaroff (1997) demonstrated that 12% of patients returned to an entirely normal life after 8.5 years of follow-up. Most patients improve over the first several years after diagnosis, but long-term prognosis is unknown (Salit, 1996). Saltzstein et al. (1998) reported that among women in a primary care setting, maintaining relationships with their physicians, employers, and family members, as well as engaging in spiritual activities, reflected healthy coping strategies. No controlled studies have provided convincing evidence for the efficacy of any treatment for CFS (Komaroff, 1997). Nonsteroidal anti-inflammatory drugs (NSAIDs) can be used to treat musculoskeletal complaints. Low-dose tricyclic antidepressants have been used, and beneficial and rapid effects on symptoms have been noted anecdotally. Letters describing the efficacy of various antidepressants underscore the variety of treatments available for mood and anxiety disorder symptoms.

Goodnick and Sandoval (1993) reviewed available studies and found that serotonergic treatments were more successful in alleviating pain than in lessening depression, and that catecholaminergic compounds seemed effective for symptoms of associated depression. Since then, two randomized controlled studies have been performed examining fluoxetine and phenelzine. Fluoxetine (Vercoulen et al., 1996) was found to have no beneficial effect in depressed or nondepressed patients with CFS, whereas phenelzine (Natelson et al., 1996) resulted in improvement in nondepressed patients with CFS.

Clinical experience suggests it is important to individualize treatment, starting with low doses of antidepressant medications to avoid side-effect-induced discontinuation of the drugs. Titration of doses should be gradual but aggressive. Frequent, regular, support-ive contacts assist in enhancing adherence to medications prescribed. Cognitive-behavior-al and supportive therapies are also utilized.

Clear, frequent communication between mental health and primary care practitio-ners is essential to address all issues that may arise. The primary goals of treatment are symptom relief and reduction of disability.

FIBROMYALGIA

FM is a complex syndrome characterized by pain amplification, musculoskeletal discom-fort, and systemic symptoms. Exaggerated tenderness to palpation has been described in medical literature since the mid-1800s. Multiple terms have been used over the past 150 years to describe this syndrome, including "fibrositis" and "neurathesthenia myasthenic syndrome."

In 1990, the American College of Rheumatology (Wolfe et al., 1990) established cri-teria for the diagnosis of FM.

> These criteria include: 1) A history of widespread pain. Pain is considered widespread when all of the following are present: pain in the left side of the body, pain in the right side of the body, pain above the waist, and pain below the waist. 2) In addition, there must be axial skel-etal pain (cervical spine or anterior chest or thoracic spine or low back must be present). In this definition, shoulder and buttock pain is considered a pain for each involved side. "Low back" pain is considered lower segment pain. The pain must be present at least 3 months. In addition to widespread pain, pain must be present in 11 of 18 tender point sites on digital pal-pation as seen in Figure [22.1]. (Quoted in Wolfe & Smythe, 1990)

This definition is highly useful in establishing research protocols. Clinical diagnosis may not be as rigid. Fatigue, which can be prominent, is not universal and not required for di-agnosis.

Women with FM can have a wide variety of symptoms other than pain, including leg cramps, dizziness, hearing loss, interstitial urethritis, irritable bowel, migraine headache, allergies, sleep problems, endometriosis, and temporomandibular dysfunction (Bennett, 1998). There also appears to be significant overlap with functional gastrointestinal disor-ders, migraine, and major depression (Chang, 1998; Nicolodi & Sicuteri, 1996; Hudson & Pope, 1996). Burkhardt et al. (1994) noted significant depressive symptoms in half of the population that they examined.

FM as defined by the American College of Rheumatology affects 2% of the popula-tion, with a breakdown of 3.4% in women and 0.5% in men (Wolfe et al., 1995). Of those afflicted, 80–90% are women, with a mean age in the mid-40s. The etiology of FM is unknown. It is not uncommon for patients with FM to report the onset of pain after an injury, emotional trauma, illness, or steroid withdrawal.

The etiology of FM remains unknown. Biopsies of tender points have revealed no clear differences between patients and controls (Yunus & Kalyan-Raman, 1989). There is increasing evidence that the problem in FM is disordered sensory processing. Patients ex-perience pain from nociceptive stimuli that are usually below the pain threshold. Pain perception is normal, but pain tolerance is decreased. Serotonin deficiency, increased Sub-

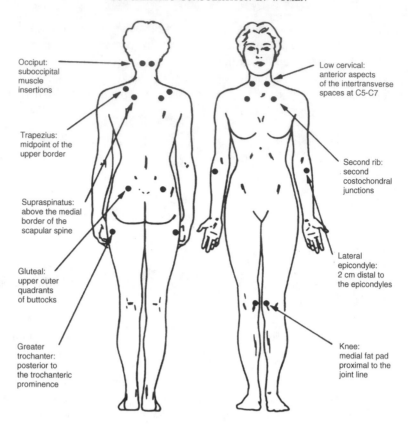

FIGURE 22.1. Location of specific tender points in fibromyalgia. From Freundlich and Leventhal (1993). Copyright 1993 by the Arthritis Foundation. Reprinted by permission.

stance P levels in the neurologic system, and abnormalities in nervous system amino acid levels have been found in patients with FM (Wallace, 1997; Olin et al., 1998; Russell et al., 1992). Symptoms of fatigue have been associated with disruption of deep sleep in patients with FM (Moldofsky, 1989).

The reproductive cycle in relation to FM has been studied. Ostensen et al. (1997) found that pregnancy resulted in worsening of FM symptoms, with the final trimester being the worst period in all women interviewed. Increased functional impairment and disability were the rule in this cohort. The premenstrual period was also noted to worsen symptoms in three-quarters of patients.

There is no specific diagnostic test for FM, and it can be a challenge to diagnose this syndrome, given its multiple clinical manifestations. The clinical criteria, however, can help in diagnosis. FM does not need to be a diagnosis of exclusion.

The clinician should fully evaluate the clinical symptoms experienced by patients with FM, as well as their psychological distress and disruptions of functional abilities. Providing educational literature and access to support groups can confirm that FM is a real disorder and may alleviate anxiety. An interdisciplinary team approach, including physicians, mental health professionals, and physical/occupational therapists, is appropriate. Granges et al. (1994) documented that about half of a community sample of individuals with FM showed resolution of the illness 2 years after diagnosis, and remission was noted in about a quarter.

There are multiple pharmacological interventions available. NSAIDs prescribed by many, are of minimal benefit. Local trigger point injection can interrupt peripheral nociceptive input to the central control mechanism (Wallace, 1997). Narcotic analgesics do not seem to improve systems and should be used with caution (Alarcón & Bradley, 1998). Low doses of tricyclic antidepressants, taken 2–3 hours before bedtime, can decrease depression and relax muscles; their use is discussed in a review by Godfrey (1996).

There are numerous reports of positive treatment response for FM with a variety of antidepressant agents. Dwight et al. (1998) reported that the presence of any lifetime psychiatric disorder predicted a positive response to venlafaxine. Hannonen et al. (1998) found that low-dose amitriptyline improved general health pain and sleep parameters. Goldenberg et al. (1996) demonstrated that both fluoxetine and amitriptyline improved patients' well-being, and that the combination worked better than either alone.

Nonpharmacological therapies, such as behavior and cognitive-behavioral therapies and exercise-based programs (particularly cardiovascular training), may also lead to short-term improvements in pain and other symptoms (Alarcón & Bradley, 1998; Nielson et al., 1992; Granges et al., 1994).

SYSTEMIC LUPUS ERYTHEMATOSUS

SLE is a multisystemic inflammatory disease characterized by highly varied clinical manifestations in association with antinuclear antibody production (Pisetsky et al., 1997). The term "lupus" is derived from the Latin word meaning "wolf," and it has been used since medieval times to describe an erythematous ulcer of the face (Hay, 1995).

The American College of Rheumatology has published the following criteria for the classification of SLE:

> At least 4 of the following are needed for diagnosis: malar rash (fixed erythema, flat or raised, over the malar emininces); discoid rash (erythematosus raised patches with adherent kerototic scaling and follicular plugging); photosensitivity; oral ulcers observed by a physician; nonerosive arthritis involving two or more peripheral joints, characterized by tenderness, swelling or effusion; pleuritis or pericarditis documented by electrocardiology or rub or evidence of pericardial effusion; proteinuria 0.5gm/day or 3+, or cellular casts; neurologic disorders such as unexplained seizures or psychosis; hematologic disorders such as hemolytic anemia or leukopenia (mg/mm^3) or lymphopenia (mm^3); immunologic disorders such as positive lupus erythematosus (LE) cell preparation, or anti-DNA or anti-Sm antibodies, or false positive serologic test for syphilis; or an abnormal antinuclear antibody titer by immunoflorescence or an equivalent assay at any time in the absence of drugs known to induce ANAs. (Tan et al., 1982)

Some of these criteria, such as LE cell test and discoid lupus, are better able to predict the likelihood of SLE than others, such as arthritis, oral ulcers, or nasal ulcers (Somogyi et al., 1993).

SLE occurs primarily in young women, with peak incidence between the ages of 15 and 40. In a general outpatient population, SLE affects 1 in 2,000 individuals. In the

United States, black and Hispanic individuals have a higher incidence of SLE than whites (Fessel, 1974). The ratio of women to men afflicted is 9:1 (Lahita, 1996).

Glomerulonephritis occurs in 60–70% of patients with SLE (Pisetsky et al., 1997). Immune complexes in the kidney appear to be the inciting event for the development of lupus nephritis. Glucocorticoids and cytotoxic drugs such as cyclophosphamide are the mainstay of treatment. These medications may have critical cardiac complications, such as valvular heart disease and accelerated atherosclerosis (Boumpas et al., 1995a).

Acute and chronic pulmonary complications are seen, including acute lupus pneumonitis and alveolar hemorrhage, interstitial lung disease, and pulmonary hypertension. Autoimmune thrombocytopenia may occur in 25% of patients with SLE (Boumpas et al., 1995a). The antiphospholipid antibody syndrome consists of the presence of antiphospholipid antibody identified by enzyme-linked immunosorbent assay for (IgG or IgM) anticardiolipin antibody, or by a positive test for lupus anticoagulant, and the occurrence of appropriate clinical events (such as recurrent venous or arterial clotting or fetal losses).

It has not been established that hormonal variation or pregnancy induces SLE clinical worsening or "flares" (Boumpas et al., 1995a). However, flares are common during pregnancy and appear to be more likely if the disease has been active recently (Petrie, 1994). Although SLE does not affect fertility, the rate of fetal loss is increased. Exogenous estrogens, such as oral contraceptives and hormonal replacement therapy, are not known to be harmful to patients with SLE (Boumpas et al., 1995 b). Various medications have been known to induce SLE. These include hydralazine, procainamide, chlorpromazine, methydopa, D-penicillamine, quinidine, and isoniazid. Discontinuance of the medication usually results in disease remittance (Sims & Smith, 1996).

Because SLE is so varied in its clinical presentation and severity, treatment must be based upon a detailed assessment of the individual and should be done in consultation with a rheumatologist. NSAIDs, antimalarials, and steroids can be used to treat specific manifestations of the illness.

SLE often presents with psychological symptoms. These may range from subtleties to severe psychosis and coma. Omdal et al. (1995) reported that half of the patients with SLE they examined had nonpsychotic disorders. When psychological symptoms are considered to be related to a flare, MRI should be used to assess for active disease. Aggressive medical therapy, rather than psychotropic medication alone, is needed to minimize the potential of progressive cognitive impairment in these individuals. Women with chronic active SLE involvement of the brain may develop dementia syndromes that worsen with the duration of the disease.

Dobkin et al. (1998) and Da Costa et al. (1999) found that stress, poor social support, and psychological distress are associated with poorer health in SLE. Waterloo et al. (1998) demonstrated an association between emotional disturbances and skin and joint complaints, which suggests additional etiologies for psychological dysfunction, rather than a direct CNS effect. The presence of more profound organ damage in women of low socioeconomic status, mediated by more severe depression (Lotstein et al., 1998), underscores the importance of treating mood disorders aggressively when they occur.

Women with SLE who require treatment for psychiatric symptoms should be given agents with low CNS toxicity. Despite being relatively young, many of these women are at risk for drug-induced side effects and delirium due to chronic cumulative brain insults and should be treated with the same caution given the elderly.

Person-centered counseling has been reported to be beneficial (Maisiak et al., 1996) as an adjunct therapy. Supportive therapy and case management services are also beneficial for individuals with cognitive impairment.

RHEUMATOID ARTHRITIS

RA is a systemic autoimmune disorder characterized by chronic, symmetric, and erosive synovitis of peripheral joints. The diagnosis of RA is a clinical diagnosis based on the features of the history, physical exam, laboratory tests, and radiological tests. The American Rheumatism Association criteria presented below were established in 1987 to assure uniformity in research definitions and were not intended for use in establishing the diagnosis in individual patients. Diagnosis should be made by clinical judgment.

> At least 4 of these 7 criteria must be filled in order to make a diagnosis of RA: 1. Morning stiffness. 2. Arthritis of 3 or more joint areas. 3. Arthritis of the hand joints. 4. Symmetric arthritis. 5. Rheumatoid nodule. 6. Serum rheumatoid factor. 7. Radiographic changes. Criteria 1–4 must be present for at least 6 weeks. (Arnett et al., 1988)

From 1% to 2% of the adult population around the world is afflicted with RA. The prevalence of RA increases with age; the peak onset is between the fourth and sixth decades. The overall ratio of men to women is about 1:2.5–4 (Wilder, 1993; Lahita, 1996).

The causative etiology of RA is unknown. There is a strong component of genetic predisposition rendering individuals susceptible to the disease. Twin studies have shown a 34% concordance for monozygotic twins. The HLA-DR4 haplotype is associated with the development of RA (Wilder, 1993).

Although the immunomodulatory effects of estrogen have been hypothesized to affect the course of disease, no clear link has been made. Oral contraceptives appear to decrease the risk of RA; pregnancy is associated with remissions, and the postpartum period with exacerbations (Goemaere et al., 1990).

The most common history is the insidious development of polyarthritis over several weeks. Intermittent attacks of monoarthritis lasting 3–5 days may also occur. Pain and stiffness of the cervical spine, constitutional symptoms, and low-grade fevers may also occur. In long-standing disease, disfiguring deformities of the hands, feet, wrists, and ankles can occur. Extra-articular manifestations of RA may involve the skin, heart, lungs, blood, and peripheral nervous system. One study reports that women describe more severe symptoms than men do, presumably because their disease is more severe (Katz & Criswell, 1996).

Rheumatoid factor, which consists of antibodies reactive to the Fc domain of IgG, is found in the serum of about 85% of patients with RA (Singer & Plota, 1956). Its presence tends to correlate with severe unremitting disease, nodules, and extra-articular lesions of RA in population studies. Rheumatoid factor is also associated with a number of other diseases, including other rheumatological diseases, infectious diseases, and other noninfectious conditions. The prevalence of rheumatoid factor increases with age. A positive rheumatoid factor in the absence of appropriate history and physical findings does not establish the diagnosis of RA.

Elevated ESR and C-reactive protein levels are often used to monitor inflammation and may be markers for progressive disease (Alarcón, 1997). Other factors associated with worse disease prognosis include extra-articular involvement, subcutaneous nodules, numerous affected joints, genetic markers, radiographic evidence of bone erosions, cartilage loss, and early functional decline.

NSAIDs are commonly used in the treatment of RA for their analgesic and anti-inflammatory effects. Gastritis and renal toxicity are the most common side effects. Corticosteroids are also commonly used. The adverse effects of steroids, including myopathy, glucose intolerance, cataracts, glaucoma, hypothalamic–pituitary–adrenal axis dysfunction, gastrointestinal bleeding, and osteoporosis, impede their use.

Disease-modifying antirheumatic drugs such as hydroxychloroquine, methotrexate, auranofin, injectable gold, sulfasalazine, D-penicillamine, cyclosporine, azathioprine, and cyclophoshamide are also used alone or in combination with the above-described agents. Bone marrow suppression and immunosuppression represent the major adverse effects of these agents. Because of the various toxicities of treatment, close follow-up with a rheumatologist or internist is needed. In recent years, these medications are being used more aggressively at earlier stages in the disease (Jain & Lipsky, 1997).

Among patients with RA, women report higher levels of depression than men do. Dowdy et al. (1996) found that quality of emotional support, passive pain coping, and functional impairment could only partially explain the differences noted. Smedstad et al. (1996) determined that patients with RA rated their mental health as poorer than controls rated theirs, but when pain, disability, and fatigue were controlled for, there was no difference from controls. In addition, dissatisfaction with illness-related disabilities has been found to exacerbate psychological distress (Blalock et al., 1998).

Interpersonal factors accounted for twice as much of the variance seen in depression as disease activity did when individuals with RA and osteoarthritis were compared (Zautra et al., 1994). Immune-stimulating hormones such as prolactin and estradiol were also positively correlated with interpersonal conflicts, depression, and clinician ratings of disease activity, suggesting that RA is psychologically and physiologically more reactive than osteoarthritis to interpersonal stressors.

Hawley (1995) reported that psychoeducational interventions do not alter physical functioning, but have a beneficial effect on self-efficacy. In this review, benefits seen were generally greater for patients with osteoarthritis than for patients with RA in the areas of pain, depressive symptoms, coping abilities, and disease self-management behaviors. Maisia et al.'s (1996) study examining person-centered counseling found no benefit for individuals with RA.

When individuals with RA require treatment for psychiatric symptoms, caution needs to be used, and treatment should be instituted with the knowledge and support of the rheumatologist or primary care provider treating the patient. Psychotropic agents that have minimal effect on bone marrow should be selected and used; treatment should start with low doses and gradually be titrated according to effect.

This population is also at risk for delirium and adverse side effects from commonly used medications. Frequent follow-up to assure that medications are tolerated, and attention to the potential for drug–drug interactions, are important.

CONCLUSION

Rheumatological disorders are syndromes rather than concise disease entities; therefore, the diagnostic criteria presented here are generally used for research purposes. The diagnosis of such a disorder is generally a clinical one, based on the patient's presentation and the clinicians diagnostic sense.

These disorders occur in both men and women, but are much more common in women. Reproductive hormones play a variable role in the expression and disability attributed to these illnesses, and more research is needed to better understand their role.

Gruber et al. (1996) have eloquently described the relationship between rheumatological diseases and major depression. These disorders appear to benefit in varying degrees from treatment with antidepressant medications, implying that there may be a link at some point in their etiology.

Psychological symptom severity varies from individual to individual, as does the potential for CNS involvement, which may complicate treatment with psychotropic medications. It is generally recommended that patients with these disorders be treated with the same care that one would use with geriatric patients in selection and dosing of medications. More controlled trials are needed to make confident recommendations regarding particular agents to treat the mood and anxiety disorders that are so common in rheumatological disorders.

Attention to psychotherapy is also important, as many individuals have ongoing issues related to the functional disability and deformity that may accompany these illnesses. Controlled trials of various interventions are needed in this area to clearly identify which modalities are most beneficial.

Above all, it is important to recognize these illnesses when they occur. Treatment options are evolving, and the future may hold more definitive therapies. At present, it may be helpful for women who have been told that their symptoms are "all in their heads" to learn that they have a recognized syndrome that others share. The general decline in overall functional status attributable to rheumatological diseases, and the high rates of psychiatric comorbidity, compel the involvement of mental health practitioners in the comprehensive care of these women.

REFERENCES

Alarcón, G. S. (1997). Predictive factors in rheumatoid arthritis. *The American Journal of Medicine, 130*(6A), 19S–23S.

Alarcón, G. S., & Bradley, L. A. (1998). Advances in the treatment of fibromyalgia; Current status and future directions. *The American Journal of the Medical Sciences, 315*(6), 397–404.

Anderson, R. J. (1993). Rheumatoid arthritis: Epidemiology, pathology, and pathogenesis. In H. R. Schumacher (Ed.), *Primer on the rheumatologic diseases* (pp. 91–95). Atlanta, GA: Arthritis Foundation.

Arnett, F. C., Edworthy, S. M., Bloch, D. A., et al. (1988). The American Rheumatism Association 1987 revised criteria for the classification of rheumatoid arthritis. *Arthritis and Rheumatism, 31*, 315–324.

Bates, D. W., Schmitt, W., Buchwald, D., et al. (1993). Prevalence of fatigue and chronic fatigue syndrome in a primary care practice. *Archives of Internal Medicine, 153*, 2759–2765.

Bennett, R. (1998). Fibromyalgia, chronic fatigue syndrome and myofascial pain. *Current Opinion in Rheumatology, 10*, 95–103.

Blalock, S. J., Orlando, M., Mutran, E. J., et al. (1998). Effect of satisfaction with one's abilities on positive and negative affect among individuals with recently diagnosed rheumatoid arthritis. *Arthritis Care Research, 11*(3), 158–165.

Boumpas, D. T., Austin, H. A., Fessler, B. J., et al. (1995a). Systemic lupus erythematosus:

Emerging concepts. Part 1. Renal, neuropsychiatric, cardiovascular, pulmonary and hematologic disease. *Annals of Internal Medicine, 122*(12), 940–950.

Boumpas, D. T., Austin, H. A., Fessler, B. J., et al. (1995b). Systemic lupus erythematosus: Emerging concepts. Part 2. Dermatologic and joint disease, the antiphospholipid antibody syndrome, pregnancy and hormonal therapy, morbidity and mortality, and pathogenesis. *Annals of Internal Medicine, 123*(1), 42–53.

Buchwald, D., Umali, P., Umali, J., et al. (1995). Chronic fatigue and chronic fatigue syndrome. *Annals of Internal Medicine, 123*, 81–88.

Burkhardt, C. S., O'Reilly, C. A., Wiens, A. N., et al. (1994). Assessing depression in fibromyalgia patients. *Arthritis Care Research, 7*(1), 35–39.

Cathebras, P. J., Robbins, J. M., Kirmayer, L. J., et al. (1992). Fatigue in primary care: Prevalence, psychiatric co-morbidity, illness behavior and outcome. *Journal of General Internal Medicine, 7*(3), 276–286.

Chang, L. (1998). The association of functional gastrointestinal disorders and fibromyalgia. *European Journal of Surgery, 583*, 32–36.

David, A., Pelosi, A., McDonald, E., et al. (1990). Tired, weak, or in need of rest: Fatigue among general practice attenders. *British Medical Journal, 301*, 1199–1202.

Da Costa, D., Clarke, A. E., Dobkin, P. L., et al. (1999). The relationship between health status, social support and satisfaction with medical care among patients with systemic lupus erythematosus. *International Journal for Quality in Health Care, 11*(3), 201–207.

Demitrack, M. A., Dale, J. K., Straus, S. E., et al. (1991). Evidence for impaired activation of the hypothalamic–pituitary–adrenal axis in patients with chronic fatigue syndrome. *Journal of Clinical Endocrinology and Metabolism, 73*, 1224–1234.

Dobkin, P. L., Fortin, P. R., Joseph, L., et al. (1998). Psychosocial contributors to mental and physical health in patients with systemic lupus erythematosus. *Arthritis Care Research, 11*(1), 23–31.

Dowdy, S. W., Dwyer, K. A., Smith, C. A., et al. (1996). Gender and psychological well-being of persons with rheumatoid arthritis. *Arthritis Care Research, 9*(6), 449–456.

Dwight, M. M., Arnold, L. M., O'Brien, H., et al. (1998). An open clinical trial of venlafaxine treatment of fibromyalgia. *Psychosomatics, 39*(1), 14–17.

Fessel, W. J. (1974). Systemic lupus erythematosus in the community: Incidence, prevalence, outcome, and first symptoms. The high prevalence in white women. *Archives of Internal Medicine, 134*, 1027–1035.

Freundlich, B., & Leventhal, L. (1993). The fibromyalgia syndrome. In H. R. Schmacher (Ed.), *Primer on the rheumatologic diseases* (p. 247–249). Atlanta, GA: Arthritis Foundation.

Fukuda, K., Straus, S. E., Hickie, I., et al. (1994). The chronic fatigue syndrome: A comprehensive approach to its definition and study. *Annals of Internal Medicine, 121*(12), 953–959.

Godfrey, R. G. (1996). A guide to understanding and use of tricyclic antidepressants in the overall management of fibromyalgia and other chronic pain syndromes. *Archives of Internal Medicine, 156*(10), 1047–1052.

Goemaere, S., Ackerman, C., Goethals, K., et al. (1990). Onset of symptoms of rheumatoid arthritis in relation to age, sex, and menopausal transition. *Journal of Rheumatology, 17*, 1620–1622.

Goldenberg, D., Mayskiy, M., Mossey, C., et al. (1996). A randomized, double-blind crossover trial of fluoxetine and amitriptyline in the treatment of fibromyalgia. *Arthritis and Rheumatism, 39*(11), 1852–1859.

Goodnick, P. J., & Sandoval, R. (1993). Psychotropic treatment of chronic fatigue syndrome and related disorders. *Journal of Clinical Psychiatry, 54*(1), 13–20.

Granges, G., Zilko, P., & Littlejohn, G. O. (1994). Fibromyalgia syndrome: Assessment of the severity of the condition 2 years after diagnosis. *Journal of Rheumatology, 21*(3), 523–529.

Greco, A., Tannock, C., Brostoff, J., et al. (1997). Brain MR in chronic fatigue syndrome. *American Journal of Neuroradiology, 18*(7), 1265–1269.

Gruber, A. J., Hudson, J. I., & Pope, H. G., Jr. (1996). The management of treatment resistant depression in disorders on the interface of psychiatry and medicine: Fibromyalgia, chronic fatigue syndrome, migraine, irritable bowel syndrome, atypical facial pain, and premenstrual dysphoric disorder. *Psychiatric Clinics of North America, 19*(2), 351–369.

Hannonen, P., Malminiemi, K., Yli-Kerttula, U., et al. (1998). A randomized, double-blind, placebo-controlled study of meclobamide and amitriptyline in the treatment of fibromyalgia in females without psychiatric disorder. *British Journal of Rheumatology, 37*(12), 1279–1286.

Hawley, D. J. (1995). Psycho-educational interventions in the treatment of arthritis. *Baillières Clinical Rheumatology, 9*(4), 803–823.

Hay, E. M. (1995). Systemic lupus erythematosus. *Baillière's Clinical Rheumatology, 9*(3), 437–470.

Hudson, J. I., & Pope, H. G. (1996). The relationship between fibromyalgia and major depressive disorder. *Rheumatic Diseases Clinics of North America, 22*(2), 285–303.

Jain, R., & Lipsky, P. E. (1997). Treatment of rheumatoid arthritis. *Medical Clinics of North America, 81*(1), 57–84.

Katz, P. P., & Criswell, L. A. (1996). Differences in symptom reports between men and women with rheumatoid arthritis. *Arthritis Care Research, 9*(6), 441–448.

Komaroff, A. L. (1997). A 56-year-old woman with chronic fatigue syndrome. *Journal of the American Medical Association, 278*(14), 1179–1185.

Lahita, R. G. (1996). The connective tissue diseases and the overall influence of gender. *International Journal of Fertility, 41*, 156–165.

Lotstein, D. S., Ward, M. M., Bush, T. M., et al. (1998). Socioeconomic status and health in women with systemic lupus erythematosis. *Journal of Rheumatology, 25*(9), 1720–1729.

Maisiak, R., Austin, J. S., West, S. G., et al. (1996). The effect of person centered counseling on the psychological status of persons with systemic lupus erythematosus or rheumatoid arthritis: A randomized, controlled trial. *Arthritis Care Research, 9*(1), 60–66.

Manu, P., Lane, T. J., & Matthews, D. A. (1993). Chronic fatigue and chronic fatigue syndrome: Clinical epidemiology and aetiological classification. *Ciba Foundation Symposium, 173*, 23–31.

McCluskey, D. R. (1993). Pharmacological approaches to the therapy of chronic fatigue syndrome. *Ciba Foundation Symposium, 173*, 287–297.

Moldofsky, H. (1989). Sleep and fibrositis syndrome. *Rheumatic Diseases Clinics of North America, 15*, 90–103.

Natelson, B. H., Cheu, J., Paraja, J., et al. (1996). Randomized, double blind, controlled placebo-phase in trial of low dose phenelzine in chronic fatigue syndrome. *Psychopharmacology (Berlin), 124*(3), 226–230.

Natelson, B. H., Cohen, J. M., Brassloff, I., et al. (1993). A controlled study of brain magnetic resonance imaging in patients with the chronic fatigue syndrome. *Journal of the Neurological Sciences, 120*, 213–217.

Nicolodi, M., & Sicuteri, F. (1996). Fibromyalgia and migraine, two faces of the same mechanism: Serotonin as the common clue for pathogenesis and therapy. *Advances in Experimental Medicine and Biology, 398*, 373–379.

Nielson, W. R., Walker, C., & McCain, G. A. (1992). Cognitive behavioral treatment of fibromyalgia syndrome: Preliminary findings. *Journal of Rheumatology, 19*(1), 98–103.

Olin, R., Klein, R., & Berg, P. A. (1998). A randomised double-blind 16–week study of ritanserin in fibromyalgia syndrome: Clinical outcome and analysis of antibodies to serotonin, gangliosides and phospolipids. *Clinical Rheumatoligy, 17*(2), 89–94.

Omdal, R., Husby, G., & Mellgren, S. I. (1995). Mental health status in systemic lupus erythematosus. *Scandinavian Journal of Rheumatology, 24*(3), 142–145.

Ostensen, M., Rugelsjoen, A., & Wigers, S. H. (1997). The effect of reproductive events and alterations of sex hormone levels on the symptoms of fibromyalgia. *Scandinavian Journal of Rheumatology, 26*(5), 355–360.

Petrie, M. (1994). Systemic lupus erythematosus and pregnancy. *Rheumatic Diseases Clinics of North America, 20*(1), 86–119.

Pisetsky, D. S., Gilkeson, G., & St. Clair, E. W. (1997). Systemic lupus erythematosus: Diagnosis and treatment. *Medical Clinics of North America, 81*(1), 113–128.

Price, R. K., North, C. S., Wessely, S., et al. (1992). Estimating the prevalence of chronic fatigue syndrome and associated symptoms in the community. *Public Health Reports, 107,* 514–522.

Rowe, P. C., & Calkins, H. (1998). Neurally mediated hypotension and chronic fatigue syndrome. *American Journal of Medicine, 105*(3A), 15S–21S.

Russell, I. J., Michalek, J. E., Vipraio, G. A., et al. (1992). Platelet 3H-imipramine uptake receptor density and serum serotonin levels in patients with fibromyalgia/fibrositis syndrome. *Journal of Rheumatology, 19*(1), 104–109.

Salit, I. E. (1996). The chronic fatigue syndrome: A position paper. *Journal of Rheumatology, 23*(3), 540–544.

Salit, I. E. (1997). Precipitating factors for the chronic fatigue syndrome. *Journal of Psychiatric Research, 31,* 59–65.

Saltzstein, B. J., Wyshak, G., Hubbuch, J. T., et al. (1998). A naturalistic study of the chronic fatigue syndrome among women in primary care. *General Hospital Psychiatry, 20*(5), 307–316.

Sims, G. N., & Smith, H. R. (1996). Outpatient management of systemic lupus erythematosus. *Cleveland Clinic Journal of Medicine, 63*(2), 94–100.

Singer, J. M., & Plota, C. M. (1956). The latex fixation test: Application to the serologic diagnosis of rheumatoid arthritis. *American Journal of Medicine, 21,* 888.

Smedstad, L. M., Moum, T., Vaglum, P., et al. (1996). The impact of early rheumatoid arthritis on psychological distress: A comparison between 238 patients with RA and 116 matched controls. *Scandinavian Journal of Rheumatology, 25*(6), 377–382.

Somogyi, L., Cikes, N., & Marusic, M. (1993). Evaluation of criteria contributions for the classification of systemic lupus erythematosus. *Scandinavian Journal of Rheumatology, 22,* 58–62.

Strickland, P., Morris, R., Wearden, A., et al. (1998). A comparison of salivary cortisol in chronic fatigue syndrome, community depression and healthy controls. *Journal of Affective Disorders, 47*(1–3), 191–194.

Tan, E. M., Cohen, A. S., Fries, J. F., et al. (1982). The 1982 revised criteria for the classification of systemic lupus erythematosus. *Arthritis and Rheumatism, 25,* 1271–1277.

Theorell, T., Blomkvist, V., Lindh, G., et al. (1999). Critical life events, infections, and symptoms during the year preceding chronic fatigue syndrome (CFS): An examination of CFS patients and subjects with nonspecific life crisis. *Psychosomatic Medicine, 61*(3), 304–310.

Tirelli, U., Chierichetti, F., Tavio, M., et al. (1998). Brain positron emission tomography in chronic fatigue syndrome: Preliminary data. *American Journal of Medicine, 105*(3A), 54S–65S.

Vercoulen, J. H., Swanik, C. M., Zitman, F. G., et al. (1996). Randomised, double-blind, placebo-controlled study of fluoxetine in chronic fatigue syndrome. *Lancet, 347*(9005), 858–861.

Wallace, D. J. (1997). The fibromyalgia syndrome. *Annals of Medicine, 27,* 9–21.

Waterloo, K., Omdal, R., Husby, G., et al. (1998). Emotional status in systemic lupus erythematosus. *Scandinavian Journal of Rheumatology, 27*(6), 410–414.

White, P. D., Thomas, J. M., Amess, J., et al. (1995). The existence of a fatigue syndrome after glandular fever. *Psychological Medicine, 25,* 907–916.

Whiteside, T. L., & Friberg, D. (1998). Natural killer cells and natural killer cell activity in chronic fatigue syndrome. *American Journal of Medicine, 105*(3A), 27S–34S.

Wilder, R. L. (1993). Rheumatoid arthritis: Epidemiology, pathology, and pathogenesis. In H. R. Schumacher (Ed.), *Primer on the rheumatologic diseases* (pp. 86–90). Atlanta, GA: Arthritis Foundation.

Wolfe, F., Ross, K., Anderson, J., et al. (1995). The prevalence and characteristics of fibromyalgia in the general population. *Arthritis and Rheumatism, 38,* 19–28.

Wolfe, F., Smythe, H. A., Yunus, M. B., et al. (1990). The American College of Rheumatology 1990 criteria for the classification of FM: Report of the multicenter Criteria Committee. *Arthritis and Rheumatism, 33,* 160–172.

Yunus, M. B., & Kalyan-Raman, U. P. (1989). Muscle biopsy findings in primary fibromyalgia and other forms of non-articular rheumatism. *Rheumatic Diseases Clinics of North America, 15,* 115–133.

Zautra, A. J., Burleson, M. H., Matt, K. S., et al. (1994). Interpersonal stress, depression, and disease activity in rheumatoid arthritis and osteoarthritis patients. *Health Psychology, 13*(2), 139–148.

23

Endocrine Disorders

JENNIFER S. BRASCH
GLENDA MacQUEEN
RUSSELL JOFFE

Homeostasis, growth, development, and reproduction are regulated by the interactions of the endocrine and nervous systems. Most endocrine secretions are controlled directly or indirectly by the brain, and virtually all hormones influence brain activity. It is not surprising, then, that endocrine diseases are associated with a wide array of psychiatric manifestations. This chapter reviews these relations, and emphasizes points where these interactions are particularly relevant to women's mental health.

HYPOTHALAMIC–PITUITARY DISORDERS

Pituitary function is regulated by three interacting elements—hypothalamic neurosecretions, feedback effects of circulating hormones, and paracrine and autocrine secretions of the pituitary itself. The posterior lobe secretes oxytocin, which acts on the breasts and uterus, and arginine vasopressin, which regulates water conservation by the kidneys. The anterior pituitary gland regulates endocrine organs by integrating signals from the brain and feedback effects of peripheral hormones to stimulate intermittent hormone release by specific glands. Hormones secreted by the anterior pituitary include thyroid-stimulating hormone (TSH), andrenocorticotropic hormone (ACTH), growth hormone (GH), prolactin (PRL), and the gonadotropins luteinizing hormone (LH) and follicle-stimulating hormone (FSH) (Reichlin, 1998).

A pituitary tumor can present with symptoms of a mass lesion, an endocrine dysfunction, or both. The endocrine abnormality can be hyperfunction, hypofunction, or a combination. The manifestations of a sellar mass include headache and symptoms secondary to compression of adjacent tissues or intracranial nerves, including visual field disturbances, ophthalmoplegia, or facial pain from trigeminal nerve compression. The most common symptom in both men and women is secondary hypogonadism because of primary LH and FSH deficiency or secondary to hyperprolactinemia (Thorner et al., 1998). Women with hypothalamic disease can experience a wide range of behavioral abnormalities, including antisocial behavior, attacks of rage, laughing and crying, disturbed sleep, hypersexuality, eating disturbances, and hallucinations (Reichlin, 1998).

Lynch et al. (1994) compared 41 adults with established hypopituitarism and GH deficiency to adults with another chronic medical illness (diabetes mellitus). Forty-six percent of the hypopituitarism group had a psychiatric disorder, compared with 24% of the diabetes group. Major depression and dysthymia were common in the adults with hypopituitarism, but this did not show a clear relationship to illness duration, biochemical indices of illness severity, or the dosage of steroid replacement therapy. Differences between males and females were not described.

DIABETES MELLITUS

Diabetes is one of the leading causes of disability in the United States among people over 45 years of age. In Type I diabetes, hyperglycemia results from a lack of insulin production from autoimmune destruction of pancreatic β cells, whereas Type II diabetes is characterized by insulin resistance in peripheral cells. Management of diabetes requires blood sugar monitoring, specific dietary constraints, regular exercise, and use of exogenous insulin or oral hypoglycemic agents. Blood sugar control is essential, since chronic hyperglycemia leads to complications such as peripheral neuropathy, autonomic neuropathy, retinopathy, and nephropathy (Unger & Foster, 1998).

Psychosocial Issues

Although some studies suggest that psychosocial problems for persons with diabetes are more severe than in other chronic illnesses, the best-designed studies indicate that this is not the case (Rubin & Peyrot, 1992). Nevertheless, individuals with diabetes are at increased risk for reduced physical and emotional well-being, which justifies attention to psychosocial issues and intervention when appropriate.

The period immediately following diagnosis is generally regarded as a time of psychosocial crisis for individuals with diabetes, but this is based predominantly on cross sectional studies of children and their parents, with few studies including longitudinal follow-up (Rubin & Peyrot, 1992). Kovacs (1985) reported that 64% of children studied with new-onset diabetes suffered mild symptoms such as sadness and social withdrawal after the diagnosis, while 36% had symptoms severe enough to meet criteria for a psychiatric disorder. All children returned to normal levels of psychological functioning within 9 months of diagnosis. A similar pattern of adaptation was apparent in mothers of affected offspring. Mothers who experienced the greatest distress immediately after diagnosis were most likely to remain distressed over an extended period (Kovacs et al., 1990). Jacobson et al. (1997) followed an onset cohort of 57 young adults with Type I diabetes for 10 years and found that they were as psychologically well adjusted as a group of young adults without a chronic illness.

High levels of stress are associated with poor glycemic control in adults and adolescents (Gill, 1991), and the subjective experience of many people with diabetes supports the view that stress affects glycemic control (Rubin & Peyrot, 1992). Wrigley and Mayou (1991) reported that adults requiring admission for poorly controlled diabetes experienced more stressful life events (unrelated to diabetes) in the 6 months prior to admission and more chronic difficulties than an outpatient control group did. Numerous studies have found that psychological distress and poor glycemic control are associated for both adults and children (Rubin & Peyrot, 1992). Interventions such as relaxation training, coping skills training, and group psychotherapy have been shown to improve stress tolerance and glycemic control (Rubin & Peyrot, 1992).

Several reports have found that poor glycemic control and psychological disturbance are associated with poor family functioning (Rubin & Peyrot, 1992). Bobrow et al. (1985) assessed 50 mother–daughter pairs in which the female adolescents had diabetes. Emotionally charged mother–daughter interactions were associated with poor treatment adherence. Poorly adherent adolescents had difficulty discussing feelings, problems, and concerns with their mothers, and believed less strongly that adherence would delay/avoid complications. Family therapy to facilitate adaptation to life with diabetes has been strongly recommended.

Medical Complications

Acute complications of poor glycemic control include diabetic ketoacidosis (a state of hyperglycemia) and hypoglycemia. Herskowitz Dumont et al. (1995) followed a cohort of 61 children and adolescents with Type I diabetes. Girls were at much greater risk for single or recurrent episodes of diabetic ketoacidosis, whereas boys were more likely to have one or more episodes of hypoglycemia. In girls, recurrent diabetic ketoacidosis was associated with higher ratings for behavior problems; lower levels of social competence; higher levels of family conflict; and lower levels of family cohesion, expressiveness, and organization. If these associated factors are assessed, it may be possible to identify girls at increased risk for recurrent diabetic ketoacidosis early in the course of illness.

The psychological sequelae of long-term medical complications in diabetes have not been well studied, especially in women. Two areas that have received some attention are sexual dysfunction and visual impairment. Increased risk of retinopathy is related to illness duration, poor glycemic control, and duration of comorbid depressive illness (Kovacs et al., 1995). Several researchers have documented increased feelings of anger, depression, and hostility in persons with diabetes who have fluctuating visual impairments as well as poorer social functioning, compared to those with more severe but stable impairments (Rubin & Peyrot, 1992). In depressed patients, depression onset antedates the detection of retinopathy by 7 years on average, but gender has not been identified as a risk factor.

Although erectile dysfunction is a recognized complication of diabetes in males, disproportionately few studies of sexual dysfunction in females with diabetes have been reported. Leedom et al. (1986) found that over one-third of women with diabetes had complete anorgasmia, which was significantly above the rate reported by medically ill women and healthy controls. Wrigley and Mayou (1991) found that women with poorly controlled diabetes complained of loss of libido more frequently than women with well-controlled diabetes did. Interestingly, Schreiner-Engel et al. (1987) reported that women with Type I diabetes had normal levels of sexual responsiveness and marital satisfaction, whereas women with Type II diabetes had impaired sexual desire, orgasmic capacity, lubrication, sexual satisfaction, and sexual activity, and less satisfaction in relationships. Of note, women were required to be in a relationship to enter this study, and women with Type I diabetes severe enough to have interfered with formation of stable sexual relationships would have been excluded by this criterion. Furthermore, these differences may be accounted for in part by the fact that women with Type I diabetes who do enter into committed relationships do so with the nature and prognosis of their illness known to them and their partners. In contrast, women with Type II diabetes (which generally has a later onset) may develop the illness after marrying, when it introduces a new stress to the relationship. Overall, there is a lack of published information regarding the effects of diabetes on female sexual function and the psychosocial correlates of this complication. No specific treatment is available, but counseling, vaginal lubricants, topical estrogen creams, hormone replacement therapy, and treatment of concomitant depression are recommended (Lunt, 1996).

Psychiatric Disorders in Patients with Diabetes

Diabetes is a significant risk factor for psychiatric illness. Contributing factors include the stresses associated with a chronic medical condition, the demanding and continuous nature of diabetic self-care, and the threat of future medical complications.

Prevalence

Popkin et al. (1988) found that 51% of individuals with diabetes had one or more psychiatric disorders. Lifetime prevalence of major depression was comparable for females (11 of 48) and males (7 of 27) with diabetes, but there was a higher prevalence of anxiety disorders among females than among males or controls. Lustman et al. (1986) reported that 71% of 114 patients with diabetes had a lifetime history of psychiatric illness; mood and anxiety disorders were the most common diagnoses, with no differences between men and women. Blanz et al. (1993) found a threefold increase of psychiatric illness in adolescents with diabetes, but again no sex-specific differences. In a study of youths with diabetes, however, Kovacs et al. (1997) found that young women with diabetes were at nine times greater risk for recurrent depression than their male counterparts. Furthermore, the duration of depressive episodes in patients with diabetes was longer than in a control group, and the risk of recurrence was greater.

Lustman et al. (1986) reported that patients who described symptoms consistent with a psychiatric disorder in the previous 6 months had higher mean glycosylated hemoglobin levels, more symptoms of poor glucose control, and more overall distress than those with lifetime diagnoses. In addition, La Greca et al. (1987) assessed adolescents with diabetes; they found that girls had poorer metabolic control than boys, and that glycemic control was significantly related to symptoms of depression and anxiety. These studies suggest that the presence of psychiatric illness may constitute a chronic stressor that leads, via direct metabolic or indirect behavioral pathways, to poor glucose control.

In contrast to studies assessing psychiatric disorders in patients with diabetes, Dixon et al. (2000), reviewed the prevalence and correlates of diabetes in national schizophrenia samples. They found that rates of diagnosed diabetes exceeded general population statistics well before the widespread use of atypical antipsychotics, and that women with schizophrenia were 2.1 times more likely to have Type II diabetes than men. Risk factors for diabetes were similar to those observed for the general population. In addition, Cassidy et al. (1999) evaluated 345 patients with bipolar disorder and found a 9.9% prevalence of diabetes, significantly greater than expected from national norms (3.4%, Harris et al., 1987). Again, more female patients (13.6%) than males (8.9%) had diabetes, but the difference was not statistically significant. This study replicated Lilliker's (1980) report of a 10% prevalence of diabetes in the manic–depressive population.

Antipsychotic medications may also be a risk factor for diabetes. Henderson et al. (2001) followed 82 patients, including 22 women, treated with clozapine for 5 years. Thirty patients (36.6%) were diagnosed with diabetes during the 5-year follow-up, but sex was not a risk factor. Patients experienced significant weight gain but it was not associated with the risk of developing diabetes. The authors recommend that patients taking clozapine be screened every 6 months for diabetes and lipid abnormalities. Other atypical antipsychotic medications, especially olanzapine, have also been associated with new-onset diabetes (Gellenberg, 1999; Rigalleau et al., 2000).

Depression and Suicidal Ideation

Gavard et al. (1993) reviewed 20 studies to determine the prevalence of depression in adult diabetic populations. The prevalence ranges for current depression were 8.5–23.3% in controlled studies and 11.0–19.9% in uncontrolled studies—rates at least three times the prevalence of major depression in the general adult population. An increased prevalence of depression in diabetes relative to other somatic illnesses remains unproven. Of the controlled studies reviewed, only one (Popkin et al., 1988) examined sex-specific prevalence estimates; they found that females with diabetes had a significantly greater prevalence of depression than females without diabetes, and that females with diabetes had a higher rate of depression than males with diabetes. In uncontrolled studies of patients with diabetes, females had an elevated prevalence of current depression compared with males in all four studies reviewed, although differences were significant in only one study.

Haire-Joshu et al. (1994) found that depressive symptomatology was more prevalent and severe among persons with diabetes who smoked, compared to nonsmokers. Interestingly, 40% of the women studied were smokers, compared to 51% of the men.

Goldston et al. (1994) studied suicidal ideation among adolescents with diabetes (39 girls and 52 boys). The rate of suicidal ideation among these adolescents was higher than expected (13.2% 1-year prevalence, 24% lifetime), but the rate of suicide attempts was comparable with that reported for the general population. Gender was not a risk factor for suicide attempts, but psychiatric disorder was, with a prevalence of 38.5% in the youths with diabetes. The adolescents with suicidal thoughts appeared to be at substantially increased risk for another form of self-destructive behavior: nonadherence to the medical regimen.

Eating Disorders

Several investigators have reported a relation between diabetes and eating disorders. Abnormal eating attitudes, intentional insulin omission, and diagnosable eating disorders are associated with high glycosylated hemoglobin levels, impaired metabolic control, and retinopathy (Affenito et al., 1997; Crow et al., 1998; Stancin et al., 1989; Steel et al.,

1989). Women with diabetes are far more likely to have an eating disorder than men, with the onset of diabetes preceding the eating disorder in the vast majority of cases (Daneman et al., 1998). The frequency of reported insulin omission varies widely, but tends to be higher than the rate of diagnosable eating disorders (Crow et al., 1998; Pollock et al., 1995). Rydall et al. (1997) followed 91 women with Type I diabetes for 4 years and found that pathological behaviors such as insulin omission, dieting, and self-induced vomiting became more common over the period. In this sample, 85% of women with highly disordered eating at baseline had some degree of retinopathy at 4-year follow-up, compared to 43% in women with moderately disordered eating and 24% in those with normal eating habits.

Daneman et al. (1998) have proposed a model of the interactions among eating psychopathology, diabetes management, and outcome in young women with Type I diabetes. They identify several factors, including the fact that preceding the diagnosis of diabetes there is often a period of weight loss. With initiation of insulin treatment, the weight is regained, and in susceptible individuals this may heighten weight and body shape concerns. Furthermore, food preoccupation and dietary restraint are integral parts of the nutritional management of diabetes. Girls with Type I diabetes frequently discover a unique and extremely potent means of purging—insulin omission or underdosing—to induce glycosuria and promote weight loss. Finally, a chronic illness such as diabetes may interfere with normal developmental processes, leading to poor self-esteem and impaired ego development and body image. In young females, the dietary focus necessary in diabetes may trigger or augment the typical body dissatisfaction and drive for thinness that may precede eating disturbances.

Early identification of abnormal eating patterns is clearly important, as it may decrease the risk of both long-term diabetes-related microvascular complications and progression to a full-blown eating disorder. Women with Type I diabetes and eating-disordered behavior are often well informed about the potential risks and complications. Health care professionals should routinely inquire about weight and shape preoccupation, dieting, bingeing, insulin omission for weight loss purposes, and the frequency and treatment of hypoglycemia (Daneman et al., 1998). Warning signs include the persistence of poor metabolic control, recurrent diabetic ketoacidosis, dieting, binge eating, and insulin omission.

Educational efforts should be directed toward themes typically addressed in eating disorder treatment, including information on societal attitudes about shape and weight, the role of dietary restriction as a precipitant of binge eating, and the biological determinants of body weight (Crow et al., 1998). Treatment is usually best delivered through the coordinated efforts of the diabetes care team, including a mental health professional. It is unclear to what extent interventions important to diabetic care potentially contradict treatment strategies effective in treating eating disorders. Perhaps excessive focus on dietary restraint—the cornerstone of diabetes care—may contribute to the development of eating disorders, and Daneman et al. (1998) have suggested that a preferable approach may be to deemphasize diet and dietary restraint, to promote healthy eating, and to decrease the focus on food.

In summary, diabetes is a common, chronic illness that causes both physical and psychiatric impairment. Compared to men with diabetes, women with this illness appear to face increased risks for recurrent depression and ketoacidosis in adolescence. Clinicians should ask their female patients with diabetes about sexual dysfunction and eating disorders.

HYPOTHALAMIC–PITUITARY–THYROID AXIS DISORDERS

Thyroid hormones play a crucial role in metabolism. They increase protein synthesis in all body tissues, and oxygen consumption in the liver, kidneys, heart, and skeletal muscles. The levels of triiodothyronine (T3) and thyroxine (T4) are influenced by TSH from the anterior pituitary. TSH levels are regulated by thyroid-releasing hormone (TRH) from the hypothalamus and the negative feedback effects of T3 and T4. Psychiatric symptoms are well-recognized components of hypo- and hyperthyroidism, with mood changes, anxiety, irritability, and cognitive dysfunction being common in thyroid disease. These—together with symptoms such as weight gain or loss, and increased or decreased energy—can be mistaken for symptoms of a primary mood disorder. Attention must always be paid to rule out thyroid disease in patients presenting with mood or anxiety symptoms.

Women have an increased vulnerability to thyroid disease, with risk periods particularly significant at times of hormonal fluctuations such as the postpartum (Wieck, 1989). Thyroid illness commonly induces mood symptoms (Whybrow & Prange, 1981)—a fact that has led to considerable study of the associations among depression, sex, and thyroid function.

Differential TRH Response in Women and Men

Some depressed patients have a reduced TSH response to TRH stimulation (Prange et al., 1972; Kastin et al., 1972). Studies have generally demonstrated that 25–30% of patients with major depressive disorder have a blunted TSH response, compared to about 5% of nonpsychiatric controls. The biological underpinnings of this blunting remain unknown, but one major hypothesis to explain the reduced TSH response in depression is that TRH receptors are down-regulated secondary to TRH hypersecretion by the hypothalamus.

Depressed women and men may differ in their responses to TRH stimulation, with reports that men are more likely to demonstrate a blunted response. Some (Kirkegaard et al., 1981; Roy et al., 1988), but not all (Unden et al., 1987), studies have found that depressed women also demonstrate a blunted TSH response to TRH stimulation. Most studies, however, have not reported the sex of the patients (Gold et al., 1977) or have not rigidly controlled for and compared this variable (Extein et al., 1982; Kirkegaard et al., 1977; Kirkegaard & Faber, 1986; Langer et al., 1986; Levy & Stern, 1987; Unden et al., 1986; Wolkin et al., 1984).

TRH stimulates the release of both TSH and PRL. Differences have been reported between men and women in TRH-induced PRL responses. Garbutt et al. (1994) reported that both men and women with depression had a reduced TSH response compared with age- and sex-matched controls across a range of protirelin doses, but only depressed men had a corresponding reduction in TRH-induced PRL response compared to control men. Sex differences in the PRL response parallel those in TSH blunting, with men more reliably demonstrating a reduced PRL response. Garbutt et al. (1994) suggested that one possible reason for the failure to find PRL blunting in depressed women may be that there is greater variation in PRL responses in women, making it less likely that statistical significance will be obtained at any given sample size. To date, no clear biological hypothesis has been put forth to account for these differential findings in men and women.

Thyroid Changes at Times of Reproductive Endocrine Fluctuations

Premenstrual Period

Premenstrual dysphoric disorder (PMDD) has been linked to depressive symptoms and to thyroid dysfunction. Most studies, however, have not found significant thyroid abnormalities in women with PMDD (Roy-Byrne et al., 1987; Schmidt et al., 1993).

Postpartum

The hypothalamic–pituitary–thyroid (HPT) axis undergoes a greater change during pregnancy than during any other nonpathological state (Pederson et al., 1993), and these changes generally return to normal within 6 weeks postpartum—the same time period during which women are at greatest risk of psychiatric morbidity (Hopkins et al., 1984; Inwood, 1985; Paffenbarger, 1982).

A number of studies have specifically examined the thyroid indices of symptomatic and asymptomatic women in the postpartum period, to determine whether thyroid abnormalities are correlated with postpartum mood changes. Stewart et al. (1988) found that women with early (less than 4 weeks postdelivery) postpartum psychosis were more likely to have higher free T4 indices and lower TSH levels than postpartum women without psychiatric symptoms, although the thyroid indices were within normal levels even for the women with psychosis. Similarly, Harris et al. (1989) found that thyroid dysfunction occurred at a higher rate in postpartum women with major depression. In a pilot study, Pedersen et al. (1993) reported that women with a history of prior depression had higher levels of T3, T4, TSH, and cortisol during the puerperium. They suggested that the abnormalities observed during this typical period of reequilibration unmask vulnerabilities toward an abnormal balance between central drive and negative feedback in the HPT and hypothalamic–pituitary–adrenocortical (HPA) axes in women with prior depression.

Menopause

Early studies suggested that psychological symptoms were prominent in menopause, and these symptoms were incorporated into menopausal screens (e.g., the Kupperman Menopausal Index; Kupperman et al., 1959). However, general population surveys have not upheld this impression (Thompson et al., 1973; McKinlay & Jefferys, 1974; Wood, 1979), and it appears that risk of onset of depression is not increased during menopause. Whether thyroid changes occur reliably at the time of menopause has also been the subject of investigation; one study found that T3, but not T4, was significantly lower in immediately premenopausal women than in women who were 1–4 years postmenopause (Ballinger et al., 1987). Ballinger et al. (1987) also found higher levels of TSH in immediately postmenopausal women than in either premenopausal women or late postmenopausal women (more than 5 years past their last menstrual cycle). They further compared the thyroid indices with depression scores and found that depressed women in the premenopausal group had evidence of higher TSH levels and higher T3 levels than nondepressed women. There was no association between depression and circulating levels of gonadal hormones, suggesting that mood symptoms in the perimenopausal period may be related to changes in thyroid rather than gonadal hormones.

Thyroid Hormones and Treatment of Depression

Antidepressant Acceleration with T3

A few studies were performed about 20–30 years ago to address the possibility that the addition of T3 at the time of tricyclic antidepressant initiation could accelerate the antidepressant response.

Prange et al. (1969) were the first to use T3 to accelerate response to antidepressants. They postulated that the efficacy of T3 as an accelerating agent for imipramine was greater in women than in men, but were clear that they could not demonstrate this differential effect statistically. Subsequent papers (Coppen et al., 1972; Wheatley, 1972; Wilson et al., 1979; Goodwin et al., 1982) reported similar findings with trends for greater improvement in women compared to men. Overall, this series of small studies suggests that T3 acceleration of antidepressant action may be more efficacious in women than men.

Antidepressant Augmentation with T3

In interesting contrast to the data suggesting a benefit to women for T3 acceleration of tricyclic antidepressants, the more extensive data on T3 augmentation of antidepressants do not support a differential effect between the sexes. A number of studies, including three double-blind trials, have examined the efficacy of T3 augmentation; overall, it appears that approximately 55% of men and women will improve when T3 is added to antidepressant therapy, generally within 2–3 weeks of T3 initiation and at doses of 25–50 Mg of T3 (Joffe, 1988; Joffe & Singer, 1990).

In summary, women appear particularly vulnerable to thyroid abnormalities, with times of hormonal fluctuation (such as the postpartum) being periods of increased risk. As thyroid disease commonly presents with mood, anxiety, and cognitive symptoms, it is important to rule out thyroid illness when investigating psychiatric symptoms.

HYPOTHALAMIC–PITUITARY–ADRENAL (HPA) AXIS DISORDERS

The HPA axis is the classic stress-responsive axis. The adrenal cortex produces androgen, glucocorticoids (including cortisol), and mineralocorticoids (aldosterone). Cortisol affects glucose metabolism, lipolysis, inflammation, and immune responses. Aldosterone causes sodium and water retention. Its secretion is regulated by the renin–angiotensin system. Isolated hypersecretion of aldosterone is rare, but more common in women (Orth & Kovacs, 1998).

Among depressed patients, women are more likely than men to have abnormalities in HPA axis regulation, with female patients demonstrating significantly higher mean plasma cortisol concentrations than matched controls (Young & Korszun, 1999). Studies suggest that ovarian steroids, particularly progesterone, influence the HPA axis response to stress by modulating sensitivity to negative feedback of glucocorticoids on ACTH secretion, which may contribute to the increased incidence of stress-related psychiatric disorders in women (Young & Korszun, 1999).

The dexamethasone suppression test measures HPA axis functioning. It has been extensively studied as a biological marker of depression, but despite its high specificity, it has not proved useful because of low sensitivity. Reproducible differences in suppression rates between men and women have not been described (American Psychiatric Association Task Force, 1987).

Glucocorticoid Disorders

Glucocorticoid Excess

Cushing's syndrome results from a chronic excess of cortisol, which may be either ACTH-dependent or independent, as in a cortisol-secreting tumor. Starkman and Schteingart (1981) studied the neuropsychiatric manifestations of hypercortisolemia in Cushing's syndrome. Patients reported symptoms of fatigue (100%), irritability (86%), memory problems (83%), weight gain (80%), depressed mood (77%), sleep disorder (69%), difficulty concentrating (66%), sexual dysfunction (69%), anxiety (66%), and crying (63%). Perceptual distortions were reported in 11% of patients, and paranoid thoughts in 9%. Overall neuropsychiatric disability rating was related to cortisol and ACTH levels. Atypical depressive disorder is the most common psychiatric disorder in untreated Cushing's syndrome, and improves gradually with time after correction of hypercortisolism (Dorn et al., 1997).

Factitious Cushing's syndrome involves the surreptitious administration of glucocorticoids. Although it is rarely reported, Cizza et al. (1996) reviewed 6 cases of factitious Cushing's syndrome from 860 patients evaluated for hypercortisolism at the National Institutes of Health Clinical Center. Five of the six cases were women; all had a history of multiple surgeries unrelated to Cushing's syndrome, as well as a history of depression or anxiety. High-pressure liquid chromatography analysis of urine steroids is recommended whenever there is clinical suspicion of glucocorticoid abuse.

In contrast to elevated levels of endogenous cortisol, administration of exogenous glucocorticoids to persons with normal adrenal function may be followed by elevated mood, irritability, increased motor activity, sleeplessness, and even psychosis (Pearson Murphy, 1991). Pope and Katz (1994) diagnosed mania, hypomania, or major depression in 23% of men using steroids for muscle and strength building; no women were interviewed in this study.

Glucocorticoid Deficiency

Glucocorticoid, mineralocorticoid, and androgen deficiencies are present in Addison's disease. Symptoms include weakness, fatigue, weight loss, and gastrointestinal complaints. Anorexia, hyperpigmentation, hypotension, and electrolyte disturbances are also common.

Psychiatric symptoms in patients with chronic adrenal insufficiency can include impaired memory, psychosis, and depression (manifested by apathy, poverty of thought, and lack of initiative). These manifestations may occur early in the disease and may predate other physical findings (Orth & Kovacs, 1998). Addison's disease, with vomiting, weight loss, dehydration, and weakness, can be mistaken for anorexia nervosa in young women (Blaustein et al., 1998); however, body image distortion, fat phobia, and preoccupation with weight loss are not seen.

Pheochromocytoma

A pheochromocytoma is a tumor that produces catecholamines; 80% of them are found in the adrenal medulla. These are rare tumors, but fatal if misdiagnosed or improperly treated. They are slightly more common in women than in men (Orth & Kovacs, 1998). Presenting manifestations include sustained hypertension resistant to conventional treatment; hypertensive crisis with malignant hypertension; or paroxysmal attacks suggestive of seizure disorder, anxiety attacks, or hyperventilation. The characteristic paroxysm is the consequence of catecholamine release. Symptoms are variable and may include headache, excessive sweating and palpitations, apprehension with a sense of impending doom, chest pain, nausea, vomiting, flushing, and hypertension.

In summary, glucocorticoids have profound psychiatric manifestations, causing depression and cognitive impairment in both excess and deficiency syndromes, whereas pheochromocytoma may mimic panic attacks.

GH (SOMATOSTATIN) DISORDERS

GH acts on the growth plates to stimulate bone growth, as well as at multiple sites in the body to alter carbohydrate and lipid utilization. Its secretion from the anterior pituitary is regulated by GH-releasing hormone from the hypothalamus.

Acromegaly

Excess GH usually results from a primary pituitary adenoma. Patients with acromegaly have an insidious onset of symptoms and signs, which include thickening and oiliness of the skin; facial changes, including thick lips and exaggerated nasolabial folds; and thickening and folding of the scalp. The hands and feet enlarge, head size increases, the mandible grows, acanthosis nigrans apppears, and joint pain and stiffness may occur. The vocal cords thicken, resulting in a characteristically deep and resonant voice. The overall appearance and deep voice give women with acromegaly a somewhat masculinized appearance. Galactorrhea and menstrual irregularities are common (Thorner et al., 1998).

Psychopathology in GH excess is poorly understood. It appears that patients suffer a loss of initiative and spontaneity with marked fluctuations in mood. Impairment in self-esteem is seen, as are body image distortion, disruption in interpersonal relations, and social withdrawal. The diagnosis is often difficult to make, and women may be initially diagnosed with depression, "stress," or a somatoform disorder (Furman & Ezzat, 1998).

GH Deficiency

The manifestations of GH deficiency in children depend on the age of onset and include short stature and reduced growth velocity. In adult-onset GH deficiency, symptoms include decreased muscle strength and exercise tolerance, emotional lability, a sense of social isolation, and diminished libido (Thorner et al., 1998).

Nicholas et al. (1997) found that whereas 38% of adults treated with GH during childhood had social phobia, only 10% of short adults without GH deficiency did, suggesting that the high prevalence of social phobia in GH-deficient adults was not explained by short stature alone. GH-deficient females scored higher on a measure of inhibition and avoidance of aversive stimuli than the GH-deficient males and short-stature males and females. The authors suggest that GH-deficient adults may have higher rates of social phobia because of the effects of chronic illness in childhood on psychosocial development. Higher rates of depressive illnesses are also seen in GH-deficient adults (Lynch et al., 1994). GH deficient adults are more likely to be unemployed and unmarried than members of the general population (Sartorio et al., 1996).

Children with GH deficiency are reported to have educational deficits, specifically learning disabilities and attention-deficit/hyperactivity disorder. The psychological effect of long-term GH treatment in these children remains controversial. Patients with GH deficiency who have been treated at centers that include psychological counseling as an integral component of the treatment program are better adjusted in early adult life (Sartorio et al., 1996). GH receptors are found in discrete areas of the brain, although the functions these receptors mediate have not been fully elucidated (Nyberg, 2000).

Overall, the psychiatric manifestations of GH excess or deficiency are poorly characterized, but studies suggest that GH deficiency is associated with anxiety and depressive disorders.

GONADAL HORMONES DISORDERS

Secretion of estrogen and progesterone from the ovaries is stimulated by LH and FSH excreted by the anterior pituitary. The reproductive hormones gave been discussed in detail by Steiner and Born (Chapter 3, this volume). Androgens are secreted by the adrenal glands and converted to testosterone and 5-α-dihydrotestosterone in peripheral tissues. Peripheral conversion contributes significantly to circulating testosterone levels in women, while the ovaries produce a small fraction of the circulating androgens.

Adrenogenital Syndrome/Polycystic Ovaries

Polycystic ovarian (PCO) syndrome is the association of hyperandrogenism with chronic anovulation in women without specific underlying diseases of the adrenal or pituitary glands (Franks, 1995). Hyperandrogenism is characterized by hirsutism, acne, androgen-dependent alopecia, and elevated serum concentrations of androgens (particularly testosterone and androstenedione); obesity is common but not universal. PCO syndrome is likely if oligomenorrhea is present with one or more of these three features: polycystic ovaries on ultrasonography, hirsutism, or hyperandrogenemia. Pituitary or adrenal disease must be excluded.

Bruce-Jones et al. (1993) described a case series of 10 women with PCO syndrome; anxiety, mood, and somatoform disorders were common. PCO syndrome was not diagnosed until after the onset of psychiatric symptoms in 7 of the 10 cases. Derogatis et al. (1993) assessed 20 women referred for idiopathic hirsutism. Correlations between unbound fractions of testosterone (free and biologically active testosterone) and symptoms of depression were found. There was no correlation between degree of hirsutism and mood symptoms, suggesting that depression among hirsute women appears more likely to have its basis in a disturbed neuroendocrine mechanism than in psychosocial causes.

PARATHYROID HORMONE DISORDERS

Parathyroid hormone is a peptide hormone that controls the minute-to-minute levels of ionized calcium in the blood and extracellular fluids. It is secreted by the parathyroid glands in response to decreases in serum calcium levels. Hypocalcemia presents with symptoms of neuromuscular irritability, including perioral paresthesias, tingling of the fingers and toes, and spontaneous or latent tetany (Bringhurst et al., 1998).

Primary hyperparathyroidism is a common endocrine disturbance with a reported incidence of between 26 and 146 cases per 100,000 people per year (Davies, 1992). It is more common in females, particularly after menopause. Hypercalcemic symptoms consisting of thirst, polyuria, constipation, nausea, lethargy, weakness, and sometimes dyspepsia are seen only in the more severe forms of primary hyperparathyroidism. Parathyroidectomy is the treatment of choice for these patients. Mild hypercalcemia is often diagnosed during routine biochemical screening when patients are asymptomatic, and management is usually conservative. However, patients with mild hypercalcemia have significantly more psychiatric symptoms than controls (Joborn et al., 1989).

Prolactin (PRL) Disorders

Most biological functions of PRL are associated with the metabolic and behavioral adaptations to parenthood and inhibition of sexual behaviour (Sobrinho, 1998). The major effects of hyperprolactinemia in women are amenorrhea, cessation of normal cyclic ovarian function, reduced libido, occasional hirsutism, and increased long-term risk of osteoporosis. Dopamine regulates PRL release from the posterior pituitary by acting as a powerful inhibitor, whereas serotonin stimulates PRL release (Nicholas et al., 1998). PRL secretion is normally increased by sleep, exercise, pregnancy, nursing, estrogens, stress, opiates, oral contraceptives, TRH, and some medical illnesses (De La Fuente & Rosenbaum, 1981). Typical antipsychotics also promote PRL release by blocking tonic dopamine inhibitory action at pituitary receptor sites (Nicholas et al., 1998), which can result in secondary infertility. Typical antipsychotics can also cause galactorrhea (Windgassen et al., 1996). PRL has been implicated in schizophrenia, mood disorders, premenstrual syndrome, and alcohol abuse and dependence, but the direct actions of PRL on the human brain require further study (De La Fuente & Rosenbaum, 1981).

Kellner et al. (1984) assessed psychiatric symptoms in women with hyperprolactinemia. These women had symptom scores that were similar to those of psychiatric patients: They were significantly more hostile, depressed, and anxious, and had more feelings of inadequacy, than either family practice patients or nonpatient employees.

Prolactinomas are the most common adenomas of the pituitary, affecting no more than 2 in 1,000 of the female population. The clinical onset often follows an important life event. Intriguingly, most women with prolactinomas or idiopathic hyperprolactinemia have backgrounds characterized by paternal deprivation in childhood (Sobrinho, 1998). Prolactinomas are associated with the psychiatric symptoms seen in hyperprolactinemia, including depression, anhedonia, and decreased libido (Sobrinho, 1998).

CONCLUSIONS/FUTURE DIRECTIONS

Many endocrine diseases have significant psychiatric manifestations. More research is needed to better understand the interrelationships between hormones and mood, cognition, and psychosis. Even less is understood about the differing psychological and psychiatric effects of endocrine disorders on men and women.

It is important for clinicians to consider the possibility of an endocrine disorder when evaluating women who present with psychiatric symptoms. When indicated, a careful review of systems, physical examination, and laboratory screening are necessary to rule out endocrine disorders such as hypothyroidism or diabetes. Conversely, women with recognized endocrinological disorders will often experience psychiatric sequelae as either direct or indirect results of the primary illness. Such psychiatric symptoms should be explored, and treatment should be offered if the symptoms are causing distress or functional impairment.

REFERENCES

Affenito, S. G., Backstrand, J. R., Welch, G. W., et al. (1997). Subclinical and clinical eating disorders in IDDM negatively affect metabolic control. *Diabetes Care, 20*(2), 182–184.

American Psychiatric Association Task Force on Laboratory Tests in Psychiatry. (1987). The dexamethasone suppression test: An overview of its current status in psychiatry. *American Journal of Psychiatry, 144*, 1253–1262.

Ballinger, C. B., Browning, M. C. K., & Smith, A. H. W. (1987). Hormone profiles and psychological symptoms in peri-menopausal women. *Maturitas, 9*, 235–251.

Blanz, B. J., Rensch-Riemann, B., Fritz-Sitmund, D. I., et al. (1993). IDDM is a risk factor for adolescent psychiatric disorders. *Diabetes Care, 16*(12), 1579–1587.

Blaustein, S. A., Golden, N. H., & Shenker, I. R. (1998). Addison's disease mimicking anorexia nervosa. *Clinical Pediatrics, 37*, 631–632.

Bobrow, E. S., AvRuskin, T. W., & Siller, J. (1985). Mother–daughter interaction and adherence to diabetes regimens. *Diabetes Care, 8*(2), 146–151.

Bringhurst, F. R., Demay, M. B., & Kronenberg, H M. (1998). Hormones and disorders of mineral metabolism. In J. D. Wilson & D. W. Foster (Eds.), *Williams textbook of endocrinology* (9th ed., pp. 1155–1209). Philadelphia: Saunders.

Bruce-Jones, W., Zolese, G., & White, P. (1993). Polycystic ovary syndrome and psychiatric morbidity. *Journal of Psychosomatic Obstetrics and Gynaecology, 14*, 111–116.

Cassidy, F., Ahearn, E., & Carroll, B. J. (1999). Elevated frequency of diabetes mellitus in hospitalized manic–depressive patients. *American Journal of Psychiatry, 156*(9), 1417–1420.

Cizza, G., Nieman, L. K., Doppman, J. L., et al. (1996). Factitious Cushing syndrome. *Journal of Clinical Endocrinology and Metabolism, 81*(10), 3573–3577.

Coppen, A., Whybrow, P. C., Noguera, R., et al. (1972). The comparative antidepressant value of L-tryptophan and imipramine with and without attempted potentiation by liothyronine. *Archives of General Psychiatry, 26*, 234–241.

Crow, S. J., Keel, P. K., & Kendall, D. (1998). Eating disorders and insulin-dependent diabetes mellitus. *Psychosomatics, 39*(3), 233–243.

Daneman, D., Olmsted, M., Rydall, A., et al. (1998). Eating disorders in young women with Type I diabetes: Prevalence, problems and prevention. *Hormone Research, 50*(Suppl. 1), 79–86.

Davies, M. (1992). Primary hyperparathyroidism: Aggressive or conservative treatment? *Clinical Endocrinology, 36*, 325–332.

De La Fuente, J. R., & Rosenbaum, A. H. (1981). Prolactin in psychiatry. *American Journal of Psychiatry, 138*(9), 1154–1159.

Derogatis, L. R., Rose, L. I., Shulman, L. H., et al. (1993). Serum androgens and psychopathology in hirsute women. *Journal of Psychosomatic Obstetrics and Gynaecology, 14*, 269–282.

Dixon, L., Weiden, P., Delahanty, J., et al. (2000). Prevalence and correlates of diabetes in national schizophrenia samples. *Schizophrenia Bulletin, 26*, 903–912.

Dorn, L. D., Burgess, E. S., Friedman, T. C., et al. (1997). The longitudinal course of psychopathology in Cushing's syndrome after correction of hypercortisolism. *Journal of Clinical Endocrinology and Metabolism, 82*(3), 912–919.

Extein, I., Pottash, A., & Gold, M. (1982). Thyroid stimulating response to thyrotropin-releasing hormone response to thyrotropin-releasing hormone in mania and bipolar depression. *Psychiatry Research, 6*, 161.

Franks, S. (1995). Polycystic ovary syndrome. *New England Journal of Medicine, 333*(13), 853–861.

Furman, K., & Ezzat, S. (1998). Psychological features of acromegaly. *Psychotherapy and Psychosomatics, 67*, 147–153.

Garbutt, J. C., Mayo, J. P., Little, K. Y., et al. (1994). Dose-response studies with protirelin. *Archives of General Psychiatry, 51*, 875–883.

Gavard, J. A., Lustman, P. J., & Clouse, R. E. (1993). Prevalence of depression in adults with diabetes: An epidemiological evaluation. *Diabetes Care, 16*(8), 1167–1178.

Gelenberg, A. J. (1999). Weight gain, diabetes, and related adverse effects of antipsychotics. *Biological Therapies in Psychiatry Newsletter, 22*(10), 41–44.

Gill, G. (1991). Psychological aspects of diabetes. *British Journal of Hospital Medicine, 46*, 301–305.

Gold, P., Goodwin, F., & Wehr, T. (1977). Pituitary thyrotropin response to thyrotropin-releasing hormone in affective illness: Relationship to spinal fluid amine metabolites. *American Journal of Psychiatry, 134*, 1028.

Goldston, D. B., Kovacs, M., Ho, V. Y., et al. (1994). Suicidal ideation and suicide attempts among youth with insulin-dependent diabetes mellitus. *Journal of the American Academy of Child and Adolescent Psychiatry, 33*(2), 240–246.

Goodwin, F. K., Prange, A. J., Post, R. M., et al. (1982). Potentiation of antidepressant effects by L-triiodothyronine in tricylcic nonresponders. *American Journal of Psychiatry, 139*, 34–38.

Haire-Joshu, D., Heady, S., Thomas, L., et al. (1994). Depressive symptomatology and smoking among persons with diabetes. *Research in Nursing and Health, 17*, 273–282.

Harris, B., Fung, H., Johns, S., et al. (1989). Transient post-partum thyroid dysfunction and thyroid antibodies and postnatal depression. *Journal of Affective Disorders, 17*, 243–249.

Harris, M. I., Hadden, W. C., Knowler, W. C., et al. (1987). Prevalence of diabetes and impaired glucose tolerance and plasma glucose levels in U.S. population aged 20–74 yr. *Diabetes, 36*, 523–534.

Henderson, D. C., Cagliero, E., Gray, C., et al. (2001). Clozapine, diabetes mellitus, weight gain, and lipid abnormalities: A five-year naturalistic study. *American Journal of Psychiatry, 157*, 975–981.

Herskowitz Dumont, R., Jacobson, A. M., Cole, C., et al. (1995). Psychosocial predictors of acute complications of diabetes in youth. *Diabetic Medicine, 12*, 612–618.

Hopkins, J., Marcus, M., & Campbell, S. B. (1984). Postpartum depression: A critical review. *Psychological Bulletin, 95*, 498–515.

Inwood, D. G. (1985). The spectrum of postpartum psychiatric disorders: In D. G. Inwood (Ed.), *Recent advances in postpartum psychiatric disorders* (pp. 1–18). Washington, DC: American Psychiatric Press.

Jacobson, A. M., Hauser, S. T., Willett, J. B., et al. (1997). Psychological adjustment to IDDM: 10-year follow-up of an onset cohort of child and adolescent patients. *Diabetes Care, 20*(5), 811–818.

Joborn, C., Metta, J., Lind, L., et al. (1989). Self-rated psychiatric symptoms in patients operated on because of primary hyperthyroidism and in patients with longstanding mild hypercalcemia. *Surgery, 105*, 72–78.

Joffe, R. T. (1988). Triiodothyronine (T3) and lithium potentiation of tricyclic antidepressants. *American Journal of Psychiatry, 145*, 1317–1318.

Joffe, R. T., & Singer, W. (1990). A comparison of triiodothyronine and thyroxine in the potentiation of tricyclic antidepressants. *Psychiatry Research, 32*, 241–252.

Kastia, A. J., Ehrensing, R. T., Schalch, D. S., et al. (1972). Improvement in mental depression with decreased thyrotropin release after administration of thyrotropin-releasing hormone. *Lancet, 2*, 740–742.

Kellner, R., Buckman, M. T., Fava, G. A., et al. (1984). Hyperprolactinemia, distress, and hostility. *American Journal of Psychiatry, 141*(6), 759–763.

Kirkegaard, C., Bjorum, N., & Cohn, D. (1977). Studies on the influence of biogenic amines and psychoactive drugs on the prognostic value of the TRH stimulation test in endogenous depression. *Psychoneuroendocrinology, 2*, 131.

Kirkegaard, C., & Faber, J. (1981). Altered serum levels of thyroxine, triiodothyronines and dilodothyroninas in endogenous depression. *Acta Endocrinology, 96*, 199–207.

Kirkegaard, C., & Faber, J. (1986). Influence of free thyroid levels on the TSH response to TRH in endogenous depression. *Psychoendocrinology, 11*, 491.

Kovacs, M., Drash, A., Mukerji, P., et al. (1995). Biomedical and psychiatric risk factors for retinopathy among children with IDDM. *Diabetes Care, 18*(12), 1592–1599.

Kovacs, M., Feinberg, T. L., Paulaushas, S., et al. (1985). Initial coping responses and psychosocial characteristics of children with insulin-dependent diabetes mellitus. *Journal of Pediatrics, 106*, 927–834.

Kovacs, M., Goldston, D., Obrosky, D. S., et al. (1997). Major depressive disorder in youths with IDDM: A controlled prospective study of course and outcome. *Diabetes Care, 20*(1), 45–51.

Kovacs, M., Iyengar, S., Goldston, D., et al. (1990). Psychological functioning among mothers of children with insulin-dependent diabetes mellitus: A longitudinal study. *Journal of Consulting and Clinical Psychology, 58*(2), 189–195.

Kupperman, H. S., Wetchler, B. B., & Blatt, M. H. G. (1959). Contemporary therapy of the menopausal syndrome. *Journal of the American Medical Association, 171*, 1627–1637.

La Greca, A. M., Madigan, S., & Klemp, S. (1987). Gender differences in adolescents coping with IDDM. *Diabetes, 36*(Suppl. 1), 87A.

Langer, G., Koinig, G., & Hatzinger, R. (1986). Response to thyrotropin and thyrotropin-releasing hormone as predictor of treatment outcome. *Archives of General Psychiatry, 43*, 861.

Leedom, L. J., Procci, W. P., Don, D., et al. (1986). Sexual dysfunction and depression in diabetic women. *Diabetes, 35*(Suppl. 1), 23A.

Levy, A., & Stern, S. (1987). DST and TRH stimulation test in mood disorder subtypes. *American Journal of Psychiatry, 111*, 472.

Lilliker, S. L. (1980). Prevalence of diabetes in a manic–depressive population. *Comprehensive Psychiatry, 21*(4), 270–275.

Lunt, H. (1996). Women and diabetes. *Diabetic Medicine, 13*, 1009–1016.

Lustman, P. J., Griffith, L. S., Clouse, R. E., et al. (1986). Psychiatric illness in diabetes mellitus: Relationship to symptoms and glucose control. *Journal of Nervous and Mental Disease, 174*(12), 736–742.

Lynch, S., Merson, S., Beshyah, S. A., et al. (1994). Psychiatric morbidity in adults with hypopituitarism. *Journal of the Royal Society of Medicine, 87*, 445–447.

McKinlay, S. M., & Jefferys, M. (1974). The menopausal syndrome. *British Journal of Preventive and Social Medicine, 28*, 108–115.

Nicholas, L. M., Dawkins, K., & Golden, R. N. (1998). Psychoneuroendocrinology of depression: Prolactin. *Psychiatric Clinics of North America, 21*(2), 341–359.

Nicholas, L. M., Tancer, M. E., Silva, S. G., et al. (1997). Short stature, growth hormone deficiency, and social anxiety. *Psychosomatic Medicine, 59,* 372–375.

Nyberg, F. (2000). Growth hormone in the brain: Characteristics of specific brain targets for the hormone and their functional significance. *Frontiers in Neuroendocrinology, 21,* 330–348.

Orth, D., & Kovacs, W. J. (1998). The adrenal cortex. In J. D. Wilson & D. W. Foster (Eds.), *Williams textbook of endocrinology* (9th ed., pp. 517–664). Philadelphia: Saunders.

Paffenbarger, R. A. (1982). Epidemiological aspects of mental illness associated with childbearing. In I. F. Brockington & R. Kumar (Eds.), *Motherhood and mental illness.* New York: Grune & Stratton.

Pearson Murphy, B. E. (1991). Steroids and depression. *Journal of Steroid Biochemistry and Molecular Biology, 38*(5), 537–559.

Pedersen, C. A., Stern, R. A., Pate, J., et al. (1993). Thyroid and adrenal measures during late pregnancy and the puerperium in women who have been major depressed or who become dysphoric postpartum. *Journal of Affective Disorders, 29,* 201–211.

Pollock, M., Kovacs, M., & Charron-Prochownik, D. (1995). Eating disorders and maladaptive dietary/insulin management among youths with childhood-onset insulin-dependent diabetes mellitus. *Journal of the American Academy of Child and Adolescent Psychiatry, 34*(3), 291–296.

Pope, H. G., Jr., & Katz, D. L. (1994). Psychiatric and medical effects of anabolic–androgenic steroid use: A controlled study of 160 athletes. *Archives of General Psychiatry, 51,* 375–382.

Popkin, M. K., Callies, A. L., Lentz, R. D., et al. (1988). Prevalence of major depression, simple phobia, and other psychiatric disorders in patients with long-standing type I diabetes mellitus. *Archives of General Psychiatry, 45,* 64–68.

Prange, A. J., Lara, P. P., Wilson, I. C., et al. (1972). Effects of thyrotropin releasing hormone in depression, *Lancet, ii,* 999–1002.

Prange, A. J., Wilson, I. C., Rabon, A. M., et al. (1969). Enhancement of imipramine antidepressant activity by thyroid hormone. *American Journal of Psychiatry, 126,* 39–51.

Reichlin, S. (1998). Neuroendocrinology. In J. D. Wilson & D. W. Foster (Eds.), *Williams textbook of endocrinology* (9th ed., pp. 165–248). Philadelphia: Saunders.

Rigalleau, V., Gatta, B., Bonnaud, S., et al. (2000). Diabetes as a result of atypical anti-psychotic drugs—A report of three cases. *Diabetic Medicine, 17,* 484–486.

Roy, A., Karoum, F., & Linnoila, M. (1988). Thyrotropin releasing test in unipolar depressed patients and controls: Relationship to clinical and biological variables. *Acta Psychiatrica Scandinavica, 77,* 155–160.

Roy-Byrne, P. P., Rubinow, D. R., Hoban, M. C., et al. (1987). TSH and prolactin responses to TRH in patients with premenstrual syndrome. *American Journal of Psychiatry, 144,* 480–484.

Rubin, R. R., & Peyrot, M. (1992). Psychosocial problems and interventions in diabetes: A review of the literature. *Diabetes Care, 15*(11), 1640–1657.

Rydall, A. C., Rodin, G. M., Olmsted, M. P., et al. (1997). Disordered eating behaviour and microvascular complications in young women with insulin-dependent diabetes mellitus. *New England Journal of Medicine, 336*(26), 1849–1854.

Sartorio, A., Conti, A., Molinari, E., et al. (1996). Growth, growth hormone and cognitive functions. *Hormone Research, 45,* 23–29.

Schmidt, P. J., Grover, G. N., Roy-Byrne, P. P., et al. (1993). Thyroid function in women with premenstrual syndrome. *Journal of Clinical Endocrinological Metabolism, 76,* 671–674.

Schreiner-Engel, P., Schiavi, R. C., Vietorisz, D., et al. (1987). The differential impact of diabetes type on female sexuality. *Journal of Psychosomatic Research, 31*(1), 23–33.

Sobrinho, L. G. (1998). Emotional aspects of hyperprolactinemia. *Psychotherapy and Psychosomatics, 67,* 133–139.

Stancin, T., Ling, D. L., & Reuter, J. M. (1989). Binge eating and purging in young women with IDDM. *Diabetes Care, 12*(9), 601–603.

Starkman, M. N., & Schteingart, D. E. (1981). Neuropsychiatric manifestations of patients with Cushing's syndrome: Relationship to cortisol and adrenocorticotropic hormone levels. *Archives of Internal Medicine, 141,* 215–219.

Steel, J. M., Young, R. J., Lloyd, G. G., et al. (1989). Abnormal eating attitudes in young insulin-dependant diabetics. *British Journal of Psychiatry, 155,* 515–521.

Stewart, D. E., Addison, A. M., Robinson, G. E., et al. (1988). Thyroid function in psychosis following childbirth. *American Journal of Psychiatry, 145,* 1579–1581.

Thompson, B., Hart, S. A., & Durno, D. (1973). Menopausal age and symptomatology in a general practice. *Journal of Biosocial Sciences, 5,* 71–82.

Thorner, M. O., Vance, M. L., Laws, E. R., et al. (1998). The anterior pituitary. In J. D. Wilson & D. W. Foster (Eds.), *Williams textbook of endocrinology* (9th ed., pp. 249–340). Philadelphia: Saunders.

Unden, F., Ljunggren, J.-G., & Kjellman, B. (1986). Twenty-four-hour serum levels of T4 and T3 in relation to decreased TSH serum levels and decreased TSH response to TRH in affective disorders. *Acta Psychiatrica Scandinavica, 73,* 358.

Unden, F., Ljunggren, J.-G., & Kjellman, B. (1987). Unaltered 24 h serum PRL levels and PRL response to TRH in contrast to decreased 24 h serum TSH levels and TSH response to TRH in major depressive disorder. *Acta Psychiatrica Scandinavica, 75,* 131.

Unger, R. H., & Foster, D. W. (1998). Diabetes mellitus. In J. D. Wilson & D. W. Foster (Eds.), *Williams textbook of endocrinology* (9th ed., pp. 973–1059). Philadelphia: Saunders.

Wheatley, D. (1972). Potentiation of amitryptilene by thyroid hormone. *Archives of General Psychiatry, 26,* 229–233.

Whybrow, P., & Prange, A. J. (1981). A hypothesis of thyroid–catecholamine–receptor interaction: Its relevance to affective illness. *Archives of General Psychiatry, 38,* 106–113.

Wieck, A. (1989). Endocrine aspects of postnatal disorders. *Ballière's Clinical Obstetrics and Gynecology, 3,* 857–877.

Wilson, I. C., Prange, A. J., McClane, T. K., et al. (1996). Thyroid hormine enhancement of imipramine in non-retarded depressions. *New England Journal of Medicine, 282,* 1063–1067.

Windgassen, K., Wesselmann, U., & Schulze Monking, H. (1996). Galactorrhea and hyperprolactinemia in schizophrenic patients on neuroleptics: Frequency and etiology. *Neuropsychobiology, 33,* 142–146.

Wolkin, A., Peselow, E., & Smith, M. (1984). TRH test abnormalities in psychiatric disorders. *Journal of Affect Disorders, 6,* 273.

Wood, C. (1979). Menopausal myths. *Medical Journal of Australia, 1,* 496–499.

Wrigley, M., & Mayou, R. (1991). Psychosocial factors and admission for poor glycaemic control: A study of psychological and social factors in poorly controlled insulin dependent diabetic patients. *Journal of Psychosomatic Research, 35*(2–3), 335–343.

Young, E., & Korszun, A. (1999). Women, stress, and depression: Sex differences in hypothalamic–pituitary–adrenal axis regulation. In E. Leibenluft (Ed.), *Gender differences in mood and anxiety disorders: From bench to bedside* (pp. 31–52). Washington, DC: American Psychiatric Press.

24

Cardiovascular Disease

SHERRI HANSEN

Cardiovascular disease is generally thought to occur in and kill mostly men. However, cardiovascular disease is also the leading cause of mortality in women and occurs equally in men and women after age 50 (Chiamvimonvat & Sternberg, 1998). Each year, over 500,000 women die from cardiac disease, twice as many as from all cancers combined (National Center for Health Statistics, 1995). One-third of women will die from cardiovascular disease, compared to 4% from breast cancer (Redberg, 1998). African American women experience mortality rates from coronary artery disease (CAD) that are double those of European American women, and CAD is the leading cause of death in African American women aged 30–39 years (Jairath, 2001). Despite these sobering statistics, an American Heart Association study found that only 8% of women consider cardiovascular disease a personal health threat (American Heart Association, 1997).

This chapter first provides a review of differences between men and women in the occurrence and treatment of cardiovascular disease, prefaced by a discussion of the fact that few research data on women and cardiac disease were available until recently. The chapter then describes various psychosocial and psychological risk factors for cardiac disease in women. Finally, an overview of situations that a consulting psychiatrist will commonly encounter is presented.

MALE–FEMALE DIFFERENCES AND TREATMENT OF CARDIAC DISEASE

Representation of Women in Cardiac Studies

Until recently, most data on cardiovascular disease in both men and women were derived from studies involving only men. The U.S. Food and Drug Administration (FDA) policy through the early 1990s prohibited women in their childbearing years from participating in Phase 1 drug trials, which test the efficacy, safety profiles, and dosages of new drugs. Guidelines also prevented women from participating in the more advanced Phase 2 trials. However, once a new drug was approved and placed on the market, physicians prescribed these drugs to women as well as men. It was assumed that women and men would require similar dosages, and that both the beneficial and adverse effects would be the same. Most studies on cardiovascular disease have excluded women for two reasons. One was a concern regarding birth defects after the thalidomide tragedy in the 1950s and 1960s. Another concern was that women who were postmenopausal, who had undergone a hysterectomy, or who were using estrogen replacement therapy would show variations in estrogen and progesterone levels, which could affect the efficacy of the trial drugs (Merkatz et al., 1993). The National Institutes of Health (NIH) and the FDA have recently revised policies regarding the inclusion of women in clinical trials. The new NIH guidelines now require women and minorities to be included, and an analysis of gender and racial differences to be performed. The FDA also now requires women and men to be included in clinical trials if both will receive the drug when it is marketed. (For a more detailed discussion, see Merkatz et al., Chapter 36, this volume.)

Physical Risk Factors and Presentation

Many women are not aware of their potential risks for cardiovascular disease. Compared to men, more women have diabetes, hypertension, hypercholesterolemia, and a family history of cardiovascular disease. Cardiovascular death rates are three to seven times higher in women with diabetes than in women without it (Barrett-Connor & Wingard, 1983). Other risk factors that affect women include smoking and obesity. Sixty percent of American women have a sedentary lifestyle, rendering physical inactivity the most prevalent coronary risk factor for women (Hennekens, 1998). Multiple studies have shown that women who engage in mild to moderate levels of exercise have significantly reduced levels of blood lipids, triglycerides, and glucose, as well as lower blood pressure (Thomas & Braus, 1998). Women with existing cardiac disease who exercise regularly, follow a low fat diet, and undergo stress management training also have a significant reduction in risk of myocardial infarction (MI) (Toobert, 2000). Rates of cigarette smoking have declined more slowly in women (from 34% to 23%) than in men from 52% to 28%) (National Center for Health Statistics, 1992). The rate of daily smoking among high school girls is also greater than that for boys (Lamkin & Houston, 1998). New studies are also demonstrating that low bone mass at menopause is a risk factor for increased mortality, especially from cardiovascular disease as well as osteoporosis (Von der Recke et al., 1999), and that higher calcium intake is associated with reduced ischemic heart disease (Bostick et al., 1999).

Women have been found to present differently than men with cardiovascular symptoms. Women are relatively protected against heart disease until after menopause, and thus present with cardiac symptoms approximately 10 years later than men. Cardiac symptoms in women are also more likely to be atypical. Women may complain initially of nonexertional chest pain, or pain in other locations, such as in the jaw, arms, shoulder, back, and epigastric area. Women are also more likely to complain of dyspnea, palpitations, and presyncope, as well as nausea and fatigue, than men are. Symptoms of arthritis or osteoporosis, which are more common in women, may also obscure the diagnosis of CAD (Redberg, 1998).

MI Mortality

A number of studies have shown that women have higher mortality rates from MI than men do (Hanratty, Lawlor, et al., 2000; Hennekens, 1998; Hochman et al., 1999). One reason for this is that, women often present to medical attention later after the onset of symptoms than men do. Women also may not acknowledge the seriousness of their symptoms initially and may use a variety of coping mechanisms and self-treatment behaviors to reduce the threat and maintain control over the situation. Women are also more likely to seek care from primary care providers than from cardiologists and may not be referred for appropriate treatment on a timely basis.

Several studies have compared psychosocial well-being and adjustment after a nonfatal MI in both women and men (Brezinka & Kittel, 1996). Most of the studies suggest that women do not cope as well physically and psychologically as men after MI. Their quality of life is more impaired, and they score higher on psychosomatic symptoms, anxiety and sleep disturbances than their male counterparts.

A number of studies have focused on differences in women's responses to standard treatments for MI. Several studies have found that women have a higher incidence of serious bleeding complications following use of thrombolytics (Fibrinolytic Therapy Trialists Collaborative Group, 1994). Women also have been found to receive thrombolytics less frequently. The International Studies of Infarct Survival (ISIS) have found aspirin to be slightly less effective in women (ISIS-2 Collaborative Group, 1988; ISIS-3 Collaborative Group, 1992). However, there is evidence that ß-blockers may be more effective in women when used early (ISIS-1 Collaborative Group, 1986; Hjalmarson, 1997). The reasons for these findings stem from the fact that the average woman with cardiac disease is approximately 10 years older than the average man with cardiac disease. Her advanced age is considered to be the most significant factor in increased cardiac mortality, decreased efficacy of thromobolytics and aspirin, and a tendency toward the underuse of these medications in women (Nohria et al., 1998).

Coronary Revascularization

Women who are referred for percutaneous transluminal coronary angioplasty are likely to be older than men and more likely to have a history of heart failure and unstable angina, but less likely to have had a prior MI. Women are also more likely to have hypertension, hyperlipidemia, and diabetes. Although the initial success rate is similar for both men and women, women experience less symptomatic relief and decreased long-term survival (Weintraub et al., 1996).

Women are less likely than men to undergo coronary artery bypass grafting (CABG). They also have a higher in-hospital mortality rate—13% for women compared to 6% for men (Maynard et al., 1992). Advanced age, late referral into treatment, severity of angina, comorbid diabetes mellitus, concurrent illnesses, number of diseased vessels, and decreased body surface area are thought to be reasons. When all of these variables are taken into account, female gender is no longer considered statistically significant. However, other studies have found CABG to be less effective in women (Aaronson et al., 1995). Many studies suggest that the differences may result from greater frequency of urgent or emergent surgery, smaller coronary arteries, and less frequent use of an internal mammary artery graft (O'Connor et al., 1996). Recurrent angina, perioperative MI, congestive heart failure (CHF), incomplete revascularization, and early and late graft reocclusion are more prevalent in women. Also, some studies suggest that women may gain less symptomatic relief from angina following CABG (Sjoland et al., 1997).

Congestive Heart Failure

The earliest study on the prevalence of CHF in women was a study conducted in the early 1960s in North Carolina and Vermont. The study reported that women were more likely to develop CHF than men, and that hypertension was the more common cause in women with CAD (Gibson et al., 1966). The risk of developing CHF in the 10 years after an MI is higher in women than in men (Kannel, 1989). Diabetes was also found to be a stronger risk factor and smoking was found to be less common for the development of CHF in women (Ho et al., 1993). Women survived longer after diagnosis of CHF (3.17 years vs. 1.66 years), with a 5-year survival rate of 28% in women and 25% in men (Petrie et al., 1999). Other studies, however, have found higher morbidity and mortality from CHF in women than in men (Linmacher & Yusuf, 1993). As noted above, though, women have been grossly underrepresented in most large studies, and more studies are needed to clarify this.

Cardiac Transplant

In 1993, 2,298 cardiac transplants were performed, with women making up 21.5% of the total (Beneson, 1994). The most likely explanation for the lower number of female transplant candidates is their more advanced age at transplantation. A study by Randall (1993) also found that women were more likely to refuse cardiac transplants. When refusals were added to the numbers of those who had the transplants, the gender bias disappeared. Aaronson et al. (1995) also found that the underrepresentation of females among transplant candidates resulted from a sex difference in patients' treatment preference and not a physician selection bias. Why might women be more inclined to refuse cardiac transplants? There are no clear answers, but one hypothesis from Travis et al. (1993) is that men may approach their physicians with a "fix it" attitude, and women may view cardiac disease as something to which they must adapt.

Survival of cardiac transplantation now approaches 85% at 1 year, with survival and quality of life nearly equivalent in both men and women (Kobashigawa et al., 1993). Other studies, however, refute this finding and show a higher incidence of rejection and risk of death in women (Sharples et al., 1991). As more transplant patients survive longer and can expect to lead productive lives, an interesting area that is emerging in transplant medicine is pregnancy. Few case series have documented pregnancy outcomes. A case series of 10 pregnancies in France documented the incidence of hypertension in 9 of the pregnancies and severe preeclampsia in 2 patients (Troche et al., 1998). Another case series of 30 pregnancies from around the world also revealed a frequent rate of complications, including chronic hypertension in 48%, preeclampsia in 24%, preterm labor in 28%, and a cesarean section rate of 32% (Scott et al., 1993). These limited case studies demonstrate that although the rate of complications is increased in heart transplant recipients, a successful outcome is possible. There are ethical issues, however, related to the possibility of a woman's giving birth to a child she may not live to raise.

Cardiac Rehabilitation

Cardiac rehabilitation is an important component of recovery from coronary revascularization and maintenance of cardiac function. However, studies of the demographics of participants of cardiac rehabilitation programs show that women are 20% less likely to enroll in such programs than men are (Ades et al., 1992). There are a variety of reasons for this finding. Women are more likely to have an increased burden of physical illness and are more likely to be unemployed and unmarried or widowed. Women may be unable to or unwilling to drive alone, and are more likely to be living alone without someone to drive them to appointments.

Women may also feel more obliged to return to prior household responsibilities, and therefore may not enroll in cardiac rehabilitation. One study by Brezinka and Kittel (1996) found that women who entered cardiac rehabilitation had a higher degree of psychosocial impairment and a lower level of physical functioning than their male counterparts. Women may also have different motivations for participation in cardiac rehabilitation as compared to men. Moore and Kremer (1996) found that women's preferences for a cardiac program featured feeling safe while exercising, being monitored, being able to exercise without being tired, having exercise options other than a cycle or a treadmill, desiring more social interaction during exercise sessions, and receiving emotional support from the staff. Other factors, such as commute time, transportation availability, and scheduling to avoid interference with other activities, have also been cited as being important for compliance.

Suggestions that might be useful to enhance compliance in women include offering a high component of social interaction. This could be met by increasing group activities and including friends and spouses/partners. Exercise programs may also be kept more interesting by increasing the use of games and avoidance of regimented exercise, such as calisthenics. Background music is likewise considered desirable. Staff should provide positive reinforcement, and should develop progress charts to stimulate self-monitoring and goal achievement (Linmacher, 1998).

Sexual Activity Following MI or CABG

Little is known regarding the sexual activity of women with CAD (Brezinka & Kittel, 1996). In a study by Papadopoulos et al. (1983), of 130 women who had survived an MI, 30% of women who were sexually active before an MI developed concerns with the safety of sexual activity, 27% did not resume such activity, and 44% decreased it. Another study (Baggs & Karch, 1987) of women's post-MI sexual activity reported that 20% of the women expressed fear about sexual intercourse, and only 33% of the women stated they received some information about return to sexual activity during hospitalization. Other studies, however, have not shown significant differences in sexual activity in men and women following MI or CABG (Rankin, 1990; Hamilton & Seidman, 1993). The data on sexual activity in women with cardiac disease are sparse, and there is a strong need for further research. Health care professionals, however, should stress the importance of sexual counseling for both men and women recovering from MI or CABG.

Effects of Reproductive Hormones on Cardiac Disease

Much concern has been voiced over the effects of oral contraceptives on cardiac disease risk factors. Previously, high estrogen and progesterone oral contraceptives increased cardiovascular disease by promoting thrombosis. Most oral contraceptive preparations today utilize low-dose estrogen and progesterone, and the risks are much lower (Mann et al., 1975). However, there is a clear link among cigarette smoking, high-estrogen contraceptives, and risk of MI, especially in women over the age of 35 (Hennekens et al., 1979).

Much has been written regarding the effects of estrogen in postmenopausal women. Estrogen has many physiological effects that contribute to delay in the onset of cardiovascular disease. Estrogen has many effects on lipids; it increases high-density lipoprotein (HDL) cholesterol by an average of 10–15%, while lowering low-density lipoprotein (LDL) cholesterol. However, estrogen does increase triglyceride levels. Transdermal preparations of estrogen are not as effective as oral preparations but cause less increase in triglycerides. Also, estrogen lowers glucose levels, lowers insulin levels, decreases insulin resistance, and lowers fibrinogen levels. Estrogen also provides a more favorable distribution of body fat, delineated by a smaller waist–hip ratio.

Traditionally, it has been thought that estrogen reduces cardiac risk factors (Menolio et al., 1993). Multiple studies have demonstrated reduction in cardiac disease with estrogen use (Stampfer et al., 1991; Henderson et al., 1991; Ettinger et al., 1996). Estrogen may reduce the risk of developing Alzheimer's disease and osteoporosis, which are also leading causes of morbidity and mortality. However, emerging studies are challenging the assumptions that postmenopausal estrogen use reduces the risk of developing coronary artery disease (Kuller, 2000; Giarelina, 2000). Estrogen can also have other detrimental effects. Estrogen used alone increases the rate of endometrial cancer, although this risk is significantly decreased with the addition of progesterone. An increased risk of breast cancer in women who use estrogen replacement has been described in many studies, but has been refuted in others (Grady et al., 1995; Bieber & Barnes, 2001; Stanford et al., 1995).

Given these concerns, it is not surprising that women are skeptical about long-term estrogen use. Women are generally more concerned about breast cancer than about cardiac disease, so part of their reluctance to use estrogen stems from the negative publicity regarding increased breast cancer risk. In the United States, the utilization of hormone replacement is greater in women aged 40–60 (35%) than in women aged over 65 (15%) (Carr, 1996). Demographic studies of women who take estrogen have found that such women are likely to be healthier, to be better educated, to have higher total household incomes, and to have better access to health care than women who do not use estrogen (Rossouw, 1996). They are also more likely to have a regular primary care physician, to use calcium supplementation, and to exercise regularly (Keating et al., 1999). However, they are also more worried about their appearance and developing illness. A history of hypertension, smoking, and a family history of cardiovascular disease or hyperlipidemia are not correlated with estrogen use.

So why don't more women use hormone replacement? A study by Salamone et al. (1996) found that the main reason women never started estrogen replacement in the first place came from a fear that the medication was harmful (38.1%) or a feeling that they did not need it (29.5%). The North American Menopause Society's 1997 Menopause Survey found that relief of physical symptoms was mentioned as the most common reason to begin hormone replacement therapy (Kaufert et al., 1998). The news media and physicians are the sources of information most often used by American women for information regarding hormone replacement, and more educational efforts by both of these sources may be useful to encourage larger numbers of women to consider hormone replacement therapy.

PSYCHOSOCIAL AND PSYCHOLOGICAL RISK FACTORS FOR CARDIAC DISEASE IN WOMEN

Personality

Much has been written about a link between Type A behavior and cardiovascular disease. The Type A personality has not been well researched in women. In a study of the 20 year incidence of CAD, Eaker et al. (1989) found no relationship between Framingham Type A behavior and the development of CAD in women. Furthermore, other studies now dispute the connection between Type A personality and CAD in men (Shekelle et al., 1985).

Of the characteristics of Type A behavior, however, only hostility has been consistently linked to the development of CAD (Smith, 1992). A prospective study found that women who reported high trait anger, a history of withholding their anger, having hostile attitudes, and being aware of themselves in social situations had a higher intima media thickness (IMT) (Matthews et al., 1998). A high IMT is considered an early marker for the development of CAD. Other studies, however, dispute this; for instance, one angiography study found no significant positive associations for either hostility or coronary occlusion (Helman et al., 1991). Sloan et al. (1994) have proposed that autonomic arousal secondary to chronic hostility and altered phasic autonomic responses to stressful life circumstances underlie at least a part of the association between hostility and CAD. They demonstrated reductions in tonic vagal cardiac modulation and a shifting of autonomic balance in the direction of sympathetic predominance in hostile young adults compared with a nonhostile comparison group.

Social Supports

Studies on the impact of social supports on the incidence and recovery from CAD have been conflicting, with associations that differ between age groups, races, and socioeconomic classes, and with most studies including only small numbers of women. Many studies have found that women with the least number of social connections had the highest mortality rates, and that nonmembership in social or community groups was linked to death from cardiovascular disease (Berkman & Syme, 1979; Wingard & Cohn, 1997). Other studies, however, have not found a significant relationship after controlling for risk factors (Schoenbach et al., 1986). Women do appear to activate their social support system more effectively than men after MI, which may help with recovery, but women are also more likely to be widowed and living alone.

Social Class, Multiple Roles, and Employment

Education appears to play a role in the risk of development of CAD. A study by Matthews et al. (1989) found that less education in women was associated with a more atherogenic risk factor profile. In women with less education, systolic blood pressure, LDL cholesterol, glucose, and body mass index were all found to be increased. Women who attained lower levels of education were also more likely to report cigarette smoking, low levels of physical exercise, and poor diets. Socioeconomic status also plays a role, in that women married to men in manual occupations have been found to experience twice the standardized mortality ratio from coronary disease than women married to men in higher socioeconomic occupations (Marmot et al., 1987).

Women are engaged in multiple roles that can precipitate stress. A study by Palmer et al. (1992) found that the number of children a woman bore had an effect on cardiac disease risk. They also showed that women who had five or more live births had a risk of heart attacks 1.6 times greater than that of nulliparous women and 1.4 times greater than that of parous women who had borne fewer children; this result was independent of educational achievement. Other studies, however, have shown that women who occupy a greater number of roles have lower rates of physical and mental stress (Rodin & Isckovics, 1990).

Work itself has not been found to promote CAD. The Framingham Heart Study found that neither employment status nor occupational level was associated with a 20-year increased incidence of MI or coronary death in women (Eaker et al., 1989). However, as women enter the work force, social class may become more ambiguous, as women whose families have high total incomes may take lower-paying jobs in order to fulfill family obligations. The nature of the work itself, rather than whether a woman is employed, may be the ultimate determinate of job and role stress. The combination of high psychological job demands and low freedom to make job decisions has been found to relate to depression, exhaustion, and job dissatisfaction (Karasek et al., 1988). Indeed, women are more likely to withdraw from the work force within 2 years after an MI than are men. However, women who returned to paid employment following an MI experienced an early survival advantage over women who quit their jobs (Chirikos & Nickel, 1984).

Clearly, the impact of multiple roles in women's lives must be considered, but it is uncertain at this time. Particular attention should be focused on measurements of low job control (see below), and demands on women at both work and home should be investigated simultaneously (LaCroix, 1994).

Other Psychosocial Factors

Other psychosocial factors may also influence the development of cardiac disease in women. Seven psychosocial variables were found to have the greatest impact on the incidence of CAD among homemakers: tension, symptoms of anxiety, a belief that one is more likely to suffer a heart attack than other women are, trouble falling asleep, housework badly affecting health, being lonely during the day, and taking infrequent vacations (Eaker et al., 1989). When all seven variables were entered together into one equation with the standard risk factors, only loneliness, infrequent vacations, and belief in one's proneness to heart disease were still significant predictors of the development of heart disease. These characteristics do not reflect a coronary-prone personality but rather a coronary-prone situation, in which women may feel isolated and may not have the latitude or perceived options available to resolve a tense situation. Eaker et al. (1989) suggest that subordination and social isolation may be instrumental in predicting the development of definite coronary disease in women.

Hopelessness and Depression

Depression is a risk factor for the development of CAD and also for increased morbidity and mortality. Several studies of patients with acute MI have reported a prevalence rate of major depressive illness of approximately 20% (Shapiro, 1996; Anda et al., 1993). Glassman and Shapiro (1998) found that the risk of developing a fatal MI with severe to moderate levels of hopelessness was increased. However, this study did not separate out gender. Multiple studies have shown that patients with preexisting cardiac disease and depression experienced acceleration of their cardiac disease. A study by Frasure-Smith et al. (1993) demonstrated that major depression in patients hospitalized following an MI was a risk factor for mortality at 6 months. This risk remained after prescription medications and severity of heart disease were controlled for. Depression was also associated with a lack of close friends.

Many theories have been postulated as to how depression may interact with cardiac disease. Depressed patients may be less likely to adhere to cardiac treatment and may be less likely to take medications, exercise, stop smoking, and change eating habits (Anda et al., 1990). Studies have focused on the fact that depression increases the likelihood of nicotine use (Glassman et al., 1990). However, even when smoking is controlled for, a link between depression and CAD continues to exist. Depression may also precipitate a decline in physical functioning, which may complicate cardiac disease.

Depressed patients with cardiac disease also have decreased cardiac rate variability (Carney et al., 1988). There is evidence that patients with decreased heart rate variability measured over a 24-hour period have a negative prognosis following MI (Kleiger et al., 1987). A study by Dalack and Roose (1990) suggests that depression may cause changes in the sympathetic–parasympathetic balance. Such changes could place depressed patients with MI at greater risk for fatal arrhythmias. Serotonin, which plays a major role in the neurobiology of depression, also plays a role in amplifying the platelet response to thrombogenesis (Meltzer & Lowy, 1987; Musselman et al., 1996). Preliminary evidence suggests that this response is enhanced in depressed patients (Frasure-Smith et al., 1995a; DeSilva, 1993), and that patients who are depressed following MI are at increased risk for thrombogenic events (Anda et al., 1990).

Anxiety

Anxious patients frequently describe chest pain as part of their symptoms, but there is no evidence that this represents a prodrome of coronary disease (Shapiro, 1996). Anxiety, however, can provoke a variety of arrhythmias. A study by DeSilva (1993) estimated that 20% of the half million cases of sudden cardiac death in the United States each year may be associated with acute psychological stress. There is evidence that panic disorder is associated with a small increase in sudden death longitudinally (Haines et al., 1987). High levels of phobic anxiety are associated with an increased risk of sudden cardiac death, presumably owing to reduced vagal modulation of cardiac rate and increased ventricular tachyarrhythmias. In the Health Professionals Study, phobic anxiety was associated with an increase in fatal MI, but not nonfatal MI (Kawachi et al., 1994). Induced psychological stress has been shown to cause reduction in left ventricular function and coronary artery spasm in patients with established CAD (Rozanski et al., 1991). Recent clinical observations have found an association between anxiety and the risk of unstable angina (Frasure-Smith et al., 1995b).

PSYCHIATRIC CONSULTATION IN WOMEN WITH CARDIOVASCULAR DISEASE

The heart is crucial to one's identity and social function. It is not surprising that normal emotional reactions to the development of cardiac disease include shock, fear, anger, guilt, sadness, and grief. The onset of illness is often felt as a narcissistic injury. Patients may have to confront issues of dependency and loss of control. They may become less able to continue at their occupations, which may lead to financial stress and feelings of inadequacy. Sexual functioning may be adversely affected, which may further contribute to loss of self-esteem. Cigarette and alcohol use, failure to exercise, and noncompliance with diet and medications may have contributed to the development of illness and result in feelings of guilt.

Patients with cardiac disease may complain of neurovegetative symptoms that mimic depression, including loss of energy, appetite, concentration, and sleep. Patients with panic disorder may present with chest pain that may be confused with pain from angina pectoris. The psychiatrist must evaluate all such patients with attention to history, physical signs, and laboratory data to establish psychiatric diagnoses. Commonly used medications such as antihypertensive drugs, including ß-blockers, can exacerbate mood states. Medication toxicity can also produce symptoms that mimic depression. Metabolic disturbances such as hyponatremia, uremia, hypoxia, and liver failure can produce mental status changes that may be confused with depression and anxiety. Symptoms such as hopelessness, helplessness, self-deprecating thoughts, and suicidal ideation are more likely to occur in cardiac patients with a depressive illness than in those without depression.

A psychiatrist also needs to be aware of issues between a patient and the medical team, issues with the patient's family and support systems, and the impact of cardiac disease on the patient's sense of self. Denial of illness is also an issue that occurs in acute care settings. Denial in the short run may be an important and normal defense mechanism against anxiety, and healthy denial may help patients to cope with symptoms and to recuperate. However, maladaptive denial may lead to a patient's inability to accept treatment recommendations and make lifestyle changes.

It was once commonplace to give patients admitted to coronary care units benzodiazepines in order to reduce anxiety, and thus to reduce circulating catecholamines and the potential for further ischemia and cardiac arrhythmias. In the absence of significant anxiety, there does not appear to be a justification for this practice. However, in patients with significant anxiety, short-acting benzodiazepines such as lorazepam may be useful for insomnia and anxiety.

Delirium is a common complication of cardiac surgery. Multiple etiologies are often responsible and include sedative medications, hypoxia, renal and hepatic impairment, and infection. Management is generally supportive and relies on correcting the underlying causes of the delirium.

CONCLUSIONS

In conclusion, cardiac disease is the most serious threat to women's health. Most research to date has overwhelmingly studied men only, and data on women's risk and course of illness are scarce. Emerging data suggest that women have different levels of risk and different responses to treatment; more research in these areas is clearly needed. Several ongoing studies should begin to provide answers to these questions. The most ambitious study is the Women's Health Initiative Study, the purpose of which is to evaluate the effectiveness of calcium replacement therapy, vitamin D therapy, a low-fat diet, and estrogen replacement therapy against osteoporosis, CAD, breast cancer, and other diseases in women. It plans to follow 1,400 women and should be completed in 2004. Other studies include the Angiographic Trial in Women and the Estrogen Replacement and Atherosclerosis Study, both of which will assess the efficacy of hormone replacement therapy in altering the course of CAD in women. Another trial, the Evaluation of Ischemic Heart Disease in Women, will attempt to determine whether diagnostic testing in women can be improved. Greater awareness on the part of both the lay public and health care professionals is needed if professionals are to identify women at risk for developing cardiac disease and to help them make good use of preventative measures. Professionals also need to make efforts to educate and counsel women regarding the risks of cardiac disease.

REFERENCES

Aaronson, K. D., Schwartz, J. S., & Goin, J. E. (1995). Sex differences in patient acceptance of cardiac transplant candidacy. *Circulation, 91*(11), 2753–2761.

Ades, P. A., Waldmann, M. L., et al. (1992). Referral patterns and exercise responses in the rehabilitation of female coronary patients aged >62. *American Journal of Cardiology, 69*(17), 1422–1425.

American Heart Association. (1997). *Take charge: A woman's guide to fighting heart disease.* Dallas, TX: Author.

Anda, R., Williamson, D., Jones, D., et al. (1993). Depressed affect, hopelessness, and risk of ischemic heart disease in a cohort of US adults. *Epidemiology, 4*(4), 285–294.

Anda, R. F., Williamson, D. F., Escobedo, L. G., et al. (1990). Depression and the dynamics of smoking: A national perspective. *Journal of the American Medical Association, 264*(12), 1541–1543.

Baggs, J. G., & Karch, A. M. (1987). Sexual counseling of women with coronary heart disease. *Heart and Lung, 16*(2), 154–159.

Barrett-Connor, E., & Wingard, D. L. (1983). Sex differential in ischemic heart disease mortality in diabetics: A prospective population-based study. *American Journal of Epidemiology, 118*(4), 489–498.

Beneson, E. (Ed.). (1994). *UNOS Update, 10*(6). Richmond, VA: United Network for Organ Sharing.

Berkman, L. F., & Syme, L. (1979). Social networks, host resistance, and mortality: A nine-year follow-up study of Alameda County residents. *American Journal of Epidemiology, 109*(2), 186–204.

Bieber, E. J., & Barnes, R. B. (2001). Breast cancer and HRT—What are the data? *International Journal of Fertility and Women's Medicine, 46*(2), 73–78.

Bostick, R. M., Kushi, L. H., Wu, Y., et al. (1999). Relation of calcium, vitamin D, and dairy food intake to ischemic heart disease mortality among postmenopausal women. *American Journal of Epidemiology, 149*(2), 151–161.

Brezinka, V., & Kittel, F. (1996). Psychosocial factors of coronary heart disease in women: A review. *Social Science and Medicine, 42*(10), 1351–1365.

Carney, R. M., Rich, W. Z., TeVelde, A., et al. (1988). The relationship between heart rate, heart rate variability, and depression in patients with coronary artery disease. *Journal of Psychosomatic Research, 32*(2), 159–164.

Carr, B. R. (1996). HRT management: The American experience. *European Journal of Obstetrics, Gynecology, and Reproductive Biology, 64*(Suppl.), 517–520.

Chiamvimonvat, V., & Sternberg, L. (1998). Coronary artery disease in women. *Canadian Family Physician, 44*, 2709–2717.

Chirikos, T. N., & Nickel, J. L. (1984). Work disability from coronary heart disease in women. *Women's Health, 9*(1), 55–71.

Dalack, G. W., & Roose, S. P. (1990). Perspectives on the relationship between cardiovascular disease and affective disorder. *Journal of Clinical Psychiatry, 51*(Suppl.), 4–9.

DeSilva, R. A. (1993). Cardiac arrhythmias and sudden cardiac death. In A. Stoudemire & B. S. Fogel (Eds.), *Medical-psychiatric practice* (Vol. 2). Washington, DC: American Psychiatric Press.

Eaker, E. D., Abott, R. D., & Kannel, W. B. (1989). Frequency of uncomplicated angina pectoris in Type A compared to Type B persons (the Framingham Study). *American Journal of Cardiology, 63*(15), 1042–1045.

Ettinger, B., Friedman, G. P., Bush, T., et al. (1996). Reduced mortality associated with long-term postmenopausal estrogen therapy. *Obstetrics and Gynecology, 87*(1), 6–12.

Fibrinolytic Therapy Trialists (FTT) Collaborative Group. (1994). Indications for fibrinolytic therapy in suspected acute myocardial infarction: Collaborative overview of early mortality and major morbidity results from all randomized trials of more than 1000 patients. *Lancet, 343*(8893), 311–322.

Frasure-Smith, N., Lesperance, F., & Talajic, M. (1993). Depression following myocardial infarction: Impact on six-month survival. *Journal of the American Medical Association, 270*(15), 1819–1825.

Frasure-Smith, N., Lesperance, F., & Talajic, M. (1995a). Depression and 18-month prognosis after myocardial infarction. *Circulation, 91*(4), 999–1005.

Frasure-Smith, N., Lesperance, F., & Talajic, M. (1995b). The impact of negative emotions on prognosis following myocardial infarction: Is it more than depression? *Health Psychology, 14*(5), 388–398.

Giardina, E. G. (2000). Heart disease in women. *International Journal of Fertility and Women's Medicine, 45*(6), 350–357.

Gibson, T. C., White, K. L., & Klainer, L. M. (1966). The prevalence of congestive heart failure in two rural communities. *Journal of Chronic Disease, 19*(2), 141–152.

Glassman, A. H., & Shapiro, P. A. (1998). Depression and the course of coronary artery disease. *American Journal of Psychiatry, 155*(1), 4–11.

Glassman, A. H., Heltzer, J. E., Covey, L. S., et al. (1990). Smoking, smoking cessation, and major depresion. *Journal of the American Medical Association, 264*(12), 1546–1549.

Grady, D., Gebratsadik, T., Kerlikowke, K., et al. (1995). Hormone replacement therapy and endometrial cancer risk: A metaanalysis. *Obstetrics and Gynecology, 85*(2), 304–313.

Haines, A. P., Imerson, J. D., & Meade, T. W. (1987). Phobic anxiety and ischaemic heart disease. *British Medical Journal, 295*(6593), 297–299.

Hamilton, G. A., & Seidman, R. N. (1993). A comparison of the recovery period for women and men after an acute myocardial infarction. *Heart and Lung, 22*(4), 308–315.

Hanratty, B., Lawlor, D. A., Robinson, M. B., et al. (2000). Sex differences in risk factors, treatment and mortality after acute myocardial infarction: An observational study. *Journal of Epidemiology and Community Health, 54*(12), 912–916.

Helman, D. C., Ragland, D. R., & Syme, S. L. (1991). Hostility and coronary artery disease. *American Journal of Epidemiology, 133*(2), 112–122.

Henderson, B. E., Paganini-Hill, A., & Ross, R. K. (1991). Decreased mortality in users of estrogen replacement therapy. *Archives of Internal Medicine, 151*(1), 75–78.

Hennekens, C. H. (1998). Risk factors for coronary heart disease in women. *Cardiology Clinics, 16*(1), 1–8.

Hennekens, C. H., Evans, D. A., Castelli, W. P., et al. (1979). Oral contraceptive use and fasting triglycerides, plasma cholesterol, and HDL cholesterol. *Circulation, 60*(3), 486–489.

Hjalmarson, A. (1997). Effects of beta blockers on sudden cardiac death during acute myocardial infarction and the postinfection period. *American Journal of Cardiology, 13*, 355–395.

Ho, K. K., Pinsky, J. L., Kannel, W. B., et al. (1993). The epidemiology of heart failure: The Framingham Study. *Journal of the American College of Cardiology, 22*(4, Suppl. A), 6A–13A.

Hochman, J. S., Tamis, J. E., Thompson, T. D., et al. (1999). Sex, clinical presentation, and outcome in patients with acute coronary syndromes: Global use of strategies to open occluded coronary arteries in acute coronary syndromes IIb investigators. *New England Journal of Medicine, 341*(4), 226–232.

ISIS-1 (First International Study of Infarct Survival) Collaborative Group. (1986). Randomized trial of intravenous atenolol among 16,027 cases of suspected acute myocardial infarction: ISIS-1. *Lancet, ii*(8498), 57–66.

ISIS-2 (Second International Study of Infarct Survival) Collaborative Group. (1988). A randomized trial of intravenous streptokinase, oral aspirin, both, or neither among 17,187 cases of suspected acute myocardial infarction: ISIS-2. *Lancet, ii*(8607), 349–360.

ISIS-3 (Third International Study of Infact Survival) Collaborative Group. (1992). ISIS-3: A randomized comparison of streptokinase vs. tissue plasminogen activator vs. antistreplase and of aspirin plus heparin vs. aspirin alone among 41,299 cases of suspected acute myocardial infarction. *Lancet, 399*(8796), 753–770.

Jairath, N. (2001). Implications of gender differences on coronary artery disease risk reduction in women. *AACN Clinical Issues, 12*(1), 17–28.

Kannel, W. B. (1989). Epidemiological aspects of heart failure. *Cardiology Clinics, 7*(1), 1–9.

Karasek, R. A., Theorell, T., Schwartz, J. E., et al. (1988). Job characterisitcs in relation to the prevalence of myocardial infarction in the US Health Examination Study (HANES). *American Journal of Public Health, 78*(8), 910–918.

Kaufert, P., Boggs, P. P., & Ettinger, B. J. (1998). Women and menopause: Beliefs, attitudes, and behaviors. The North American Menopause Society 1997 Menopause Survey. *Menopause, 5*(4), 197–202.

Kawachi, I., Colditz, G. A., Ascherio, A., et al. (1994). Prospective study of phobic anxiety and risk of coronary heart disease in men. *Circulation, 89*(5), 1992–1997.

Keating, N. L., Cleary, P. D., Ross, A. S., et al. (1999). Use of hormone replacement therapy by post-menopausal women in the United States. *Annals of Internal Medicine, 130*(7), 545–553.

Kleiger, R. E., Miller, J. P, Bigger, J. T., Jr., et al. (1987). Decreased heart rate variability and its association with mortality after myocardial infarction. *American Journal of Cardiology, 59*(4), 256–262.

Kobashigawa, J., Kirklin, J., Naftel, D., et al. (1993). Pretransplantation risk factors for acute rejection after heart transplantation: A multiinstitutional study. The Transplant Cardiologist Research Database Group. *Journal of Heart and Lung Transplantation, 12*(3), 355–366.

Kuller, L. H. (2000). Hormone replacement therapy and coronary heart disease: A new debate. *The Medical Clinics of North America, 84*(1), 181–198.

LaCroix, A. Z. (1994). Psychosocial factors and risk of coronary heart disease in women: An epidemiologic perspective. *Fertility and Sterility, 62*(Suppl. 6), 133S–139S.

Lamkin, L. P., & Houston, T. P. (1998). Nicotine dependency and adolescents: Preventing and treating. *Primary Care, 25*(1), 123–125.

Linmacher, M. C. (1998). Exercise and rehabilitation in women. *Cardiology Clinics, 16*(1), 27–36.

Linmacher, M. C., & Yusuf, S. (for the SOLVD Investigators). (1993). Gender differences in presentation, morbidity, and mortality in the studies of left ventricular dysfunction (SOLVD): A preliminary report. In N. K. Wenger, L. Speroff, & B. Packard (Eds.), *Cardiovascular health and disease in women.* Greenwich, CT: Le Jacq Communications.

Mann, J. I., Vessey, M. P., Thorogood, M., et al. (1975). Myocardial infarction in young women with special reference to oral contraceptive practice. *British Medical Journal, ii*(5965), 241–245.

Marmot, M. G., Kogevinas, M., & Elston, M. A. (1987). Social/economic status and disease. *Annual Review of Public Health, 8,* 111–135.

Matthews, K. A., Owens, J. F., Kuller, L. H., et al. (1998). Are hostility and anxiety associated with carotid atherosclerosis in healthy postmenopausal women? *Psychosomatic Medicine, 60*(5), 633–638.

Matthews, K. A., Kelsey, S. F., Meilahn, E. N., et al. (1989). Educational attainment and behavioral and biologic risk factors for coronary heart disease in middle-aged women. *American Journal of Epidemiology, 129*(6), 1132–1144.

Maynard, C., Litwin, P. E., Martin, J. S., et al. (1992). Gender differences in the treatment and outcome of acute myocardial infarction: Results from the Myocardial Infarction Triage and Interventional Registry. *Archives of Internal Medicine, 152*(5), 972–976.

Meltzer, H. Y., & Lowy, M. T. (1987). The serotonin hypothesis of depression. In H. Y. Meltzer (Ed.), *Psychopharmacology: The third generation of progress.* New York: Raven Press.

Menolio, T. A., Furberg, C. D., Shermanski, L., et al. (1993). Association of postmenopausal estrogen use and its risk factors in older women. *Circulation, 88*(Pt. 1), 2163–2171.

Merkatz, R., Temple, R., Sobel, S., et al. (1993). Women in clinical trials of new drugs. *New England Journal of Medicine, 329*(4), 292–296.

Moore, S. M., & Kremer, F. M. (1996). Women's and men's preferences for cardiac rehabilitation program features. *Journal of Cardiopulmonary Rehabilitation, 16*(3), 163–168.

Musselman, D. L., Tomer, A., Manatunga, A. K., et al. (1996). Exaggerated platelet reactivity in major depression. *American Journal of Psychiatry, 153*(10), 1313–1317.

National Center for Health Statistics. (1992). *Health United States.* Hyattsville, MD: Author.

National Center for Health Statistics. (1995). *Monthly Vital Statistics Report, 43*(1).

Nohria, A., Vaccarino, V., & Krumholtz, H. M. (1998). Gender differences in mortality after myocardial infarction. Why women fare worse than men. *Cardiology Clinics, 16*(1), 45–57.

O'Connor, N. J., Morton, J. R., Birkmeyer, J. D., et al. (1996). Effects of coronary artery diameter in patients undergoing coronary bypass surgery: Northern New England Cardiovascular Disease Study Group. *Circulation, 93*(4), 652–655.

Palmer, J. R., Rosenberg, L., & Shapiro, S. (1992). Reproductive factors and risk of myocardial infarction. *American Journal of Epidemiology, 136*(4), 408–416.

Papadopoulos, C., Beaumont, C., Shelley, S. I., et al. (1983). Myocardial infarction and sexual activity of the female patient. *Archives of Internal Medicine, 143*(8), 1528–1530.

Petrie, M. C., Dawson, N. F., Murdoch, D. R., et al. (1999). Failure of women's hearts. *Circulation, 49*(17), 2334–2341.

Randall, T. (1993). The gender gap in selection of cardiac transplantation candidates: Bogus or bias? *Journal of the American Medical Association, 269*(21), 2718–2720.

Rankin, S. H. (1990). Differences in recovery from cardiac surgery: A profile of male and female patients. *Heart and Lung, 19*(5, Pt. 1), 481–485.

Redberg, R. F. (1998). Preface to heart disease and women. *Cardiology Clinics, 16*(1), xii.

Rodin, J., & Isckovic, J. R. (1990). Women's health: Review and research agenda as we approach the 21st century. *American Journal of Psychology, 45*(9), 1018–1034.

Rossouw, J. E. (1996). Estrogens for prevention of coronary heart disease: Putting the brakes on the bandwagon. *Circulation, 94*(11), 2982–2985.

Rozanski, A., Bairey, C. N., Krantz, D. S., et al. (1988). Mental stress and the induction of silent myocardial ischemia in patients with coronary artery disease. *New England Journal of Medicine, 318*(16), 1005–1012.

Rozanski, A., Krantz, D. S., & Bairey, C. N. (1991). Ventricular responses to mental stress in patients with coronary artery disease. *Circulation, 83*(4, Suppl. II), II137–II144.

Salamone, L. M., Pressman, A. R., Seeley, D. G., et al. (1996). Estrogen replacement therapy: A survey of older women's attitudes. *Archives of Internal Medicine, 24*(12), 1293–1297.

Schoenbach, V. J., Kaplan, B. H., Fredman, L., et al. (1986). Social ties and mortality in Evan County, Georgia. *American Journal of Epidemiology, 123*(4), 577–591.

Scott, J. R., Wagoner, L. E., Olsen, S. L., et al. (1993). Pregnancy in heart transplant recipients: Management and outcome. *Obstetrics and Gynecology, 82*(3), 324–327.

Shapiro, P. A. (1996). Psychiatric aspects of cardiovascular disease. *Psychiatric Clinics of North America, 19*(3), 613–629.

Sharples, L. D., Caine, N., Mullins, D., et al. (1991). Risk factor analysis for the major hazards following heart transplantation, rejection, infection, and coronary occlusive disease. *Transplantation, 52*(2), 244–252.

Shekelle, R. B., Gale, M., & Norusis, M. (1985). Type A score (Jenkins Activity Survey) and risk of recurrent coronary heart disease in the Aspirin Myocardial Infarction Study. *American Journal of Cardiology, 56*(4), 221–225.

Sjoland, H., Caidahl, K., Karlson, B. W., et al. (1997). Limitation of physical activity, dyspnea, and chest pain before and two years after coronary artery bypass grafting in relation to sex. *International Journal of Cardiology, 61*(2), 123–133.

Sloan, R. P., Shapiro, P. A., Bigger, J. T., et al. (1994). Cardiac autonomic control and hostility in healthy subjects. *American Journal of Cardiology, 74*(3), 298–300.

Smith, T. W. (1992). Hostility and health: Current status of a psychosomatic hypothesis. *Health Psychology, 11*(3), 139–150.

Stampfer, M. J., Colditz, G. A., Willet, W. C., et al. (1991). Postmenopausal estrogen therapy and cardiovascular disease: Ten-year follow-up from the Nurses' Health Study. *New England Journal of Medicine, 325*(11), 756–762.

Stanford, J. L., Weiss, N. S., Voight, L. F., Daling, J. R., Habel, L. A., & Rossing, M. A. (1995). Combined estrogen and progestin hormone replacement therapy in relation to risk of breast cancer in middle-aged women. *Journal of the American Medical Association, 274*(2), 137–142.

Thomas, J. L., & Braus, P. A. (1998). Coronary artery disease in women: A historical perspective. *Archives of Internal Medicine, 158*(4), 333–337.

Toobert, D. S., Glasgow, R. E., & Radcliffe, S. V. (2000). Physiologic and related behavioral outcomes from the women's Lifestyle Heart Trial. *Annals of Behavioral Medicine, 22*(1), 1–9.

Travis, C. B., Gressley, D. L., & Phillippi, R. H. (1993). Medical decision making, gender, and coronary heart disease. *Journal of Women's Health, 2*(3), 269–279.

Troche, V., Ville, Y., & Fernandez, H. (1998). Pregnancy after heart or heart–lung transplantation: A series of 10 pregnancies. *British Journal of Obstetrics and Gynecology, 105*(4), 454–458.

Von der Recke, P., Hansen, M. A., & Hassager, C. (1999). The association between low bone mass at the menopause and cardiovascular mortality. *American Journal of Medicine, 106*(3), 273–278.

Weintraub, W. S., Kosinski, A. S., & Wenger, N. K. (1996). Is there a bias against performing coronary revascularization? *American Journal of Cardiology, 78*(10), 1154–1160.

Wingard, D. L., & Cohn, B. A. (1997). Coronary heart disease mortality among women in Alameda County, 1965–1973. In E. D. Eaker, B. Packard, & N. K., Wenger (Eds.), *Coronary heart disease in women.* New York: Haymarkey Doyma.

25

Gastrointestinal Disorders

THOMAS N. WISE
CATHERINE C. CRONE

Preoccupation with one's gastrointestinal system is a fundamental health concern. Individuals have always focused upon what they eat, what they excrete, and the subjective status of their gastrointestinal system. Purgatives were among the first medications utilized in ancient medicine. An early Egyptian medical treatise, dated at 1750 B.C., is devoted primarily to gastrointestinal difficulties. The Egyptian Pharaohs even appointed a court physician, named "Shepherd of the Anus," to treat their gastrointestinal difficulties (Wise, 1992). In modern medicine, gastrointestinal complaints are among the most common reasons individuals seek medical care. Clinicians must tolerate ambiguity in assessing gastrointestinal complaints in their patients, and must recognize that patients can have somatization phenomena as well as objective physiological dysfunction (Hyman, 2001). Many gastrointestinal complaints do not have clear organic etiologies, and the dichotomy between organic and psychological causes is often blurred. Kroenke and Mangelsdorff (1989) reported that only 16% of primary care patients with a new complaint were eventually documented to have an organic cause for their complaint, while only 10% were given a psychiatric diagnosis. Eleven percent of these patients presented with abdominal pain. Concurrently, more than 40% of gastroenterologists' patients are diagnosed with nonorganic or functional etiologies. Most of these patients have subthreshold psychiatric diagnoses (Mitchell & Drossman, 1987). Women have consistently been demonstrated to report more gastrointestinal symptoms than their male counterparts in ambulatory settings, even when one controls for the fact that women utilize more health services than males. Such gender disparities may be augmented by increased somatization phenomena in women. Wool and Barsky (1994) have reviewed possible explanations for such gender differences in somatization which include a somatization as an idiom for psychosocial distress. Women also appear to admit somatic discomfort more readily than men, and are more willing to seek medical attention. Furthermore, psychiatric disorders such as depression often present with prominent somatic symptoms (e.g., abdominal pain, constipation, or diarrhea) that involve the gastrointestinal tract, and many of these disorders are found more commonly in women. A higher prevalence of sexual abuse in women may also help to explain the difference. Finally, women, more than men, utilize the context and situation in which bodily sensations occur to judge how serious or dangerous a bodily symptom may be. Such contextual judgments may allow women to amplify such bodily sensations and give negative attributions to innocuous functional symptoms, and thereby may foster increased health care utilization.

Gender differences in gastrointestinal disorders vary. Irritable bowel syndrome (IBS) as well as gastroesophageal reflux disease (GERD) are more commonly reported in women, whereas rates of peptic ulcer disease appear equal between the genders (Ter, 2000). This chapter discusses common gastrointestinal disorders and reviews physiological, psychological, and treatment aspects, with particular attention to women's health.

DISORDERS OF TASTE AND SWALLOWING

Disorders of taste are increasingly recognized as conditions for which individuals seek medical or dental evaluations. Although there are no data indicating a gender bias, loss of taste perception increases with age and can be a result of normal aging, but it may also be caused by specific conditions (e.g., Alzheimer's disease or depression) that can modify one's sense of taste (Hoffman et al., 1998). Pernicious anemia or zinc deficiencies can alter gustatory perception as well. Drugs that cause taste difficulties include certain antibiotics, alcohol, flurazepam, and triazolam (Ackerman & Kasbekar, 1997). Due to anticholinergic effects, patients taking tricyclic antidepressants may experience dry mouth to such a degree that their sense of taste is compromised. Levenson (1985) has suggested that "dysgeusia," or abnormal taste sensations, may also be a conditioned adversive phenomenon. Specifically, if certain foods and tastes are paired with bouts of extreme nausea and vomiting, a protracted food aversion may develop. This phenomenan may occur when chemotherapy is introduced. Frequently, patients are told that they will experience extreme nausea and vomiting and are urged to have a meal of their favorite foods before such treatments are initiated, as they will not feel like eating for a number of weeks after therapy. This may well condition the patients to become nauseated whenever they have foods that they previously enjoyed. To best manage such situations, patients should be instructed to eat bland meals prior to the onset of any chemotherapy course that will induce nausea and vomiting.

The persistent belief that one has bad breath may indicate a serious psychological disorder. Goldberg et al. (1985) reported that psychological stressors, such as loss and separation, may be factors in patients with delusions of bad breath.

"Glossodynia," a burning sensation in the tongue, is a symptom that presents to both physicians and dentists. Glossodynia has been associated with personality traits of alexithymia and introversion, both of which complicate psychiatric management, since such patients often refuse to accept psychological factors that could complicate their medical situation (Miyoaka et al., 1996).

Although not confined to women, the fear of choking is a common complaint that may lead to avoidance of solid foods, pills, or fluids. McNally (1994) reviewed the literature on this disorder and found that two-thirds of such patients are women. The disorder may be found in patients with panic disorder and responds to antipanic medication, but it may also be a symptom of obsessive–compulsive disorder or social phobia. Fear of choking differs from globus hystericus, which is the sensation of a lump in the throat often found in generalized anxiety disorder. Either symptom may present to a gastroenterologist as "dysphagia," which denotes difficulty swallowing. Individuals who fear choking can swallow without difficulty unless they are swallowing the specific foods or pills. In patients with more generalized dysphagia, swallowing with an empty mouth is difficult.

GASTROESOPHAGEAL REFLUX DISEASE

Gastroesophageal reflux disease (GERD) is a common complaint characterized by substernal discomfort, commonly called "heartburn," which occurs postprandially and may also include bitter regurgitation. Generally, the condition is merely annoying, but persistent esophagitis due to gastric reflux may cause strictures or premalignant epithelial change. Bleeding due to such esophageal erosions and perforation may occur, though rarely. The syndrome may be caused by abnormal esophageal motility, hypotonicity of the lower esophageal sphincter, or delayed gastric emptying. If sufficiently symptomatic, GERD will affect an individual's quality of life. A recent report utilizing the Medical Outcome Study 36-Item Short-Form Health Survey found that both men and women with GERD had diminished levels of psychological well-being and physical and social functioning (Revicki et al., 1998).

Emotional stress and anxiety may alter esophageal sphincter tone, as well as motility of esophageal smooth muscles. The clinical result is that anxiety disorders are often found with symptoms suggestive of GERD. Clouse (1991) found that 84% of patients with esophageal motility disorders referred for esophageal testing had psychiatric disorders, most of which were anxiety disorders. The linkage between the two entities may be found in the neurochemical link between the central nervous system and neural pathways to the gastrointestinal tract. Low-dose trazodone was found to be helpful in these patients (Clouse, 1994).

Although GERD is found more commonly in men, women are especially vulnerable to the disorder during pregnancy or when they are taking oral contraceptives, which can lower esophageal sphincter tone. All hormonal contraceptives have been reported to lower sphincter tone. When GERD symptoms arise in a woman taking estrogen replacement therapy, the addition of progesterone may diminish the risk of reflux symptoms (van Thiel, 1979). During pregnancy, GERD symptoms occur in two-thirds of women and increase throughout the pregnancy (Borum, 1998; Chavan & Katz, 2001) A prior history of GERD appears to be a risk. Drug treatment is complicated by the potential for teratogenic effects upon the fetus. Thus treatment during pregnancy should initially emphasize nonpharmacological interventions. Medications must be carefully utilized. Antacids appear to be safe except for magnesium-containing preparations during the latter part of pregnancy, since the magnesium many slow down labor. H_2 blockers, such as cimetidine and ranitidine, may also be cautiously prescribed during the first trimester. Prokinetic drugs such as cisapride are not recommended in pregnancy unless all other methods fail.

The treatment of GERD includes nonpharmacological modifications of the patient's lifestyle, such as elevation of the head of the bed; smoking cessation; and dietary modifications to promote a low-fat, high-protein diet while avoiding acidic irritants, such as citric juices. The medical therapy includes use of promotility drugs that increase esophageal sphincter tone. Drugs such as cisapride may interact with psychotropic agents due to cytochrome P450 3A4 (CYP3A4) interaction, which could result in elevated levels of the prokinetic agent (Epstein et al., 1993). A variety of other medications should be avoided because they reduce esophageal sphincter tone and may promote esophageal reflux; these include anticholinergics, calcium channel blockers, theophylline, and nitrates.

Esophageal disorders may also be due to motility abnormalities (Clouse, 1997). Nonspecific spastic motility of the esophagus is often labeled "nutcracker esophagus" if there is an increase in contraction wave amplitudes during manometry. Symptoms of nutcracker esophagus may be similar to GERD, but are less predictable and not always linked with food or posture. These spastic disorders are linked with anxiety and mood disorders and respond to low doses of antidepressants such as trazodone or imipramine. The mechanism may be due to pain reduction rather than improvement of anxiety or depression.

OBESITY

Common in contemporary America, obesity is an independent risk factor for cardiovascular disease, diabetes, and premature mortality in both men and women. For women, the pursuit of thinness may be greater than for men, due to the cultural focus on the svelte feminine figure. The relationship between obesity and psychopathology in women continues to be debated. Epidemiological studies reveal no significant psychopathology in cohorts of individuals with obesity, while others find associations between elevated central fat distribution (particularly in the gluteofemoral area) and measures of psychopathology (such as depression, anxiety, psychotropic medication utilization, and sleep difficulties) (Wooley & Garner, 1994; Rosmond & Bjorntorp, 1998).

In contradistinction to large-scale epidemiological data, however, many studies find that individuals seeking weight reduction demonstrate frequent emotional disturbances. Whether obesity is the cause or the effect of these disturbances is not clear. Individuals with obesity are often viewed as lacking discipline or as awkward, and other studies have revealed that such individuals are less likely to be accepted into prestigious colleges or to achieve executive positions in their employment situations (Pargaman, 1969). A woman who is overweight may well be vulnerable to psychological distress, including depression, anxiety, low self-esteem, and continued abnormal body image perception, even when she is able to achieve and maintain a normative body weight (Brownell, 1984). A recent study suggests that women who are overweight feel more uncomfortable about seeking medical care for routine health maintenance, because they are sensitive about undressing or having their bodies observed. This discomfort may put them at increased risk for not receiving necessary breast examinations or gynecological follow-up, such as Pap smears (Fontaine et al., 1998). In a culture where pursuit of thinness is the norm, body image difficulties are common and may lead to bulimic behavior, as well as to anorexia nervosa.

Dieting is a ubiquitous phenomenon in America, with approximately 50% of women reporting that they are trying to lose weight at any given time (Williamson, 1996). Dieting may promote irritability, but also has obvious beneficial effects. Among the aspects of obesity management are the psychological consequences of dieting, weight loss, and subsequent regaining of weight (Foster et al., 1996). When individuals regain weight, depression, hopelessness, and despair may appear.

Pharmacotherapy for obesity has been particularly challenging. Recent serotonin-based anorexants, such as fenfluramine, demonstrate the inherent dangers of such drugs (Wadden et al., 1998). A new lipase inhibator, orlistat, may offer another strategy. However, the side effects of gastrointestinal complaints and frequent diarrhea may be particularly difficult for some individuals to manage. To date, restrained eating is the most reliable method of weight control, but may well have its own inherent stresses that can alter a woman's mental health.

Other issues in the treatment of weight gain that affect mental health include habituation to anorexant medication, such as dexedrine, that may concurrently treat a depressive disorder. Furthermore, the weight gain associated with commonly utilized antidepressants such as paroxetine or fluoxetine, may lead women to stop taking their medication and relapse into a depressive episode (Sussman & Ginsberg, 1998).

NAUSEA AND VOMITING

Queasiness, nausea, and vomiting are common symptoms in primary care among both men and women. Nausea during pregnancy is unique to women. Morning sickness occurs in 50–80% of pregnant women, and is thought to be caused by hormonal changes early in pregnancy (Broussard & Richter, 1998). In a small subset of women, however, prolonged and repeated emesis evolves into a serious condition termed "hyperemesis gravidarum." The symptoms of this syndrome include continual nausea and repeated vomiting, and create an inability to maintain a proper nutritional balance. This can lead to electrolyte imbalance, ketosis, and acetonuria, which if untreated may lead to renal or liver damage (goodwin, 1998). The onset of the disorder occurs in the first trimester, and it may recur in subsequent pregnancies. The differential diagnosis includes urinary tract infection, uremia, endocrine disorders, and other gastrointestinal conditions (such as peptic ulcer disease and pancreatitis). Vomiting may also be secondary to drugs, particularly iron supplements, which are abrasive to the gastric lining. The pathogenesis of hyperemesis has been attributed to both physiological and psychological factors (Frigo & Lang, 1998). Human chorionic gonadotropin has been demonstrated to stimulate the thyroid in patients with hyperemesis. Progesterone and cortisone have also been suggested as etiological factors. Esophageal dysmotility has been cited as a provocative factor (Torbey & Richter, 1995). Psychological theories have also been suggested to play a role in the syndrome (Fairweather, 1968). Ambivalence toward the pregnancy, and a stressful marriage/relationship or poor communication with the husband/partner, have been reported to be more frequent in women with hyperemesis. Furthermore, individuals with eating disorders, such as anorexia nervosa or bulimia nervosa, have also been found to be more likely to vomit frequently during pregnancy, although the association is not definitive (Fairburn et al., 1988).

The treatment of the disorder demands correction of metabolic imbalance, administration of intravenous fluids if necessary, and dietary behavioral modification utilizing frequent bland feedings (Nelson-Piercy, 1998). Thiamine and pyridoxine should also be utilized. Antiemetics will modify vomiting, but their benefits must be weighed against the risks of teratogenesis. Fortunately, dopamine antagonists such as metoclopramide, or histamine H_1 receptor blockers such as promethazine, are helpful. Recently methyl-prednisolone has been cited as potentially helpful in the treatment of hyperemesis (Safari et al., 1998). Psychological treatments are also useful as an adjunct to nutritional and metabolic supports. Behavioral therapy and hypnotherapy have been reported to be effective (Lub-Moss & Eurelings-Bontekow, 1997). Supportive therapy should include significant others with whom the patient lives. Often conflict with the spouse/partner or family aggravate the hyperemesis and malaise.

PEPTIC ULCER DISEASE

Approximately 10% of the U.S. population will develop peptic ulcer disease during their lifetimes (Lowe & Wolfe, 2001). Duodenal ulcers, associated with excess secretion of hydrochloric acid, differ from gastric ulcers, which have been linked to delays in gastric emptying. Duodenal ulcers are more frequent in males, whereas gastric ulcers have equal gender distribution (Chiba et al., 1998). Peptic ulcer disease, once believed to be the classic psychosomatic disorder, is now considered an infectious process due to *Helicobacter pylori*. Thus the connection between psychosocial issues and gastric or duodenal ulceration has received less recent research or clinical interest. In addition to *Helicobacter pylori*, other etiological factors include a genetic vulnerability to ulcer disease, as seen in those with blood group O (who have increased levels of pepsinogen, Type 1) and postprandial hypergastrinemia. Hyperpepsinogenemia, Type 1, has been thought to be transmitted via autosomal dominance, but recently there is a suggestion that *Helicobacter pylori* elevates serum pepsinogen levels, and the role of genetic transmission has been questioned (Raiha et al., 1998). Other factors include smoking, psychosocial stress, and increased use of analgesics. Gender differences for these stressors reveal that analgesic use is a greater vulnerability factor for men than for women (Ashley, 1997).

Despite organic factors in duodenal ulcer pathogenesis, there is increasing evidence that psychosocial issues remain a potential vulnerability factor (Levenstein, 1998). *Helicobacter pylori* infection is prevalent in many patients without ulcer disease and suggests a multiplicity of etiological factors, among which psychosocial issues are important. Levenstein et al. (1997) have demonstrated that lower socioeconomic status, lower education level, and psychological stress contribute to duodenal ulceration. In women, psychosocial stress may well mediate the potential for duodenal ulceration. A recent study demonstrates that depression and hostility continue to be associated with the presence of peptic ulcer disease, whereas anxiety has been linked to poor ulcer healing (Ashley, 1997). Treatment issues become important in such cases, as many of the standard medical treatments for ulcers may interact with psychotropic medication (Epstein et al., 1993). Cimetidine may elevate tricyclic levels, whereas ranitidine has no reported effects on tricyclic metabolism. Omeprazole may impair plasma clearance of benzodiazepines and thus elevate blood levels; this could foster drowsiness and limit fine motor skills for driving.

INFLAMMATORY BOWEL DISEASE

Inflammatory bowel disease is partitioned into two disorders: (1) ulcerative colitis, and Crohn's disease or regional enteritis. Women may develop Crohn's disease more frequently than men, whereas males develop ulcerative colitis as often as or more often than women (Tragnone et al., 1996). Although there are often mixed states, ulcerative colitis is generally limited to the mucosal and submucosa lining of the large intestine, with primary symptoms of diarrhea and bloody stools. In Crohn's disease, the process is transmural and may affect both large and small intestines. Intestinal obstruction, fistulae, and abscesses are common; these can lead to abdominal pain, infection, and severe weight loss. Crohn's disease has a chronic course with remissions and exacerbations, whereas ulcerative colitis may be "cured" following colectomy (Harpaz & Talbot, 1996). The risk of colonic cancer is elevated in both disorders.

There are few data to suggest that psychological issues are etiological factors in inflammatory bowel disease. Nevertheless, there is a significant prevalence of psychiatric disorders in patients with either Crohn's disease or ulcerative colitis. Helzer et al. (1982, 1984) found that in a cohort of patients with regional enteritis, 36% were depressed and 6% reported obsessive–compulsive symptoms. Drossman et al. (1989) found that the severity of the regional enteritis positively correlated with the psychiatric distress reported by the patients. Although reports were conflicting, these researchers also found that a comorbid psychiatric disorder affected recovery in patients with Crohn's disease, but not in patients with ulcerative colitis.

There is no evidence that a specific personality is linked to either ulcerative colitis or Crohn's disease. The special problems for both genders with inflammatory bowel disease are often secondary to the symptoms themselves, such as pain, malaise, arthritis, and malnutrition. The abdominal pain, vomiting, diarrhea, or nausea that leads to such malnutrition may create demoralization and adjustment reactions. Frequent hospitalizations may impair function and utilization of support systems at school or work. Various medications utilized for inflammatory bowel disease also have psychiatric effects. Corticosteroids have a dramatic effect on mood and can lead to either depression or euphoria, as well as insomnia. Concurrently, weight gain and cushingoid features can foster negative body image and lower self-esteem (Brydolf & Segesten, 1996). Nausea and vomiting, common symptoms in sulfasalazine therapy, can lead to malnutrition and malaise, and thus to demoralization. Higher doses of sulfasalazine and cyclosporine may cause delirium (Skeith & Russell, 1988). Finally, antibiotics are often utilized in inflammatory bowel disease; ciprofloxacin may impede the metabolic clearance of caffeine and thereby foster anxiety from increased caffeine levels. In cases of severe malnutrition, total parenteral nutrition is necessary. In such settings, vitamin deficiencies may cause organic brain syndromes that can present as depression or apathy.

Surgery is often necessary in severe inflammatory bowel disease. For ulcerative colitis, a single operation may be remarkable in eradicating the disease, whereas sufferers from regional enteritis may require multiple surgeries due to exacerbations of their illness. Such procedures may result in either an ileostomy or a colostomy. Patients may have difficulty managing such a change in their body image and react with shame, depression, and anger (Druss et al., 1972). Concerns about leakage or odor can lead to ruminative fears. Studies of psychological reactions to ostomies report that women experience more shame about their ostomies and avoid allowing their spouses/partners to view them (Druss et al., 1968). Sexual functioning can be compromised if vaginal fistulae occur with or without surgery. It is often useful for ostomy therapists to visit patients prior to surgery. Organizations such as the United Ostomy Association and the National Ileitis and Colitis Foundation offer education and support for patients with ostomies. These organizations can be important adjuncts to medical treatment, as they provide patient advocacy from individuals who have had personal experience with their own ostomies and can aid new patients in managing issues such as leakage, skin breakdown, and fear of odor. Newer surgical techniques, such as a continent ilestomy or anal pull-through, have improved the quality of life for patients with such procedures (Kennedy, 1988). Finally, it is essential for women who are facing such surgery to include their spouses/partners in preoperative consultation, if possible.

How to manage fertility and pregnancy is an important issue for women with inflammatory bowel disease (Korelitz, 1998). Women with inflammatory bowel disease are as fertile as those without such disorders (Hanan, 1998). Early reports suggesting subfertility in patients with ulcerative colitis or regional enteritis did not consider lowered libidinal factors, such as lack of desire for intercourse due to ability, perianal fistulae, or other factors. Drug therapy may also affect fertility in such patients; for example, sulfasalazine may lower sperm count and alter sperm motility, thereby inhibiting male fertility. Its effects on fertility in women are unknown.

Pregnancy does not appear to be affected by inflammatory bowel disease. Most women with these disorders are able to complete normal full-term pregnancies (Fonager et al., 1998). However, drugs commonly used for inflammatory bowel disease may complicate pregnancy (Modigliani, 1997). Corticosteroids do not seem to affect the fetus, although stopping this medication may lead to a recurrence of the inflammatory bowel disease. Sulfasalazine is also safe but may cause folate malabsorption; therefore, supplemental folate should be given. New oral formulations, such as mesalazine or asacol, appear to be safe at doses lower than 2 g per day. Immunosuppresive drugs, such as azathioprine, cross the placenta and can produce fetal abnormalities; therefore, such medicines are contraindicated during pregnancy. For women requiring total parenteral nutrition, the use of fat emulsions is controversial due to concern that the fat may embolize the placenta, resulting in either prematurity or miscarriage.

Another issue for patients with inflamatory bowel disease is the fear that the condition will be passed to their offspring. The lifetime risk of ulcerative colitis in the offspring of a parent with the disease is 11%, whereas for Crohn's disease the transmission rate varies from 0% to 15.8%. Individuals who are Jewish appear to have even higher rates. If both parents have inflammatory bowel disease, the risk is significantly higher (Parkes et al., 1997).

In summary, women with inflammatory bowel disease are at great risk for psychological difficulties. These difficulties stem from the direct effects of the disease, in that pain, diarrhea, abscesses and fistulae, and malnutrition will challenge one's mood and self-esteem. The treatments themselves may also either cause or provoke psychological symptoms. The clinician must address each of these issues and look at the various lifestyle changes each patient may make. For example, an adolescent girl who is facing an ostomy may have serious concerns about dating, whereas a very private older woman may find discussing issues such as changing ostomy appliances difficult in a group setting. Each will have unique challenges to her emotional equilibrium. It is essential that the clinician understand the disease, the patient, and her psychological issues.

IRRITABLE BOWEL SYNDROME

IBS is a common gastrointestinal condition, which accounts for 30–50% of patients in gastroenterology practices. Since many individuals with symptoms similar to IBS never seek medical treatment, those seen by physicians may have different illness behaviors and beliefs that foster help seeking. Women seek care for this syndrome two to three times more often than their male counterparts (Drossman et al., 1993). The disorder is characterized by alternating bowel habits, with abdominal pain relieved by defecation (Drossman, 1994). Abdominal bloating is frequently present. Sexual dysfunction has also been reported to be more common in those with IBS (Fass et al., 1998). Diminished drive and dyspareunia may create problems with significant others, as well as diminish quality of life. Thompson (1997) has studied gender differences in IBS and found that women report more mucus discharge, a sensation of incomplete evacuation, and abdominal distention than males do. Concurrent with such symptoms, women with IBS often complain of gastroesophageal reflux or lower pelvic pain that may suggest gynecological disorders (Walker et al., 1996). Abdominal pain is often a presenting complaint of IBS. Ectopic endometriosis may also cause abdominal complaints and may lead to misdiagnosis. The diagnosis is made when abdominal symptoms are routinely worse several days prior to the onset of menstrual flow. Individuals with IBS often report that certain foods make their symptoms worse and may view themselves as lactose-intolerant. Recent investigations have demonstrated that there is no increased incidence of lactose intolerance or other food allergies in those with IBS (Mascolo & Saltzman, 1998; Shaw & Davies, 1999).

Etiological factors in IBS include both physiological and psychological issues (Simren, Abrahamsson, et al., 2001). There is increasing evidence of a brain–gut connection that links the anterior cingulate gyrus and locus coeruleus to various gastroenteric nervous plexes (Cassileth & Drossman, 1993). This may explain the increased sensitivity of patients with IBS to fecal volume in the colon, as well as their altered gastric motility. Such connections may also explain why patients with panic disorder have higher rates of IBS, since the locus coeruleus is the neuroanatomical area involved in both panic disorder and IBS (Naliboff et al., 1998). Surveys of individuals with IBS demonstrate elevated rates of both anxiety and mood disorders (Lydiard et al., 1993). Individuals with IBS also have increased rates of sexual abuse; up to 50% of patients evaluated in tertiary care settings for IBS report early life physical or sexual trauma (Leserman et al., 1997). Life issues also may be important in the etiology and maintenance of IBS. Life stressors have been documented to increase rates of diarrhea and abdominal pain (Olden, 1998).

Treatment of patients with IBS must emphasize that minimizing the symptoms and coping with residual discomfort are the proper strategies (Gaynes & Drossman, 1999). Appropriate management mandates the investigation of the effects of irritable bowel upon the individual's life (Drossman & Thompson, 1992). Frequent diarrhea may foster social anxiety. Behavioral management of IBS symptoms, and attention to Axis I comorbidities, are strategies for treatment. These include behavioral diaries, with monitoring of the food ingested and the circumstances leading to increased symptomatology, as well as judicious psychopharmacology for anxiety and depressive disorders. Thus comorbidity with anxiety or depression can complicate the course of IBS and limit full functioning (Wise, 1992). Cognitive factors, such as a sense of helplessness, have been demonstrated to predict poor health outcomes (Drossman et al., 1998). Dietary interventions include increased fiber in the diet and avoidance of caffeine products and other foods known to cause symptoms. Psychotherapy that includes support and education can be delivered either in a primary care or a specialist setting. Mental health referrals are appropriate when a patient becomes dysfunctional or when the comorbid psychiatric disorder is serious.

Depending upon the symptoms, certain medications may be useful. For diarrhea-predominant syndromes, anticholinergic agents such as cyclomine and hyoscyamine can be used. Prokinetic medications, such as metoclopramide and cisapride, may help with constipation. Metoclopramide may cause lethargy that mandates dose reduction. Psychotropic agents can help not only with comorbid disorders, but with the abdominal pain associated with IBS. Tricyclics have been demonstrated to be helpful in diarrhea-predominant syndromes (Greenbaum et al., 1987). Serotonin reuptake inhibitors may also help decrease abdominal pain, but evidence has been limited to case reports. Benzodiazepines must be carefully administered because of their potential for abuse; however, buspirone may be useful due to its minimal effects upon gastrointestinal motility (Noyes et al., 1990).

LIVER DISEASE

Liver disease often presents with fatigue, malaise, nausea, and a sense of depression (if not overt depressed mood). Viral hepatitis is equally distributed between genders, although hepatitis E has a higher mortality among pregnant women. Agents utilized in treating viral hepatitis may cause psychiatric symptoms. Lamivudine can cause depression as a side effect, while α-2-interferon may cause depression or delirium. Acute fatty liver of pregnancy presents with nausea, vomiting, and abdominal pain, and can evolve into fulminate liver failure. The treatment is supportive, and drugs that are toxic to the liver must be avoided.

The liver is the organ that metabolizes many drugs. Thus the clinician must be aware of potential issues involved in drug–drug interactions that may elevate or lower medication levels, as well as drugs that may be toxic to the liver. For women, the drug interactions between oral contraceptives and a variety of drugs are very important (Back & Orme, 1990). Many antiepileptics, such as phenobarbital, phenytoin, and carbamazepine, may lower contraceptive levels and mandate higher doses or alternative modes of contraception (Chang & McAuley, 1998). Other medications (such as rifampin, an antituberculous drug) may also cause lowered contraceptive levels (Grange et al., 1994). Sodium valproate and gabapentin do not affect contraceptive steroid levels and can be used safely (Natsch et al., 1997).

Drug–drug interactions between antidepressants have been the topic of debate and the subject of many reviews (Owen & Nemeroff, 1998; Nemeroff et al., 1996). Sertraline and citalopram appear to have the least potential for interactions with other psychotropics, while venlafaxine, mitazepine, and bupropion appear to have minimal CYP450 interactions with most psychotropics as well as other medications. Nefazodone potently inhibits CYP3A4, and thus may raise cisapride levels as well as aprazolam levels (Alderman et al., 1997). Many psychotropic drugs are potentially toxic to the liver—either directly, in that they produce dose-related liver necrosis, or indirectly, in that the toxicity is idiopathic (Stoudemire et al., 1991). Carbamazepine may cause mild elevations of liver enzymes in 5–10% of patients, but also has been reported to cause allergic reactions (Vittorio & Muglia, 1995). Valproate also causes mild transaminase elevations in 12–12% of patients; this is usually dose-dependent (Konig et al., 1994) and occurs 2–3 months after therapy is initiated. Thus liver enzyme monitoring is necessary with both of these mood stabilizers, especially if patients have preexisting liver disease. Among the neuroleptics, chlorpromazine is the most hepatotoxic. The incidence of cholestatic jaundice induced by chlorpromazine is estimated at 0.5–2.0% (Stoudemire, 1995). Rare reports of antidepressant-induced liver damage exist. Tranylcypromine may rarely cause a hepatitis-like reaction. Tricyclics have been reported to raise transaminases, with rare cases of overt liver disease occurring.

CONCLUSIONS

Women who suffer from gastrointestinal disorders will have multiple factors that may cause or augment psychiatric disorders (Wise, 1974). The psychiatrist must partition the *impersonal* factors of the illness (such as the pain and discomfort of a disorder itself), from the *intrapsychic* variables (such as shame, regression, and mood changes) that are reactions or comorbid states. Finally, the *interpersonal* dimension may modify the individual's relationship with others. For example, a young woman with an ostomy may suffer from skin breakdown and irritation due to leakage of the ostomy (an impersonal issue), but may also experience depression from an altered self-image (an intrapsychic factor) and isolate herself from others due to fear of ostomy odor (an interpersonal dimension). It is the task of the physician to integrate all three of these issues into a comprehensive assessment of the patient and to develop a treatment plan that addresses them.

REFERENCES

Ackerman, B. H., & Kasbekar, N. (1997). Disturbances of taste and smell induced by drugs. *Pharmacotherapy, 17,* 482–496.

Alderman, J., Preskorn, S. H., Greenblatt, D. J., et al. (1997). Desipramine pharmacokinetics when coadministered with paroxetine or sertraline in extensive metabolizers. *Journal of Clinical Psychopharmacology, 17,* 284–291.

Ashley, M. J. (1997). Smoking and diseases of the gastrointestinal system: An epidemiological review withspecial reference to sex differences. *Canadian Journal of Gastroenterology, 11,* 345–352.

Back, D. J., & Orme, M. L. (1990). Pharmocokinetic drug interactions with oral contraceptives. *Clinical Pharmocokinetics, 18,* 472–484.

Borum, M. L. (1998). Gastrointestinal diseases in women. *Medical Clinics of North America, 82,* 21–50.

Broussard, C. N., Richter, J. E. (1998). Nausea and vomiting of pregnancy. *Gastroenterology Clinics of North America, 27,* 123–151.

Brownell, K. D. (1984). The psychology and physiology of obesity: Implications for screening and treatment. *Journal of the American Dietetic Association, 84,* 406–414.

Brydolf, M., & Segensten, K. (1996). Living with ulceratuve colitis: Experiences of adolescents and young adults. *Journal of Advanced Nursing, 23,* 39–47.

Cassileth, B. R., & Drossman, D. A. (1993). Psychosocial factors in gastrointestinal illness. *Psychotherapy and Psychosomatics, 59,* 131–143.

Chang, S. I., & McAuley, J. W. (1998). Pharmacotherapeutic issues for women of childbearing age with epilepsy. *Annals of Pharmacotherapy, 32,* 794–801.

Charan, M., & Katz, P. O. (2001). Gastroesophageal reflux disease in pregnancy. *Current Treatment Options in Gastroenterology, 4,* 73–81.

Chiba, N., Lahaie, R., Fedorak, R. N., (1998). *Helicobacter pylori* and peptic ulcer disease: Current evidence for management strategies. *Canadian Family Physician, 44,* 1481–1488.

Clouse, R. E. (1991). Psychiatric disorders in patients with esophageal disease. *Medical Clinics of North America, 75,* 1081–1096.

Clouse, R. E. (1994). Antidepressants for functional gastrointestinal syndromes. *Digestive Diseases and Sciences, 39,* 2352–2363.

Clouse, R. E. (1997). Spastic disorders of the esophagus. *Gastroenterologist, 5,* 112–127.

Drossman, D. A. (1994). Irritable bowel syndrome. *Gastroenterologist, 2,* 315–326.

Drossman, D. A., Li, Z., Andruzzi, E., et al. (1993). U.S. householder survey of functional gastrointestinal disorders: Prevalence, sociodemography, and health impact. *Digestive Diseases and Sciences, 38,* 1569–1580.

Drossman, D. A., Li, Z., Leserman, J., et al. (1997). Association of coping pattern and health status among female GI patients after controlling for GI disease type and abuse history: A prospective study. *Gastroenterology, 112,* 724.

Drossman, D. A., McKee, D. C., Sandler, R. S., et al. (1988). Psychosocial factors in the irritable bowel syndrome: A multivariate study of patients and nonpatients with irritable bowel syndrome. *Gastroenterology, 95,* 701–708.

Drossman, D. A., Patrick, D. L., Mitchell, C. M., et al. (1989). Health-related quality of life in inflammatory bowel disease. Functional status and patient worries and concerns. *Digestive Diseases and Sciences, 34,* 1379–1386.

Drossman, D. A., & Thompson, W. G. (1992). The irritable bowel syndrome: Review and a graduated multicomponent treatment approach. *Annals of Internal Medicine, 116,* 1009–1016.

Druss, R. G., O'Connor, J. F., Prudden, J. F., et al. (1968). Psychologic response to colectomy. *Archives of General Psychiatry, 18,* 53–59.

Druss, R. G., O'Connor, J. F., & Stern, L. O. (1972). Changes in body image following ileostomy. *Psychoanalytic Quarterly, 41,* 195–206.

Epstein, S. A., Wise, T. N., & Goldberg, R. L. (1993). Gastroenterology. In A. Stoudemire & B. S. Fogel (Eds.), *Psychiatric care of the medical patient* (pp. 611–626). New York: Oxford University Press.

Fairburn, C. G., Stein, A., & Jones, R. (1988). Eating habits and eating disorders during pregnancy. *Psychosomatic Medicine, 54,* 665–672.

Fairweather, D. V. (1968). Nausea and vomiting in pregnancy. *American Journal of Obstetrics and Gynecology, 102,* 135–175.

Fass, R., Fullerton, S., Naliboff, B., et al. (1998). Sexual dysfunction in patients with irritable bowel syndrome and non-ulcer dyspepsia. *Digestion, 59,* 79–85.

Fonager, K., Sorensen, H. T., Olsen, J., et al. (1998). Pregnancy outcome for women with Crohn's disease: A follow-up study based on linkage between national registries. *American Journal of Gastroenterology, 93,* 2426–2430.

Fontaine, K. R., Faith, M. S., Allison, D. B., et al. (1998). Body weight and health care among women in the general population. *Archives of Family Medicine, 7,* 381–384.

Foster, G. D., Wadden, T. A., Kendall, P. C., et al. (1996). Psychological effects of weight loss and regain: A prospective evaluation. *Journal of Consulting and Clinical Psychology, 64,* 752–757.

Frigo, P., Lang, C., Reisenberger, K., et al. (1998). Hyperemesis gravidarum associated with *Helicobacter pylori* seropositivity. *Obstetrics and Gynecology, 91,* 615–617.

Gaynes, B. N., & Drossman, D. A. (1999). The role of the mental health professional in the assessment and management of irritable bowel syndrome. *CNS Spectrums, 4,* 19–30.

Goldberg, R. L., Buongiorno, P. A., & Henkin, R. I. (1985). Delusions of halitosis. *Psychosomatics, 26,* 325–331.

Goodwin, T. M. (1998). Hyperemesis gravidarum. *Clinical Obstetrics and Gynecology, 41,* 597–605.

Grange, J. M., Winstanley, P. A., & Davies, P. D. (1994). Clinically significant drug interactions with antituberculosis agents. *Drug Safety, 11,* 242–251.

Greenbaum, D. S., Mayle, J. E., & Vanegeren, L. E. (1987). The effects of desimipramine on IBS compared with atropine and placebo. *Digestive Diseases and Sciences, 32,* 257–266.

Hanan, I. M. (1998). Inflammatory bowel disease in the pregnant woman. *Comprehensive Therapy, 24,* 409–414.

Harpaz, N., & Talbot, I. C. (1996). Colorectal cancer in idiopathic inflammatory bowel disease. *Seminars in Diagnostic Pathology, 13,* 339–357.

Helzer, J. E., Chammas, S., Norland, C. C., et al. (1984). A study of the association between Crohn's disease and psychiatric illness. *Gastroenterology, 86,* 324–330.

Helzer, J. E., Stillings, W. A., Chammas, S., et al. (1982). A controlled study of the association between ulcerative colitis and psychiatric diagnoses. *Digestive Diseases and Sciences, 27,* 513–518.

Hoffman, H. J., Ishii, E. K., & MacTurk, R. H. (1998). Age-related changes in the prevalence of smell/taste problems among the United States adult population: Results of the 1994 disability supplement to the National Health Interview Survey (NHIS). *Annals of the New York Academy of Sciences, 855,* 716–722.

Hyman, P. E. (2001). Functional gastrointestinal disorders and the biopsychosocial model of practice. *Journal of Pediatric Gastroenterology and Nutrition, 32,* S5–S7.

Kennedy, H. J. (1988). Quality of life in patients with an ileostomy. *International Disability Studies, 10,* 175–176.

Konig, S. A., Siemes, H., Blaker, F., et al. (1994). Severe hepatotoxicity during valproate therapy: An update and report of eight new fatalities. *Epilepsia, 35,* 1005–1015.

Korelitz, B. I. (1998). Inflammatory bowel disease and pregnancy. *Gastroenterology Clinics of North America, 27,* 213–224.

Kroenke, K., & Mangelsdorff, A. D. (1989). Common symptoms in ambulatory care: Incidence, evaluation, therapy, and outcome. *American Journal of Medicine, 86,* 262–266.

Leserman, J., Li, Z., Drossman, D. A., et al. (1997). Impact of sexual and physical abuse dimensions on health status: Development of an abuse severity measure. *Psychosomatic Medicine, 59,* 152–160.

Levenson, J. L. (1985). Dysosmia and dysgeusia presenting as depression. *General Hospital Psychiatry, 7,* 171–173.

Levenstein, S. (1998). Stress and peptic ulcer: Life beyond *Helicobacter. British Medical Journal, 316,* 538–541.

Levenstein, S., Kaplan, G. A., & Smith, M. W. (1997). Psychological predictors of peptic ulcer incidence in the Alameda County study. *Journal of Clinical Gastroenterology, 24,* 140–146.

Lowe, R. C., & Wolfe, M. M. (2001). Acid-peptic disorders, gastritis, and *Hericobacter pylori.* In J. Noble (Ed.), *Textbook of primary care medicine* (3rd ed., p. 910). St. Louis, MO: Mosby.

Lub-Moss, M. M., & Eurelings-Bontekoe, E. H. (1997). Clinical experience with patients suffering from hyperemesis gravidarum (severe nausea and vomiting during pregnancy): Thoughts about subtyping of patients, treatment and counseling models. *Patient Education and Counseling, 31,* 65–75.

Lydiard, R. B., Fossey, M. D., Marsh, W., et al. (1993). Prevalence of psychiatric disorders in patients with irritable bowel syndrome. *Psychosomatics, 34,* 229–234.

Mascolo, R., & Saltzman, J. R. (1998). Lactose intolerance and irritable bowel syndrome. *Nutrition Reviews, 56,* 306–308.

McNally, R. J. (1994). Choking phobia: A review of the literature. *Comprehensive Psychiatry, 35,* 83–89.

Mitchell, C. M., & Drossman, D. A. (1987). Survey of the AGA membership relating to patients with functional gastrointestinal disorders. *Gastroenterology, 92,* 1282–1284.

Miyoaka, H., Kamijima, K., Katayama, Y., et al. (1996). A psychiatric appraisal of "glossodynia." *Psychosomatics, 37,* 346–348.

Modigliani, R. (1997). Drug therapy for ulcerative colitis during pregnancy. *European Journal of Gastroenterology and Hepatology, 9,* 854–857.

Naliboff, B. D., Munakata, J., Chang, L., et al. (1998). Toward a biobehavioral model of visceral hypersensitivity in irritable bowel syndrome. *Journal of Psychosomatic Research, 45,* 485–492.

Natsch, S., Hekster, Y. A., Keyser, A., et al. (1997). Newer anticonvulsant drugs: Role of pharmacology, drug interactions and adverse reactions in drug choice. *Drug Safety, 17,* 228–240.

Nelson-Piercy, C. (1998). Treatment of nausea and vomiting in pregnancy: When should it be treated and what can be safely taken? *Drug Safety, 19,* 155–164.

Nemeroff, C. B., DeVane, C. L., & Pollock, B. G. (1996). Newer antidepressants and the cytochrome P450 system. *American Journal of Psychiatry, 153,* 311–320.

Noyes, R. J., Cook, B., Garvey, M., et al. (1990). Reduction of gastrointestinal symptoms following treatment for panic disorder. *Psychosomatics, 31,* 71–75.

Olden, K. W. (1998). Are psychosocial factors of aetiological importance in functional dyspepsia? *Baillière's Clinical Gastroenterology, 12,* 557–571.

Owen, J. R., & Nemeroff, C. B. (1998). New antidepressants and the cytochrome P450 system: Focus on venlafaxine, nefazodone, and mirtazapine. *Depression and Anxiety, 7*(Suppl. 1), 24–32.

Parkes, M., Satsangi, J., & Jewell, D. Mapping susceptibility loci in inflammatory bowel disease: Why and how? *Molecular Medicine Today, 3,* 546–553.

Raiha, I., Kemppainen, H., Kaprio, J., et al. (1998). Lifestyle, stress, and genes in peptic ulcer disease: A nationwide twin cohort study. *Archives of Internal Medicine, 158,* 698–704.

Revicki, D. A., Wood, M., Maton, P. N., et al. (1998). The impact of gastroesophageal reflux disease on health-related quality of life. *American Journal of Medicine, 104,* 252–258.

Rosmond, R., & Bjorntorp, P. (1998). Psychiatric ill-health of women and its relationship to obesity and body fat distribution. *Obesity Research, 6,* 338–345.

Safari, H. R., Fassett, M. J., Souter, I. C., et al. (1998). The efficacy of methylprednisolone in the treatment of hyperemesis gravidarum: A randomized, double-blind, controlled study. *American Journal of Obstetrics and Gynecology, 179,* 921–924.

Shaw, A. D., & Davies, G. J. (1999). Lactose intolerance: Problems in diagnosis and treatment. *Journal of Clinical Gastroenterology, 28,* 208–216.

Simren, M., Abrahamsson, H., Svedlund, J., et al. (2001). *Scandinavian Journal of Gastroenterology, 36,* 545–552.

Skeith, K. J., & Russell, A. S. (1988). Adverse reaction to sulfasalazine. *Journal of Rheumatology, 15,* 529–230.

Stoudemire, A. (1995). Expanding psychopharmacologic treatment options for the depressed medical patient. *Psychosomatics, 36,* S19–S26.

Stoudemire, A., Moran, M. G., & Fogel, B. S. (1991). Psychotropic drug use in the medically ill: Part II. *Psychosomatics, 32,* 34–46.

Sussman, N., & Ginsberg, D. (1998). Weight gain associated with SSRIs. *Primary Psychiatry, 4,* 28–38.

Ter, R. B. (2000). Gender differences in gastroesophageal reflux disease. *Journal of Gender Specific Medicine, 3,* 42–44.

Thompson, W. G. (1997). Gender differences in irritable bowel symptoms. *European Journal of Gastroenterology and Hepatology, 9,* 299–302.

Torbey, C. F., & Richter, J. E. (1995). Gastrointestinal motility disorders in pregnancy. *Seminars in Gastrointestinal Diseases, 6,* 203–221.

Tragnone, A., Corrao, G., Miglio, F., et al. (1996). Incidence of inflammatory bowel disease in Italy: A nationwide population-based study. Gruppo Italiano per lo Studio del Colon e del Retto (GISC). *International Journal of Epidemiology, 25,* 1044–1052.

Van Thiel, D. H., Gavaler, J. S., & Stremple, J. F. (1979). Lower esophageal sphincter pressure during the normal menstrual cycle. *American Journal of Obstetrics and Gynecology, 134,* 64–67.

Vittorio, C. C., Muglia, J. J. (1995). Anticonvulsant hypersensitivity syndrome. *Archives of Internal Medicine, 155,* 2285–2290.

Wadden, T. A., Berkowitz, R. I., Silvestry, F., et al. (1998). The fen–phen finale: A study of weight loss and valvular heart disease. *Obesity Research, 6,* 278–284.

Walker, E. A., Gelfand, A. N., Gelfand, M. D., et al. (1996). Chronic pelvic pain and gynecological symptoms in women with irritable bowel syndrome. *Journal of Psychosomatic Obstetrics and Gynecology, 17,* 39–46.

Williamson, D. F. (1996). "Weight cycling" and mortality: How do the epidemiologists explain the role of intentional weight loss? *Journal of the American College of Nutrition, 15,* 6–13.

Wise, T. N. (1974). The emotional reactions of chronic illness. *Primary Care, 1,* 373–382.

Wise, T. N. (1992). Psychiatric management of functional gastrointestinal disorders. *Psychiatric Annals, 22,* 1–6.

Wool, C. A., & Barsky, A. J. (1994). Do women somatize more than men?: Gender differences in somatization. *Psychosomatics, 35,* 445–452.

Wooley, S. C., & Garner, D. M. (1994). Controversies in management: Should obesity be treated? Dietary treatments for obesity are ineffective. *British Medical Journal, 309,* 655–656.

26

HIV/AIDS

SARAH E. HERBERT
PAMELA BACHANAS

Psychiatric consultation can be a vital and essential part of care for the HIV-infected woman. Physicians who treat women with HIV/AIDS may request psychiatric consultation for a number of reasons. Patients may be overwhelmed by grief at the diagnosis of HIV/AIDS or the progression of the disease. Individuals previously diagnosed with major mood disorders, psychoses, or substance use disorders may experience an exacerbation of symptoms when told of their condition or when their medical condition worsens. Treatment of these psychiatric disorders may be necessary in order to facilitate optimal medical management of the HIV disease. Psychiatric disorders that may be consequences of the disease, such as AIDS-related dementia or organic mood/psychotic disorders, require diagnosis and appropriate treatment as well. In addition, assistance may be sought from the psychiatric consultant in evaluating the impact of dementia or psychiatric illness on a patient's cognitive abilities, her ability to care for herself or her children, or her capacity to give informed consent for treatment.

EPIDEMIOLOGY OF HIV/AIDS IN WOMEN

Women represent an increasing proportion of AIDS cases. The proportion of all AIDS cases reported among adult and adolescent women more than tripled from 7% in 1985 to 23% in 1999 (Centers for Disease Control and Prevention [CDC], 2001). The annual incidence of AIDS in women began to decline in 1996, most likely due to the efficacy of antiretroviral drugs (CDC, 2001). Reported AIDS cases, however, do not give a clear picture of the extent of the epidemic. The time from infection with HIV until the development of AIDS may extend 10 years or longer. The incidence of HIV infection and the prevalence of women who are seropositive are important statistics that will provide information on the extent of the epidemic among women, but this is more difficult information to collect.

Injection drug use (IDU) appeared to be the largest risk factor for women in the initial surveillance of the AIDS epidemic, accounting for more than 40% of women with AIDS. The significance of this risk factor has declined; from July, 1998 to June, 1999 only 29% of AIDS cases in females were attributed to IDU (CDC, 2000a; see Figure 26.1). The percentage of women diagnosed with AIDS during this same time period who were infected through heterosexual contact was 40%. The percentage attributed to hemophilia (<1%) and infected blood or blood products (1%) has always been quite low (CDC, 2000b). There was a large group of women (31%) for whom the exposure category was unknown or not yet identified; this commonly occurs in newly reported cases (CDC, 2000a; see Figure 26.1). In order to deal with this phenomenon, an estimated AIDS incidence was calculated based on historical patterns of risk distribution and reclassification due to delays in reporting. The chart on the right in Figure 26.1 is considered to be a more accurate depiction of the AIDS incidence by risk category (CDC, 2000a). Heterosexual contact is considered to be a much more substantial risk factor, accounting for an estimated of 62% of newly diagnosed cases of AIDS. IDU is also estimated to account for a larger percentage of cases (36%), but substantially less than heterosexual contact. This estimate reduced the unidentified or other category of risk to 1%. Thus, the greatest increase in AIDS incidence rates by mode of transmission has been that attributable to heterosexual contact, particularly among the group of women who were in their middle to late teens in the late 1980s (Wortley & Fleming, 1997).

There are striking differences in the rates of AIDS among adult/adolescent women in the United States based on race and ethnicity (CDC, 2000a, 2000b, 2001; see Table 26.1). A fact sheet on HIV/AIDS among U.S. women (CDC, 2001) reported that African American and Hispanic women accounted for more than three-fourths of AIDS cases reported through 1999 in this country, and yet together they represented fewer than one-

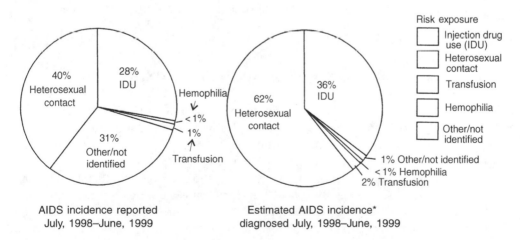

FIGURE 26.1. AIDS cases in adult/adolescent women, reported July, 1998–June, 1999, and estimated AIDS incidence, diagnosed July, 1998–June, 1999, by risk exposure, United States. *Data adjusted for reporting delays and estimated proportional redistribution of cases initially reported without risk. Data reported through March, 2000. From CDC (2000a).

TABLE 26.1. AIDS Cases and Rates in Adult/Adolescent Women, by Race/Ethnicity, Reported in 1999, United States

Race/ethnicity	Number	Percent	Rate per 100,000
White, not Hispanic	1,924	18	2
Black, not Hispanic	6,784	63	49
Hispanic	1,948	18	15
Asian/Pacific Islander	63	1	1
American Indian/Alaska Native	40	< 1	5
Total[a]	10,780	100	9

Note. From CDC (2000a).
[a]Includes 21 women of unknown race/ethnicity.

fourth of all U.S. women. The rate reported in 1998 for white, non-Hispanic women is 2 per 100,000, significantly below the rate of 50 per 100,000 for Black non-Hispanic women, and 17 per 100,000 for Hispanic women (CDC, 1999). The number of AIDS cases and rates per 100,000 women are lowest among Asian/Pacific Islanders and American Indian/Alaskan natives.

In addition to race/ethnicity, geographic location also contributed to very different rates of AIDS in women, with the highest percentages occurring in the Northeast and the South and much lower percentages occurring in the Midwest and West. CDC surveillance data (CDC, 2000b, 2001) suggest that the number of AIDS cases in women, especially in those from the South, in those infected heterosexually, and in women of color will continue to grow. Young women from these groups will be at risk for HIV infection as they reach adolescence and young adulthood. It is also important for mental health clinicians to recognize that homeless persons with mental illness are becoming another at-risk category (Kalichman et al., 1994). Severely mentally ill individuals who live in New York City and other urban areas have a high prevalence of HIV seropositivity. Up to 23% of homeless mentally ill persons who also use substances are HIV-infected (Otto-Salaj et al., 1998).

MEDICAL ASPECTS OF HIV/AIDS IN WOMEN

AIDS-related deaths among women are now decreasing due to advances in treatment of the disease, but HIV/AIDS still remains one of the leading causes of death for U.S. women in the age group 25–44 years. Among African American women in this same age group, AIDS is the third leading cause of death (Hader et al., 2001).

Manifestations of HIV infection in women and the course of the disease have not been as systematically studied as they have been for homosexual or bisexual men. However, the available literature suggests that many of the manifestations of HIV/AIDS and AIDS-defining conditions are similar for men and women, particularly when mode of transmission and race/ethnicity are controlled for (Hader et al., 2001). There is some evidence that access to care and survival times may be different for women and men. In addition, there do not appear to be significant gender differences in the progression of the disease from HIV infection to AIDS. The data on survival time are more equivocal. Some studies have found shortened survival times for women, but others have not, particularly when efforts have been made to control for confounding variables (Smith & Moore, 1996). The confounding variables that may explain differences in survival times have included differences in the quality of care received by men and women. Women are often diagnosed late in the illness and are less likely to use early intervention therapies. Since women with HIV/AIDS often come from minority communities living in poverty, there may be a lack of access to early intervention therapies. As noted later in the chapter, however, they may not be using early intervention therapies due to the multiple other responsibilities in their lives that receive higher priority than their health care.

Medical issues involving female reproductive function are significant for HIV-positive women. These include gynecological conditions such as vaginal candidiasis, human papillomavirus (HPV) infection, and cervical dysplasia. HPV lesions in HIV-positive women are more prevalent, more persistent, and found in multiple locations (vagina, cervix, vulva), thus making them more difficult to treat than in HIV-negative women (Hader et al., 2001; Kuhn et al., 1999; Smith & Moore, 1996; Sun et al., 1997). Invasive cervical carcinoma is the one AIDS-defining condition specific to women. It was included because of the high prevalence of HPV infections and cervical intraepithelial neoplasia among HIV-positive women, and the known association between these and cervical cancer. In the data initially available, increased rates of invasive cervical cancer or death had not been found among HIV-positive women (Smith & Moore, 1996). Now there does appear to be evidence emerging to suggest there are increased rates of cervical cancer among HIV-positive women (Del Mistro et al., 2001; Hader et al., 2001; Serraino et al., 1999).

The severity and location of mucosal candidiasis in women appears to be correlated with the degree of immunosuppression due to HIV disease. Women with early HIV infection may have recurrent and chronic vaginal candidiasis, compared to the episodic type found in uninfected women. Oral candidiasis may be associated with moderate immunosuppression in women, and esophageal candidiasis with marked immunosuppression (Smith & Moore, 1996).

Childbearing is another vitally important issue for HIV-positive women and their health care providers. Women with HIV who become pregnant may transmit the virus to their children. Early reports estimated that the rate of mother-to-child transmission of HIV was in the 14–40% range (Blanche et al., 1989). The results of Pediatric AIDS Clinical Trials Group Protocol 076, which assessed the impact of zidovudine on transmission rates, reported a significant decline in transmission when women were given zidovudine during pregnancy and delivery, and zidovudine was given postpartum to newborns (Sperling et al., 1996). The increased use of zidovudine and other antiretroviral therapies during pregnancy, delivery, and the postpartum period, combined with changes in the conduct and management of labor and delivery in HIV-infected pregnant women (Lindsay & Nesheim, 1997), have resulted in a significant decline in transmission rates. Furthermore, it is now known that advanced maternal disease (e.g., development of clinical symptoms, decreased CD4 count, and increased viral burden) correlates with transmission (European Collaborative Study, 1992). The effect of pregnancy on HIV disease progression was initially of concern, since women normally experience a mild form of immunosuppression in pregnancy. There does not appear, however, to be an independent effect of pregnancy worsening HIV disease (Smith & Moore, 1996).

MENTAL HEALTH ISSUES

Psychiatric consultation is often sought when emotional distress or psychiatric symptoms suggest the need for evaluation and treatment. Psychiatrists and other mental health clinicians can assist in the identification of disorders of affect, behavior, and cognition, and can evaluate their impact on an individual's functioning. They can make recommendations for appropriate treatments that incorporate biopsychosocial strategies (Halman, 1999). Finally, psychiatrists can consult with primary care providers regarding the utilization of antiretrovirals to address deficits in brain function.

Psychiatrists can play an important role in the care of patients with HIV/AIDS who have neuropsychiatric complications. Since HIV is a neurotropic virus that enters the central nervous system (CNS) soon after the initial infection, some neuropsychiatric symptoms are clinical manifestations of this viral infection (McDaniel et al., 1997; Perry, 1990). Opportunistic infections or neoplasms of the CNS are also seen in immuno-compromised individuals, and these medical conditions characteristic of patients with HIV/AIDS may initially present with neuropsychiatric symptoms. In addition, side effects of the medications used to treat HIV/AIDS include symptoms of mood disorders, such as mania (Atkinson & Grant, 1994). Neurocognitive syndromes associated with HIV include minor motor cognitive disorder, HIV-associated dementia, and delirium.

Differential Diagnoses

Careful consideration must be given to differential diagnoses, both medical and psychiatric. The psychiatric consultant is faced with the complex task of distinguishing among preexisting psychiatric illness, the emotional reaction seen in response to the diagnosis or manifestations of HIV/AIDS, substance-induced symptoms, medication side effects, psychiatric symptoms associated with opportunistic infections or neoplasms of the CNS, systemic and metabolic complications, and neurocognitive disorders. Appropriate workups should be undertaken to rule out medical etiologies for symptoms. Delirium may result from any number of systemic or metabolic complications (e.g., sepsis, fever, hypoxia, and hepatic encephalopathy), but it may also result from substance misuse or medication-induced alterations in mental status. Major depressive disorder and HIV-associated dementia may resemble each other, since apathy, anhedonia, withdrawal, anergia, inattention, and dysphoria can be associated with either diagnosis. Distinguishing between the two is important, since one would treat major depressive disorder differently and expect a more positive outcome than for HIV-associated dementia. Psychosis may be a primary psychiatric disorder; it may be secondary to the effects of HIV; it may be due to other infections or lesions in the CNS; or it may be a complication of antiretroviral medications. Once the etiology of psychiatric symptoms has been determined, appropriate intervention should be instituted promptly. This will improve the chance that neuropsychiatric symptoms will resolve and women with HIV/AIDS will have a better quality of life.

Stage of Illness

The individual's stage of HIV disease may affect both the presentation and etiology of symptoms. For example, symptoms that occur when the individual is first diagnosed may be related to a lack of knowledge about the disease. Women who are not well informed may experience an overwhelming sense of grief and loss, along with the expectation that their death is imminent. Patients who have had knowledge of their seropositive status for many years may only experience the emotional impact of the diagnosis and have an emotional crisis when physical symptoms become manifest, or when their medical condition suggests a need to begin antiretroviral therapy. At end stage, women may experience distress over their loss of functioning or impending death, or they may experience changes in mood or mental status due to advanced HIV disease. Psychiatric management of these symptoms becomes critical in maintaining optimal quality of life for women with AIDS.

Psychiatric Disorders

Initially, little attention was paid to the psychological functioning of women with HIV/AIDS. The earliest reports on the prevalence of psychiatric disorders had small numbers of women subjects, were convenience samples, and did not generally have an HIV-negative control group (Brown & Rundell, 1990; James, 1988). As women have begun to make up a larger percentage of HIV-positive individuals, more attention has been paid to the prevalence of psychiatric disorders in this group, but data are still limited (McDaniel et al., 1995; Siegel et al., 1998). Thus it has been difficult to generalize from small samples to the population of women with HIV/AIDS as a whole.

Mood Disorders

Mood disorders, especially depressive disorders, appear to be the most prevalent psychiatric disorders among individuals with HIV/AIDS (Perkins et al., 1994; Rabkin et al., 1999). Since the prevalence of depression is high for women in general, one would expect to see a high rate of depression among women with HIV. Recent evidence suggests that HIV-infected women in fact show a higher than expected rate of depressive symptoms, compared to women in general (Siegel et al., 1998). Bipolar and depressive disorders have been associated with HIV as primary major mood disorders or as mood disorders secondary to HIV (Lyketsos et al., 1993; McDaniel et al., 1997; Perry, 1990). Manic syndromes may affect as many as 8% of patients with AIDS. They tend to occur late in the course of the illness, may be associated with significant cognitive and motor impairment, and generally indicate the need for aggressive intervention (McDaniel et al., 1997). Mood disorders may also commonly be associated with dependence on or abuse of substances. HIV seropositivity appears to be an additional risk factor for the known association between mood disorders and substance dependence. Rabkin et al. (1997) found an elevated rate of mood disorders among HIV-positive men and women with IDU, compared to an HIV-negative control group. Use of antiretroviral medications has been associated with symptoms of a mood disorder as well (Atkinson & Grant, 1994). In particular, zidovudine has been associated with the development of manic symptoms (Janicak, 1995; Whitaker, 1999).

Psychotic Disorders

Psychosis in a person with HIV/AIDS may be due to a preexisting mental illness, or it may be related to HIV/AIDS itself. Chronically mentally ill individuals engage in behaviors that lead to increased risk for HIV infection, such as using condoms less frequently;

engaging in sexual activity while abusing substances; having sex with individuals who engage in IDU; and bartering sex for food, clothing, or shelter (Kalichman et al., 1994; Otto-Salaj et al., 1998). Consequently, a large number of individuals with chronic mental illness are also HIV-infected. The prevalence of HIV seropositivity varied from 4% to 23% when psychiatric patients in the northeastern United States were studied (American Psychiatric Association Commission on AIDS, 1999). The onset of psychotic symptoms in individuals with no previous evidence of psychiatric illness has been described as a manifestation of AIDS, presumably due to the CNS effects of HIV (Atkinson & Grant, 1994; Harris et al., 1991; Sewell et al., 1994a). The appearance of psychotic symptoms tends to occur later in the course of the illness and is considered a poor prognostic sign (Sewell et al., 1994a). There are case reports, however, in which psychotic symptomatology has been the first manifestation of AIDS. There are few or no data about the vulnerability of women to psychosis in comparison to men.

HIV-Associated Neurocognitive Disorders: Dementia, Delirium, and Minor Motor Cognitive Disorder

Dementia associated with HIV disease is the most frequent neurological complication of AIDS, especially in the later stages of the illness. A prevalence of 60% had initially been described, but more recent prospective data suggest a prevalence of 15% by the time of death (Halman, 1999; McArthur et al., 1993; McDaniel et al., 1997). It is not known whether the prevalence of dementia and risk factors for developing this condition are the same in men and women.

HIV-related dementia is a subcortical dementia that presents as a slowing down process with impairments in affect, behavior, cognition, and motor function. Affective changes include dysphoria, apathy, and anergia. Behavior may be either withdrawn or (in some cases) disinhibited. Cognitive effects may be manifested as inattention and poor new learning. Dyscontrol is present in motor function (Halman, 1999). The most common presenting symptoms are memory impairment, mental slowing, depressive symptoms, and difficulty walking. Late manifestations of HIV-associated dementia involve much more severe symptomatology (e.g., mutism, aphasia, global cognitive dysfunction, ataxia, seizures, coma) (Perry, 1990). In order to make the diagnosis of HIV-associated dementia, there should be no confounding medical etiology and no evidence of delirium. Early mortality may be predicted by the onset of HIV-associated dementia (Atkinson & Grant, 1994).

Minor cognitive motor disorder or milder neuropsychological impairment is considered to have a much higher prevalence—45–60% (Halman, 1999). It is a mild syndrome of motor and/or cognitive dysfunction that results in minimal impairment in functioning.

Delirium must be a prime consideration for HIV-infected individuals, as it is for other patients with serious medical illnesses requiring multiple medications. The impact of HIV on the CNS is thought to contribute additional vulnerability to delirium (Atkinson & Grant, 1994).

Substance Use Disorders

Initially, a fairly high percentage of the women who developed AIDS were individuals with a history of IDU (CDC, 1998). That rate has decreased (44% cumulative, 32% in

of cognitive impairment (McDaniel et al., 1997; Whitaker, 1999). Stimulants can act quickly, appear to be well tolerated, and are especially useful where lethargy or cognitive slowing are major symptoms (Whitaker, 1999). Since these medications have abuse potential, the patient's substance use history should be considered prior to prescribing them.

Mood stabilizers such as carbamazepine and valproic acid are metabolized by the liver and thus should be used with caution in individuals taking protease inhibitors. Monitoring drug levels carefully is advisable. Since lithium is not metabolized by the liver, there is less concern about its use in HIV-positive patients on protease inhibitors, but it can present problems for patients with HIV-related gastrointestinal problems such as diarrhea. In patients with acute mania, low-dose neuroleptics or benzodiazepines may be the first choice of medication, followed by initiation of a mood stabilizer (lithium, carbamazepine, valproic acid, or clonazepam).

Anxiety symptoms are prevalent in this group of patients. It has been recommended that benzodiazepines not be used in combination with protease inhibitors, as the pharmacological effect is an expected increased area under the curve, and there are potential clinical effects of extreme sedation and respiratory depression (Preston & Stein, 1997). If a benzodiazepine is needed, lorazepam or oxazepam would be the best choices, due to their different route of metabolism and shorter half-lives (Janicak, 1995). Antidepressants would be the treatment of choice for patients with panic disorder or anxiety symptoms associated with depression. A clinician may also want to use antidepressants to avoid potential dependence on benzodiazepines in patients for whom substance abuse has been an ongoing issue.

Treatment strategies for psychosis in HIV/AIDS involve the use of antipsychotic medications, or a mood stabilizer if there is evidence of a manic psychosis (Janicak, 1995; McDaniel et al., 1997; Sewell et al., 1994b). Like the medications noted previously, antipsychotics should be used with caution for patients on protease inhibitors. Clozapine is considered a drug that should not be used with a protease inhibitor, due to the narrower therapeutic window and potential for seizures (Preston & Stein, 1997). Other antipsychotics may be used with caution. Since patients with HIV/AIDS may be exquisitely sensitive to extrapyramidal side effects or neuroleptic malignant syndrome, it is best to avoid high-potency antipsychotics, and to begin with lower doses and titrate these up slowly. Atypical antipsychotics such as risperidone or olanzapine should be considered for use due to their favorable side effect profiles (McDaniel et al., 1997; Whitaker, 1999).

Treatment options for HIV-associated dementia include use of antiretroviral agents or medications to treat the cognitive symptoms. Antiretroviral agents that penetrate the CNS include zidovudine, stavudine (d4T), and nevirapine (Atkinson & Grant, 1994; McDaniel et al., 1997). Recent research has shown objective evidence of improvement in the HIV cognitive motor–complex with the use of highly active antiretroviral therapy (Chang et al., 1999). Symptomatic improvement without treatment of the underlying pathology has been gained with the use of psychostimulant and antipsychotic medications (Atkinson & Grant, 1994; McDaniel et al., 1997; Whitaker, 1999).

Treatment of delirium in HIV is much the same as in other medical conditions. Diagnosing and treating the underlying medical problem is the most efficacious method of resolving a delirium. If psychopharmacological interventions are used, low doses of antipsychotic medications are better than benzodiazepines. In addition, the standard interventions that one would recommend for patients with delirium (e.g., assisting with orientation to place and time, decreasing confusing stimuli) would be applicable here as well.

Psychotherapy

Individual, family, and group psychotherapy have been effective in helping women cope with their diagnosis of HIV infection, cope with issues that arise over the course of their illness, and address the grief and loss that comes with the end stages of AIDS. As noted throughout this chapter, the issues and challenges HIV-positive women face change over the course of their illness. For example, at the time of initial diagnosis with HIV infection, many women experience an acute emotional crisis. They feel shock, disbelief, anger, and fear of impending death. Many women also experience suicidal ideation at this time, due to the fear and dread of facing this devastating disease, fear of social stigma, and fear of rejection by loved ones. As mental health providers help women cope with this acute crisis, they must also address issues of disclosure and partner notification, and assess the potential for domestic violence when the women's status is disclosed. In addition, mental health providers should help individuals identify available support systems in their families, friends, or communities that can help them cope with their illness.

Over the course of HIV disease, many women struggle to find ways to get on with their lives and set new goals for themselves in the face of living with their illness. The effects of HIV on their relationships with sexual partners, family members, and children are issues frequently discussed in therapy. How, when, and what to tell others about their disease are sources of anxiety and distress for many women with HIV. Coping with illness symptoms, side effects of medication, and opportunistic infections (OIs) is difficult for women who are single mothers and have minimal help or support in caring for their children. The first appearance of an OI or the initiation of HIV medications is often an acute emotional crisis, as it signifies the reality of HIV disease progression. Many women cope with these challenges and the stress associated with poverty by resorting to alcohol and drug use, which complicates their medical treatment and social situation. Ongoing substance use treatment and relapse prevention are important aspects of mental health care for many HIV-infected women.

Compliance with complicated medication regimens of 10–30 pills per day is a continuing struggle for most HIV-infected women, as they have multiple competing caretaking demands. In addition, many women have chaotic home environments, ongoing substance abuse, or evidence of cognitive impairment. Mental health providers are frequently consulted to help address adherence issues in women who need treatment for their HIV disease. Management of premorbid psychiatric illnesses is also part of ongoing mental health care, which should be done in conjunction with medical care providers as noted previously.

As women approach the end of their illness, they experience multiple losses: loss of independence, loss of previous levels of functioning, loss of family members, and loss of their hopes and dreams for their own and their children's futures. They must face the painful processes of planning for the children they will leave behind and making decisions about quality versus quantity of life for themselves. Many women experience organic mood disorders, psychotic disorders, sleep disorders, or cognitive impairments during the end stage of their illness, which complicate the processes of making independent choices for themselves regarding their care and of saying good-bye to their children and other loved ones. Psychiatric management of these symptoms in conjunction with psychotherapy has been very helpful for many women.

We have found that individual therapy, family therapy, and group therapy have all been beneficial in helping women face these challenges. There are many times when family members will need to participate in the therapeutic process, in order to be educated about the etiology and treatment of the symptoms their HIV-infected relative is exhibiting (e.g., psychosis, dementia). Many family members have not resolved old conflicts, and thus family therapy may be effective in bringing issues out into the open, so that the family can move forward and address the new crisis of an ill member. Involving children in family therapy sessions is an important part of work with HIV-infected women. Many women need the therapist's help in disclosing their HIV status to their children and explaining the illness and prognosis to children at developmentally appropriate levels. Group therapy for HIV-infected women is also an important source of education and support. Including food (e.g., snacks or lunch) and on-site child care may be critical for support groups to succeed. Spirituality or religion is an important factor in helping many individuals and families cope with the stress of HIV infection and should be taken into consideration by therapists in their work with individuals and families (Biggar et al., 1999).

General Considerations

As noted above, a multidisciplinary approach to mental health care for HIV-infected women is critical. Psychotherapy, medication management, and case management from social workers to address housing, transportation, and other assistance are all core components of mental health intervention. Many mental health contacts will be crisis-oriented and brief; short-term therapy is the norm in many clinics. Consultation and liaison with medical care providers are critical for the ongoing care of women with HIV/AIDS. The medical care providers need to be aware of each individual's psychosocial and mental status when making treatment decisions.

Since women of color make up a large percentage of women with AIDS, there is a need for clinicians to incorporate cultural sensitivity and competence into assessment and treatment interventions. Understanding the values of families with regard to roles, strengths, child-rearing practices, and extended family involvement is a first step. Each family's level of acculturation to the dominant culture should also be considered (Balan, 1997; Boyd-Franklin et al., 1995). Health care providers must be aware that their beliefs and values may not be the same as those of individuals from other cultures, and that such differences will have an impact on clinician–patient relationships (Boyd-Franklin et al., 1995).

For example, a mental health clinician might suggest that a Latina woman who is aware of her husband's marital infidelity initiate a conversation regarding condom use. However, it would be considered improper for a traditional Latina woman to seek out information regarding sexual matters, or to speak about sex, even with her husband (Balan, 1997). If the clinician were not aware of the cultural differences, the suggestion might impair his or her relationship with the patient, or cause him to label her behavior in more pathological terms than would be appropriate.

CONCLUSIONS

Women with HIV disease face a myriad of challenges, often with minimal social support. Mental health professionals can play a critical role in helping these women cope with a complex disease process that can drastically affect their emotional and physical health, as well as their day-to-day functioning as women and mothers. What we have learned from these courageous women who struggle with dignity to cope with a devastating disease has in turn shaped our concepts of appropriate and useful mental health interventions for women and their families.

REFERENCES

American Psychiatric Association Commission on AIDS. (1999). *HIV fact sheet: HIV and people with severe and persistent mental illness*. Washingtin, DC: American Psychiatric Association AIDS Program Office.

Atkinson, J. H., & Grant, I. (1994). Natural history of neuropsychiatric manifestations of HIV disease. *Psychiatric Clinics of North America, 17*, 17–33.

Balan, I. C. (1997). HIV and the traditional Latino woman. In L. A. Wicks (Eds.), *Psychotherapy and AIDS: The human dimension* (pp. 213–223). Washington, DC: Taylor & Francis.

Biggar, H., Forehand, R., Devine, D., et al. (1999). Women who are HIV infected: The role of religious activity in psychosocial adjustment. *AIDS Care, 11*(1), 195–199.

Blanche, S., Rouzioux, C., Moscato, M. L., et al. (1989). A prospective study of infants born to women seropositive for human inmmunodeficiency virus Type 1: HIV Infection in Newborns French Collaborative Study Group. *New England Journal of Medicine, 320*, 1643–1648.

Boyd-Franklin, N., Aleman, J., Jean-Gilles, M. M., et al. (1995). Cultural sensitivity and competence: African-American, Latino, and Haitian families with HIV/AIDS. In N. Boyd-Franklin, G. L. Steiner, & M. G. Boland (Eds.), *Children, families, and HIV/AIDS* (pp. 53–77). New York: Guilford Press.

Brown, G. R., & Rundell, J. R. (1990). Prospective study of psychiatric morbidity in HIV-seropositive women without AIDS. *General Hospital Psychiatry, 12*, 30–35.

Centers for Disease Control and Prevention. (2000a). *HIV/AIDS surveillance in women: L264 slide series (through 1999)*. [Online] Available: http://www.cdc.gov/hiv/graphics/women.htm [Accessibility verified July 23, 2001]

Centers for Disease Control and Prevention. (2000b). *HIV/AIDS Surveillance Report, 12*,(1), 1–44. [Online] Available: http://www.cdc.gov/hiv/stats/hasr1201.htm [Accessibility verified July 23, 2001]

Centers for Disease Control and Prevention. (2001). *Fact sheet—HIV/AIDS among U.S. women: Minority and young women at continuing risk*. [Online] Available: http://www.cdc.gov/hiv/pubs/facts/women.htm [Accessibility verified July 23, 2001]

Chang, L., Ernst, T., Leonido-Yee, M., et al. (1999). Highly active antiretroviral therapy reverses brain metabolite abnormalities in mild HIV dementia. *Neurology, 53*, 782–789.

Del Mistro, A., & Chieco Bianchi, L. (2001). HPB-related neoplasias in HIV-infected individuals. *European Journal of Cancer, 37*, 1227–1235.

European Collaborative Study. (1992). Risk factors for mother-to-child transmission of HIV-1. *Lancet, 339*, 1007.

Ferrando, S. J., Rabkin, J. G., de Moore, G. M., et al. (1999). Antidepressant treatment of depression in seropositive women. *Journal of Clinical Psychiatry, 60*, 741–746.

Hader, S. L., Smith, D. K., Moore, J. D., et al. (2001). HIV infection in women in the United States: Status at the millenium. *Journal of the American Medical Association, 285*(9), 1186–1192.

Halman, M. H. (1999, May 18). *AIDS training: Part 1. Clinical and neuropsychiatric dimensions of HIV disease*. Paper presented at the 152nd Annual Convention of the American Psychiatric Association, Washington, DC.

Harris, M. J., Jeste, D. V., Gleghorn, A., et al. (1991). New-onset psychosis in HIV-infected patients. *Journal of Clinical Psychiatry, 52*, 369–376.

James, M. E. (1988). HIV seropositivity diagnosed during pregnancy: Psychosocial characterization of patients and their adaptation. *General Hospital Psychiatry, 10,* 1–8.

Janicak, P. G. (1995). Psychopharmacotherapy in the HIV-infected patient. *Psychiatric Annals, 25*(10), 609–613.

Jenkins, S. R., & Coons, H. L. (1996). Psychosocial stress and adaptation processes for women coping with HIV/AIDS. In A. O'Leary & L. S. Jemmot (Eds.), *Women and AIDS: Coping and care* (pp. 33–86). New York: Plenum Press.

Kalichman, S. C., Kelly, J. A., Johnson, J. R., et al. (1994). Factors associated with risk for HIV infection among chronic mentally ill adults. *American Journal of Psychiatry, 151,* 221–227.

Kuhn, L., Sun, X. W., & Wright, T. C., Jr. (1999). Human immunodeficiency virus infection and female lower genital tract malignancy. *Current Opinion in Obstetrics and Gynecology, 11,* 35–39.

Lea, A. (1994). Women with HIV and their burden of caring. *Health Care for Women International, 15,* 489–501.

Lindsay, M. K., & Nesheim, S. R. (1997). Human immunodeficiency virus infection in pregnant women and their newborns. *Clinics in Perinatology, 24,* 161–180.

Lyketsos, C. G., Hanson, A. L., Fishman, M., et al. (1993). Manic syndrome early and late in the course of HIV. *American Journal of Psychiatry, 151,* 237–242.

McArthur, J. C., Hoover, D. R., Bacellar, H., et al. (1993). Dementia in AIDS patients: Incidence and risk factors. Multicenter AIDS Cohort Study. *Neurology, 43,* 2245–2252.

McDaniel, J. S., Fowlie, E., Summerville, M. B., et al. (1995). An assessment of rates of psychiatric morbidity and functioning in HIV disease. *General Hospital Psychiatry, 17,* 346–352.

McDaniel, J. S., Purcell, D. W., & Farber, E. W. (1997). Severe mental illness and HIV-related medical and neuropsychiatric sequelae. *Clinical Psychology Review, 17*(3), 311–325.

Nannis, E. D., Patterson, T. L., & Semple, S. J. (1997). Coping with HIV disease among seropositive women: Psychosocial correlates. *Women and Health, 25*(1), 1–22.

Nyamathi, A., Flaskerud, J., & Leake, B. (1997). HIV-risk behaviors and mental health characteristics among homeless or drug recovering women and their closest sources of social support. *Nursing Research, 46*(3), 133–137.

Otto-Salaj, L. L., Heckman, T. G., Stevenson, L. Y., et al. (1998). Patterns, predictors, and gender differences in HIV risk among severely mentally ill men and women. *Community Mental Health Journal, 34,* 175–190.

Perkins, D. O., Stern, R. A., Golden, R. N., et al. (1994). Mood disorders in HIV infection: Prevalence and risk factors in a nonepicenter of the AIDS epidemic. *American Journal of Psychiatry, 151,* 233–236.

Perry, S. W. (1990). Organic mental disorders caused by HIV: Update on early diagnosis and treatment. *American Journal of Psychiatry, 147,* 696–710.

Preston, S. L., & Stein, D. S. (1997, July). Drug interactions and adverse drug reactions with protease inhibitors. *Primary Psychiatry,* pp. 64–69.

Rabkin, J. G., Johnson, J., Lin, S., et al. (1997). Psychopathology in male and female HIV-positive and negative injecting drug users: Longitudinal course over 3 years. *AIDS, 11,* 507–551.

Rabkin, J. G., Wagner, G. J., & Rabkin, R. (1999). Fluoxetine treatment for depression in patients with HIV and AIDS: A randomized, placebo-controlled trial. *American Journal of Psychiatry, 156,* 101–107.

Schwartz, J. A. J., & McDaniel, J. S. (1999). Double-blind comparison of fluoxetine and desipramine in the treatment of depressed women with HIV disease: A pilot study. *Depression and Anxiety, 9,* 70–74.

Serraino, D., Carrieri, P., Pradier, C., et al. (1999). Risk of invasive cervical cancer among women with, or at risk for, HIV infection. *International Journal of Cancer, 82,* 334–337.

Sewell, D. D., Jeste, D. V., Atkinson, J. H., et al. (1994a). HIV-associated psychosis: A study of 20 cases. *American Journal of Psychiatry, 151,* 237–242.

Sewell, D. D., Jeste, D. V., McAdams, L. A., et al. (1994b). Neuroleptic treatment of HIV-associated psychosis. *Neuropsychopharmacology, 10*, 223–229.

Siegel, K., Karus, D., Raveis, V. H., et al. (1998). Psychological adjustment of women with HIV/AIDS: Racial and ethnic comparisons. *Journal of Community Psychology, 26*(5), 439–455.

Smith, D. K., & Moore, J. S. (1996). Epidemiology, manifestations, and treatment of HIV infection in women. In A. O'Leary & L. S. Jemmot (Eds.), *Women and AIDS: Coping and care* (pp. 1–32). New York: Plenum Press.

Sperling, R. S., Shapiro, D. E., Coombs, R. W., et al. (1996). Maternal viral load, zidovudine treatment, and the risk of transmission of human immunodeficiency virus type-1 from mother to infant. *New England Journal of Medicine, 335*, 1621–1629.

Sun, X. W., Kuhn, L., Ellerbrock, T. V., et al. (1997). Human papillomavirus infection in women infected with the human immunodeficiency virus. *New England Journal of Medicine, 337*, 1343–1349.

Whitaker, R. (1999, August). Psychopharmacological treatment issues in HIV disease. *Psychiatric Times*, pp. 24–30.

Wingood, G. M., & DiClemente, R. J. (1997). Prevention of human immunodeficiency virus infection among African-American women: Sex, gender, and power and women's risk of HIV. In D. C. Umeh (Ed.), *Confronting the AIDS epidemic: Cross-cultural perspectives on HIV/AIDS education* (pp. 117–135). Trenton, NJ: Africa World Press.

Wortley, P. M., & Fleming, P. L. (1997). AIDS in women in the United States. *Journal of the American Medical Association, 278*(11), 911–916.

27

Neurological Disorders
of Increased Prevalence in Women

Migraine, Multiple Sclerosis,
and Alzheimer's Disease

HOWARD L. FIELD
REID BRACKIN

The purpose of this chapter is to acquaint the reader with three neurological disorders of increased prevalence in women. The presentations include considerations of etiology, pathology, clinical course, effects of ovarian hormones, current treatments, and psychiatric aspects of the conditions.

MIGRAINE

Epidemiological studies in recent years reveal that more than 23 million people in the United States suffer from migraine headaches (Saper, 1997). According to Kornstein and Parker (1997), women constitute approximately 18 million of this number. Saper (1997) estimates that about 17% of all women experience migraine. Up to 25% of women have migraine during their reproductive years (Fettes, 1997). The impact of migraine on patients and society is often underestimated. Lost days of work and decreased productivity contribute heavily to the indirect costs of this disorder. Stang and Ostehaus (1993) and Stang, Cady, et al. (2001) estimate that, combined with the direct costs of medical care, the United States loses $6.5 to $17.2 billion per year in productivity to migraine. Many people with migraine do not seek medical care for their condition, believing that these are "normal" headaches. It may seem to them that everyone gets these headaches because others in their family also suffer with migraine (Longworth et al., 1997). Despite the fact

that pain complaints in women are often slighted, women are better than men at request-
ing care and are more likely to receive prescription medication for headaches (Holroyd &
Penzien, 1994).

Migraine Episodes

A migraine attack may be divided into five identifiable phases: "prodrome," "aura,"
"headache proper," "headache termination," and "postdrome." In some episodes, patients may experience all five phases; however, not every episode includes all components.
The prodrome occurs hours to days before onset of a patient's headache. The most common symptoms are photophobia, phonophobia (intolerance of ordinarily acceptable level
of sound), and osmophobia (intolerance of usually inoffensive odors), but patients may
experience psychological or autonomic symptoms as well. Some patients describe irritability, euphoria, depression of affect and mood, difficulty concentrating, food cravings,
thirst, and diarrhea as prodromal symptoms (Longworth et al., 1997). In others, the
prodrome may be manifested only as a vague feeling that a migraine is forthcoming.

Aura typically occurs in closer proximity to the headache, with visual, somato-
sensory, or motor symptoms. The aura generally develops over the course of 5 to 20 minutes, then lasts up to 1 hour. The most common visual symptom is the "scintillating
scotoma," characterized by luminous displays of objects that remain after eye closure
(Marin, 1998).

The features of the migraine headache itself may also vary. The most typical migraine headache is unilateral with a throbbing or pulsating quality. However, many individuals with migraine describe the pain as pressure-like. The pain gradually builds, pla-
teaus, wanes, and disappears over the course of 4 to 72 hours. Routine physical activity
such as climbing stairs tends to aggravate the pain. Anorexia, nausea, and/or vomiting
are highly common and are considered cardinal symptoms of the disorder. It is crucial
that these gastrointestinal symptoms be elucidated in taking a patient's history (Pryse-
Phillips et al., 1997).

Classifications

In 1988, the International Headache Society (IHS) documented a complete headache classification system. The criteria for IHS definitions of "migraine without aura" and "migraine with aura" are given in Table 27.1.

Pathogenesis

The vascular theory of migraine—with initial intracranial vasodilation causing the aura,
and subsequent extracranial vasodilation producing the characteristic pain—has been
disproven. More recently, the genesis of migraine has been attributed to a neuronal
process beginning in the dorsal raphe of the brainstem; this process involves vasomotor
activation of intracranial and extracranial blood vessels, and activation of the trigeminal
nucleus, releasing vasoactive neuropeptides (Winner, 1998). Clinically, patients have
identified many precipitating factors. Lack of food caused by fasting, insufficient quantity, or missed meals may lead to migraine. Specific foods, such as aged cheese, alcohol

dysfunction, bowel dysfunction, sexual dysfunction, fatigue, sleep disorders, depression, and pain associated with MS.

Antidepressants can be helpful in treating depression. Selective serotonin reuptake inhibitors are often used as first-line treatment. Tricyclic antidepressants may be useful for patients with concomitant bladder hyperreflexia (van Oosten et al., 1998). Psychotherapy is directed at encouraging hope, resourcefulness, and continued autonomy in the presence of increasing physical incapacity. The relationship between the psychiatrist and patient is important. The consultant must be able to maintain an attitude of realistic optimism. MS also places a heavy burden on families and other caregivers. Stress disorders, separation/divorce, and spouse/partner abuse give testimony to this burden. The psychiatric consultant must be prepared to deal with emotional problems in family members and other caregivers, as well as in the patient.

ALZHEIMER'S DISEASE

One of the most serious health concerns facing the increasing aging population in the United States is dementia. Epidemiologists suggest that this acquired cognitive loss exists in 5–10% of individuals over the age of 65 (Lerner, 1999; Flynn, 1999). The prevalence of dementia increases with advancing age: up to 47% of people aged 85 years may suffer from dementia. Alzheimer's disease (AD) is the most common cause of dementia (Francis et al., 1999). Women are more often affected by AD than men are. Data suggest that 1.5 to 3 times more women than men develop AD (Henderson, 1997b; Rochon & Gurwitz, 1996). Even with adjustments made for different survival rates, the prevalence of AD remains higher in women than in men (Henderson, 1997a).

AD is a progressive degeneration of cortical neurons, primarily involving temporal, parietal, and frontal lobes. A characteristic histopathological picture identifies the disease: neurofibrillary tangles, amyloid neuritic plaques, vacuolar degeneration, neuronal cell death, and gliosis. Plaque formation may be the initial event in the pathogenesis of AD, resulting in other neuropathological features (neurofibrillary tangles, loss of synaptic connections, and neuronal death). The chief biochemical feature is a marked reduction in the synthesizing enzyme choline acetyltransferase, resulting in acetylcholine deficiency.

Etiology

Forsyth and Ritzline (1998) note that AD has a multifactorial etiology. Age is probably most significant. Genetic predisposition to the disease is a known risk factor. This risk was initially identified in relation to chromosome 21, when it was discovered that almost all patients with Down's syndrome (trisomy 21) develop symptoms of AD after the age of 40. More recently, three genes have been identified as risk factors for the rare, early-onset, familial form of AD. Amyloid precursor proteins deriving from these genes lead to an increase in amyloid-ß peptides. This increase may contribute to the formation of the senile plaques characteristic of AD. A fourth gene appears to be linked to the more common, late-onset form of the disease as well as the early-onset form. Encoding apolipoprotein E, this gene is related to cholesterol metabolism. The E4 allele of the gene confers risk of AD, especially in the homozygous state (Bidikov & Meier, 1997). Together, these four genes do not account for all of the genetic risk in AD; additional loci related to the etiology of AD are likely to exist. Other potential risk factors for AD have been identified as well. Education may confer some protection against AD. Positive family history of AD, history of head injury with loss of consciousness, and exposure to heavy metals and toxins are possible risk factors.

Findings suggest that estrogen deficiency and menopause are related to AD. The incidence of AD increases after menopause, but ERT significantly reduces this risk (Henderson, 1997a). In significant concentrations, estrogen appears to benefit neurons. Estrogen has been shown to protect neurons from oxidative stress-induced cell death *in vitro*, to stimulate nerve growth factor activity, and to modulate neurotransmitter systems and glucose utilization. Estrogen may also reduce serum apolipoprotein E and slow the deposition of senile plaques (Calaf i Alsina, 1997; Giacobini, 1998; Brinton, 1999). Investigations suggest benefits of ERT in treatment of AD (Flynn, 1999; see below).

Clinical Features

Clinically, progressive irreversible dementia is the symptom central to the profile of patients with AD. From the onset of clinical symptoms, AD has a mean duration of 8.5 years until death (Francis et al., 1999). The clinical diagnosis is not absolute until confirmed by histological findings; nevertheless, history, examination, and imaging findings can give considerable certainty to the clinician. The physician must rule out other causes of dementia, and it is particularly important to search for reversible causes, such as drug use, metabolic disorders, nutritional problems, and tumors (Forsyth & Ritzline, 1998). Diagnosis of probable AD includes establishing dementia by clinical examination and neuropsychological tests. Deficits in two or more areas of cognition, progressive deterioration of memory, and onset between the ages of 40 and 90 are necessary for diagnosis. There should be no disturbance in consciousness or any other disorder causing progressive deficits in memory and cognition. Diagnosis is supported by specific findings such as aphasia, apraxia, agnosia, impaired activities of daily living, and altered behavior patterns. Disturbances in executive function may arise, resulting in difficulty with planning, abstraction, and judgment. Last to go are long-term memory, motor skills, and social skills. Emotional manifestations of AD may include depression, agitation, aggression, delusions, and hallucinations. Anxiety syndromes, sleep disorders, and purposeless behaviors are common. The patient with AD is easily disturbed by even slight physical and environmental changes, which can sometimes result in delirium. The agitated, bewildered, newly admitted elderly patient is a familiar problem to the general hospital psychiatrist. Afternoon and evening confusion, subsumed under the rubric of "sundowning," is common.

Management

Pharmacological approaches to the memory loss of AD have been directed toward correcting acetylcholine deficits. Some results have been achieved with cholinesterase inhibitors, which slow the breakdown of acetylcholine. Cholinesterase inhibitors currently available include tacrine and donepezil, but many drugs of this class are being evaluated. Both tacrine and donepezil are indicated for patients with mild to moderate AD, but response to therapy ranges from notable improvement to no change (Gauthier, 1999; Pryse-Phillips, 1999). Hepatotoxicity is a danger; significant elevation of serum alanine aminotransaminase has been shown in up to 45% of patients receiving tacrine (Flynn, 1999). Patients with severe AD are not recommended for pharmacotherapy, as they are unlikely to benefit.

A number of other medications are being investigated for potential beneficial effects in preventing or treating AD. For example, NSAIDs may decrease the development of AD by reducing inflammatory processes associated with amyloid plaques and neurofibrillary tangles. Increasing levels of nerve growth factor or other neurotrophic factors may enhance neuronal survival and improve cognitive function. Nootopics (neural stimulant drugs) that may improve cognitive function in AD are also being researched. Other potential targets for pharmacology include drugs or dietary substances to decrease free radicals associated with neuronal degeneration, and calcium channel blockers to prevent calcium influx leading to neuronal death (Flynn & Ranno, 1999).

The management of secondary symptoms poses a considerable problem for the psychiatrist. Agitation, hallucinations, and delusions often respond to low doses of antipsychotics. The newer, atypical antipsychotics have been particularly useful because of their more benign side effect profile. The drug treatment of depression can also be helpful. Selective serotonin reuptake inhibitors are less likely to precipitate delirium than tricyclic antidepressants. Sedating antidepressants such as trazodone may be helpful for insomnia. Benzodiazepines should be used with caution in the elderly population because of their tendency to disturb balance, resulting in falls.

Psychiatric management of patients with AD should incorporate compassionate counseling, social service, and good supportive care. Constant sympathetic orientation, while maintaining a familiar environment and routine, can be helpful. The patient with AD who continues to live at home is extremely stressful for the caregivers. Alterations in the behavior and personality of the demented family member can be emotionally disturbing. Demands for care continue 24 hours a day, 7 days a week. Thus the psychiatrist's therapeutic scope must extend beyond the patient to the family and caregivers. Support groups and respite facilities are available in some locations. Knowledge of resources should be a part of the physician's armamentarium.

Estrogen Replacement Therapy

With the accumulating body of evidence to support the estrogen hypothesis, ERT is being considered as a treatment strategy for postmenopausal women with AD. Clinical trials thus far have shown small but significant improvements in memory, orientation, and calculation tasks (Birge, 1998; Calaf i Alsina, 1997). In addition, ERT appears to potentiate the therapeutic effects of cholinesterase inhibitors. Women with mild to moderate AD who received ERT with the cholinesterase inhibitor tacrine improved more than those receiving tacrine alone did (Schneider et al., 1996).

REFERENCES

Bansil, S., Troiano, R., Rohowsky-Kochan, C., et al. (1994). Multiple sclerosis: Pathogenesis and treatment. *Seminars in Neurology, 14*(2), 146–153.

Beatty, W. W. (1993). Cognitive and emotional disturbances in multiple sclerosis. *Neurologic Clinics, 11*(1), 189–204.

Bidikov, I., & Meier, D. E. (1997). Clinical decision-making with the woman after menopause. *Geriatrics, 52*(3), 28–36.

Birge, S. J. (1998). Hormones and the aging brain. *Geriatrics, 53*(Suppl. 1), S28–S30.

Brinton, R. D. (1999). A women's health issue: Alzheimer's disease and strategies for maintaining cognitive health. *International Journal of Fertility and Women's Medicine, 44*(4), 174–185.

Calaf i Alsina, J. (1997). Benefits of hormone replacement therapy—Overview and update. *International Journal of Fertility and Women's Medicine, 42*(Suppl. 2), 329–346.

Charcot, J. M. (1877). *Lectures on the diseases of the nervous system.* Delivered at La Salpetriere. London: The New Sydenham Society.

Compston, A. (1998). Future options for therapies to limit damage and enhance recovery. *Seminars in Neurology, 18*(3), 405–14.

Diener, H. C., Kaube, H., & Limmroth, V. (1998). A practical guide to the management and prevention of migraine. *Drugs, 56*(5), 811–824.

Ebers, G. C., & Dyment, D. A. (1998). Genetics of multiple sclerosis. *Seminars in Neurology, 18*(3), 295–299.

Fettes, I. (1997). Menstrual migraine: Methods of prevention and control. *Postgraduate Medicine, 101*(5), 67–70, 73–77.

Flynn, B. L. (1999). Pharmacologic management of Alzheimer disease: Part I. Hormonal and emerging investigational drug therapies. *Annals of Pharmacotherapy, 33*(2), 178–187.

Flynn, B. L., & Ranno, A. E. (1999). Pharmacologic management of Alzheimer disease: Part II. Antioxidants, antihypertensives, and ergoloid derivatives. *Annals of Pharmacotherapy, 33*(2), 188–197.

Forsyth, E., & Ritzline, P. D. (1998). An overview of the etiology, diagnosis, and treatment of Alzheimer disease. *Physical Therapy, 78*(12), 1325–1331.

Francis, P. T., Palmer, A. M., Snape, M., et al. (1999). The cholinergic hypothesis of Alzheimer's disease: A review of progress. *Journal of Neurology, Neurosurgery and Psychiatry, 66*(2), 137–147.

Gauthier, S. (1999). Do we have a treatment for Alzheimer disease? Yes. *Archives of Neurology, 56*(6), 738–739.

Giacobini, E. (1998). Aging, Alzheimer's disease, and estrogen therapy. *Experimental Gerontology, 33*(7–8), 865–869.

Glover, V., Jarman, J., & Sandler, M. (1993). Migraine and depression: Biological aspects. *Journal of Psychiatric Research, 27*(2), 223–231.

Granella, F., Sances, G., Zanferrari, C., et al. (1993). Migraine without aura and reproductive life events: A clinical epidemiological study in 1300 women. *Headache, 33,* 385–389.

Headache Classification Committee on the International Headache Society. (1988). Classification and diagnostic criteria for headache disorders, cranial neuralgias and facial pain. *Cephalgia, 8*(Suppl. 7), S1–S96.

Heaton, R. K., Nelson, L. M., Thompson, D. S., et al. (1985). Neuropsychological findings in relapsing–remitting and chronic progressive multiple sclerosis. *Journal of Consulting and Clinical Psychology, 53,* 103–110.

Henderson, V. W. (1997a). The epidemiology of estrogen replacement therapy and Alzheimer's disease. *Neurology, 48*(5, Suppl. 7), S27–S35.

Henderson, V. W. (1997b). Estrogen, cognition, and a woman's risk of Alzheimer's disease. *American Journal of Medicine, 103*(3A), 11S–18S.

Holm, J. E., Bury, L., & Suda, K. T. (1996). The relationship between stress, headache, and the menstrual cycle in young female migraineurs. *Headache, 36*(9), 531–537.

Holroyd, K. A., & Penzien, D. B. (1994). Psychosocial interventions in the management of recurrent headache disorders: 1. Overview and effectiveness [see comments]. *Behavioral Medicine, 20*(2), 53–63.

Kornstein, S. G., & Parker, A. J. (1997). Menstrual migraines: Etiology, treatment, and relationship to premenstrual syndrome. *Current Opinion in Obstetrics and Gynecology, 9*(3), 154–159.

Lerner, A. J. (1999). Women and Alzheimer's disease. *Journal of Clinical Endocrinology and Metabolism, 84*(6), 1830–1834.

Lisak, R. P. (1998). Intravenous immunoglobulins in multiple sclerosis. *Neurology, 51*(6, Suppl. 5), S25–S29.

Lokken, C., Holm, J. E., & Myers, T. C. (1997). The menstrual cycle and migraine: A time-series analysis of 20 women migraineurs. *Headache, 37*(4), 235–239.

Longworth, D. L., Stoller, J. K., & Skobieranda, F. G. (1997). A 30–year-old woman with headache [published erratum appears in *Cleveland Clinic Journal of Medicine*, 1997, 64(9), 460]. *Cleveland Clinic Journal of Medicine, 64*(6), 293–297.

Mannix, L. K., & Solomon, G. D. (1998). Quality of life in migraine. *Clinical Neuroscience, 5*, 38–42.

Marin, P. A. (1998). Pharmacologic management of migraine. *Journal of the American Academy of Nurse Practitioners, 10*(9), 407–412.

Mendez, M. F. (1995). The neuropsychiatry of multiple sclerosis. *International Journal of Psychiatry in Medicine, 25*(2), 123–130.

Merikangas, K. R. (1995). Association between psychopathology and headache syndromes. *Current Opinion in Neurology, 8*(3), 248–251.

Metz, L. (1998). Multiple sclerosis: Symptomatic therapies. *Seminars in Neurology, 18*(3), 389–395.

Miller, A. (1998). Diagnosis of multiple sclerosis. *Seminars in Neurology, 18*(3), 309–316.

Minden, S. L. (1992). Psychotherapy for people with multiple sclerosis. *Journal of Neuropsychiatry and Clinical Neurosciences, 4*(2), 198–213.

Minden, S. L., & Schiffer, R. B. (1990). Affective disorders in multiple sclerosis: Review and recommendations for clinical research. *Archives of Neurology, 47*, 98–104.

Neuhaus, O., Forina, C., Wekerle, H., et al. (2001). Mechanisms of ochons of glateramer ocetate in multiple sclerosis. *Neurology, 56*(6), 702–708.

Noseworthy, J. H. (1998). Multiple sclerosis clinical trials: Old and new challenges. *Seminars in Neurology, 18*(3), 377–388.

Pine, D. S., Douglas, C. J., Charles, E., et al. (1995). Patients with multiple sclerosis presenting to psychiatric hospitals. *Journal of Clinical Psychiatry, 57*, 297–306.

Poser, C. M., Paty, D. W., Scheinberg, L., et al. (1983). New diagnostic criteria for multiple sclerosis: Guidelines for research protocols. *Annals of Neurology, 13*(8), 227–231.

Pryse-Phillips, W. (1999). Do we have drugs for dementia? No. *Archives of Neurology, 56*(6), 735–737.

Pryse-Phillips, W. E., Dodick, D. W., Edmeads, J. G., et al. (1997). Guidelines for the diagnosis and management of migraine in clinical practice. Canadian Headache Society [see comments] [published erratum appears in *Canadian Medical Association Journal*, 1997, 157(10), 1354]. *Canadian Medical Association Journal 156*(9), 1273–1287.

Rochon, P. A., & Gurwitz, J. H. (1996). Geriatrics: The age of women. *Lancet, 348*(Suppl. 2), S118.

Saper, J. R. (1997). Diagnosis and symptomatic treatment of migraine. *Headache, 37*(Suppl. 1), S1–S14.

Schneider, L. S., Farlow, M. R., Henderson, V. W., et al. (1996). Effects of estrogen replacement therapy on response to tacrine in patients with Alzheimer's disease. *Neurology, 46*, 1580–1584.

Silberstein, S. D. (1995). Migraine and women: The link between headache and hormones. *Postgraduate Medicine, 97*(4), 147–153.

Silberstein, S. D., Armellino, J. J., Hoffman, H. D., et al. (1999). Treatment of menstruation-associated migraine with the nonprescription combination of acetaminophen, aspirin, and caffeine: Results from three randomized, placebo-controlled studies. *Clinical Therapeutics, 21*(3), 475–491.

Skaer, T. L. (1996). Clinical presentation and treatment of migraine. *Clinical Therapeutics, 18*(2), 228–245.

Skegg, K. (1993). Múltiple sclerosis presenting as a pure psychiatric disorder. *Psychological Medicine, 23,* 909–914.

Sorensen, T. L., & Ransohoff, R. M. (1998). Etiology and pathogenesis of multiple sclerosis. *Seminars in Neurology, 18*(3), 287–294.

Stang, P., Cady, R., Batenhorst, A., et al. (2001). Workplace productivity: A review of the impact of migraine and its treatment. *Pharmacoeconomics, 19*(3), 231–244.

Stang, P. E., & Osterhaus, J. T. (1993). Impact of migraine in the United States: Data from the National Health Interview survey. *Headache, 33,* 29–35.

Sugar, C., & Nadell, R. (1942). Mental symptoms in multiple sclerosis: A study of 28 cases with review of the literature. *Journal of Nervous and Mental Disease, 98,* 267–280.

Thompson, A. J. (1998). Symptomatic treatment in multiple sclerosis. *Current Opinion in Neurology, 11*(4), 305–309.

Tselis, A. C., & Lisak, R. P. (1999). Multiple sclerosis: therapeutic update. *Archives of Neurology, 56*(3), 277–280.

van Oosten, B. W., Truyen, L., Barkhof, F., et al. (1998). Choosing drug therapy for multiple sclerosis: An update. *Drugs, 56*(4), 555–569.

Weinshenker, B. G. (1998). The natural history of multiple sclerosis: Update 1998. *Seminars in Neurology, 18*(3), 301–307.

Winner, P. K. (1998). Migraine: Diagnosis and rational treatment. *International Journal of Fertility and Women's Medicine, 43*(2), 104–110.

Young, W. B., Silberstein, S. D., & Dayno, J. M. (1997). Migraine treatment. *Seminars in Neurology, 17*(4), 325–333.

28

Cosmetic Surgery

DAVID B. SARWER
MICHAEL J. PERTSCHUK

The American Society of Plastic and Reconstructive Surgeons (ASPS), which represents 97% of all physicians certified by the American Board of Plastic Surgery, reported that its membership performed over 1.3 million cosmetic procedures in 2000. This number represented an increase of 95% since 1996 and 228% since 1992 (ASPS, 2001) (See Table 28.1). Approximately 90% of these procedures were performed on women (ASPS, 2001). This is an underestimation of the actual number of cosmetic procedures performed each year, as increasing numbers of physicians in other specialties now perform cosmetic surgery. The most common procedures span the face and body—liposuction (fat removal), breast augmentation, blepharoplasty (eyelid surgery), rhytidectomy (facelift), and rhinoplasty (nose reshaping). Newer procedures, such as laser skin resurfacing and botox injections to treat unwanted wrinkle lines, are equally popular. Almost every bodily feature can now be altered by cosmetic surgery.

The increase in both the number of procedures performed and the number of physicians performing them reflects the American public's increased acceptance of cosmetic surgery as a means of self-improvement. Cosmetic surgery is no longer just for middle-aged women with disposable incomes, as was once thought; women from a variety of age, racial, and socioeconomic groups now seek cosmetic surgery. These procedures, however, have the potential for physical (from the risks associated with surgery) and perhaps psychological (from disappointment with the postoperative result) harm (Institute of Medicine, 1999). Coupling this with its increasing popularity, cosmetic surgery is quickly becoming a significant women's health concern. The popularity of cosmetic surgery also increases the likelihood that mental health professionals will encounter women who have undergone, or are interested in undergoing, cosmetic surgery. (For brevity's sake, both these groups of women are referred to in this chapter as "cosmetic surgery patients"; preoperative–postoperative status is clarified when necessary.)

This chapter provides an overview of cosmetic surgery for women. The chapter be-

TABLE 28.1. National Cosmetic Surgery Statistics

Procedure	1992	1996	1998	2000
Breast augmentation	32,607	87,704	132,378	187,755
Breast implant removal	18,297	3,013	32,262	37,984
Breast lift	7,963	16,097	31,525	45,537
Breast reduction in men	4,997	6,045	9,023	9,199
Buttock lift	291	774	1,246	1,356
Cheek implants	1,741	2,257	2,864	3,304
Chemical peel	19,049	42,628	66,002	68,198
Chin augmentation	4,115	4,797	4,795	7,087
Collagen injection	41,623	34,091	45,851	62,839
Dermabrasion	13,457	7,975	8,069	N/A
Ear surgery (otoplasty)	6,371	7,192	8,069	9,911
Eyelid surgery (blepharoplasty)	59,461	76,242	120,001	172,244
Facelift (rhytidectomy)	40,077	53,435	70,947	70,882
Fat injections	7,865	13,654	25,437	24,810
Fibril injections	357	164	1,463	1,790
Forehead lift	13,501	22,864	36,777	41,668
Laser skin resurfacing	N/A	46,263	55,623	48,038
Liposuction	47,212	109,353	172,079	229,588
Male-pattern baldness	1,955	4,042	2,146	1,958
Nose reshaping (rhinoplasty)	50,175	45,977	55,953	50,617
Retin-A treatment	23,520	74,382	106,862	99,017
Thigh lift	1,023	2,114	3,785	5,096
Tummy tuck	16,810	34,235	46,597	58,463
Upper arm lift	434	1,614	1,939	N/A
Wrinkle injections	357	164	1,463	N/A
Total	412,901	696,912	1,045,815	1,355,793

Note. All figures are projected based on a survey of American Society of Plastic Surgeons (ASPS) members only. ASPS membership includes 97% of the plastic surgeons certified by the American Board of Plastic Surgery. Data from ASPS (1992, 1996, 1998, 2001).

gins with a review of the psychological studies of cosmetic surgery patients, with an emphasis on recent investigations of body image. The relationship between cosmetic surgery and specific forms of psychopathology is then discussed. The chapter concludes with a discussion of procedures for psychiatric consultation with plastic surgery patients.

PSYCHOLOGICAL STUDIES OF COSMETIC SURGERY PATIENTS

Interview Investigations

Although the first psychological reports of cosmetic surgery patients occurred in the 1940s, a collaboration of psychiatrists and plastic surgeons at Johns Hopkins University School of Medicine in the 1950s and 1960s produced the first significant body of research. These investigations were undertaken primarily to identify patients who were most likely to benefit from cosmetic surgery. For the most part, these studies relied on clinical interviews that were conducted by psychoanalytically trained psychiatrists. Regardless of the type of surgical procedure, the majority of patients were seen as having significant psychopathology (Edgerton et al., 1960, 1961, 1964; Meyer et al., 1960; Webb et al., 1965). The most common diagnoses were personality disorders, with smaller

BDD, although any area of the body may be the focus of concern (Phillips, 1996; Phillips & Diaz, 1997; Phillips et al., 1993). Given the nature of these concerns, it is likely that persons with BDD are overrepresented in cosmetic surgery, dermatology, and other medical practices that address appearance-related issues. A study of women who sought cosmetic surgery found that 7% met diagnostic criteria for BDD (Sarwer et al., 1998e). BDD may not be limited to persons concerned with "slight" appearance defects. A study of individuals with visible appearance deformities undergoing reconstructive surgery found that 16% reported emotional distress and preoccupation with their appearance consistent with the diagnosis (Sarwer et al., 1998f). Other studies have found women with obesity frequently report a level of distress, preoccupation, and impairment consistent with BDD (Rosen et al., 1995; Sarwer et al., 1998c). Whether individuals with imagined or visible defects such as these should be diagnosed with BDD is controversial.

BDD may be particularly difficult to diagnose in cosmetic surgery patients (Sarwer, 1997; Sarwer et al., 1998e). Given the newness of BDD to American psychiatry (it was first introduced in the *Diagnostic and Statistical Manual of Mental Disorders*, third edition, revised [DSM-III-R] in 1987), many cosmetic surgeons are unfamiliar with the diagnosis. In addition, the objective of cosmetic surgery—to improve the appearance of a person with a "normal" appearance—may make diagnosis difficult. Cosmetic surgery patients frequently seek to improve slight defects in their appearance. Such slight defects, however, are frequently judged as observable and correctable by the surgeon. As a result, judgment of a defect as "slight" becomes highly subjective. We have suggested that the degree of emotional distress and behavioral impairment, rather than the size or nature of the physical defect, may be more accurate indicators of BDD in plastic surgery patients (Sarwer, 1997, 2001; Sarwer et al., 1998e).

Preliminary clinical reports have found that the vast majority of persons with BDD do not benefit from cosmetic surgery (Phillips & Diaz, 1997; Phillips et al., 1993). Following surgery, they often remain focused on the same feature or become focused on a different feature. There is also some concern that these individuals may become violent toward themselves or their surgeons. These reports suggest that BDD may contraindicate cosmetic surgery (Grossbart & Sarwer, 1999; Sarwer, 1997; Sarwer, 2001).

Psychotic Disorders

Cosmetic surgery patients with schizophrenia and other psychotic disorders have been of particular interest to cosmetic surgeons. There have been anecdotal reports of individuals who have suffered from a loss of identity following cosmetic surgery (e.g., Edgerton et al., 1991; Knorr, 1972). Plastic surgeons frequently fear that individuals with psychotic disorders are the ones most likely to threaten or become violent following unsuccessful cosmetic surgery. The presence of an active psychotic disorder is commonly thought to contraindicate cosmetic surgery (Sarwer, 1997, 2001; Sarwer et al., 1998b).

Edgerton et al. (1991) have suggested a different approach to treating patients with significant psychopathology. They reviewed the records of 100 cosmetic surgery patients with a variety of psychiatric diagnoses (including some who were described as psychotic, and several who may have had BDD). Eighty-seven patients underwent surgery, ranging from common procedures such as rhinoplasty and facelifts to dramatic facial restructuring. Eighty-three percent were judged to have experienced a successful psychological outcome. These results led Edgerton et al. (1991) to conclude that cosmetic surgery can have psychological benefits for patients with psychiatric conditions that are often considered "absolute contraindication(s)" to surgery, given that such patients are vigilantly managed by the surgeon and a mental health professional.

This is almost certainly a minority view. Most cosmetic surgeons will not operate on a patient who is actively psychotic or is experiencing other forms of significant psychopathology. However, probably very few surgeons provide these patients with referrals to mental health professionals. As a consequence, these patients continue to "surgeon-shop" until they find a surgeon willing to operate (a likely occurrence, given the number of physicians who now perform cosmetic procedures). Thus many may never receive appropriate psychiatric care.

Eating Disorders

Given the overemphasis on body image held by women with anorexia nervosa and bulimia nervosa, these disorders may be disproportionately represented among cosmetic surgery patients. There are case reports of women with both disorders who have experienced an exacerbation of symptoms following breast augmentation, rhinoplasty, and chin augmentation (McIntosh et al., 1994; Yates et al., 1988). Interestingly, a report on breast reduction patients indicated that four of five women experienced a dramatic improvement in their eating disorder symptoms postoperatively (Losee et al., 1997).

Eating disorders may be a particular concern for women interested in liposuction. Willard et al. (1996) described two cases of women with bulimia nervosa who underwent liposuction in an attempt to lose weight, only to experience an exacerbation of their bulimic symptoms postoperatively. Although liposuction is the mostly commonly performed cosmetic procedure (see Table 29.1), it may be the procedure most misunderstood by the lay public. Liposuction is commonly thought to be used to remove excess fat from the torso; however, it is frequently used to remove fat from areas throughout the face and body. Another misconception is that liposuction results in weight loss. The removal of fat cells during liposuction typically results in little if any change in body weight; thus it is not an accepted treatment for weight reduction. Eating disorders also may be a concern for women interested in breast augmentation surgery. Breast augmentation patients are frequently of below-average weight, leading to speculation that they are at risk for eating disorders (Meyer & Ringberg, 1987; Sarwer et al., 1998a). Thus both liposuction and breast augmentation patients should be questioned about a possible history of amenorrhea, weight fluctuations, binge eating, and dieting and purging behaviors.

Anxiety Disorders

Rankin and Borah (1997) have suggested that the stress of cosmetic surgery can trigger an anxiety disorder. Panic attacks and acute stress reactions may occur either just prior to surgery or in the immediate postoperative recovery period. Cosmetic surgery, like any medical treatment, can trigger a posttraumatic stress reaction in patients who have previously experienced trauma.

Personality Disorders

As noted above, the earliest investigations of cosmetic surgery patients concluded that many prospective patients were suffering from personality disorders (e.g., Edgerton et al.,

1960; Webb et al., 1965). Unfortunately, these reports probably suffered from inter-viewer bias and failed to use widely accepted diagnostic criteria. More importantly, these reports did not provide reliable evidence that given personality types were related to a poor postoperative outcome.

A more recent investigation of cosmetic surgery patients that used DSM-III-R diag-nostic criteria reported that 70% had an Axis II disorder (predominantly narcissistic and borderline personality disorders) and 19.5% had an Axis I disorder (predominantly mood and anxiety disorders) (Napoleon, 1993). Although this study improved upon ear-lier investigations by using widely accepted diagnostic criteria, the use of an unspecified clinical interview and the absence of interrater reliability of diagnoses could account for the extremely high prevalence of Axis II diagnoses in this sample.

Summary

It is likely that all of the major psychiatric diagnoses occur in cosmetic surgery patients. However, with the exception of BDD, the prevalence of specific diagnoses is unknown. Studies that utilize widely accepted diagnostic criteria in combination with standardized assessment procedures, such as the Structured Clinical Interview for DSM-IV, are needed to establish the prevalence of psychiatric disorders in cosmetic surgery patients. Equally important are studies that investigating the relationship between psychopathology and postoperative outcome. Although conditions such as BDD, active psychotic disorders, and eating disorders appear to be related to poor postoperative results and may contrain-dicate surgery, the relationship between other psychopathology (such as major depres-sion) and cosmetic surgery is less clear.

RECONSTRUCTIVE SURGERY PATIENTS

Plastic surgeons also treat individuals with disfigured appearances. A significant body of research has documented the psychological challenges of children born with disfigured appearances (for a review, see Endriga & Kapp-Simon, 1999). These studies have sug-gested that these children are at risk for low self-esteem, increased anxiety, behavioral problems, and social interaction difficulties. Psychological functioning has been found to improve following surgery; however, it does not necessarily return to normal levels, po-tentially leaving these children at risk for psychological problems later in life (Pertschuk & Whitaker, 1988). A recent study of adults born with craniofacial disfigurement found that, compared to nondisfigured adults, these adults experienced greater body image dis-satisfaction and lower self-esteem and quality of life. More than one-third of these indi-viduals also reported discrimination in employment and social situations (Sarwer et al., 1999).

Plastic surgeons also perform reconstructive surgeries following physical insults, such as automobile accidents, burns, and cancer (see Chen & Kunkel, Chapter 21, this volume, for a discussion of the psychiatric aspects of oncological treatment). The effect of these insults on appearance can range greatly, and treatment can involve one procedure or a series of surgeries over several years. The surgical results frequently have a profound affect on the psychological functioning of disfigured patients. Perhaps because of this, many plastic surgeons devote some of their time and energy to groups such as Project Hope and Operation Smile, which work with disfigured children in underdeveloped countries, while others perform no-cost surgeries on women who are survivors of domestic abuse. The residual deformity following these surgeries, however, may be related to significant distress. Many reconstructive surgery patients may experience major depressive episodes, social anxiety, or (in the case of trauma survivors) posttraumatic stress disorder. Plastic surgeons are in an ideal position to identify these conditions and to provide mental health referrals to these individuals when needed.

PSYCHIATRIC CONSULTATION WITH PLASTIC SURGERY PATIENTS

Psychiatrists and psychologists may encounter women interested in plastic surgery in a variety of contexts. For example, women patients in a psychiatry or psychotherapy practice who have body image concerns may have considered (or have undergone) cosmetic surgery. Similarly, patients with posttraumatic stress disorder following an accident that disfigured their appearance may require reconstructive surgery. Surgeons also may ask a psychiatrist or psychologist to consult on a patient. These consultations typically occur in one of two contexts: to evaluate a patient prior to surgery, or to assess psychological functioning postoperatively.

Preoperative Consultations

The vast majority of cosmetic surgery patients are probably psychologically appropriate for surgery. Most patients typically have specific appearance concerns and realistic postoperative expectations. As a result, they do not require a mental health consultation prior to surgery. A small minority, however, may exhibit symptoms to the surgeon that warrant a psychological evaluation (Sarwer, 1997, 2001). In addition to utilizing the basic principles of general psychiatric assessment, the assessment should focus on three areas: (1) motivations and expectations for surgery, (2) psychiatric history, and (3) appearance concerns and BDD.

Motivations and Expectations

It is important to assess a prospective patient's motivations for surgery. Several researchers have attempted to categorize motivations as internal (undergoing the surgery to improve one's self-esteem or body image) or external (undergoing the surgery for some secondary gain, such as starting a new romantic relationship) (Edgerton & Knorr, 1971; Goin et al., 1980; Meyer et al., 1960). Patients often struggle to articulate their motivations for surgery, and may be reluctant to share their true motivations candidly for fear that they will not be taken seriously. In addition, a clear distinction between an internal and external motivations may be difficult; however, internally motivated patients are thought to be more likely to meet their goals for surgery (Edgerton et al., 1991). To assess the source of patients' motivations, it may be useful to ask when they first started thinking about cosmetic surgery or why they are interested in surgery at this time.

Pruzinsky (1993, 1996) has categorized postoperative expectations as surgical, psychological, and social. Surgical expectations address patients' specific concerns about their appearance (discussed below). Psychological expectations include the possible psychological benefits, such as improvements in body image or self-esteem, that may occur postoperatively. Social expectations address the potential social benefits of cosmetic surgery. Many women interested in cosmetic surgery believe that they will become more physically desirable to current or potential romantic partners. Although plastic surgery can enhance physical appearance (Cash & Horton, 1983; Kalick, 1979), it may not improve patients' romantic relationships. Thus prospective patients should be aware that an improvement in appearance (which may or may not be noticeable) probably will not result in a change in the social responses of others.

Assessing patients' postoperative expectations is also helpful. It may be useful to ask for patients' views of how their lives will be different following surgery. Patients who are internally motivated, and can articulate realistic expectations, may be more likely to be satisfied with the postoperative results.

Psychiatric Status and History

An assessment of current psychological status, as would be done in any mental health consultation, is an important part of the consultation with the plastic surgery patient (Sarwer, 2001). As noted above, it is likely that all of the major psychiatric conditions occur among the expanding population of cosmetic surgery patients. Nevertheless, particular attention should be paid to disorders with a body image component, such as eating disorders and somatoform disorders (other than BDD, which is considered separately below); mood and anxiety disorders should also be considered. The presence of any of these disorders, however, may not be an absolute contraindication for cosmetic surgery. In the absence of sound data on the relationship between psychopathology and surgical outcome, appropriateness for surgery should be made on a case-by-case basis and should include careful collaboration between the mental health professional and the surgeon.

A thorough psychiatric history should be obtained. Patients should be asked about diagnoses, both past or present. Patients with a positive psychiatric history who are not currently in treatment should be carefully assessed regarding the need for treatment. Patients currently under psychiatric care should be asked whether their mental health professionals are aware of their interest in surgery. These professionals should be contacted to confirm that cosmetic surgery is appropriate at this time. Patients who have not mentioned their interest in cosmetic surgery to their mental health professionals, or do not allow them to be contacted, should be viewed with caution. Although such secretiveness was once commonplace among cosmetic surgery patients, it also may be indicative of some form of psychopathology.

Appearance Concerns and BDD

Assessment of appearance concerns and body image is a central component of the psychiatric evaluation of plastic surgery patients. Prospective patients should be able to articulate specific concerns about aspects of their appearance that should be visible to the mental health professional with little effort. Previous studies have found no relationship between degree of physical deformity and degree of emotional distress in cosmetic surgery patients (Boone et al., 1996; Edgerton et al., 1991; Hay, 1970). Patients who are markedly distressed about slight defects that are not readily visible may be suffering from BDD.

The degree of body image dissatisfaction should also be assessed. It may be useful to ask about the amount of time patients spend thinking about or addressing their appearance. It is also important to assess the degree of disruption in functioning in terms of the avoidance of activity. In addition, measures of body image dissatisfaction and BDD, as well as measures of depressive symptoms, may provide useful information on prospective patients.

Postoperative Consultations

Mental health professionals also may be asked to consult with plastic surgery patients postoperatively. This typically occurs in one of three scenarios: (1) A cosmetic surgery patient is dissatisfied with successful surgery; (2) a reconstructive surgery patient is having difficulty coping with some residual deformity following surgery; or (3) a cosmetic or reconstructive surgery patient is experiencing an exacerbation of psychopathology that was not detected preoperatively. Patients in each of these examples often warrant psychotherapeutic care. Cognitive-behavioral models of body image psychotherapy (e.g., Cash, 1996; Rosen, 1996) are often useful with these individuals, although more diagnosis-specific treatments may also be required.

CONCLUSIONS

Interest in the psychological functioning of women who undergo cosmetic surgery has a long history. Studies in this area initially set out to identify women who were most likely to experience psychological benefit from cosmetic surgery. These studies were also undertaken to identify women who might be psychologically inappropriate for such surgery. Unfortunately, methodological problems left these issues largely unresolved. Recently body image has taken a more central role in the study of cosmetic surgery patients. Body image dissatisfaction is thought to motivate the pursuit of surgery, and preliminary findings suggest that body image improves postoperatively. In addition, there appears to be an increased incidence of persons with BDD among cosmetic surgery patients. Although this research increased our understanding of the psychological issues in cosmetic surgery, there is much more to be learned. Further studies are needed to examine the prevalence of other forms of psychopathology in cosmetic surgery patients. In addition, studies examining the psychological effects, both positive and negative, of cosmetic surgery are needed. Given its rapidly increasing popularity, coupled with the potential for both physical and psychological harm, cosmetic surgery is likely to continue to develop as a significant women's health issue.

REFERENCES

American Society of Plastic and Reconstructive Surgeons (ASPRS). (1992). *1992 plastic surgery procedural statistics*. Arlington Heights, IL: Author.
American Society of Plastic and Reconstructive Surgeons (ASPRS). (1996). *1996 plastic surgery procedural statistics*. Arlington Heights, IL: Author.
American Society of Plastic and Reconstructive Surgeons (ASPRS). (1998). *1998 plastic surgery procedural statistics*. Arlington Heights, IL: Author.

American Society of Plastic Surgeons (ASPS). (2001). *2000 plastic surgery procedure statistics.* Arlington Heights, IL: Author.

Baker, J. L., Kolin, I. S., & Bartlett, E. S. (1974). Psychosexual dynamics of patients undergoing mammary augmentation. *Plastic and Reconstructive Surgery, 53,* 652–659.

Beale, S., Lisper, H., & Palm, B. (1980). A psychological study of patients seeking augmentation mammaplasty. *British Journal of Psychiatry, 136,* 133–138.

Boone, O. B., Wexler, M. R., & Kaplan-DeNour, A. K. (1996). Rhinoplasty patients' critical self-evaluations of their noses. *Plastic and Reconstructive Surgery, 98,* 436–439.

Bull, R., & Rumsey, N. (1988). *The social psychology of facial appearance.* New York: Springer-Verlag.

Cash, T. F. (1996). The treatment of body-image disturbances. In J. K. Thompson (Ed.), *Body image, eating disorders, and obesity: An integrative guide for assessment and treatment* (pp. 83–107). Washington, DC: American Psychological Association.

Cash, T. F., & Horton, C. E. (1983). Aesthetic surgery: Effects of rhinoplasty on the social perception of patients by others. *Plastic and Reconstructive Surgery, 72,* 543–548.

Cash, T. F., & Pruzinsky, T. (Eds.). (1990). *Body images: Development, deviance, and change.* New York: Guilford Press.

Edgerton, M. T., Jacobson, W. E., & Meyer, E. (1960). Surgical-psychiatric study of patients seeking plastic (cosmetic) surgery: Ninety-eight consecutive patients with minimal deformity. *British Journal of Plastic Surgery, 13,* 136–145.

Edgerton, M. T., & Knorr, N. J. (1971). Motivational patterns of patients seeking cosmetic (esthetic) surgery. *Plastic and Reconstructive Surgery, 48,* 551–557.

Edgerton, M. T., Langman, M. W., & Pruzinsky, T. (1991). Plastic surgery and psychotherapy in the treatment of 100 psychologically disturbed patients. *Plastic and Reconstructive Surgery, 88,* 594–608.

Edgerton, M. T., Meyer, E., & Jacobson, W. E. (1961). Augmentation mammaplasty: II. Further surgical and psychiatric evaluation. *Plastic and Reconstructive Surgery, 27,* 279–301.

Edgerton, M. T., Webb, W. L., Slaughter, R., et al. (1964). Surgical results and psychosocial changes following rhytidectomy. *Plastic and Reconstructive Surgery, 33,* 503–521.

Endriga, M. D., & Kapp-Simon, K. A. (1999). Psychological issues in craniofacial care: State of the art. *Cleft Palate–Craniofacial Journal, 36,* 3–11.

Feingold, A. (1992). Good-looking people are not what we think. *Psychological Bulletin, 111,* 304–341.

Garner, D. M. (1997, January/February). The 1997 body image survey results. *Psychology Today,* pp. 30–94.

Glatt, B. S., Sarwer, D. B., O'Hara, D. E., et al. (1999). A retrospective study of changes in physical symptoms and body image after reduction mammaplasty. *Plastic and Reconstructive Surgery, 103,* 76–82.

Goin, M. K., Burgoyne, R. W., Goin, J. M., et al. (1980). A prospective psychological study of 50 female face-lift patients. *Plastic and Reconstructive Surgery, 65,* 436–442.

Goin, M. K., Goin, J. M., & Gianini, M. H. (1977). The psychic consequences of a reduction mammaplasty. *Plastic and Reconstructive Surgery, 59,* 530–534.

Goin, M. K., & Rees, T. D. (1991). A prospective study of patients' psychological reactions to rhinoplasty. *Annals of Plastic Surgery, 27,* 210–215.

Grossbart, T. A., & Sarwer, D. B. (1999). Cosmetic surgery: Surgical tools—psychosocial goals. *Seminars in Cutaneous Medicine and Surgery, 18,* 101–111.

Hatfield, E., & Sprecher, S. (1986). *Mirror, mirror . . . The importance of looks in everyday life.* Albany: State University of New York Press.

Hay, G. G. (1970). Psychiatric aspects of cosmetic nasal operations. *British Journal of Psychiatry, 116,* 85–97.

Hay, G. G., & Heather, B. B. (1973). Changes in psychometric test results following cosmetic nasal operations. *British Journal of Psychiatry, 122,* 89–90.

Hollyman, J. A., Lacey, J. H., Whitfield, P. J., et al. (1986). Surgery for the psyche: A longitudinal study of women undergoing reduction mammoplasty. *British Journal of Plastic Surgery, 39,* 222–224.

Institute of Medicine. (1999). *Safety of silicone implants.* Washington, DC: National Academy Press.

Kalick, S. M. (1979). Aesthetic surgery: How it affects the way patients are perceived by others. *Annals of Plastic Surgery, 2,* 128–133.

Kaslow, F., & Becker, H. (1992). Breast augmentation: Psychological and plastic surgery considerations. *Psychotherapy, 29,* 467–473.

Kilmann, P. R., Sattler, J. I., & Taylor, J. (1987). The impact of augmentation mammaplasty: A follow-up study. *Plastic and Reconstructive Surgery, 80,* 374–378.

Knorr, N. J. (1972). Feminine loss of identity in rhinoplasty. *Archives of Otolaryngology, 96,* 11–15.

Losee, J. E., Serletti, J. M., Kreipe, R. E., et al. (1997). Reduction mammaplasty in patients with bulimia nervosa. *Annals of Plastic Surgery, 39,* 443–446.

Marcus, P. (1984). Psychological aspects of cosmetic rhinoplasty. *British Journal of Plastic Surgery, 37,* 313–318.

McIntosh, V. V., Britt, E., & Bulik, C. M. (1994). Cosmetic breast augmentation and eating disorders. *New Zealand Medical Journal, 107,* 151–152.

Meyer, E., Jacobson, W. E., Edgerton, M. T., et al. (1960). Motivational patterns in patients seeking elective plastic surgery. *Psychosomatic Medicine, 22,* 193–202.

Meyer, L., & Ringberg, A. (1987). Augmentation mammaplasty: Psychiatric and psychosocial characteristics and outcome in a group of Swedish women. *Scandinavian Journal of Plastic and Reconstructive Surgery, 21,* 199–208.

Napoleon, A. (1993). The presentation of personalities in plastic surgery. *Annals of Plastic Surgery, 31,* 193–208.

Nordmann, J. E. (1998). [*Body image and self-esteem in women seeking breast augmentation.* Unpublished doctoral dissertation.]

Ohlsen, L., Ponten, B., & Hambert, G. (1978). Augmentation mammaplasty: A surgical and psychiatric evaluation of the results. *Annals of Plastic Surgery, 2,* 42–52.

Pertschuk, M. J., & Whitaker, L. A. (1988). Psychosocial outcome of craniofacial surgery in children. *Plastic and Reconstructive Surgery, 82,* 741–744.

Phillips, K. A. (1996). *The broken mirror: Understanding and treating body dysmorphic disorder.* New York: Oxford University Press.

Phillips, K. A., & Diaz, S. F. (1997). Gender differences in body dysmorphic disorder. *Journal of Nervous and Mental Disease, 185,* 570–577.

Phillips, K. A., McElroy, S. L., Keck, P. E., et al. (1993). Body dysmorphic disorder: 30 cases of imagined ugliness. *American Journal of Psychiatry, 150,* 302–308.

Pruzinsky, T. (1993). Psychological factors in cosmetic plastic surgery: Recent developments in patient care. *Plastic Surgical Nursing, 13,* 64–71.

Pruzinsky, T. (1996). Cosmetic plastic surgery and body image: Critical factors in patient assessment. In J. K. Thompson (Ed.), *Body image, eating disorders, and obesity: An integrative guide for assessment and treatment* (pp. 109–127). Washington, DC: American Psychological Association.

Pruzinsky, T., & Edgerton, M. T. (1990). Body image change in cosmetic plastic surgery. In T. F. Cash & T. Pruzinsky (Eds.), *Body images: Development, deviance, and change* (pp. 217–236). New York: Guilford Press.

Rankin, M., & Borah, G. L. (1997). Anxiety disorders in plastic surgery. *Plastic and Reconstructive Surgery, 100,* 535–542.

Rankin, M., Borah, G. L., Perry, A. W., et al. (1998). Quality-of-life outcomes after cosmetic surgery. *Plastic and Reconstructive Surgery, 102,* 2139–2145.

Robin, A. A., Copas, J. B., Jack, A. B., et al. (1988). Reshaping the psyche: The concurrent improvement in appearance and mental state after rhinoplasty. *British Journal of Psychiatry, 152,* 539–543.

Rodin, J., Silberstein, L. R., & Striegel-Moore, R. H. (1985). Women and weight: A normative discontent. In T. B. Sonderegger (Ed.), *Nebraska Symposium on Motivation: Psychology and gender* (pp. 267–307). Lincoln: University of Nebraska Press.

Rosen, J. C. (1996). Body dysmorphic disorder: Assessment and treatment. In J. K. Thompson (Ed.), *Body image, eating disorders, and obesity: An integrative guide for assessment and treatment* (pp. 149–170). Washington, DC: American Psychological Association.

Rosen, J. C., Reiter, J., & Orosan, P. (1995). Cognitive behavioral body image therapy for body dysmorphic disorder. *Journal of Consulting and Clinical Psychology, 63,* 263–269.

Sarwer, D. B. (1997). The "obsessive" cosmetic surgery patient: A consideration of body image dissatisfaction and body dysmorphic disorder. *Plastic Surgical Nursing, 17,* 193–209.

Sarwer, D. B. (2001) [*An investigation of the psychological characteristics of cosmetic breast augmentation patients*]. Unpublished raw data.

Sarwer, D. B. (2001). Psychological considerations in cosmetic surgery. In Goldwyn & Cohen (Eds.), *The unfavorable result in plastic surgery* (3rd ed., pp. 14–23).

Sarwer, D. B., Bartlett, S. P., Bucky, L. P., et al. (1998a). Bigger is not always better: Body image dissatisfaction in breast reduction and breast augmentation patients. *Plastic and Reconstructive Surgery, 101,* 1956–1961.

Sarwer, D. B., Bartlett, S. P., Whitaker, L. A., et al. (1999). Adult psychological functioning of individuals born with craniofacial anomalies. *Plastic and Reconstructive Surgery, 103,* 412–418.

Sarwer, D. B., Nordmann, J. E., & Herbert, J. D. (2000). Cosmetic breast augmentation surgery: A critical overview. *Journal of Women's Health and Gender-Based Medicine, 9,* 843–856.

Sarwer, D. B., Pertschuk, M. J., Wadden, T. A., et al. (1998b). Psychological investigations of cosmetic surgery patients: A look back and a look ahead. *Plastic and Reconstructive Surgery, 101,* 1136–1142.

Sarwer, D. B., Wadden, T. A., & Foster, G. D. (1998c). Assessment of body image dissatisfaction in obese women: Specificity, severity, and clinical significance. *Journal of Consulting and Clinical Psychology, 66,* 651–654.

Sarwer, D. B., Wadden, T. A., Pertschuk, M. J., et al. (1998d). The psychology of cosmetic surgery: A review and reconceptualization. *Clinical Psychology Review, 18,* 1–22.

Sarwer, D. B., Wadden, T. A., & Pertschuk, M. J. (1998e). Body image dissatisfaction and body dysmorphic disorder in 100 cosmetic surgery patients. *Plastic and Reconstructive Surgery, 101,* 1644–1649.

Sarwer, D. B., Wadden, T. A., & Whitaker, L. A. (in press). An investigation of changes in body image following cosmetic surgery. *Plastic and Reconstructive Surgery.*

Sarwer, D. B., Whitaker, L. A., & Pertschuk, M. J. (1998f). Body image concerns of reconstructive surgery patients: An under recognized problem. *Annals of Plastic Surgery, 40,* 404–407.

Sarwer, D. B., Whitaker, L. A., Wadden, T. A., et al. (1997). Body image dissatisfaction in women seeking rhytidectomy or blepharoplasty. *Aesthetic Surgery Journal, 17,* 230–234.

Schlebusch, L. (1989). Negative bodily experience and prevalence of depression in patients who request augmentation mammoplasty. *South African Medical Journal, 75,* 323–326.

Schlebusch, L., & Levin, A. (1983). A psychological profile of women selected for augmentation mammoplasty. *South African Medical Journal, 64,* 481–483.

Schlebusch, L., & Mahrt, I. (1993). Long-term psychological sequelae of augmentation mammoplasty. *South African Medical Journal, 83,* 267–271.

Shipley, R. H., O'Donnell, J. M., & Bader, K. F. (1977). Personality characteristics of women seeking breast augmentation. *Plastic and Reconstructive Surgery, 60,* 369–376.

Sihm, F., Jagd, M., & Pers, M. (1978). Psychological assessment before and after augmentation mammaplasty. *Scandinavian Journal of Plastic and Reconstructive Surgery, 12,* 295–298.

Slator, R., & Harris, D. L. (1992). Are rhinoplasty patients potentially mad? *British Journal of Plastic Surgery, 45,* 307–310.

Thompson, J. K. (Ed.). (1996). *Body image, eating disorders, and obesity: An integrative guide for assessment and treatment.* Washington, DC: American Psychological Association.

Thompson, J. K., Heinberg, L. J., Altabe, M., et al. (1999). *Exacting beauty: Theory, assessment, and treatment of body image disturbance.* Washington, DC: American Psychological Association.

Webb, W. L., Slaughter, R., Meyer, E., et al. (1965). Mechanisms of psychosocial adjustment in patients seeking "face-lift" operation. *Psychosomatic Medicine, 27,* 183–192.

Willard, S. G., McDermott, B. E., & Woodhouse, L. M. (1996). Lipoplasty in the bulimic patient. *Plastic and Reconstructive Surgery, 98,* 276–278.

Wright, M. R., & Wright, W. K. (1975). A psychological study of patients undergoing cosmetic surgery. *Archives of Otolaryngology, 101,* 145–151.

Yates, A., Shisslak, C. M., Allender, J. R., et al. (1988). Plastic surgery and the bulimic patient. *International Journal of Eating Disorders, 7,* 557–560.

Part IV

Sociocultural Issues for Women

29

Developmental Perspectives on Gender

M. BETH CASEY

When one is considering women's mental health, it is clearly important to understand the origins of gender constructs, attitudes, and behaviors. There is far from universal agreement on this question, however, for gender socialization is one of the most polarized fields within developmental psychology. This polarization reflects the strong divisions between the two sides of the nature–nurture debate. Before the controversies relating to gender socialization are addressed, it is important to discuss the empirical research on how children's complex gender-based mental structures are formed. Then the theoretical debates on gender socialization are presented. The chapter concludes with the description of a biological–environmental interaction approach that is designed to integrate these competing perspectives.

DEVELOPMENTAL CHANGES IN THE
ACQUISITION OF THE CONCEPT OF GENDER

Gender Identity

In order to understand gender socialization, it is first important to distinguish between "gender identity" and "gender role identity." Gender identity determines what sex one considers oneself to be. In contrast, gender role identity relates to the prescription of allowable behaviors and attitudes for males and females, and the application of that understanding to one's own behaviors and attitudes. For example, based on her emerging gender role identity, a young girl might insist on wearing dresses to school because "that's what girls do."

The ability to label an individual's own gender occurs by age 2 or 3 (Slaby & Frey, 1975), and there is evidence that the ability to identify the gender of others may occur at an even earlier age (Poulin-Dubois et al., 1994). Serbin and her associates (Poulin-Dubois et al., 1994) found that infants as young as 1 year of age had already learned to discriminate between male and female adults by integrating information from two modalities (as shown by direction of gaze toward male and female figures when listening to male and female voices).

Gender Constancy

These types of developing gender constructs are part of a larger cognitive construct called "gender constancy." Gender constancy involves the ability to understand that an individual's gender doesn't change. It is multifaceted, and includes (1) the ability to identify oneself as male or female (gender identity), (2) the understanding that gender does not change with age and remains stable over time (gender stability), and (3) the knowledge that gender does not switch as a function of dress or behavior (gender consistency) (Slaby & Frey, 1975). There is an age-related developmental progression, starting at age 2 with acquisition of gender identity, progressing at age 4–5 when gender stability is acquired, and ending at age 6 or 7 with gender consistency (Bjorklund, 2000). For example, a 4- or 5-year-old child who is aware that she is female may still wonder whether she might become a boy if she cut her hair very short and wore only boys' clothes. This reaction is consistent with Piaget's (Flavell, 1963) view of preoperational thinkers as strongly controlled and easily confused by highly salient physical cues. It also means that in judging gender, many children at this age are more influenced by external indicators of gender such as clothing (which is highly salient) than by more hidden cues such as the genitals (Bem, 1993).

Understanding of the genital basis of gender does not emerge until 6 or 7 years of age when most children move into the concrete operations stage of thinking (Flavell, 1963). At this point, they are able to coordinate the many diverse representations of gender into a single complex system. They are able to recognize that gender constancy applies to themselves and to others, is genitally based rather than based on external cues such as clothing, and remains constant throughout life.

The Impact of Gender Constancy on Gender-Stereotyped Behaviors

Another key question relates to the connection between the development of gender constancy and its impact on children's acquisition of gender stereotypes. There is evidence that some stereotyped behaviors do not emerge until after gender constancy concepts are in place. For example, greater selective attention to same-sex models emerges after there is an understanding that gender remains constant over time (Bjorklund, 2000). In a study by Slaby and Frey (1975), preschool children were shown a split-screen film of a man and a women performing similar activities. The high-gender-constancy children spent more time observing the same-sex model than did the low-gender-constancy children. In general, research shows that preschool children who are more advanced in gender constancy are also more likely to attend to same-sex models and to imitate them more (Bjorklund, 2000). In other words, a girl who has reached the understanding that she will not switch genders as she grows older starts spending more time watching and imitating the female figures in her environment, and at the same time she notices less what the males are doing. Thus there is a developmental progression, with children's cognitive understanding of what constitutes gender preceding their acquisition of gendered behaviors.

Gender-Based Toy Preferences

Although research has shown that children's gender-based attitudes and behaviors are often functions of their cognitive level of understanding of the concept of gender, one area of gender role behavior—toy preferences—does not show this developmental pattern. First of all, gender-based toy preferences arise earlier than 2 years of age, prior to the acquisition of early gender constancy constructs such as gender identity (Perry et al., 1984). Furthermore, preschoolers' level of understanding of gender constancy appears to be unrelated to their gender-based toy preferences (Bussey & Bandura, 1992). Finally, it appears that young children's gender-based toy preferences have little relationship to their actual understanding of which toys are considered gender-stereotyped (Bussey & Bandura, 1992; Maccoby, 1994).

In addition, there is evidence that toy preferences are acquired independently of key gender-based behaviors in preschoolers. Despite a strong preference for same-sex play partners (Maccoby, 1994), it has been shown that preference for gender-stereotyped play materials is *not* related to the degree of preference for same-sex peers (Serbin et al., 1994). Children who are more prone to segregate on the basis of gender are not necessarily the ones who show the most preference for gender-stereotyped activities. Thus a preference for gender-specific toys in preschoolers does not appear to arise out of their experiences with their same-sex peers.

Bjorklund (2000) has suggested that toy preferences may not be as strongly under the influence of the social-cognitive developmental process; instead, they may be in part biologically based (with male hormones affecting activity level, temperament, or motor skills, which in turn affect the types of toys that children prefer). This observation is consistent with a separate line of research that has examined individual differences within females, focusing in particular on girls with congenital adrenal hyperplasia (CAH), a congenital abnormality involving excess testosterone production during fetal development. The effect of CAH is to produce complete or partial male genitalia at birth, and it may also have a masculinizing effect on the female brain. If girls with CAH are discovered before age 2 and surgically changed to females, they are able to switch their gender identity fairly easily. However, they still are more likely to be tomboys (Money & Ehrhardt, 1972), with a much stronger preference for masculine-stereotyped toys than their female siblings exhibit (Berenbaum & Hines, 1972). It should be noted, however, that the majority of girls with CAH are on steroids that increase activity levels and may predispose them to boy-type activities; moreover, they and/or their parents are aware of their condition, thereby affecting the social-environmental conditions under which they are reared.

Gender Role Identity and Gender Schemas

Many researchers in the field have considered gender role identity to be primarily influenced by socialization factors (Bem, 1993; Geis, 1993). As discussed earlier, gender role identity is related to individuals' perception of which attitudes, behaviors, and beliefs are appropriate for males and which are appropriate for females. Given these stereotypes, gender role identity involves the degree to which individuals perceive themselves as having these masculine and feminine stereotyped characteristics. Several measures of gender role identity have been developed (Bem, 1981a; Spence et al., 1974), and a great deal of research has been conducted relating to this concept (Bem, 1993).

Given the influence of this and related concepts on the field of gender socialization, a brief historical analysis is useful. (See Bjorklund, 2000; Golombok & Fivush, 1994; and Ruble & Martin, 1998, for reviews of this type of developmental research on gender.) One important idea proposed by Bem (1974) in the early 1970s was that masculinity and femininity are separate constructs, rather than simply being at different ends of the same continuum. Bem (1981a) constructed a way of measuring gender role identity that reflected this separation of masculine from feminine gender role identity. The Bem Sex-Role Inventory (BSRI) measures the degree to which one self-identifies with masculine and feminine characteristics. Bem used a scale in which individuals indicate how well each of 60 personality characteristics describes themselves. These characteristics include 20 stereotypically masculine items (e.g., "ambitious," "self-reliant," "independent," "assertive"), 20 stereotypically feminine items (e.g., "affectionate," "gentle," "understanding," "sensitive to the needs of others"), and 20 neutral items (e.g., "truthful," "happy," "conceited," "unsystematic"). The separate masculine and feminine scoring systems acknowledge the two scales as separate, continuous dimensions, and make it possible to assess degree of cross-gender role identity by incorporating both gender constructs. Thus, for example, a woman completing the BSRI may (1) show cross-gender role identity (high masculine–low feminine scores); (2) obtain both high masculine and high feminine scores, thereby showing androgynous preferences and behaviors; (3) be very gender-stereotyped, with high feminine and low masculine scores; or (4) score low on both scales.

This approach allowed for the examination of individual differences in gender role identity, and in the 1970s the focus was on androgyny as the ideal form of gender role identity for females. An extensive body of research on this concept was produced, using measures by Spence et al. (1974) as well as by Bem (1981a). The goal of much of this research was to document that androgyny leads to greater mental health among females. However, by the end of the 1970s there was a shift away from the concept of androgyny, mainly based on political critiques (Bem, 1993) There was also criticism of the different gender role identity measures. For example, it was argued that the male-stereotyped characteristics on the BSRI (Bem, 1981a) were biased toward being more desirable for both genders than the female-stereotyped characteristics, and that the items used to measure the gender-stereotyped characteristics were developed using a narrow sample (college students in the 1970s).

Gender Schemas

Out of this research on gender role identity, another important gender-based cognitive construct emerged in the late 1970s. This was the concept of "gender schema." Bem (1981b) proposed that gender schemas are mental structures consisting of a set of expectations and associations relating to gender that help us to organize incoming information about our world. Thus, when we know someone is male or female, we make a whole host of assumptions about that person on the basis of his or her gender. This allows for an efficient processing of information about that person, but may also result in misconceptions and biases. Although gender schemas help us to modulate our behaviors and are useful in helping us fit within a gender-delineated social world, they also limit our possibilities.

One interesting aspect of Bem's theory is that individuals differ in the degree to which they use gender schemas as organizing principles when processing information. This has an impact not only on their judgments and reactions to others, but also on their perception of the range of acceptable behaviors open to themselves. One female teenager may frame what she chooses to do and how she judges others in terms of "what girls should do," while another may be relatively indifferent to this dimension of the world when making judgments about herself and others.

"Gender scripts" relate to the types of gender schemas that involve temporally based sequences of events relating to activities typically performed by males or females. These scripts specify what is likely to happen in a sequence of events and the order in which these events will occur. When asked to report about activities (such as buying and cooking food or fixing a car), it has been shown that preschoolers can sequence a series of pictures describing these activities more accurately for their own sex than for the opposite sex. This is particularly true for boys; there is evidence in general that boys are more gender-stereotyped than girls are and acquire these schemas at an earlier age (see Golombok & Fivish, 1994).

It has been shown that gender schemas are used by children to evaluate what is appropriate for boys to do and for girls to do, and that this knowledge increases with age. Both boys and girls seem to understand and remember better information that is gender-stereotyped for their own sex than for the opposite sex (Golombok & Fivish, 1994). However, both younger boys and girls (age 3) show less flexibility than older children (age 7) do in identifying what is acceptable behavior based on gender stereotypes (Serbin & Sprafkin, 1986).

Nevertheless, elementary-age children continue to negatively evaluate other children who show cross-gender behaviors, and increasingly segregate themselves into same-sex groupings. The trends for adolescence are not as clear, with some studies showing evidence for a shift back to less flexibility in gender stereotyping (Ruble & Martin, 1998). For both sexes, there seems to be an increasing tendency toward a preference for sex-stereotyped activities and interests (Ruble & Martin, 1998). There is also a widening of cognitive differences, as well as the perception among adolescents of cognitive differences in terms of what boys and girls "can do well." For example, gender differences favoring males in mathematics emerge during adolescence, especially among brighter children (Hyde et al., 1990).

A MAJOR FRAMEWORK FOR UNDERSTANDING SOCIALIZATION

Before the competing theories relating to acquisition of gender socialization are considered, it is useful to examine a major socialization theory that provides a wider context for considering these theories. Bronfenbrenner (1989) has provided an ecological framework consisting of dynamic systems at four levels that influence the socialization process. This model provides a means of analyzing the environment's impact on the individual at different levels (Wachs, 1992). Examples are provided of ways that gender socialization can occur within each of these four dynamic systems.

The Microsystem

The "microsystem" involves face-to-face interactions in a given setting. The home and the school are two of the most critical microsystems for developing gender socialization. Within the home, environmental influences (such as the presence or absence of brothers in the family) may be key in affecting what types of toys are available to girls (Casey et al., 1999).

Classroom environments are important incubators for acquiring gender-stereotyped behaviors. Schools have even been referred to as "gender schools," where children learn what is gender-appropriate and what is not (Baenninger & Newcombe, 1995; Crawford et al., 1995). In typical early childhood classrooms, starting at ages 3 and 4, children prefer to play in gender-segregated groupings; this effect has been found across cultures and settings (Maccoby, 1994). In many preschool settings, for example, boys play in the block area for many hundreds of hours over the school year, while most girls rarely play in that area of the room. It has been shown that initially it is preschool girls (60%) more than boys (21%) who prefer to play with same-sex peers at above chance levels (Moller & Serbin, 1996). As children grow older, the preference for same-sex peers becomes more equalized.

The Mesosystem

The "mesosystem" involves the interconnections between two or more microsystems that both contain the developing person, such as the home and school. Both frequently work toward producing gender-stereotyped behaviors. Having two major microsystems that reinforce one another makes it very unlikely that a child is going to "buck the system." Conflicts between home and school may produce interesting shifts in behavior. Children are often skillful at shifting and developing strategies for exploring their interests in socially acceptable ways. Some girls at the preschool level may use the art area to construct things in three-dimensional space, probably because it is less acceptable for them to do constructions in the block area. Meanwhile, at home they may do a lot of block building—but only if block-building materials are available in the family microsystem and if there is parental permission for this type of play among the female siblings.

The Exosystem

The "exosystem" involves the interconnections between two or more microsystems, one of which does not normally contain the developing person. For example, the mother's family environment is not directly experienced by the child. However, the mother's experience of her own family's attitudes toward cross-gender play formed her attitudes and interests. These in turn will influence both the home environment and the attitudes and interests of her child.

The Macrosystem

The "macrosystem" relates to the cultural influences on the child. These influences are often mediated through a caregiver's beliefs and values. The macrosystem includes the influences within all the lower-level systems. These systems come together to form a culture or subculture. Variations in tomboy behavior and tolerance for this type of cross-gender behavior across cultures are examples of how the macrosystem influences gender-based behaviors. Tomboy behavior in girls is found in some cultures, whereas others do not tolerate or give permission for participating in cross-gender stereotypes (Casey, 1996). One example of the macrosystem at work over time is the transformation in attitudes related to changing prohibitions against cross-gender play. Sports for girls are becoming much more socially acceptable in the United States than they were 20 years ago.

THEORETICAL CONTROVERSIES RELATING TO ACQUISITION OF GENDER-BASED BEHAVIORS

Psychoanalytic Perspectives

This section of the chapter addresses the theoretical battles that have been fought over the source of gender-based understanding, attitudes, and behaviors. Perhaps the earliest approach that tried to account for these gender differences was the psychoanalytic perspective based on Freud's Oedipal theory (Freud, 1905/1962). Nancy Chodorow (1989) has provided a more recent psychoanalytic formulation that focuses on the pre-Oedipal period and considers the fact that mothers are likely to relate to their male infants as different and separate from themselves, whereas their female infants are seen as more like themselves. Furthermore, as boys grow up, they have a need to cast themselves as different from women in general. The end result of this asymmetrical relationship is that boys grow up with a self that "denies relatedness," while girls acquire a "self-in-relation" (Chodorow, 1989, p. 15). Since this perspective is less research-based (Ruble & Martin, 1998), it is only touched upon in this chapter.

Social Learning Perspectives

In the research literature, the most frequently cited theoretical perspectives from a socialization perspective are the social learning and the gender schema approaches. Social learning explanations for gender-based behaviors provided one of the earliest approaches to the nature–nurture debate (Mischel, 1966; Bandura, 1966, 1977). These theorists focused on traditional learning theory principles to account for what they considered to be learned gender behaviors. According to this view, selective reinforcement of sex-appropriate gender-based behavior by parents, teachers, peers, and the cultural institutions is a major way that gender socialization is achieved.

To test predictions from this social learning theory perspective, Lytton and Romney (1991) published a major review of the literature examining the environmental impact of parents' effects on children's gender socialization. If a key socialization influence is the differential reinforcement of boys and girls by their parents, then differential parental treatment should relate to gender differences in behavior. Lytton and Romney examined 1,250 studies, 172 of which they could use in their meta-analysis. They divided these studies into 19 areas of socialization (e.g., achievement encouragement, verbal interaction, restrictiveness, encouragement of dependency, physical punishment). In 18 of these areas, they found no evidence of differential socialization of boys and girls by parents. In studies on populations in North America, in only one area (direct encouragement of gender-typed activities) did they find significant effects, with parental behaviors influencing gender preferences. Thus parental reinforcement of gender-based behaviors, such as aggression and dependency, does not appear to be a major source of male–female differences. These findings are consistent with an earlier review by Maccoby and Jacklin (1974). It is interesting to note, however, that the one area in which parents were found to have an impact was the encouragement of sex-typed activities and interests, including toy, game, and activity choices. This type of gender preference has been discussed earlier in the context of gender-constancy and gender segregated play. The key role of parents in affecting toy preferences may help to explain why it is formed during infancy, even prior to the development of gender identity.

In addition to differential reinforcement, the social learning theorists also consider observational learning and modeling as a critical mode through which children acquire sex-appropriate behaviors (Bandura, 1966). Carefully watching others in order to figure out the appropriate ways to behave is an important component of our socialization process. However, Maccoby and Jacklin (1974) did not find evidence to show that children learn gender-appropriate behaviors through direct modeling of their same-sex parents. Young children's gender-stereotyped behaviors (e.g., playing with dolls vs. trucks) are very different from their parents' (e.g., cooking vs. carpentry). Maccoby and Jacklin's review of observational studies showed no strong evidence that children imitate same-sex models more when given an opportunity to choose either a male or a female to imitate. Instead, more recently, Huston (1983) found that children are more likely to imitate same-sex models *if* they behave in gender-appropriate ways. The gender appropriateness of the observed behavior is more important than the sex of the model (Golombok & Fivush, 1994).

Thus it is now considered simplistic to assume that children acquire gender-typed behaviors by direct imitation of same-sex models (Golombok & Fivush, 1994). Instead, Perry and Bussey (1979) proposed a modified social learning theory in which gender-based modeling is considered more of a process of abstraction. Children conceptualize what is gender-appropriate behavior for their sex through observing many different male and female models in many different contexts, including parents, peers, and the mass media. Thus typical behavior for one's gender is cognitively abstracted from a complex array of models provided by the environment. This theoretical change is consistent with the shifting of a number of early social learning views of modeling closer to a social-cognitive perspective (e.g., see Bandura's, 1977). It should be noted that the social learning view of social cognition differs from a cognitive-developmental view (discussed below). According to the social learning theory, social cognitions are directly affected by children's experiences, and are not based on children's general stage of cognitive development. Thus, according to this view, the acquisition of gender-based behaviors is environmentally determined and is not considered to change with age in a consistent pattern.

Cognitive-Developmental Perspectives

In contrast to this social learning theory perspective is a cognitive-developmental approach (Serbin & Sprafkin, 1986; Slaby & Frey, 1975), in which gender constructs are believed to develop with age and to be dependent on more general developing thought structures (see, e.g., Piaget's stages of cognitive development; Flavell, 1963). This approach considers the stages of cognitive development to be invariant and biologically based, but it stresses the critical role of the environment in affecting individual differences within this framework. In order for children to actively construct gender concepts, they engage in a dynamic interaction with their environment. The research described at the outset of this chapter on gender constancy fits within this cognitive-developmental perspective.

One strand of the cognitive-developmental approach relates to the development of gender differences in moral reasoning and of female "ways of knowing" (Gilligan, 1982). This strand is most closely associated with Carol Gilligan, who argued that there are different developmental trajectories for males and females. This research arose out of Kohlberg's (1981) original research, which posed real-life moral dilemmas and examined the stages of moral development, based on his adaptation of Piaget's theory (Flavell, 1963). Gilligan (1982) has argued that females interpret these dilemmas by emphasizing caring, compassion, and concern for others, whereas males emphasize fairness and justice. However, though these differences exist within individuals, the literature suggests that these perspectives do not divide along gender lines (Brabeck, 1983).

In her more recent relational work, Gilligan (1996) has focused on understanding the profound shifts during adolescence, when girls often "lose their voice" and their confidence in themselves in terms of their abilities and their role in society. In this theory, individual development is understood within the context of relationships with others. According to Gilligan (1996) and her associates, the conflict arises for girls during adolescence as they become aware of the norms limiting them through the patriarchal social order. These researchers developed their theory in part through a longitudinal analysis of the narratives of private school girls who were followed for 5 years. In this work, the researchers interviewed a subset of the students over an extended period and conducted a series of retreats with women psychologists and teachers, Based on the importance of interconnectedness, Gilligan and her associates proposed that relationships with adult women can help adolescent girls to find their voices and to work through the tension of their own experience and the pressures provided by the social context in which they live. However, again the issue arises of the empirical evidence for the uniqueness of girls' and women's voices, since similar methodology was not used on equivalent samples of males, and the perspective of the interviewers may have been as important as that of the interviewees (Crawford, 1989).

Gender Schema and Gender Polarization Theories

Furthermore, Bem (1993) has argued that this celebration of female differences in Gilligan's model is just the reverse of the more historically traditional male-dominated gender polarization. She has proposed that both the androgenic and the gynecentric perspectives distort the reality of true individual variations, which have more to do with our social roles and the gender schemas arising out of these roles than with any true biological differences between males and females. If the roles truly were reversed, she contends, the behaviors of males and females would be reversed. Thus, according to Bem (1993, p. 80), both belief systems are part of gender polarization, which arises from "the ubiquitous organization of social life around the distinction between male and female."

Based on the gender schema perspective, gender is a socially constructed concept that evolves out of the tendency of humans to categorize and stereotype other people. According to Geis (1993), it is through gender-based schemas that we unconsciously interpret and guide our perceptions, inferences, memories, and treatment of men and women. This applies even to those who espouse beliefs in gender equality at the conscious level. These biases are all-pervasive and affect what we notice, infer, and remember about one another. They also produce self-fulfilling prophecies that are based on gender stereotypes.

These perspectives are part of an increasing trend among feminists to reject evidence for gender differences (Crawford et al., 1995; Bem, 1993). In fact, they reject any research that focuses on gender differences, arguing that this research agenda is based on the skewed focus on gender differences arising out of our cultural fixation with gender as the way to dichotomize our world (Bem, 1993). These researchers stress the cognitive literature that shows evidence of decreasing gender differences within the last 20 years for a range of cognitive skills (Crawford et al., 1995). They argue that with increased opportunities and interventions, these gender differences favoring males will disappear altogether.

Thus a more recent series of feminist theories has essentially argued for a total socialization perspective. Basically, the position is taken that the only biological bases for gender differences are the social roles that women are forced into by the nature of their child-rearing productive function, and that gender differences result completely from the androgenic domination of males in society (Bem, 1993). (As indicated earlier, the one exception to this view is the alternative feminist perspective proposed by Gilligan in 1982, which stresses the unique nature of females.)

From a review of the research, it appears to me that some cognitive behaviors are robust and continue to show substantial gender differences over the last 20 years, although there is evidence of a reduction in some cognitive gender differences over time. The types of cognitive skills showing stable gender effects include some types of spatial and mechanical reasoning skills, as well as performance on the Mathematics Scholastic Aptitude Test (SAT-Math) among high-ability students (Masters & Soares, 1993; Stumpf, 1995). Spatial and mechanical skills have been shown to mediate gender differences in mathematics skills (Casey et al., 2001; Gallagher et al., 2000) and in fact are stronger mediators of gender differences on the SAT-Math than either mathematics self-confidence or mathematics anxiety is (Casey et al., 1997). Gender differences on these skills may have an impact on the types of strategies used by boys and girls when solving mathematics problems. (See Casey et al., 1997, for a review of these issues.) Thus it seems premature to deny any evidence of cognitive gender differences. The danger of this approach is that it may lead to abandonment of useful intervention techniques that may make a wider range of problem-solving strategies available to both girls and boys.

Evolutionary Theories

At the other side of the nature–nurture debate is the evolutionary psychology view that accounts for gender differences in behavior in terms of male–female biological differences arising out of evolutionary pressures, adaptation, and natural selection. The evolutionary perspective draws on an animal model, and argues that those gender differences found across all cultures have developed out of differential evolutionary pressures that affect males differently from females. As our male and female ancestors coevolved, they exerted selective pressures on the opposite sex, and vestiges of those pressures remain today (Kendrick & Trost, 1993). According to this view, cultures are not just arbitrarily constructed, but arise out of the genetic proclivities of the males and females who inhabit them. One view is that males and females differ in their reproductive strategies. According to this view, females are basically monogamous, putting their energies into protecting and nurturing their children; males are essentially polygamous, putting their energies toward short-term mating, which involves finding many fertile mates (Hoyenga & Hoyenga, 1993).

One difficulty with these evolutionary theories is that it is difficult to prove them. Furthermore, they have been attacked based on disagreements as to how natural selection actually works in both humans and animals (Fausto-Sterling, 1992). One strategy is to examine male–female behaviors cross-culturally to determine whether a particular male–female difference is universally found. However, Bem (1993) has argued that this type of evidence is not conclusive, since the child-rearing requirements of females may force them into certain social roles that males might take on if they had the same physical biological limitations. Therefore, the gendered behaviors themselves may originate from sociological rather than genetic sources.

Neuropsychological Theories

Neuropsychological theories (Geschwind & Galaburda, 1987; Annett, 1985) have generally accounted for gender differences in terms of a predisposition toward different patterns of brain organization in males and females. Geschwind and Galaburda (1987) apply their theory to account for individual variations in cross-gender role behaviors in girls. These researchers posit that testosterone levels within the fetal brain are affected not only by the maternal–fetal environment, but by genetic factors affecting both hormone levels and the permeability of the brain to these hormones.

In their review, Berenbaum et al. (1995) conclude that hormones acting on the brain and behavior early in development are "organizational," because they produce permanent changes in the wiring and sensitivity of the brain. For example, evidence from a variety of human clinical conditions and normal samples suggests that moderate to high levels of androgens in the prenatal and early postnatal periods can facilitate the development of spatial abilities within females.

Geschwind and Galaburda (1987) propose that the level of testosterone entering the fetal brain affects a wide range of factors in both males and females, including (1) patterns of laterality, in terms of the organization of the left and right hemispheres; (2) handedness patterns; (3) cognitive functioning; and (4) gender-based behaviors such as degree of masculinization and feminization.

Furthermore, increased testosterone levels during fetal development are more likely to lead to increased masculinization and/or defeminization for females in particular, according to these theorists. Geschwind and Galaburda (1985) refer to findings in the literature on both nonhuman primates and humans that support this position. The research shows that the administration of testosterone in pregnancy produces "pronounced morphologic and behavioral masculinization" (1985, p. 525). Geschwind and Galaburda propose that a "masculinizing effect is one that leads to male typical behavior in the female," "A defeminizing effect is one that leads to loss of female typical traits," and "The two classes of effects can occur independently and depend on hormonal effects at different sites" (1985, p. 525). Thus they distinguish between masculinization and defeminization. This dichotomy is consistent with Bem's (1981a) use of separate subscales for the masculine and feminine dimensions in the BSRI.

According to Geschwind and Galaburda's theory, about a third of the population has a nonstandard or "anomalous" pattern of brain organization. One indicator of this more variable pattern of brain organization within families is a nonstandard handedness pattern, either in the individual or in immediate family members. (Another indicator is a predisposition to language-based learning disabilities.) Based on their view, individuals who are less strongly right-handed themselves (left-handers or ambidextrous right-handers), or those who come from families with a genetic predisposition toward atypical handedness, are likely to have higher levels of testosterone reaching the brain during fetal development. They argue that the increased testosterone levels have a major impact on the early fetal neurodevelopmental process and result in a tendency for more variable patterns of brain development among these handedness groups.

There has been criticism of Geschwind and Galaburda's wide-ranging theoretical model in terms of its testability and some of its predictions (Bryden et al., 1994). However, we have found evidence connecting atypical handedness with cross-gender behaviors, and it is difficult to see on what basis an environmental model might make equivalent predictions. We provided support for this component of the Geschwind–Galaburda theory, using the BSRI (Bem, 1981a) and a tomboy scale that distinguished between an interest in male games and activities and a rejection of female games and activities (Casey & Nuttall, 1990). We divided a female college sample into an anomalous-dominant-handedness subgroup of females (left-handed women, ambidextrous right-handed women, and women with left-handed or ambidextrous immediate family members) and compared them to women with standard dominance (right-handers with all right-handed family members). We found that the anomalous-dominant women were more likely to obtain high masculine and low feminine scores in the BSRI. This group was also more likely to reject feminine activities on the tomboy scale (but did not differ in degree of interest in boys' games and activities). The results of this study provide support for Geschwind and Galaburda's theory that handedness and family handedness are indicators of biological influences on gender role identity and gender-based behaviors in females.

A BIOLOGICAL–ENVIRONMENTAL
INTERACTION MODEL OF GENDER DIFFERENCES

As shown in this review, the nature–nurture sides of the gender debate appear to have drawn even further apart in recent years. Yet, as Bjorklund (2000, p. 28) states in his review of developmental research, "All self-respecting developmentalists believe that development is the result of an interaction between genetic/biologic factors and environmental/experiential factors. There is really no other alternative." A number of researchers (Gibson & Petersen, 1991; Halpern, 2000; Petersen, 1980; Sherman, 1978) have hypothesized that both socialization and biological factors are intricately connected in human behavior. However, only a few studies have examined this interaction (e.g., Mitchell et al., 1989; Rowe, 1982), and when these are compared to the voluminous literature on gender, it is evident there has been little research arising from an integrative perspective.

The male–female distributions are clearly overlapping even with respect to gender-stereotyped behaviors, and one way to avoid some of the more emotionally charged issues in gender research is to focus on individual differences *within* females rather than *between* males and females. In addition, it is useful to consider how environmental and biological factors might interact to produce such a wide range of gender-based behaviors within females. The following is a presentation of a biological–environmental approach that attempts to integrate both perspectives, and data consistent with this approach are presented in relation to individual differences in gender role identity.

In our research, Mary Brabeck, Ronald Nuttall, Betty Pezaris, and I have chosen to unite two perspectives: one based on neuropsychological theories, such as the theory presented by Geschwind and Galaburda (1987), and one based on the environmental framework provided by Bronfenbrenner (1989). We have taken a "bent twig" approach, originally proposed by Sherman (1978), which is based on the old adage "As the twig is bent, the tree's inclined." Our research approach has been to identify the biological factors that result in "bending the twig" toward development in a particular direction (for a review, see Casey, 1996). This predisposition is assumed to lead to development only under the appropriate socialization conditions. For example, a young girl may inherit the biological potential and predisposition to develop good spatial skills, but without the environment that nurtures this potential, this ability will not be developed. Conversely, based on our theory, unless the biological potential is there, a girl who grows up in an environment supportive of spatial interests and experiences will not develop strong spatial skills. Thus biological predisposition *plus* socialization are two essential components that interact to affect human behavior. In much of our prior research, we have successfully applied this approach to predict subgroup differences in spatial ability among females. We have used handedness patterns as a measure of biological predisposition, and spatial experiences (Casey & Brabeck, 1990), math–science majors (Casey & Brabeck, 1989), and presence of brothers in the family (Casey, Nuttall, & Pezaris, 1999) as measures of environmental factors.

We have also incorporated this biological–environmental interaction approach to predict which girls are likely to show cross-gender identity. Given the focus of this chapter, I present our "bent twig" findings relating to this latter work in more detail. As discussed earlier, we had previously found evidence, based on Geschwind and Galaburda's theory, that anomalous-dominant-handedness females showed a higher predisposition to cross-gender role identity (Casey & Nuttall, 1990). In a second study, based on the "bent twig" model, we investigated how environmental factors might interact with this biological predisposition to determine which females would show atypical gender role identity.

Given Bronfenbrenner's (1989) framework, the family microsystem should be a key environment for either fostering or squelching that biological predisposition. Consistent with our "bent twig" model, we predicted that both biological and environmental factors would be essential factors in the development of cross-gender identity, and this was supported in our new findings (Casey et al., 1995). The anomalous-dominant females who also reported strong parental permission for opposite-sex toys was the subgroup that had higher masculinity than femininity scores on the BSRI, while the reverse was true for all other subgroups of females. Thus these results indicate that biological and environmental conditions combined provide the conditions that foster cross-gender role identity. The two conditions consist of (1) anomalous brain dominance, which predisposes girls toward greater cross-gender identity; and (2) a family microsystem in which girls are able to explore their predisposition without pressure from their parents to behave in gender-stereotyped ways. It should be noted that girls' biological predispositions may also be influential in helping to create the environments they experience (Scarr, 1992). In other words, some daughters may be pressuring their parents to buy masculine-stereotyped toys as well, thereby influencing their own environment (Wachs, 1992).

CONCLUSIONS

One reason for the intensity of the dialogue with regard to gender is that personal, societal, and public policy decisions may hinge on the outcome of this research debate. By considering individual variation within females, and by studying females who are exceptions to the rules of female-gender-based behaviors, it may be possible to examine gendered behaviors in a less charged atmosphere. If we explore those at the overlapping edges between the sexes, then perhaps it may be possible to understand the ways in which individuals who cross gender lines show similarities both to their own and to the opposite sex. It is time to refocus the research in this field and move away from the all-or-none positions relating to the biological and environmental impacts on gendered behaviors. By carefully selecting subgroups based on behavioral genetic or neuropsychological models as well as on sociological/environmental models, we may develop new models that will help us understand how these two types of variables interact to produce a diverse range of gendered behaviors within females (Casey, 1996).

REFERENCES

Annett, M. (1985). *Left, right, hand, and brain: The right shift theory*. Hillsdale, NJ: Erlbaum.

Baenninger, M., & Newcombe, N. (1995). Environmental input to the development of sex-related differences in spatial and mathematical ability. *Learning and Individual Differences, 7*, 363–379.

Bandura, A. (1966). *Social foundations of thought and action: A social cognitive theory*. Englewood Cliffs, NJ: Prentice-Hall.

Bandura, A. (1977). *Social learning theory*. Englewood Cliffs, NJ: Prentice-Hall.

Bem, S. L. (1974). The measurement of psychological androgyny. *Journal of Clinical and Consulting Psychology, 42*, 155–162.

Bem, S. L. (1981a). *Bem Sex-Role Inventory: Professional manual*. Palo Alto, CA: Consulting Psychologists Press.

Bem, S. L. (1981b). Gender schema theory: A cognitive account of sex-typing. *Psychological Review, 88*, 354–364.

Bem, S. L. (1993). *The lenses of gender: Transforming the debate on sexual inequality*. New Haven, CT: Yale University Press.

Berenbaum, S. A., & Hines, M. (1992). Early androgens are related to sex-typed toy preferences. *Psychological Science, 3*, 203–206.

Berenbaum, S. A., Korman, K., & Leveroni, C. (1995). Early hormones and sex differences in cognitive abilities. *Learning and Individual Differences, 7*, 303–321.

Bjorklund, D. F. (2000). *Children's thinking: Developmental function and individual differences* (3rd ed.). Belmont, CA: Wadsworth.

Brabeck, M. (1983). Moral judgment: Theory and research on differences between males and females. *Developmental Review, 3*, 274–291.

Bronfenbrenner, U. (1989). Ecological system theories. *Annals of Child Development, 6*, 187–249.

Bryden, M. P., McManis, I. C., & Bulman-Fleming, M. B. (1994). Evaluating support for the Geschwind–Behan–Galaburda model of cerebral lateralization. *Brain and Cognition, 26*, 103–167.

Bussey, K., & Bandura, A. (1992). Self-regulatory mechanisms governing gender development. *Child Development, 63*, 1236–1250.

Casey, M. B. (1996). Understanding individual differences in spatial ability within females: A nature/nurture interactionist framework. *Developmental Review, 16*, 241–260.

Casey, M. B., & Brabeck, M. M. (1989). Exceptions to the male advantage on a spatial task: Family handedness and college major as a factor identifying women who excel. *Neuropsychologia, 27*, 689–696.

Casey, M. B., & Brabeck, M. M. (1990). Women who excel on a spatial task: Proposed genetic and environmental factors. *Brain and Cognition, 12*, 73–84.

Casey, M. B., Brabeck, M. M., & Nuttall, R. L. (1995). As the twig is bent: The biology and social-ization of gender roles in women. *Brain and Cognition, 27,* 237–246.

Casey, M. B., & Nuttall, R. L. (1990). Differences in feminine and masculine characteristics in women as a function of handedness: Support for the Geschwind/Galaburda theory of brain organization. *Neuropsychologia, 28,* 749–755.

Casey, M. B., Nuttall, R. L., & Pezaris, E. (1997). Mediators of gender differences in mathematics college entrance test scores: A comparison of spatial skills with internalized beliefs and anxi-eties. *Developmental Psychology, 33,* 669–680.

Casey, M. B., Nuttall, R., & Pezaris, E. (1999). Evidence in support of a model that predicts how biological and environmental factors interact to influence spatial skills. *Developmental Psy-chology, 35,* 1237–1247.

Casey, M. B., Nuttall, R. L., & Pezaris, E. (2001). Spatial–mechanical reasoning skills versus mathe-matics self-confidence as mediators of gender differences on mathematics subtests using cross-national gender-based items. *Journal for Research in Mathematics Education, 32,* 28–57.

Chodorow, N. J. (1989). *Feminism and psychoanalytic theory.* New Haven, CT: Yale University Press.

Crawford, M. C. (1989). Agreeing to differ: Feminist epistemologies and women's ways of know-ing. In M. C. Crawford & M. Gentry (Eds.), *Gender and thought: Psychological perspectives* (pp. 128–146). New York: Springer-Verlag.

Crawford, M. C., Chaffin, R., & Fitton, L. (1995). Cognition in social context. *Learning and Indi-vidual Differences, 7,* 341–362.

Fausto-Sterling, A. (1992). *Myths of gender: Biological theories about women and men* (2nd. ed.). New York: Basic Books.

Flavell, J. H. (1963). *The developmental psychology of Jean Piaget.* Princeton, NJ: Van Nostrand.

Freud, S. (1962). *Three essays on the theory of sexuality* (J. Strachey, Ed. & Trans.) . New York: Avon. (Original work published 1905)

Gallagher, A. M., DeLisi, R., Holst, P. C., et al. (2000). Gender differences in advanced mathemati-cal problem-solving. *Experimental Child Psychology, 75,* 165–191.

Geis, F. L. (1993). Self-fulfilling prophecies: A social psychology view of gender. In A. E. Beall & R. J. Sternberg (Eds.), *The psychology of gender* (pp. 9–54). New York: Guilford Press.

Geschwind, N., & Galaburda, A. M. (1985). Cerebral lateralization: Biological mechanisms, asso-ciations, and pathology. I. A hypothesis and a program from research. *Archives of Neurology, 42,* 521–552.

Geschwind, N., & Galaburda, A .M. (1987). *Cerebral lateralization.* Cambridge, MA: Bradford Books/MIT Press.

Gibson, E., & Petersen, A. (1991). *Brain maturation and cognitive development: Comparative and cross-cultural perspectives.* New York: Aldine de Gruyter.

Gilligan, C. (1982). *In a different voice: Psychological theory and women's development.* Cam-bridge, MA: Harvard University Press.

Gilligan, C. (1996). The centrality of relationships in human development: A puzzle, some evidence and a theory. In G. G. Noam & K. W. Fischer (Eds.), *Development and vulnerability in close relationships* (pp. 236–261). Mahwah, NJ: Erlbaum.

Golombok, S., & Fivush, R. (1994). *Gender development.* Cambridge, England: Cambridge Uni-versity Press.

Halpern, D. F. (2000). *Sex differences in cognitive abilities* (3rd ed.). Mahwah, NJ: Erlbaum.

Hoyenga, K. B., & Hoyenga, K. T. (1993). *Gender related differences: Origins and outcomes.* Needham Heights, MA: Allyn & Bacon.

Huston, A. (1983). Sex-typing. In P. H. Mussen (Series Ed.) & E. M. Hetherington (vol. ed.), *Hand-book of child psychology: Vol. 4. Socialization, personality, and social development* (4th ed., pp. 16–28). New York: Wiley.

Hyde, J. S., Fennema, E., & Lamon, S. J. (1990). Gender differences in mathematics performance: A meta-analysis. *Psychological Bulletin, 107,* 139–155.

Kendrick, D. T., & Trost, M. R. (1993). The evolutionary perspective. In A. E. Beall & R. J. Sternberg (Eds.), *The psychology of gender* (pp. 148–172). New York: Guilford Press.

Kohlberg, L. (1981). *The philosophy of moral development*. San Francisco: Harper & Row.

Lytton, H., & Romney, D. M. (1991). Parents' differential socialization of boys and girls: A meta-analysis. *Psychological Bulletin, 109*, 267–296.

Maccoby, E. E. (1994). Commentary: Gender segregation in childhood. In C. Leaper (Ed.), *Childhood gender segregation: Causes and consequences* (pp. 29–39). San Francisco: Jossey-Bass.

Maccoby, E. E., & Jacklin, C. N. (1974). *The psychology of sex differences*. Stanford, CA: Stanford University Press.

Masters, S., & Soares, M. (1993). Is the gender difference in mental rotation disappearing? *Behavioral Genetics, 23*, 337–341.

Mischel, W. (1966). A social-learning view of sex differences in behavior. In E. E. Maccoby (Ed.), *The development of sex differences* (pp. 57–81). Stanford, CA: Stanford University Press.

Mitchell, J. E., Baker, L. A., & Jacklin, C. N. (1989). Masculinity and femininity in twin children: Genetic and environmental factors. *Child Development, 60*, 1475–1485.

Moller, L. C., & Serbin, L. A (1996). Antecedents to toddler gender segregation: Cognitive consonance, sex-typed toy preferences and behavioral compatibility. *Sex Roles, 35*, 445–460.

Money, J., & Ehrhardt, A. A. (1972). *Man and woman, boy and girl*. Baltimore: Johns Hopkins University Press.

Perry, D. G., & Bussey, K. (1979). The social learning theory of sex difference: Imitation is alive and well. *Journal of Personality and Social Psychology, 37*, 1699–1712.

Perry, D. G., White, A. J., & Perry, L. C. (1984). Does early sex typing result from children's attempts to match their behavior to sex role stereotypes? *Child Development, 55*, 2114–2121.

Petersen, A. C. (1980). Biopyschosocial processes in the development of sex-related differences. In J. E. Parsons (Ed.), *The psychology of sex differences and sex roles* (pp. 31–55). Washington, DC: Hemisphere.

Poulin-Dubois, D., Serbin, L. A., Kenyon, B., et al. (1994). Infants' intermodal knowledge about gender. *Developmental Psychology, 30*, 436–442.

Rowe, D. C. (1982). Sources of variability in sex-linked personality attributes: A twin study. *Developmental Psychology, 18*, 431–434.

Ruble, D. N., & Martin, C. L. (1998). Gender development. In W. Damon (Series Ed.) & N. Eisenberg (Vol. Ed.), *Handbook of child psychology: Vol. 3. Social, emotional and personality development* (5th ed., pp. 933–1016). New York: Wiley.

Scarr, S. (1992). Developmental theories for the 1990's: Development and individual differences. *Child Development, 63*, 1–19.

Serbin, L. A., Moller, L. C., Gulko, J., et al. (1994). The emergence of gender segregation in toddler playgroups. In C. Leaper (Ed.), *New directions for child development: Vol. 65. Childhood gender segregation: Causes and consequences* (pp. 7–17). San Francisco: Jossey-Bass.

Serbin, L. A., & Sprafkin, C. (1986). The salience of gender and the process of sex typing in three- to seven-year-old children. *Child Development, 57*, 1188–1199.

Sherman, J. (1978). *Sex-related cognitive differences*. Springfield, IL: Charles C Thomas.

Slaby, R. G., & Frey, K. S. (1975). Development of gender constancy and selective attention to same-sex models. *Child Development, 46*, 849–856.

Spence, J. T., Helmreich, R. L., & Stapp, J. (1974). The Personal Attributes Questionnaire: A measure of sex-role stereotypes and masculinity–femininity. *JSAS Catalog of Selected Documents in Psychology, 4*, 43–44.

Stumpf, H. (1995). Gender differences in performance on tests of cognitive abilities: Experimental design issues and empirical results. *Learning and Individual Differences, 7*, 275–287.

Wachs, T. D. (1992). *The nature of nurture*. Newbury Park, CA: Sage.

30

Marriage and Family

MARCIA LASSWELL

The institutions of marriage and parenting have proven to be durable in spite of the enormous changes in how and when people marry, how long marriages last, and when and how many children are born. Although research describing these changes in marriage and parenting demographics is plentiful, fewer studies have focused solely on how marriage specifically affects women. Moreover, the available literature on marriage is often polarized between those who report that married women are happier and healthier because they are married, and those who make the opposite argument that marriage is detrimental to women in general. The literature on parenting and divorce does not suffer from such polarization, as it reports more uniformly that both are considerably more demanding and problematic issues for women than for men.

This chapter examines how marriage, parenting, and divorce are associated with women's physical and mental health. Numerous cultural variations are explored to reflect the changing nature of the U.S. population. Because their lives are tied so closely to marriage and parenting, women often seem to be disadvantaged by these institutions, because the woman's world within the family is largely the result of genderized social norms, laws, and other forms of social legitimization. Social policy changes in the future will be necessary to add quality to the lives of women and their families.

MARRIAGE

Marriage is certainly not a dying institution, in spite of reports to the contrary in the popular press. It is true that the number of marriages in the United States currently has recently reached its lowest level in history, but still over 90% of all Americans marry at least once in a lifetime. About 2.3 million marriage licenses are issued to couples in this country every year (Department of Health and Human Services, National Center for Health Statistics, 1998). Three-quarters of those who divorce try again. Forty-six percent of all marriages each year are remarriages. It seems obvious that there is a strong inclination to form a stable relationship through bonds of marriage, even though the possibility of divorce is always present. Race and ethnicity are important predictors of marriage rates. Statistics show that African American women's marriage rate is lower than that of European American women, with the exception of women over the age of 65; in this age group, African American women have higher marriage rates than European American women (Staples, 1993). Remarriage rates are lower among both African American and Hispanic women (Cherlin, 1996).

Studies of as-yet-unmarried women reveal that they hope for success when they marry, but are quite aware that divorce could eventually occur. They also have some realization of the sacrifices they may need to make if a marriage is to work (Debold et al., 1993).

A great deal has been written about why men marry and about the benefits marriage has for them (Fowers, 1991; Unger & Crawford, 1996; Steil, 1997; Bernard, 1972). The message in the now famous article by Judy Syfers (1972/1973), "I Want a Wife," on the benefits of having a wife gave women of the day pause to reflect on the countless unpaid services they provided. It still resonates with women today, including those in college classes that may be reading it for the first time. Study after study has reported that married men are more satisfied with being married than married women are (Amato & Booth, 1995; Levenson et al., 1993). Research continues to find that married men are less depressed than are either married women or single men, and are more satisfied with their lives than are single men (Fowers, 1991; Steil & Turetsky, 1987; Gottman, 1994).

Researchers note that stress in marriage is frequently the result of lack of interpersonal support and intimacy between the partners. It is proposed that a woman's view of her own well-being is more closely tied to the relationship than is a man's. Consequently, if there is distress in the marriage, the woman is uniquely at risk for depression (Koerner et al., 1994; Hammen, 1991). Some have reported that women's marital dissatisfaction and consequent depression are correlated with the unequal distribution of labor, which disfavors wives (Whistman & Jacobson, 1989).

Two questions merge for serious consideration after one reviews studies on the subject. First, with women's changing roles in society, are the results of early studies about the toll marriage takes on women compared to men still valid? Second, if marriage favors men and has many negative consequences for women, why do women continue to pursue matrimony?

What emerges from the current literature concerning gender differences in marital satisfaction is that there have been some significant changes in recent years, not only in the findings but also in the methodology leading to those results. These new results show movement toward a position that marriage can "work for women too" (Denmark et al., 2000). The inconsistency between the newer research and the older studies may be explained in part by the early influence of feminist scholars who noted the inequality of wives' and husbands' roles and power bases, and uncovered the basic dissatisfactions of married women. In addition, more recent studies have separated samples into "satisfied" and "dissatisfied" marriages and have concluded that gender differences in happiness, mental, and physical health are more pronounced in dissatisfied marriages (Levenson et al., 1994). Many factors in women's lives, such as education, gainful and satisfying employment, and gender role equality within the marriage, contribute to increased satisfaction in women's personal identities; this satisfaction has translated into more contentment in marriage. As women have more choices in life, it now seems that whatever they are—married or single—they are finding more satisfaction as they make changes to take care of themselves. This does not imply, however, that marriage has become an "equal playing field" for all women, or even for most women when compared to their husbands (Perry-Jenkins et al., 1992).

When it is said that marriage can "work for women too," this statement is usually based on findings of general well-being, such as better physical health and longer life for both men and women who are married. One positive effect is a higher income level with two wage earners, which correlates with better health care, more adequate housing, and access to labor-saving aids. In addition, more recent research focusing on single persons reports that, contrary to past studies, single women are not necessarily happier than married women (Wu & DeMaris, 1996). Instead, it may well be that earlier studies also included women who were delaying marriage longer in order to gain education and work skills, thus skewing the earlier results in favor of single women's being happier. And once these women eventually marry, they may have grown as individuals, contributing to sustaining their gains even in marriage. These women are less likely to have traditional marriages. One study reported that the highest levels of satisfaction in the marriages of younger couples occurred when both partners in such a couple strove for a more egalitarian relationship. In contrast, this same study reported that the lowest marital quality occurred when at least one partner wanted a traditional marriage (Weigel & Weigel, 1990).

Almost all experts agree that the increased volume of married women in the labor force has rapidly shifted women's identity from being primarily domestic supporters for their husbands to one in which they provide a more similar financial contribution and enjoy a more equitable power base. This is especially the case before and after child-rearing years. The major complaint resulting from this shift for women is "role overload," as they very often find that they are expected to have primary responsibilities for household chores and children in addition to full-time employment (Suitor, 1991).

Research continues to show that old domestic task patterns persist even as gender roles have changed in other areas of life. However, more recent research offers the promising news that husbands do perform more housework traditionally allocated to wives when they are married to women who are extensively involved in the labor force. Later age at marriage plays a significant role in women's likelihood of having work lives that promote husbands' willingness to take on these tasks (Pittman & Blanchard, 1996). However, when women continue to bear the bulk of household work—and especially when child care is added—more often than not there are negative effects on their sense of well-being, both physically and mentally (Lennon & Rosenfield, 1992).

The question of why women marry cannot be answered with great certainty if the research on whether or not marriage is healthy for them is the sole criterion. The literature is still not only inconsistent but often contradictory, and this issue continues to be the subject of much interest and probing. The fact is that no matter what the research has found or does find in the future, women do get married and probably will continue to define themselves as wives and mothers more often than men define themselves as husbands and fathers. Women are not immune to socialization, which grooms them for marriage and motherhood more than for the freedom men experience in their roles (Wood et al., 1989). They are more influenced by the popular media, which tend to romanticize love, marriage, and parenthood. Many seem not to have heard of the scholarly argument about "his" and "hers" marriages (Bernard, 1972). In fact, studies note that gendered romantic ideation borders on epidemic proportions among college-age women (Debold et al., 1993).

The end result of women's romantic and traditional ideas about family life is that even though record numbers are graduating from college, during their undergraduate years far too many still lower their career aspirations and later either let go of their ambitions or downgrade them to incorporate the roles of mothers and supporters of their husbands' careers. These decisions while still in college may lead them to choose less prestigious and lower-paying occupations—a choice that becomes especially important for their futures, considering the high divorce rate. It is as though large numbers of young women are in denial concerning the fact that women increasingly have to support themselves and their children.

The more recent research suggests that if egalitarian marriages are growing in number, women should find marriage more satisfying. Studies do reveal that as role strain in marriage decreases, women's mental and physical disorders compared to those of men also decrease (Helson & Picano, 1990; Steil & Turetsky, 1987). Some experts have suggested that heterosexual couples can learn a good deal from lesbian and gay couples about equality in relationships. There is a great deal more equality in most homosexual relationships than in most heterosexual unions (Kurdek, 1989). Lesbian couples tend to be less sex-typed and to do less role playing than heterosexual couples do. Lesbian partners are more likely to divide household work on the basis of each partner's interests and skills. Choice is believed to play a major part in reports of greater relationship satisfaction, since the division of work is not a gendered assumption (Kurdek & Schmidt, 1986). Of course, their unions are not legally recognized, so the genderized norms affecting legally wed couples do not have the same weight. It is interesting to speculate but impossible to predict whether or not legal marriage status would make changes in the more egalitarian nature of such relationships. As it is now, lesbian relationships are characterized by particularly high relationship satisfaction, and this is believed to be at least partly, a function of less stereotyped roles and more equal distribution of power and workload (Greene & Herek, 1994). (For a fuller discussion of lesbian relationships, see Klinger, Chapter 33, this volume.)

PARENTING

The effects of parenting on women's lives are much more clear-cut than is the issue of whether marriage is or is not to their advantage. For both fathers and mothers, having children exacts a toll in terms of financial cost, time, energy, and others sacrifices. However, mothers especially have their lives changed in profound ways in terms of freedom, work role flexibility, and responsibility. Most experts in the field of marriage and family are of the opinion that motherhood is still the most salient and distinctive social role played by women (Hays, 1996). It is also clearly the most gendered role, even though young fathers are reported to be taking a more active part in all phases of parenting than their own fathers or grandfathers did.

Historically, women had limited control over whether or not they had children. Only in the 20th century did any kind of choice become possible, and only lately have there been real options about whether and when to become pregnant. Consequently, until the mid-1970s, having children was just what happened if a woman had sex and was fertile.

One mother, a friend of the author's, confessed that she had three children in the 1950s because three different kinds of birth control methods did not work for her. Her obstetrician was not at all sympathetic, telling her on one occasion that she had 9 months to get used to the idea of another child. Having a choice, and recognizing the toll children can take on their lives, have led an increasing number of women to decide to remain childless. Interestingly, this trend has not affected the percentage of women who have at least one child, because these voluntarily childless women have been offset by involuntarily childless women (such women are partners in about 1 in 13 American couples) who have eventually been helped to conceive by advances in fertility techniques. Consequently, the rate has stayed rather steady at about 90% of all women who bear at least one child. In addition, about 4% of Americans are adopted, indicating that if women cannot conceive or if they desire more children without bearing them themselves, a small number add to their families this way (U.S. Bureau of the Census, 1997).

Because such a large percentage of women have children, it has been suggested that there is a socially derived "motherhood mandate," which puts women on a path to motherhood from an early age and positively reinforces having children while providing negative reactions for childlessness. Motherhood takes on an idealization that consists of commonly held notions that fulfillment for women necessitates having children, and that well-adjusted women will enjoy devoting themselves to their children (Hoffung, 1995).

Logically, it might be concluded that because women now have more choice about whether or not to have children—and, if so, when and how many—that motherhood would bring more satisfaction and less stress than it did when there was far less control over fertility. To some extent this seems to be the case, although the majority of mothers still note the negative effects of children on their lives, ranging from the increased workload and physical exhaustion to social isolation and not living up to societal stereotypes of motherhood (Kitzinger, 1995). Virtually every study reports that the mother is expected to be the primary parent, even when there is an active father in the picture. Cross-cultural research on parenting indicates that this is not just the case within mainstream U.S. culture; greater involvement of mothers with children is universal (Stone & McKee, 1999). In Hispanic American, African American, and European households, mothers are shown to spend up to 20 hours a week more than fathers do interacting with their children (Hossain et al., 1995; Best et al., 1994). Nearly all studies point to the ramifications of the gendered role women assume and to fathers' expectations that this is a correct way for mothers to behave (Genevie & Margolies, 1987). Being a primary caretaker seriously limits a woman's access to choices that might be more personally rewarding and valued more highly by others. Such limitations frequently lead to stressful conditions that undermine a woman's physical and emotional health.

A major contribution to women's stress during motherhood is the reinforcement of traditional gender roles, regardless of how their lives were defined before their children were born. Even though large numbers of mothers continue to be employed, most find not only that they take major parenting responsibility, but also that their involvement in housework increases (Crogham, 1991; Douthitt, 1989). For most women, the experience of first-time motherhood is considerably different from what they were led to expect. Indeed, another major contributor to stress for mothers is that reality and romanticized notions of motherhood usually match poorly. Women not only carry the heavier workload, but are likely to be the ones blamed should anything go wrong. Many women feel guilty when they do not measure up, and others become obsessed with efforts to live up to expectations. Some of these idealistic ideas have been put to rest by the time later children arrive, although underestimating the impact on workload imposed by additional children may lead to even greater stress. In addition, mothers continue to hope for greater father involvement with each additional child, and this often does not occur.

Marital satisfaction has been shown to decline for women during the years when child care is paramount, unless they are in vital, satisfying relationships where their expectations are being met (Bryan, 1998). Much of this decline can be traced to role overload, and to wives' disappointment in their husbands' participation in household and parenting tasks. Women's employment outside the home simply adds to their shortage of time and energy but otherwise is not the major factor in dissatisfaction (Rogers, 1996). Unfortunately, some men dislike taking care of children. Many cannot believe the amount of time and energy it requires. It is common for fathers to refer to their time spent in childcare as "babysitting" their children. Women are not known to use that term, since for them being mothers is very different from being sitters.

Men who complain that they are neglected by their formerly attentive wives often do not understand or appreciate the workload mothers undertake; consequently, they may have difficulty comprehending the fatigue levels and preoccupation women exhibit. Many women complain that their husbands' demands resemble those of their children, and they feel pulled in too many directions. A frequent casualty is a couple's sex life, since a woman frequently feels pressured to have sex when she is exhausted, and a man commonly feels rejected when she refuses.

Lesbian mothers are reported to number somewhere between 1 and 5 million in the United States (Patterson, 1992). They consist primarily of women who had children within heterosexual relationships and brought them along into the lesbian relationships that followed, although increasing numbers of lesbians are adopting children or having babies by using artificial insemination or other fertility techniques while in the new lesbian relationship. There is little research on parental roles within lesbian relationships, unfortunately. One notable exception is research on the role of lesbian "stepmothers," which notes that they are more likely to share parenting tasks equally with the children's biological or birth mothers, whether or not they have adopted the children (Wright, 1998). Other studies have suggested that since domestic duties are not gendered as a rule in lesbian households, childcare follows a similar path (Mitchell, 1995; Patterson, 1992). (Again, for a fuller discussion, see Klinger, Chapter 33, this volume.)

An increasing number of women are raising children alone. There are over 1 million births to unmarried women annually in the United States (about one-third of all births) (Venture et al., 2000). In addition, millions of divorced mothers raise their children with little or no father involvement (U.S. Bureau of the Census, 1997). Even though single mothers are a very diverse group, they usually have even more burdens than married women, who usually get help from fathers even if it often is not as much as they need. The lack of economic resources and the absence of a coparent to share even a part of the workload result in particularly stressful lives for the millions of single mothers. Depression is commonly experienced by low-income single mothers with young children; ethnic minorities are particularly susceptible because of the exacerbating social factors of insufficient income and inadequate childcare (McGrath et al., 1990). African American children are nearly twice as likely to live in a one-parent home as Hispanic American children, and nearly three times as likely as European American children (U.S. Bureau of the

Census, 1996). Poverty is believed to be both a cause and an outcome of the great stress noted in most of these families.

DIVORCE

The demographic trends in the United States suggest that divorce rates have stabilized after a slight downtrend from an all-time high in 1992 (Department of Health and Human Services, National Center for Health Statistics, 1998). Divorce leaves very few women untouched at some time in their lives—whether it happens to parents, siblings, children, or themselves. For most women, the end of marriage is as traumatic an event as any they will ever face. Only the death of a child or of a beloved spouse rivals one's own divorce as a stressor. There are some women, of course, who also experience relief and report a heightened sense of self and greater companionship with their children, in spite of all of the adjustments they are forced to make (Gorlick, 1995). Most current research reports that the stress of a divorce is primarily determined by how stressful the marriage was (Wheaton, 1990). In fact, many studies indicate that the most difficult emotional period is the time before a couple's separation is final, when a woman is frequently fighting to hold the marriage together while dealing with children's questions and emotions as well as her own (Diedrick, 1991).

Interesting research on stress and adjustment comparing divorced women with widows shows that those whose identity is strongly and pervasively shaped by being a married person have the most stressful reactions to the loss (Degarmo & Kitson, 1996). It appears that the disruption of identity is usually very powerful for widows, who probably would have continued their marriages. By contrast, divorced women who were aware of the possibilities of divorce beforehand have frequently made some adjustments to prepare for the changes in identity. However, for divorced women who were taken by surprise or for whom being married is an importantly valued status, the stress is comparable to that for widows (Kitson & Holmes, 1992).

Cultural factors often come into play in adjustments to divorce (Hopper, 2001). In some societies, blame is attached to women when divorce occurs. For example, Asian American women who identify strongly with their Asian ethnicity are often put into and accept for themselves an identity of "social nonpersons" once they are not members of couples. Because they are blamed for their divorces, they receive little or no support from family, friends, or the community (Song, 1991). Having the support from others during times of loss can help immeasurably to alleviate stress. Lacking such support has been shown to be an additional stressor in and of itself (Brugha et al., 1990).

Women who have been socialized to take responsibility for relationships often feel personally to blame for what they and others deem a "failure." They may not only mourn the loss of the state of marriage and broken dreams, but also exhibit great sadness over emotional hurts they have experienced, often reliving trauma from family-of-origin rejections (Ahrons, 1994).

Increasing attention has been paid by social psychologists to depression's roots in how events are viewed. Research has found that those suffering from depressive states often perceive that they have little or no control over their circumstances, including their futures (Bruder et al., (1997). It seems little wonder that women, who are overburdened, stressed, and full of self-blame succumb to depression.

Even though historically most divorces have been obtained by women, research indicates that the decision is rarely unilateral in the beginning (Gigy et al., 1992). The legal system in the past often put women who had children in the position of being "innocent parties" which meant that they were the ones to file the action. This was tied to their receiving support and custody of the children. However, even today in the United States after divorce laws have changed, between two-thirds and three-quarters of all divorces are initiated by women (Ahrons, 1994). This does not mean necessarily that a woman starts out as the partner wanting a divorce. However, research does show that as increasing numbers of women have economic independence, they more often make the decision than do women who are financially dependent. It appears, however, that the high number of women initiators may not be due as much to financial independence as to tradition, which dies slowly.

The initiator of divorce may have an emotional advantage, because he or she has usually been doing the psychological work of separation before the partner becomes aware that a decision is being made that will change his or her life. Therapists note that spouses who have the decision about divorce made for them often exhibit pronounced mood swings, depression, anger, and physical symptoms, particularly in the early stages (Gold, 1992).

Much has been written about the financial straits most women experience following divorce. Poor women, who are often ethnic and racial minority women, appear to be hit especially hard, although custodial mothers in nearly every walk of life may be forced to make drastic cutbacks in their standard of living (Stroup & Pollock, 1994). Most current research reports that women's income is reduced by 15–30% (Ahrons, 1994). Others report that mothers' postseparation living standards are about half that of the fathers' (Bianchi et al., 1999). This is related to the fact that fathers often do not pay child support, as well as to lower earning potential for women.

The economic picture for most divorced women has been greatly affected by no-fault divorce laws. Courts have formulas by which they divide assets and debts, and award spousal and child support. The general bases of the arrangements are need and ability to earn. There is a legal assumption, however, that both partners should be treated as equals in these respects, even though that assumption is more often than not untrue. As a result, women and children are likely to be disadvantaged (Marks, 1996). A major flaw in this system is revealed by the shocking number of fathers who owe support, but pay only a part of the award or none at all (Children's Defense Fund, 1998).

Even though more recent figures have shown that the plight of divorced women is not as bleak financially as was reported by earlier studies, it is still sufficiently troublesome to create significant stress. One of the best predictors of divorced women's well-being is economic independence following the breakup (Holden & Smock, 1991).

Because a mother more often than not continues her role as the primary parent following a divorce, she quickly becomes aware that how the divorce and new family structuring are handled can make or break children's adjustment to the divorce. This puts an added burden on the mother, who may already be barely able to cope with her own changes. Many women report feeling guilty because their own stress prevents them from providing a steady environment for their children. It is frequently difficult to keep children disentangled from the conflicts between their parents, especially when there are disputes over custody, visitation, and support. Parents who are under great stress from mari-

31

Career and Workplace Issues

DIANE K. SHRIER

Until recently, research on work and career focused primarily on the experiences of men; it neglected women's work, whether paid or unpaid, as not a fit subject for serious investigation. Even fewer studies involved women's work or careers and mental health issues. However, over the past two decades an extensive and relevant literature has been written by researchers and theoreticians, primarily in the fields of management, sociology, occupational health, and psychology of women.

This chapter focuses on several major career and workplace issues that relate to women's mental health. These are the changing nature of the workplace; dual-career/dual-work families (competing or enriching commitments?); role conflicts and role overload or strain; gender discrimination, sexual harassment, tokenism, and microinequities; other work problems and sources of stress; and future directions. Practical approaches for the clinician are included.

THE CHANGING NATURE OF THE WORKPLACE AND WOMEN'S WORK

The dramatic and still-evolving changes in work and careers over the last 100 years have affected men and families, but have had their strongest impact on women (Gutek, 1993). Clinicians need to be knowledgeable about the scope and nature of these changes, in order to recognize the impact on women of different generations and to avoid imposing their own personal experiences and values.

From 1900 until World War II paid employment outside the home for women was viewed as preliminary to marriage and childbearing, if it occurred at all. Domestic service, teaching, and factory work were the primary occupations available to women (Betz & Fitzgerald, 1987). During World War II there was a temporary influx of women into the paid labor force as a patriotic duty to free up men for military service. After World

527

War II, the majority of these women returned to domestic unpaid responsibilities for home and family.

Beginning in the 1960s, as an offshoot of the civil rights and feminist movements (Friedan, 1963), there was a dramatic shift of women (including mothers of young children) into the work force, as well as a broadening of career aspirations and opportunities for girls and women. In the 1940s and 1950s only one-third of women were in the paid labor force, and two-thirds of women preferred not to work outside the home after marriage. By 1979 only 5% expressed such a preference, and currently 95% of women work outside the home for at least part of their adult lives, including two-thirds of mothers of children under 18. With the divorce rate currently at half the marriage rate and with fewer than 50% of women of childbearing age marrying, many women have sole responsibility for the financial support of their families (Unger & Crawford, 1996). The changes for women in the work force have actually occurred primarily among Caucasian women as historically most women from minority ethnic groups, especially African Americans, have by financial necessity worked in paid employment (Betz & Fitzgerald, 1987; Larwood et al., 1985).

At the same time, women's work remains associated with lower wages for comparable levels of education and work skills than is men's work (61 cents on the dollar). The female-to-male earnings ratio in 1998 was 76% overall, including 86% for Hispanics and 85% for African Americans (U.S. Department of Labor, 1999). Sex stratification and "glass ceilings" continue even for professional women, and women are underrepresented at the higher-status positions with authority to determine work conditions and policies. Although there has been a significant broadening of women's career opportunities and aspirations into a variety of work options previously closed to them, the majority of women remain employed in traditional and lower-status female-dominated occupations, such as teaching, social work, administrative support, and sales work. Women continue to carry a disproportionate share of responsibilities for household and family as a "second shift" to their paid employment (Betz & Fitzgerald, 1987). Also, for women the family role is generally allowed to intrude upon work (e.g., taking time off to care for sick children) so that "women have two *simultaneous* roles, whereas men are allowed to have *sequential* roles . . . [and generally] can defer their family roles to the evening after work" (Nieva, 1985, p. 176; emphasis in original). As opportunities for women have changed over the last several decades, considerable confusion about women's life goals, valued roles, priorities, and identities has surfaced (Lebe, 1986; Bernstein & Lenhart, 1993).

As will be noted subsequently, women who combine multiple roles tend to be among the healthiest physically and emotionally. However, the potential for role conflict and for role overload or strain; the greater likelihood of women's working in jobs where they have less autonomy and control over hours and work content; the difficulty of finding and keeping high-quality child care; and confusion over their own internalized values and roles all increase the liklihood of women's suffering from stress-related physical symptoms and emotional disorders, particularly depression and anxiety.

These changes for women have occurred in the context of other workplace and attitudinal shifts in the United States about work, separation of work and private life, leisure, and materialism (Schor, 1991; National Institute for Occupational Safety and Health [NIOSH], 1999). During the 1980s and 1990s Americans from all walks of life have begun to work increasingly longer hours, with resultant adverse effects on sleeping, meals, levels of stress, and family and leisure time. By the late 1980s, Americans were working the equivalent of 1 month more a year than two decades earlier, and 2 months more a year than their counterparts in West Germany or France where 6 weeks of annual leave had become mandatory (Schor, 1991). The new technologies have accelerated the pace of life and blurred the distinctions between private and public lives, especially for corporate workers, through making workers constantly available by cellular phones, email, pagers, call waiting, and fax machines (Fraser, 2001). The increased hours of work is closely tied to our having become a nation of shoppers and consumers with an insidious cycle of "work and spend." The average American in every income class consumes more than twice as much as Americans did 40 years ago, is saving less, spending more time shopping, and has higher consumer debt than the average resident of any other industrialized nation. Parents are also devoting less time and attention to their children. Between 1960 and 1986 the time parents had available to be with their children fell 10 hours for Caucasians and 12 hours for African Americans (Schor, 1991). But by 1997, parents (whether working outside the home or not) had increased time spent with children by 4 to 6 hours (Williams, 2000).

As a consequence of this overwork Americans, both men and women, are suffering from more stress-related emotional and physical disorders. Several recent surveys have found that 30–40% of adults surveyed feel extremely or very stressed or burned out by their work due to excessive workloads, conflicting expectations, and inadequate time for family or a personal life (NIOSH, 1999; Bond et al., 1998; Leiter & Maslach, 1998; Maslach, 1998; Zappert & Weinstein, 1985). Worker's compensation claims related to stress tripled just during the first half of the 1980s (NIOSH, 1999). In addition to general job stressors, such as work overload, affecting both sexes, women workers suffer additional sex-specific stress from discrimination (Savonson, 2000).

The situation is even worse for employed mothers. One study reported that half of all employed mothers reported feeling "a lot" to "an extreme level" of stress related to having too little time for their families. They tried to make it up to their children by taking time away from their personal leisure time and from their marriages, often compounding their level of stress (Schor, 1991). A recent survey of 1,000 workers across the country found that 88% of those surveyed indicated that the ability to balance work and family was very or extremely important—more important than health and medical coverage, job security, income, or opportunities for advancement (Heldrich, 1999).

Initially, employers' stress reduction efforts were focused on educating individual employees in stress management techniques or making referrals to employee assistance programs (EAPs). More recently, some organizations have begun to design strategies to deal with the root causes of workplace stress to enable all workers to better integrate work and family or personal life (NIOSH, 1999; Heldrich, 1999; Bailyn et al., 1997).

Sexual harassment, microinequities, and other forms of gender discrimination persist (Deal & Stevenson, 1998), though often in a more subtle and covert manner than previously, along with continuing differences in early socialization of most boys and girls (Blau & Ferber, 1985). African American women experience the double jeopardy of sex and race discrimination, while lesbians face the double jeopardy of discrimination due to gender and sexual orientation (Betz & Fitzgerald, 1987).

The asymmetry between men and women also manifests itself in career and life planning (Gutek, 1993). Males continue to view work as their primary role, with marriage and children generally having little bearing on their careers. Females, by and large, continue to consider the greater or lesser relative importance of marriage and parenthood in their life plans, as well as the possible impact of those decisions on career aspirations and timing. Women who are strongly career-oriented are less likely to marry, more likely to defer marriage or to divorce or be widowed, and to have fewer or no children than other women or than men in similar careers (Betz & Fitzgerald, 1987). Some women postpone marriage and children until they are well-established in a career; others focus on career and economic self-sufficiency, and remain single and/or childless. Some women marry young and simultaneously or sequentially establish career identities along with their roles as wives and mothers; others defer their educations, work lives, or career aspirations until their children are in school or out of the home (Bernstein & Lenhart, 1993).

DUAL-CAREER/DUAL-WORK FAMILIES: COMPETING OR ENRICHING COMMITMENTS

Rapoport and Rapoport (1969) coined the term "dual-career" couples, in which both husband and wife pursue "a professional career through choice rather than economic necessity." In "dual-work" or "dual-paycheck" couples, the "wife works out of necessity rather than choice" (Betz & Fitzgerald, 1987, p. 210).

Dual Career Families

Whereas most research on work and career has focused on men, research on combining work and family has focused almost exclusively on Caucasian, upper-middle-class women in traditionally male-dominated professions and businesses (Bickel et al., 1996; Carr et al., 1993, 1998; Gutek, 1993). Much less is known about the experiences of racial and ethnic minority women, of less financially privileged women, and of lesbian working mothers. Much of this research has searched for the assumed social and personal costs of multiple roles for women (but not men), rather than their rewards; in particular, it has raised questions about the potential detrimental (rather than beneficial) effects on the mental health of self, spouse, and children, or on the marriage (Unger & Crawford, 1996; Crosby, 1982; Gilbert, 1994).

Despite the continuing inequities for women in the work force, studies repeatedly document that paid employment is associated with *greater* mental and physical health and less psychological distress for women (and men). Employed women, including mothers, have a more positive self-image; increased power in the marital relationship, with greater influence in decision making about finances, childbearing, and childrearing; and lower levels of depression than full-time housewives (Betz & Fitzgerald, 1987). Unpaid household and family responsibilities, unfortunately, are currently devalued as not constituting a legitimate and highly skilled career option (Unger & Crawford, 1996).

There is little or no evidence, despite multiple studies and persistent societal beliefs to the contrary, that maternal (or paternal) employment has deleterious effects on children. In fact, studies document that maternal employment can have positive benefits for school-age children and adolescents. Even during the first 5 years of life, as long as stable caregiving capable of meeting a child's developmental needs is available, the effect of maternal employment is either neutral or positive. When the effects are negative, it is due to other factors, such as poor-quality day care. The need for affordable, government-subsidized, high-quality child care comparable to that available in other industrialized First

or complain about discrimination or harassment still run the risk of retaliation, though retaliation is against the law. They may be reassigned or fired; may be blackballed from obtaining other work in their field; and/or may be ostracized, discredited, or disbelieved by coworkers or employers. Over time, a target's self-esteem and professional or work identity may be undermined. Legal remedies tend to be uncertain, prolonged, and financially and emotionally very costly, and may exacerbate emotional sequelae (Lenhart & Shrier, 1996).

Psychiatrists and other mental health professionals have been misused by employers to retaliate against women who report sexual discrimination or harassment. They may be asked to provide forced fitness-to-work evaluations, unnecessary psychiatric hospitalizations, or treatments; or may deliberately or inadvertently gather information that is later misused by employers. Out of ignorance and personal prejudices or deliberately and unethically, some clinicians have provided biased assessments and stigmatizing diagnoses to the targets of discrimination/harassment; have ignored indications that women have indeed been discriminated against; have misunderstood patients' symptoms as the causes rather than the consequences of their traumatic experiences; or have communicated discriminatory attitudes about patients to the patients, employers, or legal setting (Jensvold, 1996).

Evaluation and Treatment for Targets of Sexual Harassment

A six-step evaluation and treatment framework has been developed (Bernstein & Lenhart, 1993) and expanded upon (Shrier & Hamilton, 1996). In brief, Steps 1 and 2 involve assessment of the severity of the immediate crisis, level of symptoms, and disruption of functioning. Initially, the therapist validates the patient's experience and makes efforts to establish a therapeutic alliance. For most patients a brief focused crisis intervention and active psychoeducational approach with an expectation of recovery will suffice. If indicated, a short course of psychotropic medication for sleep, depression, or anxiety may be used in combination with psychotherapy. A minority of patients may require more intensive and lengthy treatment, especially if the experience was severe and prolonged; if the symptoms have become entrenched and chronic; if there is an inadequate social support system; if the current symptoms are compounded by other current and past psychiatric problems; and there is a previous unresolved history of other severe traumatization experiences.

Steps 3 and 4 involve exploration and ventilation of common feelings of self-blame and denial within the treatment setting (but not in the workplace); anxiety, as well as realistic fears; depression and anger; and disillusionment and shattering of beliefs about fairness, justice, and loyalty. Existing adaptive coping strategies are facilitated, and the patient is helped to formulate a plan of action to reestablish a sense of control and to develop additional coping skills.

Steps 5 and 6 involve assessing and protecting against potential losses or adverse consequences. The patient is also helped to deal with actual losses of income and job, derailments from career paths, loss of ideals and belief in self and others, and other adverse impacts on personal and work relationships.

If legal action is considered, the patient needs to be helped to carefully evaluate the potential risks, which are often greater than the potential benefits (Lenhart & Shrier, 1996).

Policies and Procedures

Clinicians may be called upon to assist in the establishment of appropriate policies and procedures in the workplace or academic settings to prevent or reduce gender discrimination and sexual harassment. Written guidelines should receive conspicuous support from the highest levels of leadership in the organization, making it clear that there is a zero tolerance policy for discrimination and harassment. A range of confidential informal and formal reporting procedures should be identified, along with specific individuals trained to provide information, answer questions, and provide or refer a distressed individual reporting discrimination or harassment (or an alleged harasser) for counseling or legal advice. Educational sessions that define behaviors constituting discrimination and harassment, and that describe policies and procedures, should be mandatory and offered at regular intervals (O'Donohue, 1997; Sandler & Shoop, 1997).

OTHER WORK PROBLEMS AND SOURCES OF STRESS FOR WOMEN

Work Inhibitions

Some researchers and theoreticians (Person, 1982; Hennig & Jardim, 1977; Symonds, 1986) described a variety of primarily internally driven work inhibitions for women. These include self-devaluation, in which success is attributed primarily to luck or to relationships with others rather than to ability; fear (sometimes valid) that high achievement will lead to being seen as deviant, being rejected or retaliated against, or losing highly valued relationships; and inhibition of assertion, competition, and failure to recognize potential career opportunities, with a sense of guilt that others may be damaged or that a woman may surpass a devalued mother (Bernstein & Lenhart, 1993). Some successful women may have narrower areas of work inhibitions, such as fear of public speaking or a sense of fraudulence and fear of being exposed as a fraud. Implicit in the work of these writers is a deficit model in which women's traditional concerns about the impact of their behavior on relationships are emphasized and devalued.

Alternatively, researchers from the Stone Center at Wellesley College (Stiver, 1983; Jordan et al., 1991; Miller & Stiver, 1997) have moved from a deficit model to the concept of female development as different from traditional male development. Affiliative ties and relationships are viewed as central to women's sense of self-worth and value. In this model, rather than teach women to accept masculine workplace norms, a therapist would do better to help women find ways to integrate their affiliative skills into career and work. Recent studies from the Sloan School of Management emphasize the favorable impact of caregiving and affiliative skills developed in the private sphere (by both women and men) on the bottom line and on level of satisfaction in the workplace, along with overall reduction of stress and better balancing of work and a personal life (Bailyn et al., 1997; Fletcher, 1996).

Mixed Messages

Young women may get confusing messages from their families of origin both to be independent and achieving and to be like previous generations of nonemployed women in the family. Even women whose mothers worked or had successful careers may struggle with ambivalence about the priorities of work and family. Some researchers see a woman as often being better at "attending to the needs of others than identifying and claiming their own needs . . . especially [if she] is attempting to establish her career at a time when she is also parenting and being a wife" (Bernstein & Lenhart, 1993, p. 147; see also Lerner, 1985, 1987). Symonds (1986) And Lebe (1986) described depression in highly functioning career women who had grown up in families where their mothers rejected and devalued their daughters and idealized their sons. These women struggled with a sense of isolation and lack of entitlement and support; they suppressed their own emotional needs in order to care for others, or experienced interference with the development of emotionally intimate interpersonal relationships.

Fathers who have been very encouraging of their daughters' intellectual and career development may become ambivalent and withdraw support when their daughters become mothers. Daughters who are positively identified with their own mothers, and whose mothers had traditional feminine values and roles, may feel severe conflict about working and parenting at the same time. Alternatively, if a mother was devalued, a daughter can fear identification with her when she becomes a mother (Bernstein & Lenhart, 1993).

The Sandwich Generation

The "sandwich generation" refers to women who have primary responsibility for the care both of dependent children and of elderly relatives or in-laws, often in combination with work or careers. Responsibility, and the resultant stress, are more likely to fall on women because they traditionally value relationships and find it harder than men to compartmentalize and walk away. Bernstein and Lenhart (1993, p. 207) note that "women are especially stressed by situations that are beyond their control and by those in which they perceive themselves to be responsible for the well-being of others . . . failure causes a marked lowering of self-esteem." (See also Dohrenwend, 1973; Gilligan, 1982; Miller, 1976.)

The burden of elder care (time, emotional energy, financial strain, contagion of depression) can overwhelm a woman's mental and physical resources. It may be difficult to discriminate between realistic requirements and guilt-driven demands (Lebow & Kane, 1999). The recent increase in longevity and the reduced availability of caregivers, due to full employment and more lucrative career opportunities for women, has led to a need for assistance in making decisions for planning regarding the complex social, economic, and health needs of elderly relatives. A caregiver may feel overwhelmed and emotionally drained, and may develop their own physical health problems.

Treatment

Treatment of women's work problems and work inhibitions involves carefully evaluating the complex interplay, in each individual patient, among intrapsychic, developmental, family, sociocultural, workplace, and other environmental factors. Career life cycle issues should also be taken into account: career choice, career development, balancing career and family or personal choices, and midlife issues (Nadelson et al., 1978).

SUMMARY AND FUTURE DIRECTIONS

Women and men have very different experiences in the workplace . . .
which both reflect and perpetuate [gender differences and
discrimination].
                                    —UNGER AND CRAWFORD (1996, p. 469)

Women have dramatically increased their numbers in the work force, while men have not
similarly increased their involvement in the private sphere. As a consequence women continue to do the overwhelming majority of "housework, child care, emotional maintenance of families, and building the careers of their male partners" (Unger & Crawford,
1996, p. 469; see also Gutek, 1993). Much of women's unpaid work remains invisible,
devalued, and taken for granted.

Some women find an increased sense of well-being from juggling multiple roles and
benefit emotionally and financially from the greater opportunities available to them in
previously male-dominated occupations. Other women suffer from role conflict or role
strain/overload, or from the effects of continuing high levels of gender discrimination and
sexual harassment. Experiences of discrimination and harassment are compounded by issues of age, race, and ethnicity; sexual orientation; and prior traumatization experiences.
Men, too, though not the focus of this chapter, are under increased workplace stress; they
are often discouraged from developing the nurturing, emotional, and "growth in connection with others" aspects of themselves (Jordan et al., 1991).

When women first entered the paid labor force in significant numbers, some felt that
they could only achieve equality by adopting the competitive, achievement-oriented male
model to the work domain. Others (Kessler-Harris, 1985; Miller, 1976) took the position
that women are different from men in valuing cooperation, sharing, and relationships
over competition, and that they have special legitimate needs (for "flex-time," extended
parental leaves, child care, personal days, etc.). There was an associated risk of being designated as "special" and in need of protection, with the potential for discrimination such
as that occurring with the "mommy track."

More recently, in a era of relatively full employment and prosperity, and increasingly
overworked and stressed workers and families, there have been demands for change.
There is increasing interest in quality-of-life issues and in balancing or better integrating
personal and work lives. Some employers have tried to help individual workers deal with
workplace stress through stress management training and EAPs. Other employers have
developed packages of "family-friendly" benefits, such as flex-time, child care on site,
paid parental and family leave, sabbaticals, part-time/shared-time positions, and referrals
for elder care and child care (Muchnick-Baku, 1997).

Other employers and researchers seek ways to redesign the work setting more cre-
atively so that all workers, not just women, can better integrate work and personal life
(Fletcher, 1996; Frederiksen-Golden & Scharlach, 2001). Though not an easy task, the
approach involves challenging deeply held assumptions about what it means to be a competent, productive, effective worker, as well as redefining work–family boundaries. Organizations have valued and rewarded skills associated with the traditional, usually Caucasian, male, public domains (task mastery, technical competence, autonomous action,
competitiveness, linear reasoning) and have generally devalued skills associated with the
private, traditionally female, domain (empathy, support, interdependence, contextual rea-

soning). In order to enable workers to develop both sets of skills, the work–family boundary will need to be relaxed and work redesigned so that *all* workers can better integrate work and personal life. That means changing the traditional image of an "ideal" worker as someone with no outside responsibilities and with firm boundaries between work and personal life. It means rewarding workers who blend public and private, work and family, rational and emotional, masculine and feminine. Government policies need to support these changes (Heymann, 2000).

REFERENCES

Ayers, L., Cusack, M., & Crosby, F. (1993). Combining work and home: In *Occupational medicine: State of the art reviews* (Vol. 8, No. 4). Philadelphia: Hanley & Belfus.

Bailyn, L., Fletcher, J. K., &, Kolb, D. (1997). Unexpected connections: Considering employees' personal lives can revitalize your business. *Sloan Management Review, 38*(4), 11–19.

Bernstein, A. E., & Lenhart, S. A. (1993). *The psychodynamic treatment of women.* Washington, DC: American Psychiatric Press.

Betz, N. E., & Fitzgerald, L. F. (1987). *The career psychology of women.* Orlando, FL: Academic Press.

Bickel, J., Croft, K., & Marshall, R. (1996). *Enhancing the environment for women in academic medicine: Resources and pathways.* Washington DC: Association of American Medical Colleges.

Blau, F. D., & Ferber, M. A. (1985). Women in the labor market: The last twenty years. In L. Larwood, A. H. Stromberg, & B. A. Gutek (Eds.), *Women and work: An annual review* (Vol. 1). Beverly Hills, CA: Sage.

Bond, J. T., Galinsky, E., & Swanberg, J. E. (1998). *The 1997 national study of the changing work force.* New York: Families and Work Institute.

Carr, P. L., Ash, A. S., Friedman, R. H., et al. (1998). Relation of family responsibilities and gender to the productivity and career satisfaction of medical faculty. *Annals of Internal Medicine, 129,* 532–538.

Carr, P L., Friedman, R. H., Moskowitz, M. A., et al. (1993). Comparing the status of women and men in academic medicine. *Annals of Internal Medicine, 119,* 908–913.

Conley, F. K. (1998). *Walking out on the boys.* New York: Farrar, Straus & Giroux.

Crosby, F. J. (1982). *Relative deprivation and working women.* New York: Oxford University Press.

Crosby, F. J. (1991). *Juggling: The unexpected advantages of balancing career and home for women and their families.* New York: Free Press.

Deal, J. J., & Stevenson, M. A. (1998). Perceptions of female and male managers in the 1990s: Plus ça change ... *Sex Roles, 38*(1–2), 287–300.

Deutsch, F. M., & Saxon, S. E. (1998). Traditional ideologies, nontraditional lives. *Sex Roles, 38*(5–6), 331–362.

Dohrenwend, B. S. (1973). Social status and stressful life events. *Journal of Personality and Social Psychology, 28,* 225–235.

Elman, M. R., & Gilbert, L. A. (1984). Coping strategies for role conflict in married professional women with children. *Family Relations, 33,* 317–327.

Equal Employment Opportunity Commission. (1980). *Guidelines on discrimination because of sex.* 29 C.F.R. §1604.11 (sexual harassment)

Fletcher, J. K. (1996). A relational approach to the protean worker. In D. T. Hall & Associates (Eds.), *The career is dead—long live the career: A relational approach to careers.* San Francisco: Jossey-Bass.

Fletcher, J. K. (1999). *Disappearing acts and relational practices at work.* Cambridge, MA: MIT Press.

Fraser, J. A. (2001). *White-collar sweatshop: The deterioration of work and its rewards in corporate America.* New York: Norton.

Fredriksen-Goldsen, K. I., & Scharlach, A. E. (2001). *Families and work: New directions in the twenty-first century.* New York: Oxford University Press.

Friedan, B. (1963). *The feminine mystique.* New York: Dell.

Gilbert, L. A. (1993). *Two careers/one family: The promise of gender equality.* London: Sage.

Gilligan, C. (1982). *In a different voice.* Cambridge MA: Harvard University Press.

Gutek, B. A. (1993). Asymmetric changes in men's and women's roles. In B. C. Long & S. E. Kahn (Eds.), *Women, work and coping: A multidisciplinary approach to workplace stress.* Montreal: McGill–Queen's University Press.

Heldrich Work Trends Survey, v. 1.2; Winter 1999.

Hennig, M., & Jardim, A. (1977). *The managerial woman.* New York: Doubleday/Anchor.

Heymann, J. (2000). *The widening gap: Why America's working families are in jeopardy and what can be done about it.* New York: Basic Books.

Hochschild, A., with Machung, A. (1989). *The second shift.* New York: Viking.

Jensvold, M. F. (1996). Potential for misuse and abuse of psychiatry in workplace sexual harassment. In D. K. Shrier (Ed.), *Sexual harassment in the workplace and academia: Psychiatric issues.* Washington, DC: American Psychiatric Press.

Jordan, J. V., Kaplan, A. G., Miller, J. B., et al. (Eds.). (1991). *Women's growth in connection.* New York: Guilford Press.

Kahn, W. A., & Crosby, F. (1985). Discriminating between attitudes and discriminatory behaviors. In L. Larwood, A. H. Stromberg, & B. A. Gutek (Eds.), *Women and work: An annual review* (Vol. 1). Beverly Hills, CA: Sage.

Kessler-Harris, A. (1985). The debate over equality for women in the work place: Recognizing differences. In L. Larwood, A. H. Stromberg, & B. A. Gutek (Eds.), *Women and work: An annual review* (Vol. 1). Beverly Hills, CA: Sage.

Lebe, D. M. (1986). Female ego ideal conflicts in adulthood. *American Journal of Psychoanalysis, 46,* 22–32.

Lebow, G., & Kane, B. (1999). *Coping with your difficult older parent: Stressed-out children.* New York: Avon.

Leiter, M. P., & Maslach, C. (1998). Burnout. In H. Friedman (Ed.), *Encyclopedia of mental health* (pp. 347–357). San Diego, CA: Academic Press.

Lenhart, S. A. (1996). Physical and mental health aspects of sexual harassment. In D. K. Shrier (Ed.), *Sexual harassment in the workplace and academia: Psychiatric issues.* Washington, DC: American Psychiatric Press.

Lenhart, S. A., & Shrier, D. K. (1996). Potential costs and benefits of sexual harassment litigation. *Psychiatric Annals, 26*(3), 132–138.

Lerner, H. G. (1985). *The dance of anger.* New York: Harper & Row.

Lerner, H. G. (1987). Work and success inhibitions in women: Family systems level interventions in psychodynamic treatment. *Bulletin of the Menninger Clinic, 51,* 338–360.

Maslach, C. (1998). A multidimensional theory of burnout. In C. L. Cooper (Ed.), *Theories of organizational stress* (pp. 68–85). Oxford: Oxford University Press.

Miller, J. B. (1976). *Toward a new psychology of women.* Boston: Beacon Press.

Miller, J. B., & Stiver, I. P. (1997). *The healing connection: How women form relationships in therapy and in life.* Wellesley, MA: Stone Center, Wellesley College.

Muchnick-Baku, S. (1997). *Corporate strategies for women's health: Survey results and case studies.* Washington, DC: Washington Business Group on Health.

Nadelson, C. C., Notman, M. T., & Bennett, M. B. (1978). Success or failure: Psychotherapeutic considerations for women in conflict. *American Journal of Psychiatry, 135,* 1092–1096.

National Institute for Occupational Safety and Health. (1999). *Stress at work*(DHHS Publication No. NIOSH 99-101). Washington, DC: U.S. Government Printing Office.

Nieva, V. F. (1985). Work and family linkages. In L. Larwood, A. H. Stromberg, B. A. Gutek (Eds.), *Women and work: An annual review* (Vol. 1). Beverly Hills, CA: Sage.

O'Donohue, W. O. (Ed.). (1997). *Sexual harassment: Theory, research and treatment.* Boston: Allyn & Bacon.

Person, E. S. (1982). Women working: Fears of failure, deviance and success. *Journal of the American Academy of Psychoanalysis, 10*, 67–84.

Rapoport, R., & Rapoport, R. N. (1969). The dual-career family. *Human Relations, 22*, 3–30.

Rowe, M. P. (1990). Barriers to equality: The power of subtle discrimination to maintain unequal opportunity. *Employee Responsibilities and Rights Journal, 3*, 153–163.

Sandler, B. R., & Shoop, R. J. (1997). *Sexual harassment on campus: A guide for administrators, faculty, and students.* Boston: Allyn & Bacon.

Savonson, N. (2000). Working women and stress. *Journal of the American Medical Women's Association, 55*(2), 76–79.

Schor, J. B. (1991). *The overworked American: The unexpected decline of leisure.* New York: Basic Books.

Shrier, D. K. (Ed.). (1996). *Sexual harassment in the workplace and academia: Psychiatric issues.* Washington, DC: American Psychiatric Press.

Shrier, D. K. (1998). Sexual harassment in the workplace:Psychological issues. *Psychiatric Times, 15*(7), 59–62.

Shrier, D. K., Brodkin, A. M., & Sondheimer, A. (1993). Parenting and professionalism: Competing and enriching commitments. *Journal of the American Medical Women's Association, 18*(4), 122–124.

Shrier, D. K., & Hamilton, J. A. (1996). Therapeutic interventions and resources. In D. K. Shrier (Ed.), *Sexual harassment in the workplace and academia: Psychiatric issues.* Washington, DC: American Psychiatric Press.

Stiver, I. (1983). *Work inhibitions in women* (Work in Progress No. 82). Wellesley, MA: Stone Center, Wellesley College.

Symonds, A. (1986). The dynamics of depression in functioning women: Sexism in the family. *Journal of the American Academy of Psychoanalysis, 14*, 495–406.

Unger, R., & Crawford, M. (1996). *Women and gender: A feminist psychology* (2nd ed.). New York: McGraw-Hill.

Voydanoff, P. (1987). *Work and family life.* Newbury Park, CA: Sage.

Wharton, A. S. (1993). Women's and men's responses to sex-segregated work. In *Occupational medicine: State of the art reviews* (Vol. 8, No. 4). Philadelphia: Hanley & Belfus.

Williams, J. (2000). *Unbending gender: Why fa??? and work conflict and what to do about it.* New York: Oxford University Press.

Zappert, L. T., & Weinstein, H. M. (1985). Sex differences in the impact of work on physical and psychological health. *American Journal of Psychiatry, 142*(10), 1174–1178.

32

Trauma and Violence

BETHANY BRAND

Some incidents of violence in society have gotten a lot of attention; for example, fatal school shootings by children shock and outrage the public. Sadly, though other violent events—such as child abuse, domestic violence, and rape—take place on a daily basis throughout this country, yet they rarely reach the public eye. Women are often the victims of these hidden traumas and violence. This chapter reviews how tragically common trauma and violence involving women are, how far-reaching and enduring the damage they inflict can be, and how relatively little we as mental health professionals know about mitigating their sequelae. Unfortunately, the need for effective treatments and sufficient access to qualified clinicians who know how to implement them far exceeds the resources currently available.

The use of terms such as "survivor" versus "victim" is controversial. Some people object to either or both words. These words are used interchangeably in this chapter, although neither is entirely satisfactory. "Victim" can imply that a woman is powerless, while "survivor" can imply that being traumatized did not harm the woman. Neither implication is intended by this word choice. Although the words "trauma" and "violence" are also used interchangeably here, correctly speaking, "violence" refers to physically destructive actions that injure or infringe upon others' rights, whereas "trauma" refers to an event involving actual or perceived threat either to oneself or to another that elicits an intense emotional response. Not all traumas involve violence. For example, a husband could tell his wife that he will kill her without ever doing actual violence to her. The terror and helplessness she might experience would nonetheless be traumatizing.

THE SCOPE OF THE PROBLEM

Physical and sexual violence against women is an enormous problem in the United States and throughout the world. The perpetrators are typically males close to the women, such as intimate partners and family members. Violence puts women at risk for both short- and long-term sequelae involving their psychological, physical, and social well-being.

Broadly defined, "trauma" consists of (1) childhood sexual and physical abuse and neglect, (2) domestic violence, (3) sexual and nonsexual assault, (4) community violence, (5) war and civil conflict, and (6) natural disasters. The prevalence rates of violence and trauma vary across studies due to methodological differences. Because of space constraints, interpersonal forms of trauma are emphasized in this chapter, and a sampling of the most recent and best studies is presented.

The prevalence of violence involving women is alarming and constitutes a serious health problem. According to one study, two-thirds of American women have experienced at least one trauma (Resnick et al., 1993). This study of 4,008 randomly selected women found that 13% reported experiencing a completed rape, 14% reported other sexual assault, 10% reported physical assault, 13% reported the homicide of a family member, 36% reported some type of criminal victimization, and 33 % reported experiencing a noncriminal disaster only.

According to another study, 1 of every 20 women presenting to a primary care internal medicine practice had experienced domestic violence in the previous year (McCauley et al., 1995). Between 21% and 34% of women will be physically assaulted by their male partners during the course of their lives (Browne, 1993; Sassetti, 1993). American women are more likely to be assaulted, raped, or killed by current or former male partners than by all other types of assailants combined (Council on Scientific Affairs, American Medical Association, 1992).

As shocking as these general statistics are, the risk is even greater for some women. The research is very clear that women who were abused in childhood are much more likely to be victimized again in adulthood. Women who were sexually abused in childhood were found to be 5.12 times more likely to be raped than were women who had not experienced sexual abuse (Merrill et al., 1999). Native American women are at increased risk for violence (Robin et al., 1989). Women with serious mental illness also appear to be at increased risk for victimization (Jacobson, 1989). Women with alcoholism, too, are at higher risk; for example, they are nine times more likely to be slapped and five times more likely to be beaten by their husbands than are women without alcohol problems (Miller et al., 1989). For urban adolescent girls, it is even worse. One study found that urban adolescents, many of whom were of color, experienced between 8 and 55 different types of community and domestic violent experiences, with the average number of experiences being 28 (Horowitz et al., 1995).

The prevalence of childhood abuse is also alarming. Estimates vary according to the definition of abuse, the setting, and the methodology used. More children die from maltreatment than from car accidents each year (Putnam, 1997). Rates of child abuse appear to be growing, due to greater awareness and increased reporting of abuse. A national study found that reported physical and sexual abuse of children doubled from 1.4 million to 2.8 million between the years of 1986 and 1993 (U.S. Department of Health and Human Services, 1996). During those years, the number of children seriously injured by maltreatment almost quadrupled (from 143,000 to 570,000). Males perpetrate the vast majority of sexual abuse of females, and are typically family members. An early, yet classic, random study found that 38% of the 930 women interviewed reported a history of being sexually abused during childhood (Russell, 1983). Only 2% of the cases of intrafamilial abuse and 6% of the cases of extrafamilial abuse were reported to the police. Although these rates of abuse shock mental health professionals, these numbers include only the women who reported sexual physical contact, rather than noncontact abuse (e.g., genital exposure). If the definition of sexual abuse is broadened to include noncontact experiences, 54% of the women in Russell's (1983) study reported at least one intra- or extrafamilial sexual abuse experience.

The sexual abuse of children is not just an American tragedy. According to an international review of rates of abuse, women around the world appear to be sexually abused in childhood at 1.5 to 3 times the rate of men (Finkelhor, 1994). This study found that 7–36% of women and 3–29% of men reported having been sexually abused in childhood. For both sexes, more detailed and appropriate questions revealed higher rates of endorsement.

Overwhelmingly, women are likely to be the victims of violence and men the perpetrators. Only 1 out of 100 rapists is a woman (Greenfeld, 1997). Ninety-six percent of the perpetrators were male in Russell's (1983) study, compared to the 4% who were females, primarily mothers. Whereas nearly 30% of all female homicide victims are killed by their male partners, just over 3% of male homicide victims were killed by their female partners (Bureau of Justice Statistics, 1995).

THE EFFECTS OF TRAUMA

Traumatic life events—especially those of an interpersonal nature, such as sexual and other criminal assault—are often followed by a multitude of psychological, physical, and interpersonal sequelae. During the trauma, victims feel helplessness, terror, and horror. After the trauma, they typically experience a variety of symptoms, which are clustered into three categories: reexperiencing, avoidance, and hyperarousal symptoms. Reexperiencing symptoms include recurrent, intrusive thoughts and distressing dreams about the trauma; intense psychological and physiological reactivity and distress in response to "triggers" that resemble the event (e.g., a man who looks like one's abuser); and feeling as if the trauma were recurring (i.e., "having a flashback"). Avoidant symptoms include trying to avoid "triggers" and thoughts of the trauma; a sense of detachment from others; blunted affect; decreased interest in activities; sense of a truncated future; and an inability to recall an important aspect of the trauma. Increased arousal includes hypervigilance; heightened startle response; trouble falling or staying asleep; trouble concentrating; and irritability. If these symptoms persist for longer than 1 month, then the person is diagnosed with posttraumatic stress disorder (PTSD) according to the *Diagnostic and Statistical Manual of Mental Disorders*, fourth edition (DSM-IV; American Psychiatric Association, 1994).

Lifetime rates of PTSD in the general population range from 1% to 12.3%, depending on measurement and sampling strategies used by various researchers (for a review, see Solomon & Davidson, 1997). However, not all people who experience trauma develop PTSD or any other psychiatric disorder. For example, 1 month after being raped, 35% of women in a prospective study did not meet criteria for PTSD (Rothbaum et al., 1994). Many of these women, however, were nonetheless quite distressed and had some symptoms of PTSD even if they did not meet full diagnostic criteria for PTSD. Researchers are trying to learn what factors protect some people from the damaging effects of trauma.

Once again, there are gender differences in the rate and impact of trauma. Some studies have found that men are exposed to the same number of traumatic events as are women (Breslau et al., 1997), whereas others have found that men have slightly higher rates of trauma exposure than women (60.7% vs. 51.2%; Kessler et al., 1995). The risk for developing PTSD after exposure to trauma is twice as high for women as for men (30% vs. 13%, according to Breslau et al., 1997; about 10% vs. 5%, according to Kessler et al., 1995). Furthermore, women report experiencing different types of traumas than do men. For example, a higher proportion of women than men experienced rape, assault, or ongoing physical or sexual abuse (27% vs. 8%); men reported a higher incidence of serious childhood accidents or injuries than women (28% vs. 11%) (Breslau et al., 1997). Rape is the trauma that causes PTSD at the highest rate for both men and women, followed by sexual molestation, physical attack, being threatened with a weapon, and childhood physical abuse for women, and by combat exposure, childhood neglect, and childhood physical abuse for men (Kessler et al., 1997).

Experts differ in how they account for the sex differences in PTSD. According to some researchers (Breslau et al., 1997), the sex difference does not appear to be due to either multiple experiences of trauma or age at the time of trauma, but instead to preexisting anxiety or major depressive disorders. Breslau et al. (1997) concluded that the differences in type of trauma do not account for the gender difference because women's higher rate of PTSD occurs across nonsexual types of trauma (e.g., in their study, witnessing violence and receiving news of sudden death or injury led to PTSD in 39% of women vs. 4.5% of men). Other researchers believe that women's greater vulnerability to PTSD is due to their experiencing events that are "intrinsically more devastating in type and severity" (Solomon & Davidson, 1997, p. 7). Rape is a good example. Women are 13 times more likely to be raped than are men, yet men are somewhat more likely than women to develop PTSD after being raped (65% for men vs. 49.5% for women; Solomon & Davidson, 1997). Of the various risk factors studied, some similarities across the sexes have emerged. For example, a preexisting history of anxiety or mood disorders and early separation from parents are risk factors for PTSD in both sexes (Breslau et al., 1997). Further research is needed to clarify why women are more vulnerable to developing PTSD than are men.

Of those who are exposed to all types of trauma, about one-fourth will develop PTSD; over one third of those people will eventually develop chronic PTSD (Breslau et al., 1991). However, some types of trauma, such as sexual assault, are particularly disturbing and lead to much higher rates of PTSD. The reexperiencing, avoidance, and hyperarousal symptoms are typically most severe soon after the trauma and often decline over the next several months. Various studies show that individuals who spontaneously recover from PTSD typically do so within 3 months of the trauma; those who do not become chronic sufferers if untreated (Solomon & Davidson, 1997).

Although victims of sexual and nonsexual assault show a similar pattern of response including initially high rates of PTSD, which gradually decline over time, sexual assault seems to be particularly damaging. Rape victims, for example, are more likely to develop PTSD initially, to have more severe symptoms, and to continue to have more persistent symptoms over time (Foa & Riggs, 1993; Kilpatrick et al., 1987; Rothbaum et al., 1992). Rates of PTSD vary for rape victims from 35% in a retrospective study (Kilpatrick & Resnick, 1993) to 65% in a prospective study of women 1 month after being raped (Rothbaum et al., 1992). Prospective studies are thought to be more accurate in that they do not rely on memory, so the latter, higher rate is probably a more reliable estimate of PTSD following rape. Survivors of domestic abuse also have very high rates of PTSD (i.e.,

78%), as well as significantly higher rates of depression, substance dependence, avoidant personality disorder, and panic disorder, than do women who have not been battered (Watson et al., 1997).

An estimated 6.5 million women in United States are currently struggling to live with PTSD (Resnick et al., 1993). This is a staggering problem, especially in light of how debilitating this condition can be. For example, individuals with PTSD have been found to be up to 15 times more likely than those without PTSD to have attempted suicide (Thompson et al., 1999; Davidson et al., 1991).

Although PTSD is debilitating in its own right, it tends to be further troubling because it co-occurs with other psychiatric disorders and symptoms. For example, 79% of women with PTSD also had a history of at least one other disorder (Kessler et al., 1995). Compared to those without PTSD, people with PTSD were two to four times more likely to have a depressive disorder, an anxiety disorder, a substance use disorder, or somatization disorder (Kessler et al., 1995). An Australian study concluded that one-third of the psychiatric diagnoses in a sample of 335 women were attributable to domestic violence (Roberts et al., 1998).

Childhood and adult abuse contribute to the development of psychiatric dysfunction, just as does PTSD. Childhood abuse in females has been linked to dissociative disorders, borderline personality disorder, depression, anxiety disorders, eating disorders, somatization disorder, pseudoseizures, sexual dysfunction, self-mutilation and suicidality, low self-esteem, guilt and interpersonal problems, and substance use disorders (for a review, see Kendall-Tackett et al., 1993). Some research suggests that specific types of childhood maltreatment may be related to specific adult outcomes. For example, in women a history of childhood sexual abuse was related to maladaptive sexual behavior, whereas psychological abuse was linked with low self-esteem, and physical abuse was associated with aggression toward others (Briere & Runtz, 1990). Women who were "doubly abused," meaning that they had been abused in both childhood and adulthood, had the highest rates of psychological and physical problems (McCauley et al., 1997).

A similar pattern of sequelae characterizes women who are abused in adulthood. For example, battered women have higher levels of depression, anxiety, low self-esteem, and substance use problems, as well as higher rates of attempted suicide, than do women who are not battered (McCauley et al., 1995).

Given the pervasiveness of the effects of trauma on psychological functioning, it is imperative that mental health professionals be sensitive to the role of trauma in their clients' lives. Putnam (1997) contends that this pattern of relatively nonspecific effects of childhood abuse (which are nevertheless far-reaching for many survivors) is due to trauma's causing disturbances in four developmental domains: (1) problems with regulation of affect and emotion, (2) problems with impulse control, (3) biological dysregulation and somatization, and (4) difficulties in the development and integration of the self. Putnam (1997) reviews the literature and suggests that between 50% and 81% of patients diagnosed with borderline personality disorder report trauma histories. He concludes, along with other experts whom he cites, that borderline personality disorder is a special pattern of disturbance of affect, impulse control, biological regulation, and self that may have trauma as a factor in its origin.

Until recently, few clinicians or researchers recognized that dissociation is a common reaction to trauma. During and after a traumatic experience, many people report a sense of numbing, a feeling of estrangement or detached from their bodies and/or environments, alterations in sensory perceptions, and impairments in memory (Bremner et al., 1992; Marmar et al., 1994). For example, a woman may feel that familiar surroundings suddenly seem strange or foreign, or as if they are far away. She may feel that parts of her body are detached. Alternatively, she may view herself from a point outside of her body, "seeing" herself from a distance as might an observer. These experiences can all be classified as types of dissociation.

According to DSM-IV, dissociation is a disturbance in the normally integrated functions of identity, memory, consciousness, or environmental perception (American Psychiatric Association, 1994). Although victims of trauma often report frequent dissociative symptomatology, mild forms of dissociation are common and not linked to trauma (e.g., driving along a familiar highway and missing an exit because one was not paying attention). Traumatized women may experience symptoms of dissociation that are not sufficiently severe to merit a separate diagnosis of a dissociative disorder. Higher levels of dissociation are found in victims with higher levels of distress and PTSD (e.g., in victims of rape and nonsexual assault) (Dancu et al., 1990). The most severe forms (e.g., dissociative identity disorder [DID], known as multiple personality disorder [MPD] in older versions of the DSM) have been strongly associated with trauma. For example, 97% of 100 patients with DID reported histories of significant childhood abuse, most commonly incest (68%) (Putnam et al., 1986). The preponderance of cases of DID involve females (ratios of women to men range from 6:1 to 9:1; Putnam, 1997).

In addition to contributing to a variety of mental health problems, trauma is associated with numerous physical problems. Somatization was found to be 90 times more likely in those with PTSD than in those without PTSD (Davidson et al., 1991). Women who were being battered by their partners had more physical symptoms than women who were not being battered, according to one study of a large sample ($n = 1,952$) of women presenting to primary care internal medicine practices (McCauley et al., 1995). Patients reporting six or more symptoms were nearly five times as likely to report domestic abuse as those with no, one, or two symptoms. Symptoms were varied but included various types of pain, sleep and appetite problems, broken bones and serious cuts, fainting, gastrointestinal distress and symptoms, and tiredness. This research team also found similar patterns of significantly increased physical problems for women who reported histories of childhood abuse, compared to those who did not report abuse (McCauley et al., 1997). The physical problems appear to be compounded for poor women. Extremely poor women with PTSD report not only more bodily pain and chronic health conditions than women without PTSD; they also experience more difficulty using medical care due to problematic relationships with health care providers and perceived barriers to care (Bassuk et al., 2001).

Women who are victims of crime (sexual as well as nonsexual) have been found to be between two and five times more likely to have HIV than those who do not report criminal victimization (Kimerling et al., 1999). Victimized women also appear to have more psychological problems and poorer physical health than do HIV-positive women who have not been traumatized do (Kimerling et al., 1999). Women who reported having been sexually abused in childhood were found to have higher rates of sexually transmitted diseases and more abortions, as well as to engage in more HIV high-risk behaviors, than women who were not sexually abused (Wingood & DiClemente, 1997).

Given all of the sequelae of trauma, it is not surprising that people with PTSD symptoms are functionally impaired, including experiencing significant problems with interpersonal relationships (Cloitre et al., 1997). The only functional impairment study to date found that people with even a single PTSD symptom were more likely than those without any disorder to experience poor social support, marital difficulties, occupational problems, and lower incomes (unpublished data, cited in Breslau et al., 1991). As reviewed above, childhood abuse increases the likelihood of adult revictimization, including sexual assault and domestic violence. It appears that a history of trauma may increase the risk for criminal behavior, as evidenced by incarcerated female felons' reporting higher incidence of lifetime traumatic events than do women in the general population (Jordan et al., 1996). A particularly tragic outcome of rape, pregnancy, occurs in 5% of rape victims of reproductive age; this means that every year approximately 32,000 pregnancies result from rape, almost half of which occur in women aged 12–17 years (Holmes et al., 1996).

There is also a heavy financial cost to being victimized. Severely victimized women have been found to have double the outpatient medical expenses within a health maintenance organization (HMO), compared to control HMO members (Koss et al., 1990). It has been estimated that the direct cost of personal crime is $105 billion annually, including medical costs, lost earnings, and public program costs related to victim assistance. When intangible losses (e.g., pain, suffering, and lost quality of life, estimated by using willingness to pay and jury-awarded compensation as indicators) were taken into account, the cost of crime to victims increased to an estimated $450 billion annually (Miller et al., 1996). As astounding as these numbers are, they are surely underestimates of the actual costs due to crime, because the researchers excluded some forms of crime (e.g., drug-related and child abuse crimes).

In summary, women are subjected to an alarming amount of violence in childhood and adulthood. The effects of this violence are often profound and long-term, both for the individuals and for society. Given the prevalence of trauma and its sequelae, there is a great need for effective treatment for trauma survivors.

TREATMENT FOR TRAUMA SURVIVORS

Increasing awareness of the prevalence of trauma in women's lives has led to efforts to provide treatment for PTSD and related sequelae. Unfortunately, although there is an extensive clinical literature about treatments of trauma, there has been little research to prove the efficacy of these treatments. Much of the research to date has focused on the treatment of male combat veterans. Recent efforts directed toward the treatment of women have tended to focus on recovery from acute trauma (e.g., rape) rather than recurrent abuse or chronic PTSD. Thus research is desperately needed on the treatment of trauma-related disorders in women.

In one study, the average duration of PTSD among patients who received treatment for PTSD was 36 months, compared to 66 months for untreated patients (Kessler et al., 1995). Thus treatment may reduce the duration of illness by half.

Cases of one-time, recent trauma are generally more amenable to treatment than are more complicated cases involving multiple and/or chronic traumatization in childhood and adulthood. Often a repeatedly abused patient comes to therapy years after being traumatized and having suffered from a variety of disorders. In chronic cases of trauma, the disturbances across domains of behavior, affect, relationships, self-perception, impulse control, memory and attention, and somatization become much more difficult to treat because of their complexity, leading some experts to distinguish these disturbances as "complex PTSD" or "disorders of extreme stress" (Herman, 1992; Lubin et al., 1998; van der Kolk et al., 1993). Although research indicates that relatively simple cases of trauma respond fairly well to treatment involving cognitive and behavioral components such as exposure (i.e., encouraging the patient to describe in detail all aspects of the trauma while reexperiencing affect related to the event), relaxation, and the replacement of trauma-based cognitive distortions with more accurate beliefs (Foa, 1997), complex PTSD is less responsive to treatment (for a review, see Ford & Kidd, 1998). Patients with dissociation, for example, often decompensate during exposure therapy (Foa, 1997). As many as 25% of people with chronic, complex PTSD drop out of treatment, and only one-third eventually complete treatment showing clear benefit (Ford & Kidd, 1998). Thus the first stage of treatment for patients with dissociation and other manifestations of complex PTSD is tailored so that traumatic material and affect are contained rather than "opened up" and abreacted (Herman, 1992; Putnam, 1989). There is excellent clinical literature regarding the treatment of complex PTSD (Herman, 1992) and dissociative disorders (Chu, 1998; Putnam, 1989).

Treatment approaches for traumatized people include individual and group psychotherapy as well as medications. Individual treatment focuses on the reduction of PTSD symptoms via openly discussing trauma, whereas for the most part, group treatment for trauma survivors has focused less on trauma and more on improving self-esteem and interpersonal relationships (Lubin et al., 1998). Psychoeducational groups that take a structured, cognitive-behavioral approach to teaching patients about the effects of trauma and PTSD symptom management techniques are being more frequently used by clinicians and show promise (Courtois, 1993; Harris, 1998).

A review of the most common treatments of PTSD indicates that they all seek to help a patient achieve three goals: (1) develop a realistic appraisal of the threat experienced during the trauma; (2) overcome avoidance of internal cues and external reminders of the trauma; and (3) work through the meaning of the traumatic experience, in order to gain a sense of mastery over intrusive recollections (McFarlane, 1994). Behavioral approaches generally assume that PTSD is a "conditioned response" or avoidance of "conditioned stimuli" (i.e., reminders of the trauma) that needs to be undone. Behavioral treatments focus on exposing people to the real or imaginary feared stimuli, with the goal of eventual desensitization and reduction of anxiety. One type of exposure therapy, "prolonged exposure," entails having a patient relive the traumatic memory and recount it in detail in sessions, followed by listening to audiotaped accounts between therapy sessions. Prolonged exposure, as well as the behavioral techniques of "flooding " (extended periods of high-intensity exposure) and "systematic desensitization" (gradually increasing the intensity of exposure), show particular efficacy in reducing the intrusive symptoms of PTSD. However, patients occasionally experience severe complications from exposure treatments (Solomon et al., 1992). Some reviewers have concluded that exposure treatments do little to improve avoidance and emotional numbing (Solomon et al., 1992; Shalev et al., 1996).

Behavioral therapy may be most effective when combined with other modalities, such as cognitive therapy (Solomon et al., 1992; Shalev et al., 1996). Cognitive techniques teach patients to reduce anxiety and other symptoms by using skills to control fear and dysfunctional thinking patterns related to the trauma (e.g., assuming that all men are "bad" because one's abuser was male). Many studies have found that cognitive-behavioral techniques are useful in treating PTSD. One study of women who had been raped (Foa & Meadows, 1997) compared exposure therapy, a combination of behavioral and cognitive techniques called "stress inoculation training" (SIT), both exposure and SIT, and a control group. SIT involves teaching patients a variety of stress management techniques, including controlled breathing, progressive muscle relaxation, thought stopping, cognitive restructuring, preparation for stressors, covert modeling, and role playing. Patients receiving both treatments showed significantly reduced symptoms of depression, anxiety, and PTSD compared to the control group, even though many of the patients had histories of repeated abuse. The improvements in symptoms endured through a 10-month follow-up period. However, in this study (as in other PTSD treatment studies to date), treatments helped significantly to minimize, rather than to ameliorate, symptoms. That is, many patients did not meet full criteria for PTSD at the end of therapy, but continued to have some of the symptoms of PTSD. The same can be said for the few studies investigating the efficacy of psychodynamic therapy and hypnotherapy (Shalev et al., 1996).

A recent meta-analysis of 17 controlled treatment studies (Sherman, 1998) found that 62% of those who were treated for PTSD improved, compared to 38% of those who were not treated. After treatment, 48% no longer met criteria for PTSD, and moderate improvement was maintained at a 3-month follow-up. The reviewer concluded that although no one type of treatment was most effective, most of the treatments were moderately helpful; an exception was *in vivo* exposure-based techniques, which led to considerable decompensation.

Lastly, biological interventions also show some promise. Medications including antidepressants, anxiolytics, anticonvulsants, and mood stabilizers have been found to reduce PTSD symptoms. As in the case of psychotherapy techniques, pharmacotherapy alone has not cured PTSD. Rather, medication tends to decrease symptoms somewhat, and so is generally used as an adjunct to psychotherapy (Shalev et al., 1996; Davidson, 1997).

It is useful for patients to understand that many of their symptoms are related to trauma and may have been adaptive responses to trauma, even if they are no longer useful. For example, the biphasic nature of PTSD, in which intrusion alternates with avoidance, can be described as a way the mind tries to slow the processing of trauma by presenting the information that needs to be worked through, yet also allowing periods of reprieve in which the overwhelming material is avoided. Patients can be taught ways to manage their understandable and normal responses to what was an overwhelming and terrifying experience. Thus they can be taught ways to control, at least to some extent, the degree to which they think about or avoid traumatic material. It is relieving for women to realize that they are not "weak" or "crazy" because they continue to have problems due to trauma. For example, a woman who berates herself for feeling unreal and disconnected from her body during sexual activity can be told that this is dissociation, a common result of trauma. Furthermore, she may be comforted to learn that disconnecting from her body via dissociation during an activity that reminds her of having been raped is an adaptive attempt to protect herself from being overwhelmed. She can be taught "grounding techniques" that help her stay focused in the present and in her body, and to pace sexual contact so that she does not dissociate or experience overwhelming feelings or flashbacks. Thus therapy can still be quite helpful, even if it is not curative.

Women who have been traumatized can be helped significantly by compassionate treatment providers who are familiar with the wide range of difficulties common to trauma survivors. Clinicians interested in working with this population should seek out additional training in trauma because of the complexities that these patients present (for a training manual for clinicians, see Saakvitne et al., 1999). In particular, clinicians need to be sensitive to maintaining boundaries while remaining empathic and nonblaming. The early psychoanalytic theory that women's stories about incest are due to Oedipal fantasy is not a helpful framework with trauma survivors. Professionals need to accept that girls and women are not to blame for abuse, and that reports of trauma are much more often based in reality than in fantasy. Therapy needs to take place in a safe environment where a woman can openly reveal her feelings and discuss events that may fill her, and to some extent even the therapist, with horror, rage, sadness, terror, helplessness, and shame. Moreover, clinicians need familiarity with the dynamics common to survivors that are played out in sessions. For example, behavioral reenactments can occur that repeat sequences from earlier abuse, such as when the patient adopts a passive, helpless role in a childlike manner that forfeits her self-efficacy and power and may draw an unsuspecting therapist into an attempt to "rescue" the patient (Messler Davies & Frawley, 1994). Careful attention must be paid to the pacing of therapy and to establishing a therapeutic alliance. At times, especially early in treatment and during crises, traumatic material should not be explored because it may be severely destabilizing to the patient. Because this type of therapy can be demanding and unsettling for both the therapist and patient, it is important that professionals protect themselves from secondary traumatization and burnout (Courtois, 1988; McCann & Pearlman, 1990).

CONCLUSIONS

Violence and trauma are extremely prevalent in the lives of women, and the emotional, physical, social, and financial costs are often enduring and pervasive. The high prevalence of trauma and the chronicity of its sequelae make it imperative that effective treatments be designed for trauma survivors. Although a considerable amount is known about the impact of trauma, much less is known about how to help survivors fully recover, especially women suffering from complex PTSD. Initial studies of treatment are promising, but many of them suffer from serious methodological limitations. Much research is needed, especially controlled, prospective studies, to illuminate both normal and pathological responses to violence. Future research needs to focus on which components of treatment, in which combinations, at which times, and with which patients lead to improvement. Additional funding is sorely needed for research and treatment. In addition, in order to help the enormous number of people who have endured trauma and violence, all mental health professionals should receive training in the impact of trauma, methods of assessing for trauma, and principles of its treatment.

REFERENCES

American Psychiatric Association. (1994). *Diagnostic and statistical manual of mental disorders* (4th ed.). Washington, DC: Author.

Bassuk, E. L., Dawson, R., Perloff, J., et al. (2001). Posttraumatic stress disorder in extremely poor women: Implications for health care clinicians. *Journal of the American Medical Women's Association, 56*(2), 79–85.

Bremner, J. D., Southwick, S., Brett, E., et al. (1992). Dissociation and posttraumatic stress disorder in Vietnam combat veterans. *American Journal of Psychiatry, 149,* 328–332.

Breslau, N., Davis, G. C., Andreski, P., et al. (1991). Traumatic events and post-traumatic stress disorder in an urban population of young adults. *Archives of General Psychiatry, 48,* 216–222.

Breslau, N., Davis, G. C., Andreski, P., et al. (1997). Sex differences in posttraumatic stress disorder.. *Archives of General Psychiatry, 54*(11), 1044–1048.

Briere, J., & Runtz, M. (1990). Differential adult symptomatology associated with three types of child abuse histories. *Child Abuse and Neglect, 14,* 357–364.

Browne, A. (1993). Violence against women by male partners: Prevalence, outcomes, and policy implications. *American Psychologist, 48,* 1077–1087.

Bureau of Justice Statistics. (1995, August). *National crime victimization survey* (NCJ Publication No. 165812). Washington, DC: U.S. Government Printing Office.

Chu, J. A. (1998). *Rebuilding shattered lives: The responsible treatment of complex post-traumatic and dissociative disorders.* New York: John Wiley and Sons, Inc.

Cloitre, M., Scarvalone, P., & Difede, J. (1997). Posttraumatic stress disorder, self- and interpersonal dysfunction among sexually retraumatized women. *Journal of Traumatic Stress, 10*(3), 437–452.

Council on Scientific Affairs, American Medical Association. (1992). Violence against women: Relevance for medical practitioners. *Journal of the American Medical Association, 267,* 3184–3189.

Courtois, C. (1988). *Healing the incest wound: Adult survivors in therapy.* New York: Norton.

Courtois, C. (1993). *Workshop models for family life education: Adult survivors of child sexual abuse.* Milwaukee, WI: Families International.

Dancu, C., Rothbaum, B. O., Riggs, D., et al. (1990). *The relationship between dissociation and PTSD.* Paper presented at the 23rd Annual Convention of the Association for Advancement of Behavior Therapy, San Francisco.

Davidson, J. R. (1997). Biological therapies for posttraumatic stress disorder: An overview. *Journal of Clinical Psychiatry, 58*(Suppl. 9), 29–32.

Davidson, J. R., Hughes, D., Blazer, D., et al. (1991). Posttraumatic stress disorder in the community: An epidemiologic study. *Psychological Medicine, 21,* 713–721.

Finkelhor, D. (1994). The international epidemiology of child sexual abuse. *Child Abuse and Neglect, 19,* 409–417.

Foa, E. B. (1997). Trauma and women: Course, predictors, and treatment. *Journal of Clinical Psychiatry, 58*(Suppl. 9).

Foa, E. B., & Meadows, E. A. (1997). Psychosocial treatments for post-traumatic stress disorder: A critical review. *Annual Review of Psychology, 48,* 449–480.

Foa, E. B., & Riggs, D. S. (1993). Post-traumatic stress disorder in rape victims. In J. Oldham, M. B. Riba, & A. Tasman (Eds.), *American Psychiatric Press review of psychiatry* (Vol. 12, pp. 273–303). Washington, DC: American Psychiatric Press.

Ford, J. D., & Kidd, P. (1998). Early childhood trauma and disorders of extreme stress as predictors of treatment outcome with chronic posttraumatic stress disorder. *Journal of Traumatic Stress, 11*(4), 743–761.

Greenfeld, L. A. (1997, February). *Sex offenses and offenders: an analysis of data on rape and sexual assault* (NCJ Publication No. 163392). Washington, DC: U.S. Department of Justice.

Harris, M. (1998). *Trauma recovery and empowerment: A clinician's guide for working with women in groups.* New York: Free Press.

Herman, J. (1992). *Trauma and recovery.* New York: Basic Books.

Holmes, M. M., Resnick, H. S., Kilpatrick, D. G., et al. (1996). Rape-related pregnancy: Estimates and descriptive characteristics from a national sample of women. *American Jouranl of Obstetrics and Gynecology, 175,* 320–325.

Horowitz, K., Weine, S., & Jekel, J. (1995). PTSD symptoms in urban adolescent girls: Compounded community trauma. *Journal of the Academy of Child and Adolescent Psychiatry,* *34*(10), 1353–1361.

Jacobson, A. (1989). Physical and sexual assault history among psychiatric outpatients.. *American Journal of Psychiatry, 146,* 755–758.

Jordan, K. B., Schlenger, W. E., Fairbank, J. A., et al. (1996). Prevalence of psychiatric disorders among incarcerated women: Convicted felons entering prison. *Archives of General Psychiatry, 53*(6), 513–519.

Kendall-Tackett, K., Williams, L., & Finkelhor, D. (1993). Impact of sexual abuse on children: A review and synthesis of recent empirical studies. *Psychological Bulletin, 113,* 164–180.

Kessler, R. C., Sonnega, A., Bromet, E., et al. (1995). Posttraumatic stress disorder in the National Comorbidity Survey.. *Archives of General Psychiatry, 52*(12), 1048–1060.

Kilpatrick, D. G., & Resnick, H. S. (1993). Posttraumatic stress disorder associated with exposure to criminal victimization in clinical and community populations. In J. R. Davidson & E. Foa (Eds.), *Posttraumatic stress disorder: DSM-IV and beyond* (pp. 113–143). Washington, DC: American Psychiatric Press.

Kilpatrick, D. G., Saunders, B. E., Veronen, L. J., et al. (1987). Criminal victimization: Lifetime prevalence, reporting to police, and psychological impact. *Crime and Delinquency, 33,* 479–489.

Kimerling, R., Armistead, L., & Forehand, R. (1999). Victimization experiences and HIV infection in women: Associations with serostatus, psychological symptoms, and health status. *Journal of Traumatic Stress, 12,* 41–58.

Koss, M. P., Woodruff, W. J., & Koss, P. G. (1990). Criminal victimization among primary care medical patients: Prevalence, incidence and physician usage. *Behavior in Science and Law,* 85–96.

Lubin, H., Loris, M., Burt, J., et al. (1998). Efficacy of psychoeducational group therapy in reducing symptoms of posttraumatic stress disorder among multiply traumatized women. *American Journal of Psychiatry, 155*(9), 1172–1177.

Marmar, C. R., Weiss, D. S., Schlenger, W. E., et al. (1994). Peritraumatic dissociation and posttraumatic stress in male Vietnam theatre veterans. *American Journal of Psychiatry, 151*(6), 902–907.

McCann, I. L., & Pearlman, L. A. (1990). Vicarious traumatization: A framework for understanding the psychological effects of working with victims. *Journal of Traumatic Stress, 3*(1), 131–149.

McCauley, J., Kern, D. E., Kolodner, K., et al. (1995). The "battering syndrome": Prevalence and clinical characteristics of domestic violence in primary care internal medicine practices. *Annals of Internal Medicine, 123*(10), 737–746.

McCauley, J., Kern, D. E., Kolodner, K., et al. (1997). Clinical characteristics of women with a history of childhood abuse. *Journal of the American Medical Association, 277*(17), 1362–1368.

McFarlane, A. C. (1994). Individual psychotherapy for posttraumatic stress disorder. *Psychiatric Clinics of North America, 17,* 393–408.

Merrill, L. L., Newell, C. E., Thomsen, C. J., et al. (1999). Childhood abuse and sexual revictimization in a female Navy recruit sample. *Journal of Traumatic Stress, 12*(2), 211–225.

Messler Davies, J., & Frawley, M. G. (1994). *Treating the adult survivor of childhood sexual abuse: A psychoanalytic perspective.* New York: Basic Books.

Miller, M. A., Downs, W. R., & Gondoli, D. M. (1989). Spousal violence among alcoholic women as compared to a random household sample of women. *Journal of Studies on Alcohol, 50,* 533–540.

Miller, T. R., Cohen, M. A., & Wiersma, B. (1996). *Victim costs and consequences: A new look.* Washington, DC: U.S. Government Printing Office.

Putnam, F. W. (1989). *Diagnosis and treatment of multiple personality disorder.* New York: Guilford Press.

Putnam, F. W. (1997). *Dissociation in children and adolescents: A developmental perspective.* New York: Guilford Press.

Putnam, F. W., Guroff, J. J., Silberman, E. K., et al. (1986). The clinical phenomenology of multiple personality disorder: 100 recent cases. *Journal of Clinical Psychiatry, 47,* 285–293.

Resnick, H. S., Kilpatrick, D. G., Dansky, B. S., et al. (1993). Prevalence of civilian trauma and posttraumatic stress disorder in a representative national sample of women. *Journal of Consulting and Clinical Psychology, 61*(6), 984–991.

Roberts, G. L., Lawrence, J. M., Williams, G. M., et al. (1998). The impact of domestic violence on women's mental health.. *Australian and New Zealand Journal of Public Health, 22*(7), 796–801.

Robin, R. W., Chester, B., Rasmussen, J. K., et al. (1997). Prevalence and characteristics of trauma and PTSD in a southwestern American Indian community. *American Journal of Psychiatry, 154*(11), 1582–1588.

Rothbaum, R. O., Foa, E. B., Murdock, T., et al. (1992). A prospective examination of posttraumatic stress disorder in rape victims. *Journal of Traumatic Stress, 5,* 455–475.

Russell, D. E. (1983). The incidence and prevalence of intrafamiliar and extrafamilial sexual abuse of female children. *Child Abuse and Neglect, 7,* 133–146.

Saakvitne, K. W., Gamble, S. J., Pearlman, L. A., et al. (1999). *Risking connection: A training manual for working with survivors of childhood abuse.* Lutherville, MD: Sidran Press.

Sassetti, M. R. (1993). Domestic violence. *Primary Care, 20,* 289–305.

Shalev, A. Y., Bonne, O., & Eth, S. (1996). Treatment of posttraumatic stress disorder: A review. *Psychosomatic Medicine, 58,* 165–182.

Sherman, J. J. (1998). Effects of psychotherapeutic treatments for PTSD: A meta-analysis of controlled clinical trials. *Journal of Traumatic Stress, 11*(3), 413–435.

Solomon, S. D., & Davidson, J. T. (1997). Trauma: Prevalence, impairment, service use, and cost. *Journal of Clinical Psychiatry, 58*(Suppl. 9), 5–11.

Solomon, S. D., Gerrity, E. T., & Muff, A. M. (1992). Efficacy of treatments for posttraumatic stress disorder. *Journal of the American Medical Association, 268*(5), 633–638.

Thompson, M. P., Kaslow, N. J., Kingree, J. B., et al. (1999). Partner abuse and posttraumatic stress disorder as risk factors for suicide attempts in a sample of low-income, inner-city women. *Journal of Traumatic Stress, 12*(1), 59–72.

U.S. Department of Health and Human Services. (1996). *The third national incidence study of child abuse and neglect.* Washington, DC: U.S. Government Printing Office.

Watson, C. G., Barnett, M., Nikunen, L., et al. (1997). Lifetime prevalences of nine common psychiatric/personality disorders in female domestic abuse survivors. *Journal of Nervous and Mental Disease, 185*(10), 645–647.

Wingood, G. M., & DiClemente, R. J. (1997). Child sexual abuse, HIV risk, and gender relations of African-American women. *American Journal of Preventive Medicine, 13*(5), 380–384.

van der Kolk, B. A., Roth, S., Pelcovitz, D., et al. (1993). *Complex PTSD: Results of the PTSD field trials for DSM-IV.* Washington, DC: American Psychiatric Association.

33

Lesbian Women

ROCHELLE L. KLINGER

The fact that a chapter on lesbian women is considered an important component of a textbook on women's mental health reflects the progress of the last 30 years. Until the early 1970s, the majority of the limited psychological literature on homosexuality addressed etiology and psychopathology. In 1973, the American Psychiatric Association reviewed pioneering scientific literature to date and removed homosexuality from the list of mental disorders in the *Diagnostic and Statistical Manual of Mental Disorders*. Not surprisingly, this decision was quite controversial, but it was ultimately scientifically rather than politically based (Bayer, 1981). Over the subsequent years, a robust and growing research base on the psychology of lesbians and gay men has emerged.

Although the literature on lesbian and bisexual women is now more plentiful, much of it shares some basic limitations. First, there is the problem of obtaining a representative sample. Ongoing cultural and legal proscriptions discourage many lesbians from being open about their sexual orientation. There are few true probability samples of lesbian women. Most studies are based on convenience samples, such as women who attend lesbian events, who are active in other ways in the lesbian community, or who are willing to be visible. These women are likely to be European American, well educated, and middle-class. Fortunately, there has been a concerted effort to do more research with lesbians from diverse ethnic groups (e.g., Greene, 1997). Second, it is difficult to do the literature justice in a single summary chapter. Readers are encouraged to consult many of the excellent works referenced here for further details. Finally, it is important to realize that lesbians are a heterogeneous group of women of various ages, ethnicities, and socioeconomic levels, who may have little more in common than their sexual orientation.

RELEVANT DEFINITIONS

This chapter approaches lesbian women from a gay-affirmative perspective, which assumes that same-sex orientation is not pathological, but that unique cultural and clinical issues are relevant in working with gay men and lesbians (Malyon, 1982). This approach was initially a reaction to the pathologizing stance of some traditional psychoanalytic approaches (e.g., Socarides, 1968), and perhaps went too far in assuming that most psychopathology in gay men and lesbians resulted from internalization of societal homophobia. Most contemporary literature takes a more balanced approach: It acknowledges that lesbians and gay men have the same mental disorders as heterosexuals, but that the cultural context must be taken into account (e.g., Cabaj & Stein, 1996).

In defining sexual orientation, it is important to distinguish among several related components. These include "gender identity," the personal sense of being male or female, which is generally well established by age 3; "sex roles," characterized by how well a man or woman conforms to cultural expectations of "masculinity" or "femininity," respectively; and "sexual orientation," defined as the gender to which a person is emotionally and sexually attracted (Ryan & Futterman, 1998). The concept of "sexual orientation" can be further divided into "sexual behavior," "sexual desire," and "sexual identity," which are not necessarily consistent. For example, Laumann et al. (1994) found that although 4% of women in a national survey reported homosexual behavior as adults, only 15% of this subset of women, or less than 2% of women in the general population, reported a lesbian identity. Clinicians should keep this in mind when phrasing questions in psychotherapy or medical care. Some people have same-sex partners and may engage in intermittent same-sex behavior, but do not self-identify as lesbian (or gay). Although same-sex behavior is seen in many cultures and historical eras, the concept of a lesbian identity is a construct of 20th-century Western culture (Faderman, 1982).

Finally, clinicians treating lesbian women need to be aware of social and psychological manifestations of stigma that affect mental health and well-being. "Homophobia," as defined by Weinberg (1972), is culturally endorsed hostility or prejudice against lesbians and gay men, whereas "heterosexism" (Herek, 1984, 1995) is the denial, denigration, and stigmatization of nonheterosexual identity and behavior, often expressed in subtler forms than homophobia is. These terms have evolved over time and may ultimately be subsumed under the broader category of "sexual prejudice"; nevertheless, "homophobia," which can be cultural or individual, is often used, and the concept is always internalized to some degree by lesbians and gay men. Examples of cultural heterosexism include the lack of legal protection in employment or housing for lesbians, the inability to marry legally, and laws in many states that make it difficult for lesbians to retain custody of their children (Editors of the Harvard Law Review, 1990). Individual manifestations of homophobia can result in disgust or condemnation of lesbians, and at its most extreme can result in physical violence toward lesbians (Herek, 1990).

INCIDENCE/ORIGINS

Questions about the incidence and origins of lesbianism are fraught with controversy and politics. Lesbian activists may simplistically believe that higher numbers equal more power in a homophobic society, and the anti-gay lobby may believe the opposite. The question of origins is also a politically controversial one. Activists would like to believe that if homosexuality is proven to be genetic, then gay men and lesbians will be more readily accepted. Unfortunately, this is unlikely, as prejudice is not based on logic.

There are also technical difficulties in studying the incidence and origins of lesbianism. As noted previously, lesbians are a hidden minority who may not readily present themselves for research, or who may manifest same-sex behavior without endorsing lesbian identity. There are only a few full probability samples of same-sex behavior to date. As mentioned above, Laumann et al. (1994), in a probablity sample found that 4% of women reported same-sex behavior and 1.5% endorsed a lesbian identity. This is in contrast to Kinsey et al.'s (1953) nonprobability sample of adult women, which showed that 13% of adult women reported a lesbian sexual experience leading to orgasm.

The origins of lesbian identity have been considered from biological and psychological viewpoints. Evidence for heritability of lesbianism is decidedly less robust than that for male homosexuality (Bailey, 1995). Psychological models for lesbian identity include traditional psychoanalytic models, beginning with Freud (1905/1953, 1920/1955), which have not held up to modern scrutiny; lesbian/feminist psychodynamic models (e.g., Burch, 1997; Magee & Miller, 1997); and stage models (e.g., Cass, 1979; Coleman, 1982; Troiden, 1979). When clinicians and researchers discuss the "coming-out" process, they are generally referring to stage models. These are based on the assumption that future lesbians progress through a series of stages in adolescence or adulthood involving acknowledging, exploring and finally integrating a stigmatized lesbian identity. However, Gonsiorek (1988) suggests that the coming-out process for women is less abrupt than for men and is characterized by greater ambiguity and fluidity. In fact, it is not unusual for women to come out as lesbians later in life, or to have a series of partners of different genders (Golden, 1987). Lesbians, in contrast to gay men, often first become emotionally attached to a same-sex partner prior to engaging in actual sexual behavior (Sears, 1991).

DEVELOPMENTAL ISSUES IN THE LESBIAN LIFE CYCLE

Lesbian and Bisexual Youth

Resources are often lacking to study gay and lesbian youths, due to the myth that prepubertal children are asexual and to cultural expectations of heterosexuality. As a result, most in-depth studies of sexual minority adolescents are nonrepresentative samples, such as youths attending urban support groups. As reported retrospectively, the most common initial awareness of lesbianism may occur before puberty, a general sense of "feeling different" (Hunter & Schraecher, 1987). This may be due to gender atypicality, which is generally better tolerated in females than in males. With the onset of puberty, this feeling of difference is gradually given the meaning of being lesbian. Of note, the ages of awareness of homosexual attraction, experience, and self-identification have dropped significantly for young lesbians compared to older cohorts—to 10, 15, and 16 years, respectively (Herdt & Boxer, 1996). The coming-out process may be more difficult for ethnic minority lesbian youths, who often need to manage more than one stigmatized identity. Ethnic minority youths may also be less likely to disclose their sexual orientation to parents than European American youths are (Greene, 1994).

Most adolescents have strong desires to come out to their parents, but fear of rejection and other negative reactions hold many back (Boxer et al., 1991; D'Augelli et al., 1998). In a study of family disclosure experiences of lesbian, gay, and bisexual youths, D'Augelli et al. (1998) found that most adolescents who came out to their parents did so at about age 17 (generally following initial disclosure to friends), approximately 6 years after first awareness of same-sex attraction and 2 years after self-labeling as lesbian, gay,

or bisexual. Youths who disclosed were more likely to be "out," were more readily identified by others as being gay, had more gay and lesbian friends, felt more comfortable
about their sexual identity, and were more comfortable disclosing their identity. However,
these youths were also more likely to lose friends and to report significantly higher frequency of victimization at home and school than were youths who did not disclose their
sexual identity. Moreover, youths who came out to their parents were four times more
likely than those who did not to attempt suicide (51% vs. 12%), and two and a half times
as likely to report more frequent thoughts of suicide (30% vs. 12%); these findings suggest that coming out while youths are still dependent emotionally and financially on their
parents may have negative consequences. Herdt and Boxer (1996) found that parents of
younger children and teens had more difficulty coping with the news that their children
were gay than parents of older youths did. However, often a period of initial sadness and
disruption is followed by resumption of a satisfying parent–child relationship.

A subset of gay and lesbian adolescents have significant mental health difficulties
during the coming-out process. For example, community-based samples of lesbian and
gay youths found that 20–42% attempted suicide, some more than once (Ryan &
Futterman, 1998). Gonsiorek and Rudolph (1991) theorize from a self-psychological perspective that the process of coming out in a world that stigmatizes homosexuality is a
narcissistic injury. This may result in a loss of self-esteem. In youths who are otherwise
narcissistically injured (e.g., through childhood abuse), this may be too much to bear and
may cause significant fragmentation. Parents or clinicians who arrange for lesbian youths
to have so-called "reparative therapy"—psychotherapy aimed at changing sexual orientation to heterosexual—may contribute to mental health problems and suicide risk. Practitioners should be aware that multiple professional organizations, including the American
Academy of Pediatrics (1993) and the American Psychiatric Association (1998), have issued position papers stating that reparative therapy is ineffective and contraindicated.

Adulthood

In early adulthood, lesbian women must confront the usual developmental milestones of
establishing themselves in a social and professional context, as well as ongoing lesbian
identity consolidation. Many lesbians in the baby boomer cohort did not self-identify until their early to middle 20s, thus missing many of the dating and practicing strategies of
adolescence (Troiden, 1988). Young lesbians who come out in their teens and are fortu-
nate enough to have proper support resources may be more comfortable with their sexual
identity by the time they reach young adulthood (D'Augelli, 1996). However, the process
of coming out is a lifelong one, and is particularly salient in young adulthood. Lesbians
continually choose between self-disclosure (risking stigma, prejudice, and victimization)
and nondisclosure (which can lead to constriction and decreased self-esteem).

Research on adult midlife development has been overwhelmingly focused on heterosexual adults. Major themes at midlife include increasing awareness of health and mortality, assessment of limitations and priorities, and changing roles in regard to children and
parents (Vaillant, 1977; Bumpass & Aquilino, 1995). Limited evidence suggests that lesbians have similar health status and concerns similar to those of heterosexual women of
the same age, but may have more financial difficulties obtaining health care (Bradford &
Ryan, 1991). Most midlife lesbians studied by Sang (1991), whether childless or not, had
already been in the work force, so they did not have to cope with returning to work as
children left the home. The majority of women in Sang's study reported a satisfying and

active sex life, despite the onset of menopause. Overall, 76% reported that midlife was the best time of their lives.

Older lesbians may differ in their world view from younger women by more than age. The cohort of lesbians who came of age during and after World War II lived in a secret community of covert gatherings and fear of the repercussions of detection (Herdt & Boxer, 1992), making it harder for this group to reach out to the gay community. However, contrary to popular myths, lesbians are not destined to grow old alone. Many have support networks of friends that may extend over many decades (e.g., Strickland, 1997) and/or of family members, with 27% in one study having children (Kehoe, 1989). In addition, the challenges faced by older lesbians who successfully achieve a positive lesbian identity may actually improve their ability to deal with the challenges and uncertainties of aging (Friend, 1991). In summary, the limited research evidence to date suggests that most lesbians studied adjust well to the aging process and report a high level of life satisfaction (Reid, 1995).

Lesbians in Relationships

Lesbians form relationships for the same reasons as heterosexuals: to satisfy basic human needs for love, companionship, and sexuality. Lesbian relationships have much in common with heterosexual relationships, but they develop and are sustained without the support of social institutions. Unique legal and sociocultural challenges apply to same-sex relationships.

Surveys have indicated that between 45% and 80% of lesbians are currently involved in relationships (Peplau & Cochran, 1990). Lesbian couples are likely to endorse monogamy, with over 90% in a study of primarily European American lesbians stating that they were sexually exclusive (Kurdek, 1988, 1989). However, a study of African American lesbians revealed that 43% were in partnerships that allowed sex outside of the partnerships (Cochran & Mays, 1994; Mays & Cochran, 1988; Mays & Jackson, 1991). Like married partners, lesbian partners tend to be highly matched on demographic characteristics such as age, education, and income (Kurdek & Schmitt, 1987). In one study, interracial relationships were documented in 30% of African American lesbians, compared to 42% of African American gay men and 2% of heterosexual African American women (Taylor et al., 1990). The increased incidence of interracial gay and lesbian partnerships may be a result of limited partner choice (Mays et al., 1993).

Lesbians report a level of relationship satisfaction similar to that of gay men and heterosexuals (Kurdek, 1995). Lesbian couples show a lower frequency of genital sexual contact than heterosexual or gay male couples, but a high level of satisfaction with sexual relations (Blumstein & Schwartz, 1983; Loulan, 1988). Lesbian couples are more likely to divide household labor equally than are heterosexual couples, generally showing a high degree of masculine–feminine role flexibility (Blumstein & Schwartz, 1983; Kurdek, 1993). Lesbians generally endorse a higher degree of equality and relatedness in their relationships than gay male and heterosexual couples do (Caldwell & Peplau, 1984). This can be understood in the context of women's socialization, which favors relatedness. When two women are coupled, this tendency toward relatedness is unmitigated by the male push toward autonomy. This closeness may sometimes become too intense and lead to a maladaptive fusion in which individuality is lost (Burch, 1993). However, a degree of fusion is helpful for the healthy functioning of a lesbian couple as a defense against external homophobia and invisibility (Slater & Mencher, 1991).

Lesbians as Parents

The invisibility of many lesbian mothers makes it difficult to know how many lesbian and bisexual women have children in the home, with estimates ranging from 1 to 5 million women (Gottman, 1990; Patterson, 1992). Lesbian women are thought to be as likely to report the desire to bear children as heterosexual women are, although clearly they face many more challenges in becoming mothers and maintaining custody (Kirkpatrick, 1996). Research on children of lesbian mothers began in the 1970s with primarily divorced lesbian mothers, and has continued into the present with the reported "lesbian baby boom"—children born to or adopted by lesbians after they came out (Patterson, 1994). Research in this area is relevant from both a clinical and a legal perspective, as lesbian mothers in the United States still face the prospect of losing custody of their children in some states (Editors of the *Harvard Law Review*, 1990).

Children of divorced heterosexual and lesbian mothers have been compared on measures of gender identity, sex role behavior, sexual orientation, social and psychological functioning, and relationships with parents. None of these studies have shown significant differences in any of these areas (Kirkpatrick et al., 1981; Patterson, 1992). Research extending follow-up to adolescence and young adulthood has yielded the same results (Gottman, 1990; Huggins, 1989). Gottman's (1990) research suggested that the presence of a coparent of either gender in the household enhanced a sense of well-being in children.

The mothers of the "lesbian baby boom" (Patterson, 1994, 2001) become parents through artificial insemination, adoption, foster care and various forms of coparenting (e.g., a lesbian's having a child jointly with a gay man). Lesbian mothers and couples face the challenges of how to explain and present the role of nonbiological or nonadoptive parents to outside agencies such as schools, to their families of origin, and to the children themselves and their peers. Patterson's (1992, 2001) research revealed that children may face challenges due to peer stigma, but that this may increase resilience rather than lead to negative consequences in the long run. Several well-designed studies with well-matched samples of heterosexual controls have reached similar conclusions—namely, that children's overall adjustment and mental health are similarly robust in heterosexual and lesbian families (Patterson, 1998). Further research is continuing to follow these children as they grow into later childhood, adolescence, and adulthood.

Lesbians and Families of Origin

Much of the limited psychological literature on lesbians and their families focuses on the coming-out process. Coming out to families is often discussed in the gay and lesbian adolescent literature, but in fact lesbian women may come out to their families of origin at any stage of life. Disclosure of sexual orientation to parents generally creates a family crisis. Parents may go through stages of resistance and restructuring of expectations, usually, but not always, culminating in acceptance (Ryan & Futterman, 1998). In a sense, parents go through a grief process in mourning the loss of heterosexual expectations for the child (Robinson et al., 1989). Ethnic minority lesbians may be less likely to come out to families to avoid bringing shame on their families, even if their sexual orientation is unspoken but understood (Greene, 1997). Accurate information about lesbian and gay issues can be critical in helping families accept their lesbian members. Parents and Friends of Lesbians and Gays (PFLAG) is a national group with chapters in many cities. PFLAG offers support groups, information, and "parent-to-parent" contact.

Although little systematic research has been done in the area of long-term outcome after coming out, narrative accounts indicate that many lesbians have forged positive relationships with their families, sometimes after a period of struggle. A family's reaction to lesbianism does not occur in a vacuum, but is a function of its overall dynamics, as Laird (1998) states:

> The family's response to the daughter's lesbianism reflects its more enduring patterns of organization and the extent to which the autobiographical family narrative is available for reauthoring. Families who tend to be inflexible concerning rules for behavior and visions for their children are often inflexible about many things. Families that have difficulty talking about sensitive or controversial issues of any kind will have more trouble talking about sexual identity. Families that have difficulty allowing their children to leave or to grow up, for whatever reasons, can use the convenient red herring of lesbianism to stall their child's leaving or to insist on loyalty to traditional social, religious or political ideas.

MENTAL HEALTH TREATMENT WITH LESBIANS

Gonsiorek (1991) comprehensively reviewed the psychological literature through 1990, which showed that homosexuality is not an intrinsic mental illness and that there are no unique personality traits among gay or lesbian individuals. The National Lesbian Health Care Survey (Bradford & Ryan, 1987) of 1,925 geographically and ethnically diverse lesbians showed no difference in the incidence of mental disorders for lesbians as compared to heterosexual women. Jaffe et al. (2000) recently reviewed the literature and studied alcoholism in lesbian versus heterosexual women. They noted an 18% prevalence of alcoholism in lesbian versus 7% in heterosexual women, consistent with older studies. Substance abuse disorders are higher in lesbians. Bradford and Ryan (1987) also found that lesbians were more likely than heterosexual women to utilize mental health services because they often had less access to other sources of support (e.g., families or clergy). In their study, 73% of the subjects had received some form of counseling, half of them for less than 1 year. However, two more recent articles (Gilman et al., 2001; Sandfort et al., 2001) suggest a higher rate of mood, anxiety, and substance abuse disorders in lesbians and gay men.

Lesbians present for mental health treatment for a variety of reasons. These can be divided into (1) issues related to being lesbians, such as coming out, internalized or societal homophobia, or relationship issues; and (2) psychiatric disorders that are unrelated to sexual orientation but whose manifestation may be affected by sociocultural factors. Many of these unique issues and sociocultural factors have been discussed earlier in this chapter.

Individual Assessment and Psychotherapy

In assessing a newly referred individual, it is important not to assume heterosexuality, as many lesbians will wait to reveal their sexual orientation to a therapist until they decide whether or not he or she is trustworthy and nonjudgmental. Garnets et al. (1991) conducted a national survey of psychologists and found a presumption that clients are heterosexual to be the most common therapeutic error in working with gay men or lesbians. A presumption of heterosexuality gives a client the impression, rightly or wrongly, that a therapist is homophobic. They found another potential pitfall to be therapists' assuming that they knew what clients' sexual orientation was before the clients had completed their identity development. Therapists may also err by offering unfounded psychological explanations for lesbian orientation. Therapists should pay close attention to using nonheterosexist language and keeping an open mind to all possibilities with clients who are struggling with sexual orientation issues.

Therapists who treat lesbians are most effective when they have both factual knowledge of lesbian issues and development; and self-knowledge about their own attitudes toward homosexuality. Stein (1988) has also noted the importance of a therapist's acknowledging to him- or herself the presence of homophobia, which is ubiquitous even in gay or lesbian therapists. Without this step, Stein has cautioned, the therapist may subtly collude with a client's unexamined internalized homophobia. It is not necessary or possible for most lesbian clients to be treated by gay or lesbian therapists, but heterosexual therapists who treat lesbians must be comfortable with and accepting of their clients' orientation.

Treatment of Serious Psychiatric Disorders in Lesbians

Lesbians are as likely as individuals in the general population to have serious mental illness. Although sexual orientation has nothing to do with the etiology of serious mental illness, it can affect its manifestations and treatment. Individuals with severe and persistent mental illness are often treated as if they are asexual. In fact, 20% of women with severe and persistent mental illness in one survey reported same-sex activity, although they rarely self-identified as lesbian or bisexual (Cournos et al., 1994). Staff members of community mental health centers and other settings that deal with mentally ill individuals need to be well informed about lesbian issues and sensitive to lesbians' needs (e.g., including partners and families in discussions of treatment options).

Assessment and Treatment of Lesbian Couples and Families

A lesbian couple may seek treatment for a variety of reasons, including communication or sexual difficulties; the effects of one or both partners' substance abuse or dependence on the relationship; domestic violence; infidelity; decisions about having or raising children; and differences in progression through the coming-out process. Given the complexity of factors affecting lesbian couples, it is helpful to have a system with which to approach clinical evaluation. Cabaj and Klinger (1996) have presented a four-dimensional matrix to clarify societal and psychodynamic issues affecting gay and lesbian relationships.

The first dimension is evaluation of the individuals. The therapist's task is to assess each individual's level of maturity, cultural and ethnic factors, and any individual psychopathology. In the second dimension, lesbian development (i.e., the degree of coming out and of internalized homophobia) is evaluated for each individual. Significant mismatches in lesbian development can cause conflict. The third dimension involves "staging" the relationship—that is, assessing where the relationship is in its natural history and whether the individuals are concordant in this respect (McWhirter & Mattison, 1984). Finally, in the fourth dimension, an evaluation is made of external issues—events going on around the partners that affect them, such as illness, substance misuse, or family conflict.

Depending on the results of this evaluation, treatment strategies for the couple are recommended. Treatment of individual disorders is often paramount before a couple can successfully embark on a course of couple therapy.

It is important to assess lesbian couples for the presence of domestic violence, defined as any pattern of behavior designed to coerce, dominate, isolate, or maintain control in a relationship via threatened or actual violence (Walber, 1988). Many lesbians believe that relationships with other women are immune to domestic violence, and they are unprepared to deal with it if it occurs. At present there are no population-based studies of the incidence of lesbian domestic violence, so the true rate is unclear. Couple therapy is almost always contraindicated in the face of active domestic violence, because it may increase the risk to the victim if the perpetrator believes she is revealing information about the abuse (Frank & Houghton, 1987). Safety of the victim should be the therapist's first consideration.

After making a complete assessment of the couple as outlined above, the therapist must decide which interventions to apply. Carl (1990) has discussed the difference between symptom-oriented and relationship-oriented couple therapy for same-sex couples. Symptom-oriented therapy is more supportive in nature and deals directly with the symptoms presented by the couple (e.g., dealing with children). Relationship-focused therapy addresses interactional relationship issues in the couple. In reality, most couple therapy involves a little of both. Couple therapy may help a couple stay together in a more harmonious way, but it is also reasonable as a tool to facilitate more effective separation when a breakup is inevitable. With the proper training and attitude, any therapist, regardless of sexual orientation, can be effective and helpful in providing couple therapy to lesbian clients.

CONCLUSIONS

It is exciting but challenging to try to integrate the relevant literature on lesbian women into a coherent summary. As we begin a new millenium, there is a robust body of information on lesbians, but much more remains to be studied. It is clear that lesbianism is a normal variant of human sexual desire and that most lesbians are healthy and functional. Lesbians still face significant stigma in society, however, and this can engender violence and self-hatred. It is particularly difficult for young lesbians and those from conservative backgrounds to become comfortable with themselves as they go through the coming-out process. Lesbian women have been studied as individuals, in couples, as parents, and as members of extended families and communities. They are a vibrant and important part of all these systems.

Further research needs to be done on lesbians in their respective communities, especially ethnically diverse lesbians. Much more research is needed on the development of sexual orientation in children and adolescents. Normal and abnormal development needs to be further studied in lesbian adults throughout the life course. As stigma against lesbians begins to decrease, it will be easier to obtain research samples that truly represent the diversity of lesbians in society.

REFERENCES

American Academy of Pediatrics. (1993). Homosexuality and adolescence. *Pediatrics, 92*, 631–634.

American Psychiatric Association. (1998, December 11). *Position statement on psychiatric treatment and sexual orientation.* Washington, DC: Author.

Bailey, J. (1995). Biological perspectives on sexual orientation. In A. R. D'Augelli & C. J. Patterson (Eds.), *Lesbian, gay and bisexual identities over the lifespan* (pp. 102–135). New York: Oxford University Press.

Bayer, R. (1981). *Homosexuality and American psychiatry: The politics of diagnosis.* Princeton, NJ: Princeton University Press.

Blumstein, P., & Schwartz, P. (1983). *American couples: Money, work, sex.* New York: Morrow.

Boxer, A. M., Cook, J. A., & Herdt, G. (1991). Double jeopardy: Identity transitions and parent–child relations among gay and lesbian youth. In K. Pillemer & K. McCartney (Eds.), *Parent–child relations throughout life* (pp. 59–92). Hillsdale, NJ: Erlbaum.

Bradford, J., & Ryan, C. (1987). *National Lesbian Health Care Survey: Mental health implications* (Contract No. 86MO19832201D). Rockville, MD: National Institute of Mental Health.

Bradford, J., & Ryan, C. (1991). Who we are: Health concerns of middle-aged lesbians. In B. Sang, J. Warshow, & A. J. Smith (Eds.), *Lesbians at midlife: The creative transition* (pp. 147–163). San Francisco: Spinster Books.

Bumpass, L. L., & Aquilino, W. S. (1995). *A social map of midlife: Family and work over the middle life course.* Vero Beach, FL: MacArthur Foundation Research Network on Successful Midlife Development.

Burch, B. (1993). *On intimate terms: The psychology of difference in lesbian relationships.* Urbana: University of Illinois Press.

Burch, B. (1997). *Other women: Lesbian/bisexual experience and psychoanalytic views of women.* New York: Columbia University Press.

Cabaj, R. P., & Klinger, R. L. (1996). Psychotherapeutic interventions with lesbian and gay couples. In R. P. Cabaj & T. S. Stein (Eds.), *Textbook of homosexuality and mental health* (pp. 485–501). Washington, DC: American Psychiatric Press.

Cabaj, R. P., & Stein, T. S. (Eds.). (1996). *Textbook of homosexuality and mental health.* Washington, DC: American Psychiatric Press.

Caldwell, M. A., & Peplau, L. A. (1984). The balance of power in lesbian relationships. *Sex Roles, 10*, 587–599.

Carl, D. (1990). *Counseling same-sex couples.* New York: Norton.

Cass, V. C. (1979). Homosexual identity formation: A theoretical model. *Journal of Homosexuality, 4*, 219–236.

Cochran, S. D., & Mays, V. M. (1994). Depressive distress among homosexually active African American men and women. *American Journal of Psychiatry, 151*, 524–529.

Coleman, E. (1982). Developmental stages of the coming out process. In J. C. Gonsiorek (Ed.), *Homosexuality and psychotherapy* (pp. 31–44). New York: Haworth Press.

Cournos, F., Guido, R., Coomaraswamy, S., et al. (1994). HIV seroprevalence among patients admitted to two psychiatric hospitals. *American Journal of Psychiatry, 151*, 228–232.

D'Augelli, A. R. (1996). Lesbian, gay and bisexual development during adolescence and young adulthood. In R. P. Cabaj & T. S. Stein (Eds.), *Textbook of homosexuality and mental health* (pp. 267–288). Washington, DC: American Psychiatric Press.

D'Augelli, A. R., Hershberger, S. L., & Pilkington, N. W. (1998). Lesbian, gay and bisexual youth and their families: Disclosure of sexual orientation and its consequences. *American Journal of Orthopsychiatry, 68*, 361–371.

Editors of the Harvard Law Review. (1990). *Sexual orientation and the law.* Cambridge, MA: Harvard University Press.

Faderman, L. (1982). *Surpassing the love of men: Romantic friendship and love between women from the Renaissance to the present.* New York: Morrow.

Frank, P., & Houghton, B. (1987). *Confronting the batterer: A guide to creating the spouse abuse educational workshop.* New York: Volunteer Counseling Service of Rockland County.

Friend, R. A. (1991). Older lesbian and gay people: A theory of successful aging. In J. A. Lee (Ed.), *Gay midlife and maturity* (pp. 119–135). New York: Haworth Press.

Freud, S. (1953). Three essays on the theory of sexuality. In J. Strachey (Ed. & Trans.), *The standard edition of the complete psychological works of Sigmund Freud* (Vol. 7, pp. 125–243). London: Hogarth Press. (Original work published 1905)

Freud, S. (1955). Psychogenesis of a case of homosexuality in a woman. In J. Strachey (Ed. & Trans.), *The standard edition of the complete psychological works of Sigmund Freud* (Vol. 18, pp. 143–175). London: Hogarth Press. (Original work published 1920)

Garnets, L., Hancock, K., Cochran, S., et al. (1991). Issues in psychotherapy with lesbians and gay men: A survey of psychologists. *American Psychologist, 46*(9), 964–972.

Gilman, S. E., Cochran, S. D., Mays, U. M., et al. (2001). Risk of psychiatric disorders among individuals reporting same-sex sexual partners in the national comobidity survey. *American Journal of Public Health, 91*(6), 933–939.

Golden, C. (1987). Diversity and variability in women's sexual identities. In Boston Lesbian Psychologies Collective (Eds.), *Lesbian psychologies: Explorations and challenges* (pp. 18–34). Urbana: University of Illinois Press.

Gonsiorek, J. C. (1988). Mental health issues of gay and lesbian adolescents. *Journal of Adolescent Health Care, 9,* 114–122.

Gonsiorek, J. C. (1991). The empirical basis for the demise of the illness model of homosexuality. In J. C. Gonsiorek & J. D. Weinrich (Eds.), *Homosexuality: Research implication for public policy* (pp. 115–136). Newbury Park, CA: Sage.

Gonsiorek, J. C., & Rudolph, J. R. (1991). Homosexual identity: Coming out and other developmental events. In J. C. Gonsiorek & J. D. Weinrich (Eds.), *Homosexuality: Research implications for public policy* (pp. 161–176). Newbury Park, CA: Sage.

Gottman, J. S. (1990). Children of gay and lesbian parents. In F. Bozett & M. B. Sussman (Eds.), *Homosexuality and family relations* (pp. 177–196). New York: Harrington Park Press.

Greene, B. (1994). Ethnic minority lesbians and gay men: Mental health treatment issues. *Journal of Consulting and Clinical Psychology, 62,* 243.

Greene, B. (Ed). (1997). *Ethnic and cultural diversity among lesbians and gay men.* Thousand Oaks, CA: Sage.

Herdt, G., & Boxer, A. (1992). Introduction: Culture, history and life course of gay men. In G. Herdt (Ed.), *Gay culture in America: Essays from the field* (pp. 1–28). Boston: Beacon Press.

Herdt, G., & Boxer, A. (1996). *Children of horizons* (2nd ed.). Boston: Beacon Press.

Herek, G. M. (1984). Beyond homophobia: A social psychological perspective on attitudes towards lesbians and gay men. *Journal of Homosexuality, 10*(1–2), 1–21.

Herek, G. M. (1990). The context of anti-gay violence: Notes on cultural and psychological heterosexism. *Journal of Interpersonal Violence, 5*(3), 316–333.

Herek, G. M. (1995). Psychological heterosexism in the United States. In A. R. D'Augelli & C. J. Patterson (Eds.), *Lesbian, gay and bisexual identities over the lifespan* (pp. 321–346). New York: Oxford University Press.

Huggins, S. (1989). A comparative study of self-esteem of adolescent children of divorced lesbian mothers and divorced heterosexual mothers. *Journal of Homosexuality, 18,* 123–135.

Hunter, J., & Schraecher, R. (1987). Stresses on lesbian and gay adolescents in schools. *Social Work in Education, 9,* 180–189.

Kehoe, M. (1989). *Lesbians over sixty speak for themselves.* New York: Haworth Press.

Kinsey, A. C., Pomeroy, W. B., Martin, C. E., et al. (1953). *Sexual behavior in the human female.* Philadelphia: W. B. Saunders.

Kirkpatrick, M. (1996). Lesbians as parents. In R. P. Cabaj & T. S. Stein (Eds.), *Textbook of homosexuality and mental health* (pp. 353–370). Washington, DC: American Psychiatric Press.

Kirkpatrick, M., Smith, K., & Roy, R. (1981). Studies of a new population: The lesbian mother. In J. Howells (Ed.), *Modern perspectives in the psychiatry of middle age* (pp. 132–143). New York: Brunner/Mazel.

Kurdek, L. A. (1988). Relationship quality of gay and lesbian cohabitating couples. *Journal of Homosexuality, 15*, 93–118.

Kurdek, L. A. (1989). Relationship quality in gay and lesbian cohabitating couples: A 1–year follow-up study. *Journal of Social and Personal Relationships, 6*, 39–59.

Kurdek, L. A. (1993). The allocation of household labor in homosexual and heterosexual cohabitating couples. *Journal of Social Issues, 49*, 127–139.

Kurdek, L. A. (1995). Lesbian and gay couples. In A. R. D'Augelli & C. J. Patterson (Eds), *Lesbian, gay and bisexual identities over the lifespan* (pp. 243–261). New York: Oxford University Press.

Kurdek, L. A., & Schmitt, J. P. (1987). Partner homogamy in married, heterosexual cohabitating, gay and lesbian couples. *Journal of Sex Research, 23*, 212–232.

Laird, J. (1998). Invisible ties: Lesbians and their families of origin. In C. J. Patterson & A. R. D'Augelli (Eds.), *Lesbian, gay and bisexual identities in families* (pp. 197–228). New York: Oxford University Press.

Laumann, E. O., Gagnon, J. H., Michael, R. T., et al. (1994). *The social organization of sexuality: Sexual practices in the United States.* Chicago: University of Chicago Press.

Loulan, J. (1988). Research on the sex practices of 1566 lesbians and the clinical applications. *Women and Therapy, 7*, 221–234.

Magee, M., & Miller, D. C. (1997). *Lesbian lives: Psychoanalytic narratives old and new.* Hillsdale, NJ: Analytic Press.

Malyon, A. K. (1982). Psychotherapeutic implications of internalized homophobia in gay men. In J. C. Gonsiorek (Ed.), *Homosexuality and psychotherapy* (pp. 59–69). New York: Haworth Press.

Mays, V. M., & Cochran, S. D. (1988). The Black Woman's Relationship Project: A national survey of black lesbians. In M. Shernoff & W. A. Scott (Eds.), *A sourcebook of gay/lesbian health care* (2nd ed., pp. 54–62), Washington, DC: National Lesbian and Gay Health Foundation.

Mays, V. M., Cochran, S. D., & Rhue, S. (1993). The impact of perceived discrimination on the intimate relationships of black lesbians. *Journal of Homosexuality, 25*(4), 1–14.

Mays, V. M., & Jackson, J. S. (1991). AIDS survey methodology with black Americans. *Social Science and Medicine, 33*, 47–54.

McWhirter, D. P., & Mattison, A. M. (1984). *The male couple: How relationships develop.* Englewood Cliffs, NJ: Prentice Hall.

Patterson, C. J. (1992). Children of lesbian and gay parents. *Child Development, 63*, 1025–1042.

Patterson, C. J. (1994). Children of the lesbian baby boom: Behavioral adjustment, self-concepts and sex role identity. In B. Greene & G. M. Herek (Eds.), *Lesbian and gay psychology: Theory, research and clinical applications* (pp. 156–175). Newbury Park, CA: Sage Publications.

Patterson, C. J. (1998). Family lives of children born to lesbian mothers. In C. J. Patterson & A. R. D'Augelli (Eds.), *Lesbian, gay and bisexual identities in families* (pp. 154–176). New York: Oxford University Press.

Patterson, C. J. (2001). Families of the lesbian baby boom: Maternal mental health and child adjustment. *Journal of Gay and Lesbian Psychotherapy, 4*(3–4), 91–107.

Peplau, L. A., & Cochran, S. D. (1990). A relationship perspective on homosexuality. In D. P. McWhirter, S. A. Sanders, & J. M. Reinisch (Eds.), *Homosexuality/heterosexuality: Concepts of sexual orientation* (pp. 321–349). New York: Oxford University Press.

Reid, J. D. (1995). Development in late life: Older lesbian and gay lives. In A. R. D'Augelli & C. J.

Patterson (Eds.), *Lesbian, gay and bisexual identities over the lifespan* (pp. 215–240). New York: Oxford University Press.

Robinson, B., Walter, L. H., & Skeen, P. (1989). Response of parents to learning that their child is homosexual and their concern over AIDS: A national study. *Journal of Homosexuality, 18,* 59–80.

Ryan, C., & Futterman, D. (1998). *Lesbian and gay youth: Care and counseling.* New York: Columbia University Press.

Sandfurt, T. G. M., de Graaf, R., Bijl, R. U., & Schabel, P. (2001). Same-sex sexual behavior and psychiatric disorders. *Archives of General Psychiatry, 58,* 85–91.

Sang, B. (1991). Moving toward balance and integration. In B. Sang, J. Warshow, & A. J. Smith (Eds.), *Lesbians at midlife: The creative transition* (pp. 206–214). San Francisco: Spinster Books.

Savin-Williams, R. C. (1990). *Gay and lesbian youth: Expressions of identity.* New York: Hemisphere.

Sears, J. T. (1991). *Growing up gay in the South: Race, gender and journeys of the spirit.* New York: Harrington Park Press.

Slater, S., & Mencher, J. (1991). The lesbian family life cycle: A contextual approach. *American Journal of Orthopsychiatry, 61,* 372–382.

Socarides, C. (1968). *The overt homosexual.* New York: Grune & Stratton.

Stein, T. S. (1988). Theoretical considerations in psychotherapy with gay men and lesbians. *Journal of Homosexuality, 15*(1–2), 75–95.

Strickland, B. R. (1997). Leaving the confederate closet. In B. Greene (Ed.), *Ethnic and cultural diversity among lesbians and gay men* (pp. 39–62). Thousand Oaks, CA: Sage.

Taylor, R. J., Chatters, L. M., Tucker, M. B., et al. (1990). Development in research on black families: A decade review. *Journal of Marriage and the Family, 52,* 163–172.

Troiden, R. R. (1979). Becoming homosexual: A model of gay identity acquisition. *Psychiatry, 42,* 362–373.

Troiden, R. R. (1988). Homosexual identity development. *Journal of Adolescent Health, 9,* 105.

Vaillant, G. E. (1977). *Adaptation to life.* Boston: Little, Brown.

Walber, E. (1988). Behind closed doors: Battering and abuse in the lesbian and gay community. In M. Shernoff & W. Scott (Eds.), *Sourcebook on lesbian and gay health* (pp. 250–256). Washington, DC: National Lesbian and Gay Health Foundation.

Weinberg, G. (1972). *Society and the health homosexual.* New York: St. Martin's Press.

34

Women of Color

CHERYL S. AL-MATEEN
FRANCES M. CHRISTIAN
ASHA MISHRA
MICHELE COFIELD
TONI TILDON

As this textbook thoroughly considers the mental health needs of all women, this chapter provides an overview of the special attention that must be given to the mental health needs of women of color. Women in this category are numerous as well as heterogeneous. Despite the growing proportions of what have been called "minority" members of the U.S. population, there has not been a commensurate increase in the number of minority mental health practitioners. Therefore, it is far more likely that women of color will be treated by "majority" mental health practitioners. Regardless of their own cultural or racial group, however, all care providers must develop "cultural competence"—that is, a basis for expertise in working with women of color. In addition to the special concerns inherent in the treatment of the one "cultural" group on which this text focuses—females—many unique cultural issues that are part of the psychological development of subgroups of women of color (Al-Mateen et al., 2000). Although there are a few exceptions (Comas-Diaz & Greene, 1994; Jackson & Greene, 2000; Porter, 2000; Gutierrez & Lewis, 1999), minimal systematic attention in the mental health literature has been given to the psychological problems of women of color. It is not possible in one chapter to provide all the known information relevant to working with women in different cultural groups. Therefore, we review the basic concepts and principles necessary for the appreciation of cultural differences among subgroups of women of color.

WHO ARE WOMEN OF COLOR?

Women of color are a population that is immensely heterogeneous, both between and within groups. For example, Hispanics or Latinas are united by a common language, but may come from places as diverse as Puerto Rico, Mexico, Cuba, other Caribbean Islands, Spain, Central America, and South America. Similarly, African Americans or Blacks share ethnic origins from Africa and include African Caribbeans, but they may also represent diverse regional backgrounds in the United States. Blacks who are immigrants or refugees have different cultural backgrounds than blacks born in the United States. Native Americans are comprised of individuals from many different tribes, and these women of color also include Alaskan and Hawaiian natives. Likewise, "Asian American" is a term that subsumes a number of unique cultural groups, including women from India, China, Japan, Korea, Vietnam, and other Asian countries. 2000 U.S. Census data report indicates that Asian Americans and Hispanic/Latinas are the fastest growing ethnic groups (U.S. Bureau of the Census, 2001).

In addition to demographic diversity, there is much within-group variability: Women of color differ on factors such as age, place of residence (urban vs. rural), religion, degree of acculturation, sexual orientation, educational level, and socioeconomic status. Given these factors, a woman can belong to multiple cultures at the same time. Clearly, women of color belong to more than one minority group (women, who constitute a minority in terms of relative power if not in numbers, and their ethnic/racial minority group). Living in at least two cultural worlds, they are often forced to negotiate at times competing sets of ideals as well as to avoid internalization of sexist and racist values (Westkott, 1998). Women of color must be seen as representative of a "double minority with multiple consciousness" (Nadelson & Zimmerman, 1993, p. 509).

All of these potential differences add to the contextual complexity for women of color. Therefore, one should be cautious and not assume within-group homogeneity that simply does not exist. Despite their heterogeneity, many women of color share the common bonds of societal inequalities, oppression, discrimination, and devaluation based on their gender and race/ethnicity. Mental health professionals working with women of color must develop some understanding of culture and become culturally competent in order to treat them effectively.

CULTURE AND ITS IMPACT ON MENTAL HEALTH

"Culture" is "the matrix of belief, values, and norms that inform, give meaning to, and regulate behavior" (Westkott, 1998, p. 816). In addition to beliefs, norms, and values, culture includes the historical experiences that have resulted in a group's economic, social, and political status in the general social structure (Kaplan, 1999). These experiences have a significant impact on group members' psychological well-being. Therefore, in addition to well-accepted factors such as biology, early life experiences, and family relationships, cultural experiences such as difficulties with racism, sexism, acculturation, stress, poverty, and identity conflicts should be a routine part of treatment considerations with women of color.

Culture has objective and subjective aspects. The objective aspects are most easily observable and include clothing, food, and artifacts. Subjective components of culture are values, ideals, attitudes, roles, and norms. They are frequently bases for misunderstanding among those of different cultures and are sources of challenge in the assessment and provision of mental health care (Singh, 1996).

Therapists are generally taught about psychological development, psychopathology, and the practice of psychotherapy from the perspective of the mainstream culture in the United States—that of white, European, Christian ethnic groups and their descendants (Katz, 1985). The establishment of eye contact, control of emotions, limitation of physical contact, future orientation, and a focus on the importance of youth and the nuclear family are part of the framework of clinical supervision. These perspectives often are not shared by all cultural groups and may complicate the assessment and treatment process with women of color (Sue & Sue, 1990).

Culture and ethnicity may affect biology, identity development, and day-to-day stressors, as well as the acceptance of the need for mental health treatment. Culture affects the way a woman views her role in her family of origin, in society, as a partner in a romantic relationship, as a mother, or in her place of worship; each of these roles affects the others, as well as her perception of her therapist or other health care provider.

Intrapsychic factors such as low self-esteem and ineffective coping skills may contribute to the psychologically and physiologically stressful experiences of women of color. However, the mental health problems of these women tend to be especially related to such extrinsic factors as racism, sexism, poverty, and the daily hassles of discriminatory experiences (Christian, 1994; Porter, 2000). It is clear that the psychological problems women of color bring to the treatment situation cannot be fully understood as merely individual psychopathology or maladaptation. Clinicians will need to include consideration of the social ecology in order to provide culturally sensitive mental health services (Christian et al., 2000).

ROLES OF WOMEN OF COLOR

Before industrialization, most American women had to balance work on the family farm with motherhood and other family responsibilities. Women of color in the United States also balanced these responsibilities with additional work outside the home as farmhands, slaves, domestics, and laborers. During industrialization and wartime, European American women often worked in factories; they would resign once they married or when men were available to work after the war. In contrast, women of color often continued to work both inside and outside the home, regardless of their marital status. In the process of balancing motherhood with work and family responsibilities, women of color have had some unique hurdles to overcome while cultivating methods for coping with or resolving these issues.

Since this country's inception, African American women have held outside employment in order to help support their families, while balancing the additional stressors of being competent mothers and loving wives. When faced with the daily burden of these multiple roles, many African American women rely on their female friends, elders, "church families," and ministers to support them through difficult times. Paradoxically, African American women who achieve a measure of success may not only be isolated by their coworkers owing to cultural differences; they may also be isolated from their communities of origin owing to a shift in their social status (Christian et al., 2000). This has been especially noted in African American female athletes who struggle with the challenges of upward mobility while attending majority European American institutions (Bond, 1997).

The social stressors inherent in being a woman of color in the United States should not be underestimated. Women of color must often contend with others' assumptions about their capabilities that may be based solely on skin color, appearance, and/or perceived class level. Given the ubiquity of such experiences, it may be difficult for an individual to assess whether a superficially amiable environment is truly supportive. The "microinsults" or "microaggressions" (Pierce, 1995) often experienced as products of overt or institutional racism and sexism within the workplace add to the level of stress. As a result, when errors or conflicts arise in the workplace, women of color have the additional burden of worrying about the origins of the conflict and whether or not their race or gender is a contributing factor.

Women of color have many mechanisms with which to cope with these feelings and issues. Sometimes they live in silence, sometimes with depression; often they seek support from religious institutions, their communities, and self-styled support networks.

HELP SEEKING AND OBSTACLES

Gender is a powerful predictor for seeking psychological services. Women are more likely than men to seek professional mental health treatment (Neighbors & Howard, 1987). However, women of color must often overcome many obstacles to gain access or entrance into the mental health system. Cultural beliefs or attitudinal factors frequently play an important role in their underutilization of psychotherapeutic services (Padgett et al., 1994). Shame, stigma, and a greater tolerance for unusual behaviors than in mainstream society may inhibit women of color from seeking professional help (Mays et al., 1996; Padgett et al., 1994; Yamashiro & Matsuoka, 1997). Among Asian Americans and Pacific islanders, shame is a collective identity, as the behavior of an individual reflects upon the entire group or family (Yamashiro & Matsuoka, 1997): "The individual defers his or her desires to the family and only those behaviors that maintain and improve the family name are considered valuable" (Meston et al., 1999, pp. 139–140). This cultural attitude may prevent seeking mental health assistance from professionals and create an environment for conflict within the family and the individual herself. African Americans also have an "I am because we are" orientation that emphasizes the importance of the group over the individual. In addition, African American women tend to view seeking psychotherapy as indicating that they are personally "weak" or "broken down and couldn't take it" (Greene, 1994, p.21). Such beliefs represent internalized stereotypes of being a strong matriarch and superwoman (Greene, 1994; Olmedo & Parron, 1981; Porter, 2000). The importance of *familism*, which instills a preference to rely on a network of family members for emotional support, may impede Hispanic or Latina women from seeking mental health treatment (Henslin, 1985; Vasquez, 1994; Woodward, 1998). Other women of color have been found to share this preference to use familiar sources of help—family, friends, folk healers, and religious/spiritual leaders with knowledge of their cultural beliefs. These kinds of cultural attitudes and reliance on informal community-based institutional supports often mean that women of color delay seeking help until their problems become severe (Caldwell, 2000; Mays et al., 1996; Padgett et al., 1994; Yamashiro & Matsuoka, 1997).

Language differences, a lack of translators/interpreters, and an absence of ethnic clinicians may contribute to anticipated misunderstandings and mistrust of clinicians by women of color. They may not access or remain engaged in treatment if there is a perception of cultural insensitivity. Furthermore, aspects of the service delivery system or agency may present barriers to women of color. Waiting lists, rigid intake procedures, inconvenient hours, and inappropriate treatment modalities (Copeland, 1982), or difficulties with transportation and child care (Belle, 1984), may prevent women of color from keeping scheduled appointments. Also, managed care restrictions have jeopardized much access to mental health care. An effort to use culture-specific treatments in the community may be the most acceptable and useful approach for many women of color. However, managed mental health care efforts have been more targeted toward limiting costs by restricting visit frequency, as well as using only selected credentialed clinicians who may not be familiar with the language or cultural values. These clinicians may not practice in the local community or be located on a bus line, thus limiting the availability of services. Also, as service delivery sites in nontraditional settings (churches, storefronts, and community organizations) are being eliminated by managed care organizations, access to services is being adversely affected (Kaplan, 1999). If managed mental health care organizations do not develop and implement standards and guidelines for providing culturally competent care, then women of color are likely to be barred in the future from access to a variety of mental health treatment options.

CULTURAL IDENTITY

"Cultural identity" is the part of the individual's self-concept that derives from knowledge of membership in a social group or groups, plus the value and emotional significance attached to that membership (Phinney, 1990). It includes self-identification as a member of a group, as well as an awareness of the position of that group in the larger society (Spencer & Markstrom-Adams, 1990). This includes such factors as racism, discrimination, unequal societal distribution of power and resources, and inconsistencies in the messages and behaviors of the majority culture regarding racial and ethnic minorities.

One develops a cultural identity over time. A woman may be strongly or weakly identified with her culture and with the dominant, or majority, culture. The woman whose cultural identity is primarily with her group of origin to the exclusion of the dominant culture, is seen as "separate" or "dissociated" from the dominant culture. The woman of color who identifies with the majority culture and retains only minimal association with her own culture is referred to as "assimilated," having lost her cultural distinctiveness. The woman who feels that she belongs to neither group is seen as "marginalized," while the woman who is able to embrace and appreciate aspects of both cultures is "bicultural," adapting to both cultures. A bicultural woman is seen as having the most satisfactory level of functioning (Locke, 1992). These definitions are useful for women raised in a culture, as well as for those who have immigrated to a different culture. The cultural identity of both the therapist and the patient have an impact on the therapeutic relationship.

The initial stage of cultural identity, "conformity," happens in almost all individuals. In this stage, one does not recognize the impact of racism (overt or covert/institutional) on one's life. The child or adolescent in this stage accepts that the majority culture is superior to her own. As the denial of the stage of conformity is eroded, the stage of "dissonance" is reached. Racism is seen as affecting members of one's own and other cultural groups. However, women in this stage still do not recognize the impact of racism (overt or covert/institutional) on their lives, and they accept the majority culture as superior to their own and that of other devalued groups (Sue & Sue, 1990). In the next stage, "resistance and immersion," the young person completely rejects the superiority of the majority culture and espouses "militant" minority-supportive views, including anger toward the majority culture for historical racism and oppression of minority groups. In the stage of "introspection," the intensity of resistance and immersion becomes psychologically draining and difficult to maintain. It prevents the use of energy to further explore oneself or one's own cultural group. The views of resistance and immersion are seen as unnecessarily rigid and extreme. In the final stage, "integrative awareness," one becomes able to appreciate unique aspects of one's own as well as other cultures, with a strong commitment to eliminate the oppression of all minority cultural groups. The individual is more secure within her own sense of identity (Sue & Sue, 1990).

A woman's stage of cultural identity development is likely to affect her choice of, and relationship with, a mental health care provider. A woman in conformity is likely to prefer a provider of the majority population (Sue & Sue, 1990). A woman in dissonance may accept a majority counselor with good knowledge of the woman's own cultural group, or may prefer a minority therapist. A woman in resistance and immersion is likely to be suspicious of any therapist who has been trained in a program sanctioned by the majority culture; a therapist in the majority group will be seen as an unacceptable representative of the "Establishment," while a person of color may be seen as someone who has "sold out" to the Establishment, buying into its views. A woman who has progressed to introspection or integrative awareness is more likely to easily accept any therapist who is able to understand her world view and, as a result, her.

Similarly, there are models of white racial identity development, based on the premise of this group's being the majority and "ubiquitous veil"/"baseline" cultural group of the United States (Hardiman, 1982; Helms, 1992; Sue & Sue, 1990). In the early stage of these models, a child does not recognize the meaning of race or its impact on her life. Although the child may recognize that there are differences in skin color, there is no fear, hostility, or sense of racial superiority. An event then occurs that helps the child realize what race means in our society and how things are done, involving the superiority of the white race in our society at large. This is the "acceptance" stage, and it is similar to conformity. Acceptance may be "passive" or "active." Passive acceptance means that although there is what can be called "subtle racism," the individual does not identify herself as racist. Those in active acceptance are forthright in expressing their belief of superiority. Some may join white supremacist groups (Hardiman, 1982).

Some individuals never move beyond this stage. Should a dissonance-like reaction occur, feelings related to race and cultural issues may range from anger and disgust to guilt and embarrassment. At this time, the stage of resistance and immersion is entered. There may be awareness with little behavioral change; the woman may feel as if one person cannot make a difference in the huge race relations problem. Or she may choose not to participate in anything perceived to be racist. In active resistance, the individual realizes not only that racism exists, but also that she has been racist to some degree, because of what she has internalized while growing up.

Introspection starts when the individual realizes that her white identity has been defined by others in racist terms, and that she needs to redefine it in nonracist terms (i.e., not in terms of superiority to others). A middle ground is approached. She may choose to learn more about her ethnic group at this time. When these new values and definitions are applied to her life, and she is aware of the past and making a difference in the future, the final stage of integrative awareness is reached (Hardiman, 1982; Sue & Sue, 1990).

IMMIGRANT WOMEN OF COLOR

The United States is primarily a land of immigrants. The early European immigrants shared with all the other immigrants similar reasons for this migration and the need to succeed in a new country. However, over subsequent generations, the immigrants of European descent were able to "blend in"—assimilate and acculturate—and emerge out of this melting pot with an "American" identity. Those who could not "blend in" due to unique, identifying ethnic/racial characteristics (such as color) have remained the "minorities," despite generations of living in the United States. They continue to face oppression, racism, and exclusion. The slavery of African Americans, the Chinese Exclusion Act, the internment of Japanese Americans during World War II, and general restrictions on immigration of Asians by a 1917 act (which even allowed withdrawal of citizenship already granted and was repealed only after court battles in 1946) are all grim reminders of this bias against immigration of "minorities."

The earlier migration of "colored" people primarily involved males who immigrated involuntarily or voluntarily as slaves and/or indentured labor into this country. Migration of women was allowed at a later date for the purposes of marriage or family reunification. These women came to the United States primarily to join their spouses or as mail-order brides. They came from Africa, Central and South America, Asia, and the Middle East. They are a very heterogeneous group at various degrees of assimilation and acculturation.

When one migrates to another country, one experiences a crisis event; a certain amount of acculturation must result. Hertz (1988) and his group have described stages in this acculturation. They note that difficulties in acculturation are due to culture shock related to both intrapsychic and interpersonal factors. Differences in modes of verbal and nonverbal communication, educational systems, and other aspects of culture we have already discussed can cause difficulty.

There are three stages in the positive adjustment to immigration. The first is "preimmigration," in which the individual and/or family needs motivation for the change. There is generally a positive expectation before the move, which creates the proper emotional atmosphere for such a move. Overidealization or denial of potential difficulties can place the migrating family at risk for maladjustment. In the second stage, "coping," the reality of the move is encountered. Language barriers (with subsequent difficulty in communication) and subjective cultural differences may result in dysphoria. Emotional supports are usually located, however, and a sense of security begins to develop. This adjustment progresses during the "settlement" stage, in which the family members feel more understood by the environment and in turn feel more prepared to understand the demands of the new environment on them. A sense of belonging develops. Positive adjustment is increased by having cohesive forces in the family and ethnic group at large in the new location.

Adolescents and elderly persons are at highest risk for poor acculturation. Those who were poorly motivated to move are also at risk, as are those who used the migration to attempt to get away from inner conflicts.

Stress in the Lives of Immigrant Women

Currently, Asian and Hispanic Americans are the fastest-growing populations (Woodward, 1998; U.S. Bureau of the Census, 2001). While working full-time or part-time in lower-paying jobs, or even at the higher-paying jobs enjoyed by the small subset of women with professional and managerial positions, these women have to contend with what Hochschild has called the "second shift" (Hochschild with Machung, 1989). The entry of these women into the working world is usually not accompanied by a parallel shift in cultural understanding of marriage roles and work (Hochschild with Machung, 1989). The American dream of equal opportunities, freedom for all, and more egalitarian roles for women and men remains an even more elusive dream for these women than for others. They continue to struggle with internalized racism and oppression, as well as the traditional role expectations from their families, spouses, and society at large. At work, they deal with issues centering around assertiveness, competitiveness, and individualism; these cultural expectations are forces that run counter to their traditional upbringing. As do all women, they must also contend with discrimination and "glass ceilings" (Homma-True, 1997). At home, they are frequently carrying the burdens of the primary homemaker. Despite the geographical distance, the pressures from the extended family still living in the home country cannot be underestimated, and the responsibilities to the extended family continue to take their toll (Thara & Rajkumar, 1992; Naik et al., 1998).

Coping with the many stresses of adjusting to a new culture, frequently even having to learn a new language, while working in low-paying marginal jobs leads to tremendous strains on immigrant women. As their stress level increases, they may not have the traditional support systems of the old country in this new country.

Immigrant women who are refugees have the additional burden of the memories of traumatic experiences that they experienced in their homelands. Posttraumatic stress symptoms may be difficult to broach with outsiders, particularly in instances of sexual trauma. Refugees have little likelihood of returning home in the future; this sense of disconnection, together with the issues of security and traumatization, can negatively affect the acculturation process.

Members of the second generation of immigrant women from traditional cultures continue to struggle as well. For most of them, coming of age in this day and time, the question of egalitarian roles between men and women and the problems of identity formation are of paramount importance. U.S. society, though not gender-equal, does allow women greater choices and wider roles. Second-generation women often seem eager to denounce the male dominance of their traditional cultures and to seize new opportunities. However, it is difficult for such a woman to assert this autonomy without much inner turmoil, many anxieties, and explosive family conflicts, regardless of her age (Lessinger, 1995; Ananth & Ananth, 1995).

Many women of color are from patriarchal societies in which the threshold of tolerance for psychiatric illness in women is much lower than that for such illness in men (Naik et al., 1998). The worth of a woman is measured in terms of her usefulness to the functioning of a family. Help is sought only when her role performance becomes significantly impaired, and some psychological problems may be missed because of different presentations.

Psychiatric Illness in Immigrant Women of Color

It is the common experience of all who work with people from other cultures that those from traditional societies tend to manifest mental distress in somatic terms (Rack, 1982). There are two possible explanations for this tendency. The first is the fact that most immigrants and many other minorities do not go to the doctor unless they experience something physical, for "is this not what the doctors are for?" Furthermore, when financial resources are limited, treatment for purely psychological symptoms is often seen as something that cannot be afforded. For such distress, these women tend either to sort it out themselves or to go to friends or nonmedical healers. The second reason for such a presentation is that the somatic complaint is often a metaphor for emotional distress (Rack, 1982). Many Asian languages have a vocabulary that only expresses emotions through attribution to specific physical organs. For example, the heart, liver, spleen, and head are used to express fear, love, anxieties, and worries, in the Hindi and Urdu languages. The literal translation of symptoms, in the absence of adequate fluency in the English language, could lead to disastrous or humorous results. Expressions such as "My heart is fluttering or sinking," or "It feels like someone has pushed a dagger into my heart," with accompanying gestures could mean either bona fide cardiac symptoms or expressions of intense emotional pain or worry. The Asian languages also tend to be very rich in names for various extended family members, but poor in different names for different degrees of mood states; perhaps this is a function of the value these cultures place on families, in contrast to individual or internal experiences.

Given this inherent tendency to deny psychological distress, the symptoms of such distress are frequently ignored until impairment in role performance is evident. These negative attitudes toward seeking mental health services fortunately diminish over subsequent generations of stay in this country and begin to correspond more closely with the help-seeking behaviors of the general population (Furnham & Malik, 1994). However, given the possibility that assimilation can take place without corresponding acculturation, one could erroneously assume that the traditional values are no longer operating. It is important, therefore, to look for the typical as well as the atypical presentations of mental illnesses. These atypical presentations may present as "culture-bound syndromes" or atypical manifestations of anxiety, depression, mania, or psychosis. Conversion disorders, hysterical blindness, hysterical psychosis, and possession states all must be considered in the differential diagnoses.

Culture-Bound Syndromes in Immigrant Women

Culture-bound syndromes do not present only in exotic places. They are best considered examples of how people from particular lands may experience or explain their illness (Kleinman et al., 1978). It is not possible to include a description of all known culture-bound syndromes in this chapter. Some names are included in Table 34.1 to help readers become familiar with these syndromes. Many culture-bound syndromes have been reported in a review of the topic by Simon and Hughes (1993).

Of particular note is the issue of "possession state" in some groups of women of

TABLE 34.1. Examples of Culture-Bound Syndrome

Syndrome	Group(s) affected
Ataque de nervios	Puerto Ricans in New York City (Garrison, 1977)
Brain fag	Students from Africa (Prince, 1960)
Falling out	African Americans and African Caribbeans in the southeastern United States (Weidman, 1979)
Ghost sickness	Navajos (Kaplan & Johnson, 1964)
Hwa-byung	Koreans on the West Coast (Liu, 1986)
Taijin kyofusho	Japanese Americans (Tanaka Matsumi, 1979)
Voodoo deaths	African Americans and African Caribbeans (Snow, 1974)
Wacinko	Oglala Sioux (Lewis, 1975)
Wind illness	Chinese Americans (Eisenbruch, 1983)

color. The affected person, frequently a female, is believed to be possessed by a deity, the spirit of an ancestor, or a historical person. These states may be a manifestation of psychosis, hysteria, anxiety, phobia, depression, or neurotic states, but frequently the possession is the playing out of a socially prescribed role (Simon & Hughes, 1993; Rack, 1982). Many clinicians regard this as a culturally sanctioned form of depression, especially in Asian Indian women (Naik et al., 1998).

The Korean syndrome *hwa-byung* is viewed as a manifestation of suppressed anger or rage (Kim, 1993; Lin, 1983; Lin et al., 1992; Pang, 1990). In the United States, it has been described predominantly among married middle-aged Korean immigrant women of lower socioeconomic status. Reported symptoms include feelings of heaviness, mass in the epigastric region, headaches, muscle aches and pains, dry mouth, insomnia, palpitations, and indigestion; it may also include symptoms of depression (Kim, 1993).

Clinicians working with immigrant women of color need to consider culture-bound syndromes before ascribing patients a diagnosis of severe psychopathology, such as psychosis. Clinicians should also explore what (if any) indigenous treatments are being currently considered, used, or sought.

CULTURAL COMPETENCE

Dana (1993) describes that a culturally competent mental health professional has acquired the "ability to provide services that are perceived by the patient[s] as relevant to their problems and helpful for intervention outcomes" (p. 220). The process of striving for cultural competence involves becoming aware of one's own cultural identity, values, and biases, while respecting cultural differences that may influence the behaviors of patients. In order for mental health professionals to accurately assess women of color and provide appropriate and relevant care, the clinicians must first appreciate the impact of culture on themselves, their patients, and each clinician–patient relationship. An initial step is the clinicians' initial consideration that there may be a cultural difference between themselves and their patients. Without such consideration, no evaluation can be culturally competent. Thoughtful mental health practitioners must ask themselves whether they are biased in their interactions with any patients. Similarly, they must ask whether they are relying on past clinical information that is culturally biased. If clinicians are not already knowledgeable about a particular ethnic or cultural group, it is necessary to gather this information. Practitioners must have an understanding of each patient's ethnocultural background, the reasons for any relocation, each patient's cultural adjustment as an individual and as a member of her family, and any impact of the therapists' own ethnocultural identity on each therapeutic relationship (Jacobsen, 1988). Table 34.2 lists some questions practitioners may use to help them begin the process of ensuring that their practices are culturally competent.

Culturally competent clinicians assessing women of color are able to balance a consideration of universal human norms, individual uniqueness, and cultural group specific norms in order to determine what is normal or abnormal behavior for any particular woman of color (Lopez et al., 1989; Speight et al., 1991). They are able to apply cultural knowledge without stereotyping and be able to generate cultural hypotheses alongside other accepted theoretical explanations for human behavior (Lopez et al., 1989). If a clinician has specific cultural group knowledge and understanding for a woman of color, then appropriate individualized treatments are more likely to be recommended for and considered acceptable by the patient. Clinicians who strive to develop their cultural competence skills are open to obtaining knowledge via readings, workshops and a variety of experiential encounters, as well as to learning from their patients and their family members. Culturally skilled clinicians are also not adverse to seeking consultation from traditional healers or religious/spiritual healers in treating women of color, when such consultation is appropriate (Sue et al., 1992). Developing cultural competence skills must, then, be an ongoing process in order to stay abreast of the latest clinical knowledge and research about women of color (Lopez et al., 1989).

Cultural competence increases a clinician's confidence and credibility. Lack of sensitivity to cultural issues affects diagnosis, prognosis, compliance, patient satisfaction, and ultimately clinical outcome. Culturally skilled clinicians will be less likely to misunderstand behaviors and thus to make diagnostic errors. Although the overall incidence and prevalence of the major mental illnesses remain the same around the globe, the diagnosis of major mental illnesses can be challenging. Pitfalls in diagnosis may result from (1) linguistic difficulties, (2) lack of corresponding vocabulary to describe mood states, (3) cultural permission to focus only on somatic symptoms, and/or (4) confounding acculturation difficulties (Franks & Faux, 1990; LaFromboise et al., 1994). Women of color are likely to be misdiagnosed, overdiagnosed, or underdiagnosed due to these various factors, and ultimately to be undertreated or inadvertently mistreated. We have frequently come

TABLE 34.2. Am I Culturally Biased?

- What in this person's appearance or behavior makes me assume that what I am seeing is psychopathology? Is there another interpretation besides psychopathology?

- Am I subconsciously applying any labels to this patient? Where did those labels come from?

- What am I assuming about the patient's social class or group? What are my prejudices about that group?

- Is there evidence of cultural bias in the current chart or previous record?

Note. Adapted from Hughes (1993). Copyright 1993 by the American Psychiatric Association. Adapted by permission.

across the application of a "sicker" diagnosis (schizophrenia) to women of color suffering from depression with psychotic features; malingering as a diagnosis instead of conversion disorder in one patient and schizophrenia in another; and instances of missed assessment for domestic violence in women presenting with internalized oppression and resultant feelings of deserved abuse.

All symptoms, therefore, must be assessed in the context of patients' cultural beliefs. The *Diagnostic and Statistical Manual of Mental Disorders*, fourth edition, text revision, specifies that symptoms must be outside of cultural norms (American Psychiatric Association, 2000). Beliefs in possession states, hexes, roots, punishments for past deeds, and cultural paranoia are all realities for many women of color and must be explored actively. Specific issues centering around differences in psychopharmacological responses and variability in experience, as well as rates of adverse reactions, have to be considered as well.

EFFECTS OF ETHNICITY ON PSYCHOPHARMACOLOGY

The study of the effects of ethnicity on the effect of psychopharmacological agents is fairly recent (Chien, 1993; Sramek & Pi, 1996). Many differences in pharmacodynamics are related to the fact that many psychotropic medications are metabolized by liver processes, including acetylation and the cytochrome P450 (CYP450) isoenzymes with the different rates of metabolism that result from polymorphism (Lin et al., 1993b, 1995). It is also noted that eating habits, environment, and lifestyles affect metabolism of medications. These are cultural factors that may change as immigrants acculturate over time and over generations (Lin et al., 1995; Sramek & Pi, 1996). Lin et al. (1995) also found that "level of stress, quality and quantity of social support and personality styles all have been reported to influence significantly psychotropic response" (p. 641).

A substantial literature corroborates that Asians and Native Americans are more sensitive to the effects of alcohol than European Americans are. In their review, Lin et al. (1995) noted that Asians appear to have lower activity of the CYP2D6 isoenzyme than European Americans do. They have been found to respond to lower levels of tricyclic antidepressants (Silver et al., 1993). Those of African descent, including African Americans, appear to be more susceptible to untoward effects from lithium because of a less active sodium–lithium countertransport system. Lithium may also have a longer half-life in this population (Strickland et al., 1993). Asians may show a therapeutic response to lower lithium levels than other populations, although there is no difference in pharmacokinetics (Lin et al., 1995; Chien, 1993). Similarly, there may be a response to lower doses of benzodiazepines in both these populations (Lin et al., 1993a). African Americans and Hispanics may be more susceptible to side effects from tricyclics (Silver et al., 1993; Sramek & Pi, 1996). One group found Hispanics and Asians to respond to lower doses of antipsychotics than the general population (Collazo et al., 1996; Ruiz et al., 1996). In their review, Eastham et al. (1996) found that Asians may be less susceptible to tardive dyskinesia, and that African Americans may be more susceptible.

Given the small subject size of many studies, the numerous psychosocial confounding factors that can be culturally based, and the early nature of many of the findings, it is as necessary to avoid developing "stereotypes" about responses to medication as it is to avoid the use of stereotypes in the psychosocial aspects of mental health (Lin, 1996; Sramek & Pi, 1996). It is useful, however, to be aware of the level of knowledge that does exist. Many authors have recommended further study in this area (Chien, 1993; Collazo et al., 1996; Eastham et al., 1996; Lawson, 1996; Lin et al., 1995; Ruiz et al., 1996; Silver et al., 1993; Strickland et al., 1993; Sramek & Pi, 1996; Yoshida, 1993).

CONCLUSIONS

We have reviewed important issues regarding culture; cultural identity and its formation; and some of the stressful experiences of both American-born and Immigrant women of color in the United States. These factors all influence help-seeking and assessment processes, as well as the diagnosis and mental health treatment of women of color. An appreciation of the impact of these determinants will enable thoughtful clinicians to provide better mental health care for these women. We have also reviewed steps that clinicians may take to ensure that they are culturally competent.

Although the literature on the psychosocial aspects of culture is vast, the multicultural nature of our world continues to expand. Biracial and multiracial women have additional identity issues we have not addressed. Much research remains to be done in the area of ethnic psychopharmacology. Cross-cultural psychiatry is a rich field in which study is not yet complete.

REFERENCES

Al-Mateen, C. S., Webb, C. T., Christian, F. M., et al. (2000). Identity issues. In N. J. Burgess & E. Brown (Eds.), *African American women: An ecological perspective*. New York: Falmer Press.

American Psychiatric Association. (2000). *Diagnostic and statistical manual of mental disorders* (4th ed., text revision, pp. 15–39). Washington, DC: Author.

Ananth, J., & Ananth, K. (1995). *East Indian immigrants to the United States: Life cycle issues and adjustment*. East Meadow, NY: Indo-American Psychiatric Association.

Belle, D. (1984). Inequality and mental health: Low income and minority women. In L. E. Walker (Ed.), *Women and mental health policy* (pp. 135–150). Beverly Hills, CA: Sage.

Bond, M. A. (1997). The multitextured lives of women of color. *American Journal of Community Psychology, 25(5),* 733–743.

Caldwell, C. H. (2000). Social networks: Community-based institutional supports. In N. J. Burgess & E. Brown (Eds.), *African American women: An ecological perspective* (pp. 99–114). New York: Falmer Press.

Chien, C.-P. (1993). Ethnopsychopharmacology. In A. C. Gaw (Ed.), *Culture, ethnicity, and mental illness* (pp. 413–440). Washington, DC: American Psychiatric Press.

Christian, F. M. (1994). *Stress and coping response of African-American women*. Unpublished doctoral dissertation, Virginia Commonwealth University.

Christian, F. M., Al-Mateen, C. S., Webb, C. T., et al. (2000). Stress, coping and the mental health of African American women. In N. J. Burgess & E. Brown (Eds.), *African American women: An ecological perspective* (pp. 135–159). New York: Falmer Press.

Collazo, Y., Tam, R., Sramek, J. et al. (1996). Neuroleptic dosing in Hispanic and Asian inpatients with schizophrenia. *Mount Sinai Journal of Medicine, 63,* 310–313.

Comas-Diaz, L., & Greene, B. (Eds.). (1994). *Women of color: Integrating ethnic and gender identities in psychotherapy.* New York: Guilford Press.

Copeland, E. J. (1982). Oppressed conditions and the mental health needs of low-income black women: Barriers to services, strategies for change. *Women and Therapy, 1(1),* 13–26.

Dana, R. H. (1993). *Multicultural assessment perspectives for professional psychology.* Boston: Allyn & Bacon.

Eastham, J. H., Lacro, J. P., & Jeste, D. V. (1996). Ethnicity and movement disorders. *Mount Sinai Journal of Medicine, 63,* 314–319.

Eisenbruch, M. (1983). "Wind illness" or somatic depression? A case study in psychiatric anthropology. *British Journal of Psychiatry, 143,* 323–326.

Franks, F., & Faux, S. A. (1990). Depression, stress masking and social resources in four ethnocultural women's groups. *Research in Nursing and Health, 13,* 283–292.

Furnham, A., & Malik, R. (1994). Cross-cultural beliefs about "depression." *International Journal of Social Psychiatry, 40*(2), 106–123.

Garrison, V. (1977). The Puerto Rican syndrome in psychiatry and *espritismo.* In V. Crapazano & V. Garrison (Eds.), *Case studies in spirit possession* (pp. 383–449). New York: Wiley.

Greene, B. (1994). African American women. In L. Comas-Diaz, & B. Greene (Eds.), *Women of color: Integrating ethnic and gender identities in psychotherapy* (pp. 10–29). New York: Guilford Press.

Gutierrez, L. M., & Lewis, E. A. (1999). *Empowering women of color.* New York: Columbia University Press.

Henslin, J. M. (1985). *Marriage and family in a changing society.* New York: Free Press.

Hardiman, R. (1982). White identity development: A process oriented model for describing the racial consciousness of white Americans. *Dissertation Abstracts International, 43,* 104A. (University Microfilms No. 82–10330)

Helms, J. (1992). *A race is a nice thing to have.* Topeka, KS: Content.

Hertz, D. G. (1988). Identity—lost and found: Patterns of migration and psychological and psychosocial adjustment of migrants. *Acta Psychiatrica Scandinavica, 78*(Suppl. 344), 159–165.

Hochschild, A., with Machung, A. (1989). *The second shift.* New York: Viking.

Homma-True, R. (1997). Asian American women. In E. Lee (Ed.), *Working with Asian Americans: A guide for clinicians* (pp. 420–427). New York: Guilford Press.

Hughes, C. C. (1993). Culture in clinical psychiatry. In A. C. Gaw (Ed.), *Culture, ethnicity, and mental illness* (pp. 3–41). Washington, DC: American Psychiatric Press.

Jackson, L. C., & Greene, B. (Eds.). (2000). *Psychotherapy with African American women.* New York: Guilford Press.

Jacobsen, F. M. (1988). Ethnocultural assessment. In L. Comas-Diaz & E. E. H. Griffith (Eds.), *Clinical guidelines in cross-cultural mental health* (pp. 135–147). New York: Wiley.

Kaplan, A. (1999). Managed care and culturally diverse populations: A disconnect? *Psychiatric Times, 16*(4), 16–17.

Kaplan, B., & Johnson, D. (1964). The social meaning of Navaho psychopathology and psychotherapy. In *Magic, faith and healing: Studies in primitive psychiatry today* (pp. 203–229). New York: Free Press.

Katz, J. (1985). The sociopolitical nature of counseling. *The Counseling Psychologist, 13,* 615–624.

Kim, L. I. C. (1993). Psychiatric care of Korean Americans. In A. C. Gaw (Ed.), *Culture, ethnicity, and mental illness* (pp. 347–376). Washington, DC: American Psychiatric Press.

Kleinman, A., Eisenberg, L., & Good, B. (1978). Clinical lessons from anthropologic and cross-cultural research. *Annals of Internal Medicine, 88,* 251–258.

LaFromboise, T. D., Berman, J. S., & Sohi, B. K. (1994). American Indian women. In L. Comas-Diaz & B. Greene (Eds.), *Women of color: Integrating ethnic and gender identities in psychotherapy* (pp. 30–71). New York: Guilford Press.

Lawson, W. B. (1996). The art and science of the psychopharmacotherapy of African Americans. *Mount Sinai Journal of Medicine, 63,* 301–305.

Lessinger, J. (1998). *From the Ganges to the Hudson: Indian immigrants in New York City.* Boston: Allyn & Bacon.

Lewis, T. H. (1975). A syndrome of depression and mutism in the Oglala Sioux. *American Journal of Psychiatry, 132*(7), 753–755.

Lin, K.-M. (1983). *Hwa-byung*: A Korean culture bound syndrome? *American Journal of Psychiatry, 140,* 105–107.

Lin, K.-M. (1996). Psychopharmacology in cross-cultural psychiatry. *Mount Sinai Journal of Medicine, 63,* 283–284.

Lin, K.-M., Anderson, D., & Poland, R. E. (1995). Ethnicity and psychopharmacology. *Psychiatric Clinics of North America, 18,* 635–647.

Lin, K.-M., Lau, J. R. C., Yamamoto, J., et al. (1992). *Hwa-byung*: A community study of Korean Americans. *Journal of Nervous and Mental Disease, 180,* 386–391.

Lin, K.-M., Poland, R. E., Fleishaker, J. C., et al. (1993a). Ethnicity and differential responses to benzodiazepines. In K.-M. Lin, R. E. Poland, & G. Nakasaki (Eds.), *Psychopharmacology and psychobiology of ethnicity* (pp. 91–105). Washington, DC: American Psychiatric Press.

Lin, K.-M., Poland, R. E., & Silver, B. (1993). Overview: The interface between psychobiology and ethnicity. In K.-M. Lin, R. E. Poland, & G. Nakasaki (Eds.), *Psychopharmacology and psychobiology of ethnicity* (pp. 11–35). Washington, DC: American Psychiatric Press.

Liu, W. T. (1986). Health services for Asian elderly. *Research on Aging, 8*(1), 156–175.

Locke, D. C. (1992). *Increasing multicultural understanding: A comprehensive model.* Newbury Park, CA: Sage.

Lopez, S. R., Grover, P., Holland, D., et al. (1989). Development of culturally sensitive psychotherapists. *Professional Psychology: Research and Practice, 20,* 369–376.

Mays, V. M., Caldwell, C. H., & Jackson, J. S. (1996). Mental health symptoms and service utilization patterns of help-seeking among African American women. In H. W. Neighbors & J. S. Jackson (Eds.), *Mental health in black America* (pp. 161–176). Thousand Oaks, CA: Sage.

Meston, C. M., Heiman, J. R., Trapnell, P. D., et al. (1999). Ethnicity, desirable responding, and self reports of abuse: A comparison of European- and Asian-ancestry undergraduates. *Journal of Consulting and Clinical Psychology, 67*(1), 139–144.

Nadelson, C. C., & Zimmerman, V. (1993). Culture and psychiatric care of women. In A. C. Gaw (Ed.), *Culture, ethnicity, and mental illness* (pp. 501–513). Washington, DC: American Psychiatric Press.

Naik, U., Menon, S., & Ahmed, S. (1998). Culture and psychiatry: An Indian overview of issues in women and children. In S. Okpaku (Ed.), *Clinical methods in transcultural psychiatry* (pp. 413–435). Washington, DC: American Psychiatric Press.

Neighbors, H. W., & Howard, C. S. (1987). Sex differences in help seeking among black Americans. *American Journal of Community Psychology, 15,* 403–415.

Olmedo, E. L., & Parron, D. L. (1981). Mental health of minority women: Some special issues. *Professional Psychology, 12,* 103–111.

Padgett, D. K., Patrick, C., Burns, B. J., et al. (1994). Women and outpatient mental health services: Use by black, Hispanic, and white women in a national insured population. *Journal of Mental Health Administration, 21*(4), 347–360.

Pang, K. Y. C. (1990). *Hwa-byung*: The construction of a Korean popular illness among Korean elderly immigrant women in the United States. *Culture, Medicine, and Psychiatry, 14,* 495–512.

Phinney, J. S. (1990). Ethnic identity in adolescents and adults: Review of the research. *Psychological Bulletin, 108,* 499–514.

Pierce, C. M. (1995). Stress analogs of racism and sexism: Terrorism, torture, and disaster. In C. Willie, P. Rieker, B. Kramer, & B. Brown (Eds.), *Mental health, racism and sexism* (pp. 277–279). Pittsburgh, PA: University of Pittsburgh Press.

Porter, R. Y. (2000). Clinical issues and intervention with ethnic minority women. In J. F. Aponte & J. Wohl (Eds.), *Psychological intervention and cultural diversity* (pp. 183–199). Boston: Allyn & Bacon.

Prince, R. (1960). The *brain fag* syndrome in Nigerian students. *Journal of Mental Science, 106,* 559–570.

Rack, P. (1982). *Race, culture and mental disorder*, New York: Tavistock.

Ruiz S., Chu, P., Sramek, J., et al. (1996). Neuroleptic dosing in Asian and Hispanic outpatients with schizophrenia. *Mount Sinai Journal of Medicine, 63,* 306–309.

Silver, B., Poland, R. E., & Lin, K.-M. (1993). Ethnicity and the pharmacology of tricyclic antidepressants. In K.-M. Lin, R. E. Poland, & G. Nakasaki (Eds.), *Psychopharmacology and psychobiology of ethnicity* (pp. 61–89). Washington, DC: American Psychiatric Press.

Simon, R. C., & Hughes, C. C. (1993). Culture bound syndromes. In A. C. Gaw (Ed.), *Culture, ethnicity and mental illness* (pp. 75–94). Washington, DC: American Psychiatric Press.

Singh, N. N. (1996). Cultural diversity in the 21st century: Beyond *E pluribus unum*. *Journal of Child and Family Studies 5,* 121–136.

Snow, L. F. (1974). Folk medicine beliefs and their implications for care of patients—A review based on studies among black Americans. *Annals of Internal Medicine, 81*(1), 82–96.

Speight, S. L., Myers, L. J., Cox, C. I., et al. (1991). A redefinition of multicultural counseling. *Journal of Counseling and Development, 70,* 29–35.

Spencer, M. B., & Markstrom-Adams, C. (1990). Identity processes among racial and ethnic minority children in America. *Child Development, 61,* 290–310.

Sramek, J. J., & Pi, E. H. (1996). Ethnicity and antidepressant response. *Mount Sinai Journal of Medicine, 63,* 320–325.

Strickland, T. L., Lawson, W. B., & Lin, K.-M. (1993). Interethnic variation in response to lithium therapy among African-American and Asian-American populations. In K.-M. Lin, R. E. Poland, & G. Nakasaki (Eds.), *Psychopharmacology and psychobiology of ethnicity* (pp. 107–123). Washington, DC: American Psychiatric Press.

Sue, D. W., Arredondo, P., & McDavis, R. J. (1992). Multicultural counseling competencies and standards: A call to the profession. *Journal of Counseling and Development, 70,* 477–486.

Sue, D. W., & Sue, D. (1990). *Counseling the culturally different: Theory and practice.* New York: Wiley.

Tanaka-Matsumi, J. (1979). *Taijin Kyofusho*: Diagnostic and cultural issues in Japanese psychiatry. *Culture, Medicine and Psychiatry, 3,* 231–245.

Thara, R., & Rajkumar, S. (1992). Gender differences in schizophrenia: Results of a follow-up study in India. *Schizophrenia Research, 7,* 65–90.

U.S. Bureau of the Census. (1990). *1990 census of the population.* Washington, DC: U.S. Government Printing Office.

U.S. Bureau of the Census. (2001). *Difference in population by race and Hispanic or Latino origin for the United States: 1990 to 2000.* http://blue.census.gov/population/cen2000/ohc-t1/tab04.pdf

Vasquez, M. J. T. (1994). Latinas. In L. Comas-Diaz & B. Greene (Eds.), *Women of color: Integrating ethnic and gender identities in psychotherapy* (pp. 114–138). New York: Guilford Press.

Weidman, H. H. (1979). *Falling out*: A diagnostic and treatment problem viewed from a transcultural perspective. *Social Science Medicine, 13B,* 95–112.

Westkott, M. (1998). Culture and women's health. In E. Blechman & K. Brownell (Eds.), *Behavioral medicine and women: A comprehensive handbook* (pp. 816–820). New York: Guilford Press.

Woodward, A. M. (1998). Hispanic women and health care. In E. Blechman & K. Brownell (Eds.), *Behavioral medicine and women: A comprehensive handbook* (pp. 833–838). New York: Guilford Press.

Yamashiro, G., & Matsuoka, J. K. (1997). Help-seeking among Asian and Pacific Americans: A multiperspective analysis. *Social Work, 42*(2), 176–186.

Yoshida, A. (1993). Genetic polymorphisms of alcohol-metabolizing enzymes related to alcohol sensitivity and alcoholic diseases. In K.-M. Lin, R. E. Poland, & G. Nakasaki (Eds.), *Psychopharmacology and psychobiology of ethnicity* (pp. 169–183). Washington, DC: American Psychiatric Press.

35

Aging and Elderly Women

SUZANNE HOLROYD

As the field of geriatric psychiatry continues to progress in its understanding of mental health and mental illness in late life, relatively little attention has been paid to gender differences in geriatric disorders. This is understandable, as the field of geriatric psychiatry is a relatively new one. Nonetheless, some gender differences have already been noted in the epidemiology, presentation, and treatment of certain disorders. Although most of these differences were found incidentally, other differences have been the focus of research—for example, the effects of estrogen on mood and cognition. The purpose of this chapter is to assemble what is currently known of such gender differences within psychiatric disorders, focusing on issues pertaining to elderly women.

Perhaps the best-known gender difference among the elderly is that women have a longer life expectancy than men do in the United States. The proportion of females to males increases with age. By age 30, females outnumber men, largely due to a higher male mortality rate (Treas, 1995). By age 65, however, the ratio increases so that for every 100 females there are only 67.8 men (U.S. Bureau of the Census, 1995). It is predicted, however, that as male deaths but not female deaths from heart disease decline, the ratio will narrow in the future (Treas, 1995). It is projected, for example, that the ratio of men to women for persons aged 65 and over by the year 2025 will be 82 men to 100 women (U.S. Bureau of the Census, 1995). This change in ratios is a reminder that gender differences are not just biological; they can also be due to social, cultural, environmental, and cohort effects. Thus speaking about differences in gender does not imply that the differences will necessarily be unchanging over time, due to innate differences in having a Y versus an X chromosome. Instead, these gender differences could change or disappear, depending on cultural, cohort, and environmental changes.

Specific psychiatric symptoms and disorders are now considered.

MOOD DISORDERS AND SUICIDE

It is widely known that clinical depression and clinically significant depressive symptoms are more prevalent among women across the lifespan, as measured by a variety of epidemiological surveys, including the National Health Examination Follow-Up Study and the Epidemiologic Catchment Area (ECA) study (Robins & Regier, 1991; Zonderman & Costa, 1991). However, this difference narrows with advancing age, and some studies actually find no statistical differences in rates of depression between elderly women and men (Blazer et al., 1987; George et al., 1988) In general, however, the difference in prevalence between elderly men and women is greater when depressive symptoms are examined than when a strict diagnosis of major depression is considered. Overall, female gender is believed to be only a weak to moderate risk factor for elderly depression (George, 1994). Whether the factors placing women at increased risk for depression lessen with age is unknown, as these factors have not been adequately identified across the lifespan. Interestingly, there are no differences in the prevalence of bipolar disorder between elderly men and women (Schneider et al., 1994).

Gender differences in the presentation of depressive symptoms in elderly persons have has not been formally studied. Clinical lore has it that delusions of poverty (delusions regarding the lack of money or clothes despite proof that there is adequate money and clothes) are more common in women, whereas delusions regarding somatic concerns and cancer are more common in men. Whether there are differences in depressive symptoms due to gender, however, is currently unknown.

Depression in the elderly can present differently than in other age groups. Such atypical depressions have been described as "masked depression," because the mood or emotion of depression may be absent. Depressed women may not recognize the feeling of depression, but may complain more of anxiety and "nerves" (Blazer et al., 1989). Somatic complaints may be common or may even be the presenting symptoms (Casper et al., 1985). Chronic abdominal distress, nonlocalized pain ("I hurt all over"), and other unresponsive pain syndromes, can all be depressive equivalents. Of course, an appropriate medical workup is required for all somatic complaints. Other symptoms that are commonly reported among depressed elderly individuals include decreased life satisfaction (seen in 92%; Beck, 1967), a sense of emptiness (Goldfarb, 1974), low self esteem or poor self-attitude (Beck, 1967), and cognition/memory problems (Sternberg & Jarvik, 1976; Miller & Lewis, 1978). Memory tests requiring more effort are most likely to be affected (Weingartner et al., 1981), and severity of depression is correlated with the cognitive impairment (Cavanaugh & Wettson, 1983).

Suicide represents an area of marked differences between genders in elderly individuals. The suicide rates for elderly persons are higher than for any other age group (Meehan et al., 1991; Mellick et al., 1992). Interestingly, there is a significant difference in suicide rates between men and women. Males aged 65 and over have markedly higher suicide rates than females, with a rate for men of 45.6 per 100,000, compared with the rate for women of 7.5 per 100,000 (Meehan et al., 1991). Within the elderly age group, differences also exist among age subgroups. The absolute highest rates are those for men aged 80–84, with a rate of 58.5 per 100,000. However, the highest rates for females are for those aged 75–79, with a rate of 7.9, then dropping after age 80 to a low of 4.7 per 100,000 in the 85-and-over age group (Meehan et al., 1991). Among women, rates also differ by race. The rate of suicide among white women aged 65 and over is 6.4 per

100,000, whereas the rate for black women is only 2.6 per 100,000 (McIntosh et al., 1997).

The most frequent method of suicide for elderly women is the use of firearms, accounting for approximately 28% of female suicides; overdose is a close second, accounting for approximately 24% of all female suicides, followed by hanging and gas inhalation (Meehan et al., 1991). This is important information, as clinicians may incorrectly minimize the risk of elderly suicide, especially in women. Clinicians need to be aware of the highly lethal methods that elderly women may use. Guns should be removed from the home environments of depressed elderly individuals.

Treatment of elderly depression specifically is just starting to receive research attention; therefore, little has been done differentiating the responses of men and women, except in the area of estrogen replacement therapy (ERT). It has been noted that estrogen has mood-improving effects in depressed women inpatients and even in nondepressed postmenopausal women (Ditkoff et al., 1991; Kantor et al., 1978; Klaiber et al., 1979). Similarly, women who receive ERT when in their 60s or older have lower rates of depressive symptoms than those not on estrogen, implying that estrogen exerts protective effects against elderly depression in women (Palinkas & Barrett-Connor, 1992).

Two recent studies have examined the effect of ERT on the response to antidepressant therapy. A study examining women 60 and over with major depression in a 6-week trial of fluoxetine versus a placebo found that women receiving ERT and fluoxetine had significantly greater improvement in their depressive symptoms as compared to ERT and placebo, whereas women receiving only fluoxetine did not show improvement as compared to women receiving only placebo (Schneider et al., 1997). Similarly, a study examining women aged 60 and over with major depression in a trial of sertraline versus a placebo found that women receiving ERT showed significantly greater improvement of depressive symptoms than those receiving sertraline without ERT (Schneider et al., 1998). The results of these studies are provocative and suggest that estrogen may augment the response of antidepressant therapy in elderly women. It should be noted, however, that estrogen use was not randomized in either of these studies, and thus estrogen use may be associated with another factor that actually influences response to antidepressant therapy. Future studies of ERT and antidepressant therapy should include randomization of both ERT and the antidepressant.

DEMENTIA

"Dementia" is a term referring to a group of disorders that cause memory loss and global cognitive decline. The most prevalent dementia in the United States is Alzheimer's disease, followed by dementia of the Lewy body type and vascular dementia. The risk for acquiring dementia increases with age, but may level off after age 95 (Ritchie & Kildea, 1995). The prevalence of dementia as recorded by the ECA study showed no gender differences (George et al., 1991). Some studies indicate no differences in the incidence of Alzheimer's disease due to gender (Paykel et al., 1994), but other research suggests that the prevalence of this disorder is higher in women (Rocca et al., 1991). The presentation of dementia is generally felt to be similar between men and women, although one study of visual hallucinations in Alzheimer's disease found that the presence of visual hallucinations was associated with female gender (Holroyd & Sheldon-Keller, 1995).

Treatment and prevention of dementia, specifically in Alzheimer's disease, have recently focused on the role of estrogen. Estrogen receptors exists in multiple brain regions, including the hypothalamus, preoptic area, anterior pituitary, and hippocampus. The exact role of these receptors and their influence on neuropsychological function are unknown (McEwen & Woolley, 1994). Estrogen may decrease the risk of dementia by a variety of mechanisms, one of which is modulation of neurotransmitters. It is known that estradiol increases choline acetyltransferase in mammals (Luine, 1985), prolongs survival of cholinergic neurons (Honjo et al., 1992), and counteracts the cognitive impairments caused by cholinergic receptor blockade by scopolamine (Dohanich et al., 1994). These data suggest that estrogen may promote cholinergic activity in the brain, thus improving cognitive function. In addition, estrogen affects other neurotransmitters via monoamine oxidase, which is also postulated to be involved in neuronal pathways for memory and learning (Yaffe et al., 1998). Estrogen has also been proposed to have a direct effect on neurons by stimulating neuronal synaptic formation in hippocampal areas (Matsumoto, 1991; McEwen & Woolley, 1994). Moreover, there is evidence that estrogen may protect against cerebral ischemia by multiple mechanisms, including vasodilation of cerebral vessels, reduction of platelet aggregation, and reduction of central arterial smooth muscle injury response (Applebaum-Bowden et al., 1989; Gangar et al., 1991; Sullivan et al., 1995). Finally, there is evidence that estrogen may modulate apolipoprotein E gene expression, which has been shown to be a major genetic risk factor for development of Alzheimer's disease. Theoretically, this modulation could reduce the risk of Alzheimer's disease (Honjo et al., 1995; Srivastava et al., 1996).

A meta-analysis of studies examining the effect of postmenopausal estrogen on the risk of developing dementia demonstrated a 29% decreased risk among estrogen users (Yaffe et al., 1998). However many of the studies had significant methodological problems, and there were even conflicting results between studies. Large placebo controlled trials are clearly needed to further assess the role of estrogen in the prevention of dementia. Several large-scale studies are now in progress (Women's Health Initiative Memory Study, Women's International Study of Long Duration Oestrogen after Menopause, Preventing Postmenopausal Memory Loss and the Alzheimer's with Replacement Estrogens Study) and their results will provide much needed data in the primary prevention of Alzheimer's disease (Hendrie, 1998; Shaywitz et al., 2000).

In addition, several initial small studies of estrogen use in those with diagnosed Alzheimer's disease have yielded initial positive results of improvement in various dementia scales. However, a recent 12-month, randomized, double-blind, placebo-controlled study of 120 women with mild to moderate Alzheimer's disease, who were posthysterectomy, receiving ERT for 1 year, revealed no slowing of disease progression, nor did it improve cognitive or functional outcomes (Mulnard et al., 2000). These negative results were supported in another recent study as well (Henderson et al., 2000). At present then, ERT cannot be recommended as a potential treatment for dementia, but the possibility remains it may have a role in primary prevention of dementia in women.

PSYCHOSIS

Psychosis occurs in a variety of disorders, including schizophrenia, mood disorders, dementia, and delirium. Interestingly, it appears that female gender may be associated with higher rates of psychosis in the elderly population. An examination of the occurrence of hallucinations in the ECA study, which included 15,258 community-dwelling individuals, revealed that the incidence of visual hallucinations was slightly higher in males from ages 18 to 80 (20 per 1,000 per year for men, 13 per 1,000 per year for women); however, after age 80 the rate for females increased to a much higher level than that for men, to 40 per 1,000 per year (Tien, 1991). Similarly, elderly females were found to have higher rates of auditory, somatic, and olfactory hallucinations than males in the ECA study. Rates of hallucinations increased with aging for both men and women, and may be attributable to changes in the brain due to medical conditions associated with aging. It has already been noted that females are more likely than males to have visual hallucinations in Alzheimer's disease (Holroyd & Sheldon-Keller, 1995).

Late-onset schizophrenia is a disorder of late life characterized by bizarre delusions, often of a paranoid flavor, as well as by visual, tactile, olfactory, and auditory hallucinations (Pearlson et al., 1989). Late-onset schizophrenia has been found to be more common in females than in males (Grahame, 1984; Marneros & Deister, 1984; Rabins et al., 1984). Most studies show that 2 to 10 times more women than men develop this disorder (Jeste et al., 1991).

In addition, delusions are more common in women who have late-onset depression than in men, as revealed in a retrospective review of depressed inpatients (Meyers & Greenberg, 1986). Finally, a study of elderly patients with delusional parasitosis revealed that the typical patient was a female (Raesaenen et al., 1998).

The reasons for the higher rates of psychosis in elderly females than in elderly males are unknown. Proposed theories include gender differences in recall and reporting of such symptoms, gender-specific cultural differences, and biological differences associated with the aging process.

SUBSTANCE USE DISORDERS

Overall, little is currently known about substance use disorders in elderly persons (Abrams & Alexopoulos, 1987; Curtis et al., 1989; Johnson, 1989; Szwabo, 1993). Even less is known about substance use among elderly women. The ECA study revealed that women aged 65 and older had a rate of alcohol dependence of 1.5%, compared to 14% among men (Robins et al., 1988). The rate of alcohol dependence falls with advancing age. A study of elderly community-dwelling persons in the rural South revealed that over 20% had an alcohol use disorder and that half of these subjects were women. This study noted the difficulty in making an accurate diagnosis on initial interview without the use of outside informants and an ongoing relationship with the patients (Holroyd et al., 1997). Thus the prevalence of alcohol dependence in elderly women (and men) is most likely underestimated by large epidemiological studies.

A study of benzodiazepine use in an elderly community sample revealed that the prevalence of benzodiazepine use in women was twice that of men, and the use of other hypnotics was also higher in women (Taylor et al., 1998). As well, a study of substance use in a geriatric psychiatry clinic revealed that greater numbers of women than men had diagnoses of alcohol dependence and benzodiazepine dependence (Holroyd & Duryee, 1997). Over 87.5% of the patients with benzodiazepine dependence were women, while 58.3% of those with alcohol dependence were women. These data suggest that elderly women do suffer from substance use disorders and that the rates may be greater in clinic settings. In general, much more needs to be known about the use of substances in the elderly population. Future studies need to address the methodological difficulties in diagnosing these disorders via one-time interviews and surveys.

ANXIETY DISORDERS

Anxiety disorders usually have their onset in younger life and demonstrate a lower prevalence with aging, as demonstrated in large epidemiological studies (Regier et al., 1988). Gender differences do exist among anxiety disorders in the elderly population. Women were more likely to have an anxiety disorder in the ECA study: They had a rate of 6.8% overall, with 6.1% for phobias, 0.9% for obsessive–compulsive disorder, and 0.2% for panic disorder, whereas the rates for men were 3.6% overall, 2.9% for phobias, 0.7% for obsessive–compulsive disorder, and 0.0% for panic disorder (Regier et al., 1988). A review of eight random-sample community surveys of anxiety disorders in persons aged 60 and over suggests that agoraphobia and possibly obsessive–compulsive disorder may occur as a primary disorder for the first time in late life (Flint, 1994). Although future research is clearly needed, serious problems exist in studying anxiety in elderly persons, given the considerable overlap of depression and anxiety in the elderly population.

PERSONALITY DISORDERS

As with many psychiatric disorders, little is known about personality disorders in the elderly population, and even less is known about potential gender differences. There are many conceptual difficulties in diagnosing personality disorders in elderly individuals, including the potential age bias of diagnostic criteria, as well as the difficulty in assessing lifetime personality traits (Holroyd, 1994). The prevalence of personality disorders appears to decrease in late life, though the reasons unclear. Theories include early death of those with such disorders, maturity with aging, and diagnostic issues. The ECA study revealed that persons aged 55 and over had significantly lower rates of personality disorders than those under age 55 (10.5% vs. 6.6%). This decrease was due almost entirely to a decrease in Cluster B personality diagnoses, including antisocial, borderline, and histrionic personality disorders (Cohen et al., 1994). Although there is a reported gender difference in histrionic personality disorder, with a decline in this disorder in older men but not in older women (Nestadt et al., 1990), a meta-analysis of studies to date reveals no gender differences in diagnosed personality disorders in late life (Abrams & Horowitz, 1996).

CONCLUSIONS

Clearly, much needs to be learned about psychiatric disorders in elderly individuals, especially about gender-specific differences; however, some preliminary conclusions can be stated. Although there are minimal differences in the epidemiology of depression between elderly men and women, women have markedly lower suicide rates. ERT is promising in the prevention and treatment of depression and possibly the prevention of dementia in elderly women, although definitive studies are still needed. Women may be more prone to psychosis in late life, although the reasons are not clearly understood. The rates of substance use disorders are reported to be relatively low for elderly females, but the diagnoses of these disorders are likely to be underestimated. Much more research is needed in the areas of anxiety disorders and personality disorders in elderly women, as little exists other than large epidemiological research studies. As the field of geriatric psychiatry expands and enlarges its knowledge base, information will increase regarding psychiatric disorders specific to elderly women.

REFERENCES

Abrams, R. C., & Alexopoulous, G. S. (1987). Substance abuse in the elderly: Alcohol and prescription drugs. *Hospital and Community Psychiatry, 38,* 1285–1287.

Abrams, R. C., & Horowitz, S. V. (1996). Personality disorders after age 50: A meta-analysis. *Journal of Personality Disorders, 10,* 271–281.

Applebaum-Bowden, D., McLean, P., Steinmetz, A., et al. (1989). Lipoprotein, apolipoprotein, and lipolytic enzyme changes following estrogen administration in postmenopausal women. *Journal of Lipid Research, 30,* 1895–1906.

Beck, A. T. (1967). *Depression: Causes and treatment.* Philadelphia: University of Pennsylvania Press.

Blazer, D. G., Hughes, D. C., & Fowler, N. (1989). Anxiety as an outcome symptom of depression in elderly and middle-aged adults. *International Journal of Geriatric Psychiatry, 4,* 273–278.

Blazer, D. G., Hughes, D. C., & George, L. K. (1987). The epidemiology of depression in an elderly community population. *Gerontologist, 27,* 281–287.

Casper, R. C., Redmond, E., Katz, M. M., et al. (1985). Somatic symptoms in primary affective disorder: Presence and relationship to the classification of depression. *Archives of General Psychiatry, 42,* 1098–1104.

Cavanaugh, S. V. A., & Wettson, R. (1983). The relationship between severity of depression, cognitive dysfunction and age in medical inpatients. *American Journal of Psychiatry, 140,* 495–496.

Cohen, B. J., Nestadt, G., Samuels, J. F., et al. (1994). Personality disorders in later life: A community study. *British Journal of Psychiatry, 165,* 493–499.

Curtis, J. R., Gellar, F., Stokes, E. S., et al. (1989). Characteristics, diagnosis and treatment of alcoholism in elderly patients. *Journal of the American Geriatrics Society, 37,* 310–316.

Ditkoff, E. C., Crary, W. G., Cristo, M., et al. (1991). Estrogen improves psychological function in asymptomatic postmenopausal women. *Obstetrics and Gynecology, 78,* 991–995.

Dohanich, G. P., Fader, A. J., & Javorsky, D. J. (1994). Estrogen and estrogen-progesterone treatments counteract the effect of scopolamine on reinforced T maze alteration in female rats. *Behavorial Neuroscience, 108,* 988–992.

Flint, A. J. (1994). Epidemiology and comorbidity of anxiety in the elderly. *American Journal of Psychiatry, 151,* 640–649.

Gangar, K. E., Vyas, S., Whitehead, M., et al. (1991). Pulsatility index in internal carotid artery in relation to transdermal oestradiol and time since menopause. *Lancet, 338,* 839–842.

George, L. K. (1994). Social factors and depression in late life. In L. S. Schneider, C. F. Reynolds, B. D. Lebowitz, et al. (Eds.), *Diagnosis and treatment of depression in late life* (pp. 131–153). Washington, DC: American Psychiatric Press.

George, L. K., Blazer, D. G., & Winfield-Larid, I. (1988). Psychiatric disorders and mental health services use in late life: Evidence from the Epidemiologic Catchment Area program. In J. Brady & G. L. Maddox (Eds.), *Epidemiology and aging* (pp. 189–219). New York: Springer.

George, L. K., Landerman, R., Blazer, D. G., et al. (1991). Cognitive impairment. In L. N. Robins & D. A. Regier (Eds.), *Psychiatric disorders in America* (pp. 291–327). New York: Free Press.

Goldfarb, A. I. (1974). Masked depression in the elderly. In G. L. Lesse (Ed.), *Masked depression* (pp. 236–249). New York, Jason Aronson.

Grahame, P. S. (1984). Schizophrenia in old age (late paraphrenia). *British Journal of Psychiatry, 145,* 493–495.

Henderson, V. N., Paganini-Hill, A., Miller, B. L., et al. (2000). Estrogen for Alzheimer's disease in women: Randomized, double-blind, placebo-controlled trial. *Neurology, 54,* 295–301.

Hendrie, H. C. (1998). Epidemiology of dementia and Alzheimer's disease. *American Journal of Geriatric Psychiatry, 6,* S3–18.

Holroyd, S. (1994). Personality disorders. In W. R. Hazzard, E. L. Bierman, J. P. Blass, et al. (Eds.), *Principles of geriatric medicine and gerontology* (pp. 1131–1136). New York: McGraw-Hill.

Holroyd, S., Currie, L., Thompson-Heisterman, et al. (1997). A descriptive study of elderly community dwelling alcoholic patients in the rural South. *American Journal of Geriatric Psychiatry, 5,* 221–228.

Holroyd, S., & Duryee, J. J. (1997). Substance use disorders in a geriatric psychiatry outpatient clinic: Prevalence and epidemiologic characteristics. *Journal of Nervous and Mental Disease, 185,* 627–632.

Holroyd, S., & Sheldon-Keller, A. (1995). A study of visual hallucinations in Alzheimer's disease. *American Journal of Geriatric Psychiatry, 3,* 198–205.

Honjo, H., Tamura, T., & Matsumuto, Y. (1992). Estrogen as a growth factor to central nervous cells: Estrogen treatment promotes development of acetyl-cholinesterase-positive basal forebrain neurons transplanted in the anterior eye chamber. *Journal of Steroid Biochemistry and Molecular Biology, 41,* 633–635.

Honjo, H., Tanaka, K., Kashlwagi, T. L., et al. (1995). Senile dementia—Alzheimer's type and estrogen. *Hormone and Metabolic Research, 27,* 204–207.

Jeste, D. J., Manley, M., & Harris, M. J. (1991). Psychoses. In J. Sadavoy, L. W. Lazarus, & L. F. Jarvik (Eds.), *Comprehensive review of geriatric psychiatry* (pp. 353–368) Washington, DC: American Psychiatric Press.

Johnson, L. K. (1989). How to diagnose and treat chemical dependency in the elderly. *Journal of Gerontologic Nursing, 15,* 22–26.

Kantor, H. I., Milton, L. J., & Ernst, M. L. (1978). Comparative psychologic effects of estrogen administration on institutional and non-institutional elderly women. *Journal of the American Geriatrics Society, 26,* 9–16.

Klaiber, E. L., Braverman, D. M., Vogel, W., et al. (1979). Estrogen therapy for severe, persistent depressions in women. *Archives of General Psychiatry, 36,* 550–554.

Luine, V. N. (1985) Estradiol increases choline acetyl transferase activity in specific basal forebrain nuclei and projection areas of female rats. *Experimental Neurology, 89,* 484–490.

Marneros, A., & Deister, A. (1984). The psychopathology of "late schizophrenia." *Psychopathology, 17,* 264–274.

Matsumoto, A. (1991). Synaptic action of sex steroids in developing and adult neuroendocrine brain. *Psychoneuroendocrinology, 16,* 25–40.

McEwen, B. S., & Woolley, C. S. (1994). Estradiol and progesterone regulate neuronal structure and synaptic connectivity in adult as well as developing brain. *Experimental Gerontology, 29,* 431–436.

McIntosh, J. L., Pearson, J. L., & Lebowitz, B. D. (1997). Mental disorders of elderly men. In J. I. Kosberg & L. W. Kaye (Eds.), *Elderly men* (pp. 193–215). New York, Springer.

Meehan, P. J., Saltzman, L. E., & Sattin, R. W. (1991). Suicides among older U.S. residents: Epidemiologic characteristics and trends. *American Journal of Public Health, 81,* 1198–1200.

Mellick, E., Buckwalter, K. C., & Stolley, J. M. (1992). Suicide among elderly white men: Development of a profile. *Journal of Psychological Nursing, 30,* 29–37.

Meyers, B. S., & Greenberg, R. (1986). Late-life delusional depression. *Journal of Affective Disorders, 11,* 133–137.

Miller, E., & Lewis, P. (1978). Recognition memory in elderly patients with depression and dementia: A signal detection analysis. *Journal of Abnormal Psychology, 86,* 84–86.

Molnard, R. A., Cotman, C. W., Kawas, C., et al. (2000). Estrogen replacement therapy for treatment of mild to moderate Alzheimer's disease: A randomized and controlled trial. Alzheimer's Disease Cooperative Study. *Journal of the American Medical Association, 283,* 1007–1015.

Nestadt, G., Romanoski, A. J., Chahal, R., et al. (1990). An epidemiologic study of histronic personality disorder. *Psychological Medicine, 20,* 413–422.

Palinkas, L. A., & Bassett-Connor, E. V. (1992). Estrogen use and depressive symptoms in postmenopausal women. *Obstetrics and Gynecology, 80,* 30–36.

Paykel, E. S., Brayne, C., Huppert, F. A., et al. (1994). Incidence of dementia in a population older than 75 years in the United Kingdom. *Archives of General Psychiatry, 51,* 325–332.

Pearlson, S. P., Kreger, L., Rabins, P. V., et al. (1989). A chart review study of late-onset and early-onset schizophrenia. *American Journal of Psychiatry, 149,* 1568–1574.

Rabins, P. V., Pauker, S., & Thomas, J. (1984). Can schizophrenia begin after age 44? *Comprehensive Psychiatry, 25,* 290–295.

Raesaenen, P., Erkonen, K., Isaksson, U., et al. (1998). Delusional parasitosis in the elderly: A review and report of six cases from northern Finland. *International Psychogeriatrics, 9,* 459–464.

Regier, D. A., Boyd, J. H., Burke, J. D., et al. (1988). One-month prevalence of mental disorders in the United States. *Archives of General Psychiatry, 45,* 977–986.

Ritchie, K., & Kildea, D. (1995). Is senile dementia age-related or ageing-related?: Evidence from meta-analysis of dementia prevalence in the oldest old. *Lancet, 346,* 931–934.

Robins, L. N., Helzer, J. E., & Przybeck, T. R. (1988). Alcohol disorders in the community: A report from the Epidemiologic Catchment Area. In R. Rose & J. Barret (Eds.), *Alcoholism: Origins and outcome* (pp. 15–29). New York: Raven Press.

Robins, L. N., & Regier, D. A. (Eds.). (1991). *Psychiatric disorders in America.* New York: Free Press.

Rocca, W. A., Hoffman, A., Brayne, C., et al. (1991). Frequency and distribution of Alzheimer's disease in Europe: A collaborative study of 1980–1990 prevalence findings. *Annals of Neurology, 30,* 381–390.

Schneider, L. S., Reynolds, C. F., Lebowitz, B. D., et al. (Eds.). (1994). *Diagnosis and treatment of depression in late life.* Washington, DC: American Psychiatric Press.

Schneider, L. S., Small, G. W., & Clary, C. (1998). ERT status and antidepressant response to sertraline. *American Psychiatric Association New Research Program and Abstracts, NR426,* 182.

Schneider, L. S., Small, G. W., Hamilton, S. H., et al. (1997). Estrogen replacement and response to fluoxetine in a multicenter geriatric depression trial: The Fluoxetine Collaborative Study Group. *American Journal of Geriatric Psychiatry, 5,* 97–106.

Shaywitz, B. A., & Shaywitz, S. E. (2000). Estrogen and Alzheimer's disease: Plausible theory, negative clinical trial [editorial comment]. *Journal of the American Medical Association, 283,* 1055–1056.

Srivastava, R. A., Bhasin, N., & Srivastava, N. (1996). Apolipoprotein E gene expression in various tissues of mouse and regulation by estrogen. *Biochemistry and Molecular Biology International, 38,* 91–101

Sternberg, D. F., & Jarvik, M. E. (1976). Memory functions in depression. *Archives of General Psychiatry, 33,* 219–227.

Sullivan, T. J., Karas, R. H., Aronovitz, M., et al. (1995). Estrogen inhibits response-to-injury in a mouse carotid artery model. *Journal of Clinical Investigation, 96,* 2482–2488.

Szwabo, P. A. (1993). Substance abuse in older women. *Clinics in Geriatric Medicine, 9,* 197–208.

Taylor, S., McCracken, C. F., Wilson, K. C., et al. (1998). Extent and appropriateness of benzodiazepine use: Results from an elderly urban community. *British Journal of Psychiatry, 173*, 433–438.

Tien, A. Y. (1991). Distribution of hallucinations in the population. *Social Psychiatry and Psychiatric Epidemiology, 26*, 287–292.

Treas, J. (1995). Older Americans in the 1990's and beyond. *Population Bulletin, 50*, 1–46.

U.S. Bureau of the Census. (1995). *Statistical abstract of the United States, 1994*. Washington, DC: U.S. Government Printing Office.

Weingartner, H., Cohen, R. M., Murphy, D. L., et al. (1981). Cognitive process in depression. *Archives of General Psychiatry, 38*, 42–47.

Yaffe, K., Sawaya, G., Lieberburg, I., et al. (1998). Estrogen therapy in postmenopausal women. *Journal of the American Medical Association, 279*, 688–696.

Zonderman, A. B., & Costa, P. T. (1991). *The absence of increased levels of depression in older adults: Evidence from a national representative study*. Abstract, American Psychological Association, San Francisco.

Part V

Research and Health Policy Issues

36

Women and Mental Health Research Methodology

RUTH B. MERKATZ
CATHRYN M. CLARY
WILMA HARRISON

And the end of all our exploring
Will be to arrive where we started
And know the place for the first time.
—T. S. ELIOT, *Four Quartets*

In the past decade, pharmaceutical companies have eclipsed the National Institute of Mental Health to become the foremost funding source for mental health research. This has led to an explosion in drug treatment studies. Clinical drug trials now constitute the single biggest category of research in the mental health field, and sit at the nexus where research, commercial, regulatory, and public health interests converge. Because of their predominance, this chapter uses these trials as a convenient lens to bring some of the key issues of sex, gender and mental health research into focus.

As the previous chapters in this book have summarized in rich detail, there is no aspect of mental health in which the issues of sex and gender can safely be ignored. Several milestones in two federal agencies during the past decade reflect a growing recognition of the importance of gender. First, the Office of Research on Women's Health was established in 1990 at the National Institutes of Health (NIH), in response to concerns that women's health had been inadequately addressed as a matter of public health. This was followed by the NIH Revitalization Act of 1993, which mandated, among other requirements, proportional inclusion of women in all federally supported research. Second, the U.S. Food and Drug Administration (FDA) in 1993 reversed a long-standing policy that had virtually banned participation of women with childbearing potential from early phases of clinical trials, and issued a guideline and subsequent regulation making clear its position that women should be included in all phases of clinical drug development ("FDA Guideline . . . ," 1993; "FDA Final Rule," 1998, 2000).

In the aftermath of these initiatives, progress has certainly been made with regard to including women in research, but a recent General Accounting Office (2000) report has noted that "less progress has been made by the NIH implementing the requirement that phase III clinical trials be designed and carried out to permit the analysis of whether interventions affect women and men differently" (p. 7). We would agree; especially when it comes to psychiatric illness, where women so frequently predominate, more could be done in the design and analysis of clinical trials to improve understanding of sex and gender effects on differential clinical presentations, morbidity risk, and response trajectories. In this chapter, we attempt to provide a conceptual framework for thinking about mental health treatment research as it relates to women, and propose some tentative guidelines to assist in clinical trial design and data analysis.

We approach the topic of research and women from two vantage points: first, by highlighting how clinical trial methodology is strengthened by taking account of potential sex and gender effects in all phases of study design and implementation; and second, by summarizing the preclinical and clinical "topics" in psychopharmacology research that appear to require independent evaluation in women. These "topics" include the pharmacokinetic and pharmacodynamic properties of a drug, and sex-specific life cycle issues with a potential impact on efficacy and tolerability, such as pregnancy, nursing, menstrual cycle phase, and menopause. Given space limitations, the current chapter does not provide a systematic review. Instead, it highlights some of the key issues and principles, and provides examples that illustrate some of the more important points.

In this chapter, we use the term "sex" when referring to the neurobiological correlates of female–male differences, and "gender" when referring to the psychosocial correlates of these differences. This distinction is especially crucial when it comes to analyzing the impact of treatment on women versus men. In fact, one of the principles we attempt to establish is that studies should be designed in such a way as to reasonably permit one to identify whether treatment differences are due to sex or gender effects.

SEX/GENDER: METHODOLOGICAL ISSUES IN CLINICAL TRIALS

To conduct a treatment study, the investigators have to recruit appropriate patients, use valid and reliable diagnostic methods to confirm that they suffer from the illness under study, use valid and reliable measures to assess the severity of their illness, and implement a study design that will permit the investigators to evaluate clinical improvement, as well as the degree to which improvement can be specifically attributed to the drug under study and not to other, nonspecific factors. As we briefly summarize, every step in this process is potentially influenced by sex or gender.

Patient Recruitment

The generalizability of the results of treatment studies depends on how *representative* the sample of patients under study is when compared to patients with the same disorder, both in the community and in typical treatment settings (e.g., outpatient primary care). Beginning in 1977, FDA guidelines had effectively excluded women of childbearing potential from the early phases of clinical trials. In 1993, the FDA issued a revised "FDA Guideline for the Study and Evaluation of Clinical Differences in the Clinical Evaluation of Drugs," which called for a "reasonable" number of women to be included in clinical trials. This guideline, which was later codified through regulations ("FDA Final Rule," 1998, 2000), reversed the 1977 policy and made it clear that representative inclusion of women in clinical trials, even in the earliest phases of drug development, was a necessary goal (Merkatz et al., 1993). More ambitiously, the guideline emphasized the need to assess sex differences in pharmacokinetic parameters. Furthermore, it called for pharmacodynamic studies to assess the body's response to a given concentration of drug when efficacy, rates of adverse events, and dose–response effects differ by gender. In one stroke, the 1993 guideline pushed issues of sex and gender toward the center of drug development. The FDA guideline—together with the NIH Revitalization Act of 1993, which required evidence of efforts to ensure gender representativeness in both treatment and pathophysiology research—effectively established a benchmark for ensuring the representative inclusion of women in all phases of research. Its effect, beyond that, was more mixed. As we discuss in subsequent sections, the FDA guideline is *proactive* in terms of studying sex differences in pharmacokinetic parameters, but is *reactive* when it comes to studying sex differences in pharmacodynamic issues (i.e., it calls for study only if gross differences in efficacy and/ or tolerability have previously been identified). As a consequence, substantially more progress has been made in evaluating sex differences in pharmacokinetic than in pharmacodynamic properties of drugs.

Although representativeness of study samples is guaranteed by public policy in a *global* way, the devil, as the saying goes, is in the details. As previous chapters have summarized, females differ substantially from males in the age of onset, course of illness characteristics, clinical presentation, and comorbidity rates for many Axis I psychiatric disorders. It is also known that there are significant differences between females and males in the community in rates of medical help seeking (Leaf et al., 1985; Wells et al., 1986; Lin et al., 1996). Not well established, though, is the extent to which this difference is due to illness-related variables such as severity, comorbidity, or disability, or to illness-independent differences related to gender that influence willingness to seek medical help. Also, almost no information is available about the impact of gender on recruitment rates into studies—from initial contact, to attendance at a screening appointment, to willingness to give informed consent, to actual random assignment to a study drug. There is growing evidence that psychopharmacology research "pulls" a somewhat different type of patient than community treatment does (Aronson, 1987; Mohr & Czobor, 2000; Patten, 2000; Robinson et al., 1996; Stack et al., 1995; Sullivan & Joyce, 1994; Thompson et al., 1994; Amori & Lenox, 1989). Some of these studies specifically identify gender as one of the significant variables that exhibits bias (Robinson et al., 1996; Sullivan & Joyce, 1994). It should be noted that an attrition rate of more than 70% occurs from the earliest stages of patient inquiry and contact at a research center through to actual randomization. Yet the extent to which bias is introduced, and whether there are female–male differences in prestudy attrition, are unknown. Research on who gets into a study and why is the terra incognita of psychopharmacology research, and gender is one of the least understood factors in this recruitment process.

Study Entry

All treatment research depends on the identification of a small sample of patients in whom a valid and reliable diagnosis can be made of the illness under study. To accomplish this, studies typically require at least a clinical interview performed by an expert clinician, using a checklist of diagnostic criteria based on the *Diagnostic and Statistical Manual of Mental Disorders* (DSM). Frequently a structured interview is required. Furthermore, strict inclusion and exclusion criteria are employed to exclude other diagnoses or medical conditions that might interfere with interpreting the results of the study. Finally, a minimal level of symptom severity is typically required in order to ensure that a treatment effect can be observed.

It is well established that females exhibit higher prevalence rates and rates of comorbidity than males for many DSM Axis I illnesses, such as the majority of mood and anxiety disorders (Kessler et al., 1994; Maser & Cloninger, 1990). It has also been established (though there is less available research) that females and males differ in clinical presentation, as well as in the pattern and severity of symptoms (Leibenluft, 1996; Susser & Wanderling, 1994; Faraone et al., 1994; Häfner et al., 1994). Finally, course of illness can vary substantially for females versus males with respect to various Axis I disorders (Szymanski et al., 1995; Leibenluft, 1996; Leung & Chue, 2000). For example, women tend to have a later onset of illness in schizophrenia and frequently have a better treatment response (Leung & Chue, 2000), though they also have a differentially higher risk of developing tardive dyskinesia (Jeste & Caligiuri, 1993). In contrast, the poor-prognosis rapid-cycling subtype of bipolar disorder is more common in women (Leibenluft, 1996).

Study inclusion criteria frequently require patients to meet a minimum level of illness severity, typically based on the score achieved on one of the primary outcome measures—for example, the Hamilton Depression Rating Scale (HAM-D), the Hamilton Anxiety Rating Scale (HAM-A), or the Positive and Negative Syndrome Scale (PANSS). Study exclusion criteria frequently exclude patients based on the presence of various illness parameters (Axis I comorbidity, current or recent substance abuse or dependence, use of specific concomitant medications, etc.).

The value of these inclusion and exclusion criteria is that they define a relatively homogeneous patient sample that will permit inferences about drug efficacy to be made with greater confidence. If a patient sample is excessively heterogeneous, then it is impossible to determine, unless prohibitively large sample sizes are employed, whether clinical improvement is due to the study drug or to some other clinical or demographic variable that predisposes to response or nonresponse. The potential drawback of inclusion–exclusion criteria is that they may bias recruitment and yield a nonrepresentative patient sample. The consequence is that study results generalize only imperfectly to the "real world" of clinical practice.

Whether and how study entry criteria might lead to systematic bias in terms of female versus male study enrollment is not known. If women have greater comorbidity, or higher medical help seeking resulting in higher utilization of medications, then entry criteria designed to exclude patients on this basis will introduce a gender bias. It should be noted that the effect may not be manifested only in terms of crude proportions of males versus females. Instead, it may create a sieve effect, resulting in a study sample whose clinical characteristics differ considerably from female patients in the community; more importantly, the size of the "gap" between study sample and community sample may be different for females versus males.

In terms of symptom severity criteria, as we discuss in a subsequent section, traditional outcome measures may give disproportionate weight to certain illness features that may be more common in females than in males, or vice versa. For example, the HAM-A appears to provide much more weight to symptoms of somatic anxiety than of psychic anxiety. Similarly, the standard HAM-D seems disproportionately weighted toward insomnia and anxiety items; it also rates anorexia, while ignoring overeating. Insofar as there are sex differences in the clinical presentation of anxiety and depression, these differences in scales used to establish illness severity for study entry may also introduce a sex bias in study enrollment. For example, women may present more often than men with "atypical" depressive symptoms, such as hypersomnia and hyperphagia (Young et al., 1990; Kornstein et al., 2000). This may result in fewer women with these symptoms meeting entry criteria.

Efficacy of Study Treatment

In addition to potential effects on the recruitment process and study entry, sex and/or gender may influence the efficacy results of study treatment through at least three potential mechanisms, none of which are well studied.

The first potential mechanism consists of demographic and clinical variables, the incidence of which differs in females versus males, and which constitute prescriptive and/or prognostic predictors of differential response to treatment. "Prognostic" variables are variables that predict an overall tendency to improve or not to improve, regardless of the treatment employed. Positive symptoms of schizophrenia constitute a favorable prognostic variable, as does shorter illness duration for many mood and anxiety disorders. "Prescriptive" variables are variables that predict a *differential* tendency for an illness to respond to one class of medication over another class. For example, "atypical" depressive symptoms (e.g., oversleeping and overeating instead of insomnia and anorexia) are prescriptive predictors of more favorable response to monoamine oxidase (MAO) inhibitor antidepressants than to tricyclic antidepressants (Quitkin et al., 1993; Sotsky & Simmens, 1999).

Examples of clinical variables that have higher incidence in females *and* that may be predictors of outcome or response include comorbidity (higher rates of comorbidity are frequently associated with lower response; Schiebe & Albus, 1997; Roy-Byrne & Cowley, 1994–1995; Cowley et al., 1996), course-of-illness characteristics (e.g., rapid cycling in bipolar disorder; Kilzieh & Akiskal, 1999), and illness subtype. For example, agoraphobia in panic disorder is associated with a poorer prognosis (Slaap et al., 1995; Pollack et al., 1994) and may be a prescriptive predictor of more favorable response to antidepressants than to high potency benzodiazepines. Negative symptoms in schizophrenia have been shown in some studies (Kinon et al., 1993), but not all (Robinson et al., 1999), to be associated with a poorer response to neuroleptics.

A second putative mechanism that may influence the outcome of clinical trials is the potential for differential susceptibility to nonspecific therapeutic effects, such as expectancy effects, need for social approval, and therapeutic alliance effects or supportive variables. Nonspecific effects may contribute to elevated placebo response rates, which range on average between 25% and 40% for most Axis I disorders. Some variables that have been suggested as predictors of placebo response, such as need for social approval, are significantly higher in females than in males (Pervin et al., 1998). To date, though, sex differences in placebo response rates have not been consistently identified in the treatment of most Axis I disorders. Still, it is possible that gender-related predictor variables may be operating, but identifying them would require analysis (using regression techniques) and large, well-characterized samples.

A third mechanism through which sex may exert a differential influence on clinical response is how the drug itself acts on females versus males. The potential reasons for such differential drug action are enumerated below; they include sex-related differences in drug pharmacokinetics, pharmacodynamics, and behavioral pharmacology, as well as menstrual-hormonal and life cycle issues such as pregnancy, postpartum, and menopause. We briefly review methodological issues that relate to drug pharmacokinetics and pharmacodynamics before turning to life cycle issues.

PSYCHOPHARMACOLOGY "TOPICS" REQUIRING SPECIFIC EVALUATION IN WOMEN

Sex and Drug Effects

Pharmacokinetic Effects

Pharmacokinetics is one area in which enormous progress has been made in the past 20 years. As detailed by Brawman-Mintzer and Book in Chapter 2 of this volume, sex differences in pharmacokinetic parameters have been identified for many drugs. Partly in response to FDA requirements, pharmacokinetic evaluation by sex has become a standard expectation in new drug development, including evaluation of such parameters as bioavailability, maximal concentration of drug (Cmax), time to maximal concentration (Tmax), and elimination half-life (Harris et al., 1995). Significant sex-differences have been identified for multiple drugs in rates of absorption, first-pass elimination, protein binding, volume of distribution, and drug metabolism. It should be noted that sex-specific differences have frequently been reported preclinically for substrates of different cytochrome P450 (CYP450) enzymes; yet these differences often are not observable clinically, most likely because sex-specific differences are masked by interindividual variability in CYP450 enzyme activity. Perhaps the most common and clinically relevant sex-specific pharmacokinetic effect relates to potential drug–drug interactions. However, evaluation of drug interaction effects with female-specific medications such as oral contraceptives and estrogen is still not a standard practice in drug development.

Regarding sex-specific pharmacokinetic effects, several points are important to remember. First, drugs within a specific *pharmacodynamic* class, such as selective serotonin reuptake inhibitor (SSRI) antidepressants, benzodiazepines, triptans, or atypical neuroleptics, may behave quite differently from a *pharmacokinetic* standpoint. Second, there may be significant sex-specific differences in pharmacokinetic parameters in elderly individuals and members of various ethnic groups. The possibilities for sex–age and sex–ethnicity interactions are two of the least well-studied topics in the pharmacokinetics of psychotropic drugs.

Of course, for many psychiatric drugs there appears to be only a loose correlation between efficacy or adverse events and plasma level, so the actual clinical significance of pharmacokinetic changes is at this point largely speculative. They will unfortunately remain speculative if the clinical relevance of sex-specific pharmacokinetic effects is never systematically examined. The dearth of useful sex-specific pharmacokinetic data is especially notable in regard to long-term use of psychotropic medications. Although maintenance therapy is a frequent treatment recommendation in the majority of Axis I psychiatric disorders, almost nothing is known about fluctuations in pharmacokinetics during long-term treatment, or the clinical implications in terms of safety and efficacy of these potential changes. Points of concern include induction of CYP450 enzymes that might lead to reduced plasma levels, resulting in illness exacerbation or relapse; increased potential for drug–drug interactions with long-term therapy; and weight gain.

At the other end of the treatment spectrum, at the time of treatment initiation, little is known about sex differences in optimal starting doses of a drug or in rates of titration. This may be especially relevant for drugs that have a relatively narrow therapeutic range or window, or drugs associated with a high level of early side effects to which tolerance eventually develops. At this point, with minor adjustments based on body weight, the operant treatment philosophy is "one size fits all." And yet adverse event rates (see subsequent section) are by far the highest in the first few weeks of treatment, as are rates of drug discontinuation. Virtually no published literature has systematically examined whether there are sex-specific differences in optimal starting dose or titration rates, or whether tolerability or efficacy varies based on the time point in the menstrual cycle at which treatment is initiated.

Finally, pharmacokinetic parameters are rarely evaluated at different points in the menstrual cycle, though there is evidence for menstrual-cycle-related differences in drug absorption, protein binding, and CYP450 activity (Tanaka et al., 1999).

Pharmacodynamic Effects and Behavioral Pharmacology

It is self-evident that all central nervous system (CNS) drugs achieve their therapeutic efficacy by acting at some CNS site, either directly or indirectly. Drugs may be receptor agonists or antagonists (partial or full), such as the benzodiazepines, the triptans, or the typical or atypical neuroleptics. Other drugs may be monoamine reuptake inhibitors that act by binding to a membrane transporter protein, such as the SSRI antidepressants. Alternatively, drugs may act to inhibit an enzyme system, as the MAO inhibitor antidepressants do, or they may act on second-messenger systems or have some other as yet undefined trophic effect.

Given how well understood the mechanisms of action of so many CNS drugs are, it is perhaps surprising how little published research characterizes sex-specific differences in the CNS substrate that forms the target end organ of psychotropic drug effects. For example, it would be of interest to know the extent to which there are sex differences in the density or functional status of postsynaptic receptors, transporter proteins, or MAO-like enzymes. It also would be useful to know how each of these sex-specific differences might change over the course of the menstrual cycle, or how they might be affected by levels of estrogen and progesterone, chronic administration of oral contraceptives or hormone replacement, postmenopausal status, or ovariectomy.

The results of the growing body of research on this topic (reviewed in more detail by Brawman-Mintzer and Book in Chapter 2) suggest consistent differences across multiple systems, many of which may have clinical significance. For example, sexual dimorphisms have been identified in hemispheric lateralization (Wisniewski, 1998; Breedlove et al., 1999); CNS plasticity and response to environmental stimuli/stressors (Wisniewski,

1998; Trenerry et al., 1995); gross measures of CNS functioning .such as cortical event-related potentials, cerebral blood flow, and glucose metabolism (Ragland et al., 2000); and CNS receptor interactions (see Chapter 3 for more details). Sexual dimorphisms in CNS receptor function include steroid sex hormone effects on γ-aminobutyric acid$_A$ receptors (Perez et al., 1986), dopamine receptors (McEwen and Parsons, 1982), serotonin receptors (Rubinow et al., 1998), and MAO enzymes (Chevillard et al., 1981; Luine & Rhodes, 1983). It is also known that there are clinically relevant polymorphisms in the serotonin transporter protein, but it is not well established whether these or other polymorphisms are sex-linked.

Among patients with schizophrenia, there is evidence of significant sexual dimorphism in the underlying CNS correlates of the illness. For example, CNS imaging studies suggest structural deficits in fronto-temporal regions, and these deficits are frequently more marked in males (Cowell et al., 1996; Kopala et al., 1989). Estrogens also appear to have both dopaminergic activity and some effect on nerve growth factor, both of which may alter rates of neuronal cell death thought to be associated with the etiology of schizophrenia (Häfner et al., 1991; Toran-Allerand, 1990).

What is the clinical significance of the diverse examples of sexual dimorphism noted above? The answer is that there are multiple examples of differences in clinical response between females and males. These include, to cite only a few examples, results that suggest differential response rates for women treated for depressive disorders with various tricyclic, SSRI, and MAO inhibitor antidepressants (Kornstein et al., 2000; see Kornstein & Wojcik, Chapter 8, this volume); and differentially superior short-term response rates in women treated with neuroleptics for schizophrenia (Leung & Chue, 2000). For every example (such as the schizophrenia data) in which sex- and/or gender-specific results are relatively consistent, there are other examples (such as the depressive disorder data) in which the findings are not consistent from study to study. There is clearly a need for more systematic research.

Even where a consistent treatment response difference between women and men is found, it is still often difficult to disentangle whether differential efficacy should be more properly attributed to sex-specific pharmacodynamic effects of a drug or to sex-specific pharmacokinetic effects. It is also difficult to disentangle the impact of differential tolerability and drug discontinuation from efficacy. This is relevant whether a completer analysis or an intent-to-treat endpoint analysis is performed—though there is no consistency in how the efficacy results of these studies are reported. Finally, it is far from clear whether sex-specific differences in clinical response represent a true pharmacodynamic effect (i.e., one that is acting through a direct pharmacological mechanism) or whether the effect is indirect, due to differences in clinical presentation or other illness features associated with differential clinical response, as briefly summarized in a previous section.

The main lesson one may draw, once again, is that the whole issue of sex-specific differences in efficacy is dauntingly complex. It will yield tantalizing yet inconsistent findings that will remain refractory to understanding until and unless sex- and/or gender-specific questions help to shape a priori study hypotheses and become an explicit part of study design.

Behavioral Pharmacology

Psychotropic drugs often have clinically significant effects on neuropsychological functions (e.g., memory, cognition, vigilance, attention, etc.) and on psychomotor functions (reaction time, coordination, etc.). The behavioral pharmacology profile of these drugs can be subtle, and may not be manifested as crude differences in adverse event rates. Nonetheless, an unfavorable profile can have a profound effect on tolerability and long-term compliance. Furthermore, the degree to which symptomatic improvement (captured on such scales as the PANSS, the HAM-A, the HAM-D, the Yale–Brown Obsessive Compulsive Scale [Y-BOCS], etc.) actually translates into restoration of normal functioning and quality of life depends to a critical degree on the behavioral pharmacology of the drug under study. Elderly individuals are especially sensitive to the subtle collateral CNS effects of psychotropic drugs (Moore, O'Keeffe, et al., 1999).

The interpretation of behavioral pharmacology effects of psychotropic drugs is complicated by the fact that many Axis I disorders (e.g., depression, schizophrenia) are associated with neuropsychological impairments, so treatment response itself is associated with neuropsychological improvement, which may be simply *reduced* by treatment with drugs with an unfavorable CNS profile. An example of this is the significantly greater degree of improvement in various neuropsychological measures observed after depression treatment in elderly patients with sertraline compared to nortriptyline (Bondareff et al., 2000). Though nortriptyline is one of the least anticholinergic of all the tricyclic antidepressants, having approximately the same anticholinergic potency of the SSRI paroxetine, it still was sufficient to blunt the beneficial neuropsychological effect associated with a comparable level of improvement in depression.

Perhaps not surprisingly, sex steroids such as estrogen and progesterone have clinically significant behavioral pharmacology effects, as detailed by Brawman-Mintzer and Book in Chapter 2. Nevertheless, the sex-specific neuropsychological and psychomotor effects of psychotropic drugs at different phases of the menstrual cycle, as well as postmenopausally, have not been systematically studied.

Sleep and Circadian Rhythms

There is growing evidence that there are sex-based differences in circadian rhythms, melatonin secretion, body temperature fluctuations, and in sleep architecture (Manber & Armitage, 1999; Leibenluft, 1993). These differences vary according to the phase of the menstrual cycle. During aging, changes in sleep continue to differ between females and males (Manber & Armitage, 1999). It is also known that some CNS illnesses, such as mood disorders, are prominently associated with disruptions in various neuroendocrine circadian rhythms and sleep architecture (Duncan, 1996; Leibenluft, 1993; van Bemmel, 1997). Bipolar disorder (especially the rapid-cycling variant) and seasonal affective disorder are examples of illnesses in which women predominate and in which there are prominent disruptions in circadian rhythms. Yet very little research has focused on sex-specific differences in the effect of psychotropic drugs on either neuroendocrine rhythms or sleep architecture.

Safety and Tolerability

Data from the FDA's annual *Adverse Drug Experience Report* (Knapp et al., 1995) finds a preponderance of women among reportees by a ratio that ranges from 1.5:1 up to more than 2:1, with women of reproductive years having the highest ratio. Surveys of clinic populations (Tran et al., 1998) confirm this finding, which has also been noted for treatment with psychotropic drugs (Yonkers et al., 1992; Frackiewicz et al., 2000). Most studies, though, make no attempt to analyze the prevalence data to determine the extent to which the higher adverse event incidence in women is due to higher baseline use of concommittant medications, higher medical help seeking, or other variables.

In psychopharmacology clinical trials, treatment-emergent adverse events and laboratory abnormalities are currently analyzed by gender, but usually in a pro forma way that typically does not covary dose, differential illness severity, or other gender-based differences in either illness or patient characteristics. This is unfortunate, since differences in pharmacokinetics, pharmacodynamics, endogenous sex steroids, concomitant medication use, and incidence of medical comorbidity may all contribute significant differences in risk of treatment-emergent events. These events in turn may have a significant effect on treatment tolerability and compliance.

Two brief examples illustrate the need for greater attention to these sorts of sex-specific differences in clinical trials. The first example comes from the cardiovascular drug literature. Makkar et al. (1993) have reported that 70% of all drug-related cases of torsades de pointes in a large case series occurred in women. The incidence of this potentially serious adverse event was higher in women even after the investigators adjusted for underlying severity of coronary artery disease, electrolyte abnormalities, left ventricular function, and baseline QTc. Reasons for higher rates of torsades de pointes in women are not entirely known, but further study is ongoing (Drici et al., 1996; Ebert et al., 1998). The second example comes from the schizophrenia treatment literature and relates to the observation that women develop tardive dyskinesia at a significantly higher rate than men (Jeste & Caligiuri, 1993). Dosage ranges and titration rates for both older and newer atypical neuroleptics have been based on the results of clinical trials conducted predominantly with males. As a consequence, dosing in females may be higher than is appropriate for the underlying CNS substrate.

Sex-Specific Life Cycle Issues with a Potential Impact on Clinical Outcome

Previous chapters of this volume have detailed the importance of women's life cycle issues for an adequate understanding of psychiatric disorders and their treatment. These issues include the menstrual cycle (Steiner & Born, Chapter 3), pregnancy (Nonacs et al., Chapter 4), the postpartum period and lactation (Arnold et al., Chapter 5), and the perimenopausal, and postmenopausal periods (Ayubi-Moak & Parry, Chapter 7).

In previous sections of this chapter, we have briefly summarized the potential impact of these times in a woman's life on the conduct of psychopharmacology research. Increasingly, psychopharmacology research is making the systematic collection of data on drugs during these times a part of the overall characterization of a drug's profile. Where controlled research is not generally permissible—for example, during pregnancy—collation of large amounts of community data into registries may provide a useful substitute (Goldstein et al., 1997).

Despite these advances, the impact of sex-specific life cycle variables on treatment research is still honored primarily in the breach. Space does not permit a detailed review of the topic, some of which has already been touched on in previous chapters. Instead, in the next section we have chosen to use one example to illustrate the potential impact of women's life cycle issues on the efficacy of study treatment.

Impact of Menstrual Cycle on Assessment of Outcome

For women entering psychopharmacology treatment studies, menstrual cycle status is almost never a variable that is taken into account. The potential impact of initiating treatment at different phases of the menstrual cycle may be due to pharmacodynamic effects, as summarized in a previous section. The impact may also be due to the effect of fluctuating premenstrual dysphoric disorder (PMDD) symptomatology superimposed on primary major depression. This is not a trivial concern, because it is estimated that more than one-third of women of childbearing age who enter major depression treatment studies suffer from premenstrual syndrome (PMS) or PMDD. The impact of this superimposition is highlighted in Table 36.1, which compares a male and a female who begin a study with the same severity in their major depression, and who show the same degree of improvement in this disorder. The only difference is the timing of treatment relative to the menstrual cycle. As can be seen from the table, ignoring menstrual cycle effects can easily lead to a substantial difference in clinical outcome. The corollary of this is that neglect of this menstrual phase variable may introduce a significant confounding variable that constitutes a form of "noise," which will make it more difficult to detect the efficacy "signal" of a drug effect. Finally, it should be noted that there is some evidence that similar fluctuations in symptom severity occur in both panic disorder (Cameron et al., 1988; Basoglu et al., 2000) and schizophrenia (Hallonquist et al., 1993).

CONCLUSIONS AND FUTURE DIRECTIONS

So what can we conclude about the issue of sex and gender? Does it appear to be a clinically relevant variable in psychopharmacology treatment research? The answer is proba-

TABLE 36.1. The Effect of Comorbid PMS Symptoms on Assessment of Treatment Outcome: Modeling Two Different Menstrual Cycle Scenarios

	Screening	Baseline	Week 1	Week 2	Week 3	Week 4	Week 5	Endpoint HAM-D change score
Male HAM-D score	25	24	21	19	17	16	14	11
Female HAM-D: PMS scenario #1								
HAM-D score	29	28	21	19	20	19	14	14
Day of cycle	21	28/0	7	14	21	28/0	14	
PMS contribution	+4	+4	0	0	+3	+3	0	
Female HAM-D: PMS scenario #1								
HAM-D score	25	24	25	23	17	16	17	7
Day of cycle	7	14	21	28/0	7	14	28	
PMS contribution	0	0	+4	+4	0	0	+3	

Note. This model assumes a PMS contribution to the HAM-D score of 4 points during last 2 weeks of cycle. It also assumes partial (25%) improvement in PMS contribution (to 3 points).

bly "Yes," but the jury is still out. There is ample evidence for sexual dimorphisms in the CNS substrate, and there is ample evidence for interactions between sex steroids and monoaminergic receptor systems. There is also ample evidence for gender-related differences in Axis I psychiatric disorders—from their prevalence, clinical presentation, and rates of comorbidity to their course of illness. There is also evidence of occasional sex-specific differences in pharmacokinetic parameters. Finally, there is tentative evidence that gender-specific differences exist in patient recruitment and study entry, and that gender-related issues may subtly bias assessment.

With sex and gender operating at so many levels, the task of identifying clinically relevant determinants of treatment response is daunting. The only thing that is clear is that no consistent progress will be made until the issue of sex and gender becomes an a priori part of a treatment research program. The question then becomes this: How can drug trials be designed to detect clinically relevant sex and/or gender differences—or to evaluate whether an apparent difference in treatment response between women and men is a sex difference (relating to a pharmacokinetic, pharmacodynamic, or CNS substrate difference); or instead might be due to gender-based clinical or psychosocial dimensions?

The issues underlying this question can be summarized as follows:

1. A sex- and gender-sensitive research agenda does not consist simply of a pro forma listing of treatment-emergent adverse events by gender. Instead, such an analysis should evaluate the contribution to side effect burden of differences in menopausal and hormonal status; differences (from males) in medical and psychiatric comorbidity and illness characteristics; differences in pharmacokinetic profile; and differences in use of concomitant medications. Until these variables are analyzed as covariates, no clear understanding of sex and/or gender differences in treatment tolerability can be arrived at.

2. A gender-sensitive analysis of a mood or anxiety disorder study should routinely record menstrual cycle information that is likely to contribute significant "noise" to any assessment of efficacy.

3. In instances where female gender is known to be a significant prescriptive or prognostic variable (and per-treatment sample sizes are <100), a stratified, or even an adaptive (urn), randomization scheme might ensure the ability of subanalyses to evaluate the role of sex and/or gender effects (Yao & Wei, 1996; Rosenberger, 1999; Kernan et al., 1999).

4. Case report forms should be designed to record a minimum consensus level of information—not simply concerning cycle/reproductive/menopausal status information, but also data on relevant psychosocial variables that contribute to the transformation of sex into gender.

To begin the task of implementing such an agenda, treatment research protocols might be strengthened by undergoing a sex and gender review (in terms of study design, analysis plan, and completeness of sex- and gender-specific information). This review would be analogous to the current standard statistical review of proposed protocols.

The Institute of Medicine has recently released a report entitled *Exploring the Biological Contributions to Human Health. Does Sex Matter?* The results of this report provide compelling evidence that sex *does* matter, and that the time has come to move beyond talk to action (Wizemann & Pardue, 2001). Until and unless such a research agenda is undertaken in earnest, and refined in light of emerging data, we will not be able to realize the goal of the epigraph at the beginning of this chapter: "to arrive where we started, and know the place for the first time."

REFERENCES

Amori, G., & Lenox, R. H. (1989). Do volunteer subjects bias clinical trials? *Journal of Clinical Psychopharmacology, 9*(5), 321–327.

Aronson, T. A. (1987). A follow-up of two panic disorder–agoraphobic study populations: The role of recruitment biases. *Journal of Nervous and Mental Disease, 175*(10), 595–598.

Basoglu, C., Cetin, M., Semiz, U. B., et al. (2000). Premenstrual exacerbation and suicidal behavior in patients with panic disorder. *Comprehensive Psychiatry, 41*(2), 103–105.

Bondareff, W., Alpert, M., Friedhoff, A. J., et al. (2000). Comparison of sertraline and nortriptyline in the treatment of major depressive disorder in late life. *American Journal of Psychiatry, 157*(5), 729–736.

Breedlove, S. M., Cooke, B. M., & Jordan, C. L. (1999). The orthodox view of brain sexual differentiation. *Brain, Behavior and Evolution, 54*(1), 8–14.

Cameron, O. G., Kuttesch, D., McPhee, K., et al. (1988). Menstrual fluctuation in the symptoms of panic anxiety. *Journal of Affective Disorders, 15*(2), 169–174.

Chevillard, C., Barden, N., & Saavedra, J. M. (1981). Estradiol treatment decreases Type A and increases Type B monoamine oxidase in specific brain stem areas and cerebellum of ovariectomized rats. *Brain Research, 222*(1), 177–181.

Cowell, P. E., Kostianovsky, D. J., Gur, R. C., et al. (1996). Sex differences in neuroanatomical and clinical correlations in schizophrenia. *American Journal of Psychiatry, 153*, 799–805.

Cowley, D. S., Flick, S. N., Roy-Byrne, P. P. (1996). Long-term course and outcome in panic disorder: A naturalistic follow-up study. *Anxiety, 2*, 13–21.

Duncan, W. C., Jr. (1996). Circadian rhythms and the pharmacology of affective illness. *Pharmacology and Therapeutics, 71*(3), 253–312.

Drici, M. D., Burklow, T. R., Haridasse, V., et al. (1996). Sex hormones prolong the QT interval and downregulate potassium channel expression in the rabbit heart. *Circulation, 94*(6), 1471–1474.

Ebert, S. N., Liu, X. K., & Woosley, R. L. (1998). Female gender as a risk factor for drug-induced cardiac arrhythmias: Evaluation of clinical and experimental evidence. *Journal of Women's Health, 7*(5), 547–557.

Faraone, S. V., Chen, W. J., Goldstein, J. M., et al.(1994). Gender differences in age at onset of schizophrenia. *British Journal of Psychiatry, 164*, 625–629.

FDA Final Rule: Investigational New Drug Applications and New Drug Applications, 21 C.F.R. §§ 312, 314 (1998, February 11).

FDA Final Rule: Investigational New Drug Applications; Amendment to Clinical Hold Regulation for Products Intended for Life-Threatening Diseases and Conditions, 21 C.F.R. §§ 312, 312.42 (2000, May).

FDA Guideline for the Study and Evaluation of Gender Differences in the Clinical Evaluation of Drugs, 58 Fed. Reg. 139 (1993, July 22).

Frackiewicz, E. J., Sramek, J. J., & Cutler, N. R. (2000). Gender differences in depression and antidepressant pharmacokinetics and adverse events. *Annals of Pharmacotherapy, 34*(1), 80–88.

General Accounting Office. (2000, May). *Women's health: NIH has increased its efforts to include women in research* (Report No. GAO/HEHS-00–96). Washington, DC: Author.

Goldstein, D. J., Corbin, L. A., & Sundell, K. L. (1997). Effects of first-trimester fluoxetine exposure on the newborn. *Obstetrics and Gynecology, 89*(5, Pt. 1), 713–718.

Goldstein, J. M., & Link, B. (1988). Gender and the expression of schizophrenia. *Journal of Psychiatric Research, 22*, 141–155.

Häfner, H., Behrens, S., De Vry, J., et al. (1991). Oestradiol enhances the vulnerability threshold for schizophrenia in women by an early effect on dopaminergic neurotransmission. *European Archives of Psychiatry and Clinical Neuroscience, 241*, 65–68.

Häfner, H., Maurer, K., Löffler, W., et al. (1994). The epidemiology of early schizophrenia: Influence of age and gender on onset and early course. *British Journal of Psychiatry, 164*, 29–38.

Hallonquist, J., Seeman, M. V., Lang, M., et al. (1993). Variation in symptom severity over the menstrual cycle of schizophrenics. *Biological Psychiatry, 33*, 207–209.

Harris, R. B., Benet, L. Z., & Schwartz, J. B. (1995). Gender effects in pharmacokinetics and pharmacodynamics. *Drugs, 50*(2), 222–239.

Jeste, D. V., & Caligiuri, M. P. (1993). Tardive dyskinesia. *Schizophrenia Bulletin, 19*, 303–315.

Kernan, W. N., Viscoli, C. M., Makuch, R. W., et al. (1999). Stratified randomization for clinical trials. *Journal of Clinical Epidemiology, 52*, 19–26.

Kessler, R. C., McGonagle, K. A., Zhao, S., et al. (1994). Lifetime and 12–month prevalence of DSM-III-R psychiatric disorders in the United States: Results from the National Comorbidity Survey. *Archives of General Psychiatry, 51*, 8–19.

Kilzieh, N., & Akiskal, H. S. Rapid-cycling bipolar disorder: An overview of research and clinical experience. *Psychiatric Clinics of North America, 22*, 585–607.

Kinon, B. J., Kane, J. M., Chakos, M., et al. (1993). Possible predictors of neuroleptic-resistant schizophrenic relapse: Influence of negative symptoms and acute extrapyramidal side effects. *Psychopharmacology Bulletin, 29*, 365–369.

Knapp, D. E., Robinson, J. I., & Britt, A. L. (1995). *Adverse drug experience report.* Rockville, MD: Surveillance and Data Processing Branch, Center for Drug Evaluation and Research, U.S. Food and Drug Administration.

Kopala, L., Clark, C., & Hurwitz, T. (1989). Sex differences in olfactory function in schizophrenia. *American Journal of Psychiatry, 146*, 1320–1322.

Kornstein, S. G., Schatzberg, A. F., Thase, M. E., et al. (2000). Gender differences in chronic major and double depression. *Journal of Affective Disorders, 60*, 1–11.

Leaf, P. J., Livingston, M. M., Tischler, G. L., et al. (1985). Contact with health professionals for the treatment of psychiatric and emotional problems. *Medical Care, 23*, 1322–1337.

Leibenluft, E. (1993). Do gonadal steroids regulate circadian rhythms in humans? *Journal of Affective Disorders, 29*(2–3), 175–181.

Leibenluft, E. (1996). Women with bipolar illness: Clinical and research issues. *American Journal of Psychiatry, 153*, 163–173.

Leung, A., & Chue, P. (2000). Sex differences in schizophrenia: A review of the literature. *Acta Psychiatrica Scandinavica*, (Suppl. 401), 3–38.

Lin, E., Goering, P., Offord, D. R., et al. (1996). The use of mental health services in Ontario: Epidemiologic findings. *Canadian Journal of Psychiatry, 41*, 572–577.

Luine, V. N., & Rhodes, J. C. (1983). Gonadal hormone regulation of MAO and other enzymes in hypothalamic areas. *Neuroendocrinology, 36*(3), 235–241.

Makkar, R. R., Fromm, B. S., Steinman, R. T., et al. (1993). Female gender as a risk factor for torsades de pointes associated with cardiovascular drugs. *Journal of the American Medical Association, 270*(21), 2590–2597.

Manber, R., & Armitage, R. (1999). Sex, steroids, and sleep: A review. *Sleep, 22*(5), 540–555.

Maser, J. D., & Cloninger, C. R. (Eds.). (1990). *Comorbidity of mood and anxiety disorders.* Washington, DC: American Psychiatric Press.

McEwen, B. S., & Parsons, B. (1982). Gonadal steroid action on the brain: Neurochemistry and neuropharmacology. *Annual Review of Pharmacology and Toxicology, 22*, 555–598.

Merkatz, R. B., Temple, R., & Sobel, S. (1993). Women in clinical trials of new drugs. *New England Journal of Medicine, 329*(4), 291–296.

Mohr, P., & Czobor, P. (2000). Subject selection for the placebo- and comparator-controlled trials of neuroleptics in schizophrenia. *Journal of Clinical Psychopharmacology, 20*(2), 240–245.

Moore, A. R., & O'Keeffe, S. T. (1999). Drug-induced cognitive impairment in the elderly. *Drugs and Aging, 15*, 15–28.

National Institutes of Health Revitalization Act of 1993, Pub. L. No. 103-43 (1993).

Patten, S. B. (2000). Selection bias in studies of major depression using clinical subjects. *Journal of Clinical Epidemiology, 53*(4), 351–357.

Perez, J., Zucchi, I., & Maggi, A. (1986). Sexual dimorphism in the response of the GABAergic system to estrogen administration. *Journal of Neurochemistry, 47*(6), 1798–1803.

Pervin, L. A., Merrens, M. R., & Brannigan, G. G. (1998). *Personality: Research, assessment, and change.* New York: Wiley.

Pollack, M. H., Otto, M. W., Sachs, G. S., et al. (1994). Anxiety psychopathology predictive of outcome in patients with panic disorder and depression treated with imipramine, alprazolam and placebo. *Journal of Affective Disorders, 30*, 273–281.

Quitkin, F. M., Stewart, J. W., McGrath, P. J., et al. (1993). Columbia atypical depression: A subgroup of depressives with better response to MAOI than to tricyclic antidepressants or placebo. *British Journal of Psychiatry, 163*(Suppl. 21), 30–34.

Ragland, J. D., Coleman, A. R., Gur, R. C., et al. (2000). Sex differences in brain–behavior relationships between verbal episodic memory and resting regional cerebral blood flow. *Neuropsychologia, 38*(4), 451–461.

Robinson, D. G., Woerner, M. G., Alvir, J. M., et al. (1999). Predictors of treatment response from a first episode of schizophrenia or schizoaffective disorder. *American Journal of Psychiatry, 156*, 544–549.

Robinson, D., Woerner, M. G., Pollack, S., et al. (1996). Subject selection biases in clinical trials: data from a multicenter schizophrenia treatment study. *Journal of Clinical Psychopharmacology, 16*(2), 170–176.

Rosenberger, W. F. (1999). Randomized play-the-winner clinical trials: review and recommendations. *Controlled Clinical Trials, 20*, 328–342.

Roy-Byrne, P. P., & Cowley, D. S. (1994). Course and outcome in panic disorder: A review of recent follow-up studies. *Anxiety, 1*(4), 151–160.

Rubinow, D. R., Schmidt, P. J., & Roca, C. A. (1998). Estrogen–serotonin interactions: Implications for affective regulation. *Biological Psychiatry, 44*, 839–850.

Scheibe, G., & Albus, M. (1997). Predictors and outcome in panic disorder: A 2-year prospective follow-up study. *Psychopathology, 30*, 177–184.

Slaap, B. R., van Vlict, I. M., Westenberg, H. G., et al. (1995). Phobic symptoms as predictors of nonresponse to drug therapy in panic disorder patients (a preliminary report). *Journal of Affective Disorders, 33*, 31–38.

Sotsky, S. M., & Simmens, S. J. (1999). Pharmacotherapy response and diagnostic validity in atypical depression. *Journal of Affective Disorders, 54*(3), 237–247.

Stack, J. A., Paradis, C. F., Reynolds, C. F., 3rd, et al. (1995). Does recruitment method make a difference?: Effects on protocol retention and treatment outcome in elderly depressed patients. *Psychiatry Research, 56*(1), 17–24.

Sullivan, P. F., & Joyce, P. R. (1994). Effects of exclusion criteria in depression treatment studies. *Journal of Affective Disorders, 32*(1), 21–26.

Susser, E., & Wanderling, J. (1994). Epidemiology of nonaffective acute remitting psychosis vs. schizophrenia: Sex and sociocultural setting. *Archives of General Psychiatry, 51*, 294–301.

Szymanski, S., Lieberman, J. A., Alvir, J. M., et al. (1995). Gender differences in onset of illness, treatment response, course, and biologic indexes in first-episode schizophrenic patients. *American Journal of Psychiatry, 152*, 698–703.

Tanaka, E. (1999). Gender-related differences in pharmacokinetics and their clinical significance. *Journal of Clinical Pharmacological Therapy, 24*, 339–346.

Thompson, M. G., Heller, K., & Rody, C. A. (1994). Recruitment challenges in studying late-life depression: Do community samples adequately represent depressed older adults? *Psychology and Aging, 9*(1), 121–125.

Toran-Allerand, C. D. (1990). Interactions of estrogens with growth factors in the developing central nervous system. In R. B. Hochberg & F. Naftolin (Eds.), *The new biology of steroid hormones.* New York: Raven Press.

Tran, C., Knowles, S. R., Liu, B. A., et al. (1998). Gender differences in adverse drug reactions. *Journal of Clinical Pharmacology, 38*(11), 1003–1009.

Trenerry, M. R., Jack, C. R., Jr., Cascino, G. D., et al. (1995). Gender differences in post-temporal lobectomy verbal memory and relationships between MRI hippocampal volumes and preoperative verbal memory. *Epilepsy Research, 20*(1), 69–76.

van Bemmel, A. L. (1997). The link between sleep and depression. *Journal of Psychosomatic Research, 42*(6), 555–564.

Wells, K. B., Manning, W. G., Duan, N., et al. (1986). Sociodemographic factors and the use of outpatient mental health services. *Medical Care, 24,* 75–85.

Wisniewski, A. B. (1998). Sexually-dimorphic patterns of cortical asymmetry, and the role for sex steroid hormones in determining cortical patterns of lateralization. *Psychoneuroendocrinology, 23*(5), 519–547.

Wizeman, T. M., & Pardue, M.-L. (2001). *Exploring the biological contributions to human health. Does sex matter?* Institute of Medicine report. Washington, DC: National Academy Press.

Yao, Q., & Wei, L. J. (1996). Play the winner for Phase II/III clinical trials. *Statistics in Medicine, 15,* 2413–2423.

Yonkers, K. A., Kando, J. C., Cole, J. O., et al. (1992). Gender differences in pharmacokinetics and pharmacodynamics of psychotropic medication. *American Journal of Psychiatry, 149*(5), 587–595.

Young, M. A., Scheftner, W. A., Fawcett, J., et al. (1990). Gender differences in the clinical features of unipolar major depressive disorder. *Journal of Nervous and Mental Disease, 178,* 200–203.

37

Mental Health Policy and Women

MARY C. BLEHAR
GRAYSON NORQUIST

In the near future, basic and applied research promises to advance our understanding of the multiple biological and environmental factors that influence the onset and course of such mental disorders as schizophrenia, bipolar disorder, and depression. Within the next 10 years, the Human Genome Project should identify the majority of genes that arc expressed in the Central Nervous System, enabling clinical researchers to define more etiologically homogeneous groups of mental disorders. Epidemiological and prevention research will be able to focus on understanding environmental risk factors as they affect genetically high-risk individuals. Molecular pharmacological technologies, also benefiting from genetic findings, are likely to accelerate the process of psychotropic drug discovery.

During the past two decades, there have been major advances in diagnosis and sampling methodology, enabling researchers to establish estimates of the impact of and need deriving from mental disorders. Two population-based studies, the Epidemiologic Catchment Area program (Robins & Regier, 1991) and the National Comorbidity Survey (Kessler et al., 1994), have provided estimates in national samples. These studies also identified demographic risk factors for mental illness and intergroup disparities in the prevalence of different mental disorders. One of the most striking findings was that of large gender differences in prevalence of various disorders. In both surveys, females were found to have approximately twice the risk of mood and anxiety disorders as males, but males were found to have twice the risk of alcohol and other substance use disorders and antisocial personality disorder.

Despite these gender differences, little clinical research in mental illness has examined possible gender differences in etiological factors until relatively recently, and even less research has explored the treatment and services implications of gender differences. However, research in these areas is rapidly growing.

Material presented here does not necessarily reflect the opinions, official policy, or position of the National Institute of Mental Health.

Research on women's health at the National Institutes of Health (NIH) was expanded with the Enactment of the NIH Revitalization Act of 1993. Provisions of this act included a legislative mandate for the Office of Research on Women's Health and a mandate for the inclusion of women in clinical research. In particular, NIH-funded Phase III clinical trials, were required to include sufficient numbers of women to permit a valid analysis of outcome data for gender differences. This move toward an explicit focus on gender differences in clinical trials promises to increase our knowledge of therapeutic differences in response between men and women in the coming years.

In this chapter, we discuss the policy implications of mental health treatment and services research for women with mental illnesses. We start with a discussion of services and epidemiological research that may be used to address the issue of the public health significance of mental illnesses in women and their treatment and service needs. This information is critical for decision makers who must allocate health care resources and plan systems of health care. We then discuss issues related to the diagnosis of women with mental illnesses, the functional impact of these illnesses, intervention research on barriers to their identification and treatment, and ethical issues involved in the provision of treatments and services. Throughout we discuss the kinds of research needed to inform mental health public policy for women.

THE PUBLIC HEALTH SIGNIFICANCE OF MENTAL ILLNESS IN WOMEN

In the 1990s, the World Bank, the World Health Organization, and several private foundations jointly funded a comprehensive study of the impact of illnesses, described in the book *The Global Burden of Disease* (Murray & Lopez, 1996). A composite score (the disability-adjusted life year, or DALY) measured lost years of healthy life due to premature death or disability. For the first time ever the study provided a basis for comparing the public health burden of different physical and mental illnesses. Based on 1990 data, depression ranked first in DALYs for women age 5 and older worldwide. The top 10 sources of DALYs for these women are shown in Table 37.1.

When the measure of years lived with disability was disaggregated from the DALY

TABLE 37.1. Leading Causes of DALYs: World, Women (Ages 5 and Older)—1990

	Total (millions)	Percent of total
All causes	407.2	
1. Unipolar major depression	32.7	8.0
2. Ischemic heart disease	20.1	5.0
3. Cerebrovascular disease	18.7	4.6
4. Tuberculosis	15.3	3.8
5. Chronic obstructive pulmonary disease	12.0	3.0
6. Iron deficiency anemia	12.0	2.9
7. Other intentional injuries	11.4	2.8
8. Lower respiratory infection	11.4	2.8
9. Self-inflicted injuries	8.8	2.1
10. Road traffic accidents	8.0	2.0

Note. The data are from Murray and Lopez (1996).

score and considered alone, The *Global Burden of Disease* found that for women ages 5 and older worldwide, bipolar disorder, schizophrenia, and obsessive–compulsive disorder (OCD) were among the top 10 sources of disability. Table 37.2 shows a rank ordering of the top 10 disabling conditions.

The Developmental Epidemiology of Mental Disorders in Women

The lifetime prevalence of major depressive disorder has been studied in two U.S. epidemiological surveys (Robins & Regier, 1991; Kessler et al., 1994). For major depression, the lifetime prevalence has been estimated to vary from 10% to 25% for women and from 5% to 12% for men. The lifetime prevalence of bipolar disorder and schizophrenia is much lower, at approximately 1% of adults aged 18 and older. Equal numbers of men and women are affected. OCD has an estimated lifetime prevalence of 2.5% and occurs equally often in women and men.

Major Depression

A single untreated episode of major depression lasts an average of 8 months. Over 60% of cases of major depression recur after an initial episode, and the probability of recurrence increases with each subsequent episode. In approximately 30% of cases, depression does not fully remit. Patients with major depression may also experience a chronic course (defined as depression of 2 years' duration without prior dysthymia); major depression superimposed on dysthymia; or pure dysthymia. Women with past episodes of major depression are also at risk for the onset of postpartum and perimenopausal episodes, and they may experience exacerbation of depressive symptoms in relation to the menstrual cycle (Yonkers, 1998).

Bipolar Disorder

According to the Diagnostic and Statistical Manual of Mental Disorders, bipolar disorder is characterized longitudinally by episodes of both depression and mania. In addition to

TABLE 37.2. The Leading Causes of Disability: World (Ages 5 and Older)—1990

	Total (millions)	Percent of total
All causes	386.1	
1. Unipolar major depression	50.8	13.2
2. Other unintentional injuries	24.4	6.3
3. Iron deficiency anemia	19.2	5.0
4. Falls	16.2	4.2
5. Alcohol use	15.8	4.1
6. Chronic obstructive pulmonary disease	14.7	3.8
7. Bipolar disorder	14.1	3.7
8. Osteoarthritis	13.3	3.4
9. Schizophrenia	12.2	3.2
10. Obsessive–compulsive disorder	10.2	2.6

Note. The data are from Murray and Lopez (1996).

the clinical features of depressive episodes identified above as potential sources of functional impairment, episodes of mania also tend to be highly disruptive of interpersonal and occupational functioning. Features of manic episodes include disregard for the consequences of one's own behavior, overspending, and argumentativeness. Women with bipolar disorder are overrepresented among samples with difficult-to-treat clinical features such as rapid cycling, defined as four or more episodes of mania or depression in a 1-year period. Women with bipolar disorder are at increased risk for the onset of a severe possibly psychotic mood disorder episode in relation to recent childbirth. Less is known about the course of bipolar disorder in relation to perimenopause or menstrual cycling, but there is evidence (Blehar et al., 1998) that bipolar women have increased risk for exacerbation of mood symptoms in relation to these reproductive transitions.

Schizophrenia

Schizophrenia is the most serious of the mental disorders. The onset of florid schizophrenia is typically preceded by a prodromal phase in late adolescence or young adulthood, during which psychosocial functioning deteriorates gradually. The occurrence of a florid psychotic episode with delusions and hallucinations signals the onset of schizophrenia. Acute episodes typically resolve over time but are recurrent. Between episodes, individuals with schizophrenia often continue to show persistent negative symptoms (e.g., flattened affect, social withdrawal, and apathy), as well as deficits in cognitive functioning. These aspects of schizophrenia have profound consequences for social and occupational functioning. Onset tends to be earlier in males than in females who generally have better functional outcomes (American Psychiatric Association, 1994). It has been speculated that this disparity in outcome is due to the protective effects of estrogen against psychosis. However, women with schizophrenia may have increased vulnerability to relapse premenstrually, during the early postpartum period, and at menopause (Hoff et al., 1997).

Obsessive–Compulsive Disorder

OCD is characterized by recurrent behaviors or rituals to reduce anxiety. With typical onset in childhood or adolescence and a chronic and relapsing course, OCD causes disability by virtue of the time spent in performing disorder-related behaviors and interference with other more productive behaviors. OCD has high rates of comorbidity with depressive disorders and with other anxiety disorders. There have been few studies of clinical course differences between men and women, or of clinical course in women in relation to reproductive transitions; however, there is clinical evidence for a worsening of course during pregnancy (Shear & Mammen, 1995) and the postpartum period, as well as premenstrually.

Other Common Disorders Affecting Women

Space does not permit us to discuss the clinical course of other mental disorders in women. However, women are twice as likely as men to be diagnosed with dysthymia, panic disorder, social phobia, agoraphobia, and posttraumatic stress disorder. Eating disorders are also more likely to be diagnosed in females. All the disorders mentioned here share key clinical course features; these include early onset (typically in late adolescence or young adulthood in a majority of those affected), as well as a tendency to develop a recurrent or chronic course.

Comorbidity among the mental disorders is common and is associated with greater clinical severity. For women more than men, anxiety and mood disorders often co-occur. Comorbidity of substance use disorders with other mental disorders is less common in women than in men (Warner et al, 1995) but poses special problems in treatment, especially for pregnant substance-using women. Women with mental disorders also frequently report comorbid medical disorders. For instance there is increased prevalence of migraine and other headaches and of respiratory and gastrointestinal disorders among women with depressive disorders (Moldin et al., 1993).

Policy Implications

The implications of gender difference in clinical course and patterns of comorbidity have been little studied in the treatment or services setting. The available data, however, suggest that primary care physicians in particular should be aware of the possibility of depressive and anxiety disorders in women who present with somatic complaints. In specialized settings, women with substance use problems should be screened for the presence of other mental disorders.

The course of mental disorders, especially mood disorders, may be adversely affected by hormonal fluctuations occurring in women during pregnancy and the postpartum period, premenstrually, and at the time of the perimenopause. Primary care doctors need to be aware of this association. Especially in women with a history of mental illnesses it may be important to carefully monitor the patients and to initiate interventions early if signs of incipient onset of a recurrent episode of a disorder or worsening of a chronic condition become apparent. In other cases, it may be wise to initiate preventive interventions—for instance, in the case of women with prior histories of pregnancy-onset or postpartum-onset mood disorders. To this end, and as we discuss further below, screening of women in primary care and in obstetrics and gynecology clinical settings appears to be an important way to detect mental illnesses in women. Treatment of women in such settings may be seen as one of the most effective means currently available to reduce the disability burden of mental disorders. Finally, the inclusion of mental health care providers in the primary care and obstetrics/gynecology settings may be one way of ensuring that the assessment of women is comprehensive and integrated.

SPECIAL CONSIDERATIONS IN THE DIAGNOSIS OF WOMEN

For women, psychiatric diagnosis has often been a controversial topic. From a feminist perspective, the diagnostic activities of clinicians (and, more recently, clinical committees) are considered activities of a predominantly male psychiatric culture, wedded to a medical model and defining female personality and behavior as pathological. Diagnoses affecting only women and implicating hormonal fluctuations in onset and course, such as premenstrual dysphoric disorder, have been proposed in DSM-IV (American Psychiatric Association, 1994) as "criteria sets for further study" amid considerable controversy.

Depending on one's perspective, mood and anxiety symptoms in women may be seen as reflecting the consequences of social conditions such as inequality, discrimination, and violence against women. Women do not differ from men in the prevalence of schizophrenia and bipolar disorder, which are more putatively biologically based. Such patterns have suggested to some that culturally based gender bias is operative in the diagnostic enterprise.

It is beyond the scope of this chapter to critique the social context in which diagnoses rise and fall in psychiatry. Yet there are minimal research data on the relative contribution of various biological and psychosocial factors to gender differences in disorders. Furthermore definitional and methodological explanations for gender differences in disorders remain to be fully evaluated. Among possible explanations are that alcohol and other substance use disorders are depressive equivalents in men, so that the gender difference in prevalence of depression may be more apparent than real. A preponderance of evidence indicates that the gender difference in major depression cannot be accounted for entirely by methodological bias (Wolk & Weissman, 1995). However, methodological studies that vary the threshold for diagnosis of depression also have reported decreases in the magnitude of the gender difference in depression with decreases in the number of symptoms required for case identification (Kessler et al., 1993), although the difference did not disappear. Such work underscores the problems with current diagnostic schemes.

On the other hand, current diagnostic schemes can be used as a tool for assessing the scope of disorders in women and identifying need for treatment. Viewed in this way, the value of diagnoses, including those more prevalent in women or occurring almost exclusively in women, needs to be demonstrated in terms of the information they convey about meaningful functional outcomes and the potential impact that interventions will have on the public health burden of mental disorders in women.

DEFINING MEANINGFUL FUNCTIONAL OUTCOMES IN WOMEN

Data from the National Household Interview Survey (NHIS) showed that women were almost twice as likely to report a mental health problem (excluding substance abuse or dependence) in the past year as men. Of those women reporting anxiety or depressive symptoms, 33% reported being unable to perform their major activities. Almost 16% reported limitations in major activities, and 10% reported limitations in other activities (Willis et al., 1998). The level of functional disability among those identified with symptoms did not differ by gender.

However, in the NHIS, women who reported major role limitations due to a physical disorder also have the highest rates of severe depression (Campbell, 1999). In general, the association between depression and medical conditions is stronger for women than for men (Moldin et al., 1993). Women with disabilities or serious medical illnesses may have secondary mood and anxiety symptoms to a greater extent than men. Mental health symptoms have been shown to complicate treatment of the medical conditions and to be associated with relatively poorer outcome. There is a particular need for screening of women with physical disabilities and chronic medical conditions by primary care doctors; there is also a need for the development of rehabilitative interventions that take into account the special mental health issues of women with such conditions.

Methods for assessing functional status are of critical importance as a way of monitoring the impact of diagnosis and treatment on public health and they need to reflect gender-relevant variables and functional outcomes. For women, major tasks of young and middle adult life include the pursuit and completion of formal education, engagement in meaningful work, the establishment of intimate relationships, the formation of families, and the care of children and older family members. Differences between men and women in the amount of time spent performing various roles may mediate the gender difference in depression. Typically, women not only contribute to the economic support of the household but also have major responsibility for domestic chores, child care, and the care of aging relatives. In a national longitudinal survey of U.S. adults, working women reported typically performing almost twice as much household work as working men (Bird, 1999). This difference was correlated with higher rates of depressive symptoms in women in the study. The majority of research on functional outcomes has tended to assess performance in globally defined major roles versus subsidiary life roles, with little further refinement of assessment domains by gender of respondent. There has been little specification of gender differences in major and subsidiary roles, of possible gender differences in the value placed on different roles, or of the functional consequences of impairments in roles. Failure to consider these factors may neglect important gender differences in the functional impact of interventions. Furthermore, interventions in women have the potential to affect not only their symptoms and functional outcomes, but also their children's mental health. Outcomes in the children of affected women are rarely considered in assessments of intervention effectiveness.

From a policy perspective, there is value in considering gender differences in functional roles when measures are being developed to assess functional consequences of disorders. This is not to argue that individual women may not place the same value on work as men or may not indeed have similar functional roles. Nonetheless, average differences between men and women in role structure and the importance of different roles are likely to exist. Then the issue can be raised of the added value of assessment of different functional outcomes in women and men, or even of different schemes to weight elements in deriving a more global score of outcome.

INTERVENTION RESEARCH: IDENTIFYING WOMEN IN NEED OF SERVICES

Screening

In general, fewer than a third of people with mental disorders seek treatment and a significant number remain undetected, misdiagnosed, or suboptimally managed (Campbell et al, 1997; Robinson et al., 1997). Half of patients with depression see a primary care physician and another 20–30% see both primary care and behavioral health care providers (Katon et al.,1996). Despite this, primary care physicians are estimated to diagnose only about half the cases of major or minor depression among their patients (Eisenberg, 1992). Young single women in obstetrics and gynecology settings are reported to have high rates of mental disorders (Miranda et al., 1998). Depressive symptoms in women have also been related social variables such as three or more children at home; lack of a confiding, intimate relationship; and unemployment (Brown & Harris, 1978). Such risk factors may be overrepresented in lower socioeconomic groups such as those studied by Miranda and colleagues. There is, however, relatively little in the services research literature about the impact of screening, diagnosis and treatment of mental disorders in women seen in obstetrics and gynecology settings.

Routine screening for postnatal depression is implemented in other health care systems. A study of 121 New Zealand women (Holt, 1995) examined scores on the Edinburgh Postnatal Depression Scale (EPDS; Cox et al., 1987) at 6 weeks following delivery, to predict likelihood of major depression in the 12 months following delivery. Seven women were found to have postnatal depression, and six of these had scored over 12.5 on the EPDS. Eight women had other depressive disorders, and of these, five had also scored over 12.5. Those scoring over 12.5 had a 64% risk of some form of depressive disorder, and those scoring under 12.5 had only a 4% risk (Holt, 1995). Currently, mental health screening is not routinely done in U.S. obstetrics and gynecology settings. This is surprising in view of the fact that many women of childbearing age receive their primary medical care in such settings. The occurrence of depression in late pregnancy and postpartum is well documented (O'Hara, 1986). Furthermore, other conditions and disorders seen in gynecological settings may also be associated with increased risk for depression. These include chronic pelvic pain, severe premenstrual and perimenopausal symptoms, and treatments for infertility, and endometriosis. For more than a decade, guidelines from the American College of Obstetricians and Gynecologists have called for routine screening of women for domestic violence. In response to a survey, the majority of obstetrician–gynecologists reported screening both pregnant and nonpregnant patients for domestic violence but only when they suspected abuse (Horan et al., 1998). Universal screening may yield higher identification of women subjected to violence who are in need of services (Horan et al., 1998). A review of the literature on violence against pregnant women (Gazmararian et al., 1996) found estimates of prevalence ranging from 0.9% to 20.1%. Studies that asked about violence more than once during in-person interviews, or asked during the third trimester of pregnancy, reported higher prevalence rates. The lowest estimates were reported by women attending a private clinic and by those responding to a self-administered questionnaire (Gazmararian et al., 1996). Partner violence is also associated with increased risk for depression and anxiety disorders in women (Mazza & Dennerstein, 1996). This fact as well as the high rates of violence found in primary care settings indicates a clear need for more focus on mental health screening for women of childbearing age. Mental health screening of postpartum women at their 6-week checkup appears to be easily done, readily accepted and reliable in identifying most women with postnatal depression and other depressive disorders.

Translational Research: Tapping Behavioral Science for Gender Factors Relevant in the Clinical Setting

Mental disorders affecting women have impact throughout the critical developmental stages of young and middle adulthood. The majority of episodes of depression occur in women between the ages of 18 and 44, and peak onsets of depression occur in women between ages 25 and 44 (Burke et al., 1991). Therefore, intervention research and services focused on women in these age groups are especially important. Behavioral science is a potential source of hypotheses about differential impact of therapeutic approaches on women and men

Women have been reported to differ from men in the value they place on interpersonal relationships versus instrumentality (Feingold, 1994). This gender difference may affect their services needs and responses to different mental health care treatment and service settings. Women may also have greater vulnerability both to experience stress in response to adverse life events, and to react stressfully to a wider variety of life events than men. For instance, there is evidence that women are twice as likely as men to develop posttraumatic stress disorder following exposure to a stressor (Breslau et al., 1998). In a community study of adult men and women (Maciejewski et al., 2001), women were three times more likely than men to develop major depression following a stressful life experience. In that study, there was also evidence that women experienced depression in response to a wider range of stressful life event than did men. Event-related depression in men was found to be concentrated in events affecting their interpersonal ties to immediate loved ones. For women, event-related risk included these events but also extended to a variety of other events such as those affecting close friends, as well as personal and family problems (Maciejewski et al., 2001). Certain life events may have special salience to women. For example, in one study of couples in therapy, women were more likely to develop depression following a problem with children than were men (Nazroo et al., 1997) The authors attributed this to the greater salience of the caregiver role for women.

Personal cognitive and affective style differences between men and women in response to life events are hypothesized to underlie gender differences in rates of depression. For instance, there is evidence of gender differences in emotional and cognitive responses to stresses (Nolen-Hoeksema et al., 1999). Women are more likely to ruminate about adverse life events than men and to demonstrate lower levels of mastery behaviors than men. Nonetheless, despite the face validity of such factors as potentially important variables in clinical outcomes, they have rarely been explored in clinical research on interventions and services.

The context in which care is offered may affect its utilization by men and women in different ways. To give an example from treatment research on pregnant substance-using women (Substance Abuse and Mental Health Services Administration, 1993), such women are more likely to participate in settings that provide treatment as an integral part of their overall health care than they are in traditional specialized settings. They also prefer same-sex treatment settings to traditional settings with both men and women. An admission of a substance use problem has potentially different consequences for women than for men, since many women fear that its detection may lead to the loss of child custody. These women frequently have other complicating mental disorders that also require treatment in an integrated health care setting.

Furthermore, as noted previously, women in need of mental health intervention frequently report the occurrence of past or ongoing abuse from their male partners. Fear of retaliation for attending therapeutic sessions or for reporting domestic violence issues may be an important potential impediment to treatment seeking by women. Childhood sexual abuse is a more common occurrence in females than in males, and is a risk factor for depression and other mental disorders (Weiss et al., 1999). Attention to this risk factor needs to be incorporated into services and treatment approaches for women with mental disorders.

Women are the primary consumers of psychotropic drugs. An estimated 60–70% of antidepressant prescriptions written for depression are given to women (Agency for Health Care Policy and Research [AHCPR], 1993). Women utilize the general health care system, including mental health services, more than men do (Kessler et al., 1981). Large-scale data sets are not available to address the issue of gender differences in utilization patterns of different psychotherapeutic interventions. Yet this is an important issue, in light of the common belief that psychotherapies are more attractive to women than to men because of their greater valuation of interpersonal relationships as well as their childbearing role.

Furthermore, there has been little attention to the special rehabilitation needs of women with mental disorders beyond the acute treatment phase for mental disorders. Except for women with severe mental disorders such as schizophrenia, rehabilitative care following an acute episode of a mental disorder is rarely integrated into current health care systems. Given the demographics of mental disorders, with the majority of treated caseload consisting of women of childbearing age, there is a special need to consider rehabilitation needs in the context of the social roles of affected women.

Compliance and Adherence

Consumers of potentially effective psychotropic drugs—both men and women—often do not comply with treatment regimens. In primary care settings, it is estimated that 35% of patients diagnosed with depression discontinue their medications within the first month of treatment (Way et al., 1999). Since availability alone of efficacious treatments does not ensure their utilization, the identification of barriers to adherence is needed. Understanding patient factors related to noncompliance is important to improving health care outcomes. There is indication that side effects may have a different impact on drop out in women and men.

Clinical reports suggest that women may experience more severe side effects from drug regimens than men do, and that these may be a factor in differential dropout from efficacious treatments (Jensvold et al., 1996). Clinical reports also suggest that medication related weight gain may be a more important factor in medication discontinuation in women than in men, particularly for women who may have experienced weight gain as part of the clinical profile of their disorder (Kornstein & Wojcik, 2000). Such issues remain to be explored more thoroughly in larger-scale studies. As we also discuss below, women of reproductive age may discontinue medications if they are planning to conceive, or become pregnant. Abrupt discontinuation of medication may be a risk factor for recurrence of a mental disorder.

ETHICAL ISSUES IN TREATMENT OF WOMEN

Consideration of ethical issues in clinical intervention research on women must come to grips with the potential impact on treatment or non-treatment on their children. A December 2000 FDA/NIH Conference, "Clinical Pharmacology during Pregnancy: Addressing Clinical Needs through Science" focused on issues related to testing and administration of drugs and other biological treatments in pregnant women. A paramount concern was the need to address fetal and maternal well-being, as well as the need for more information on the effects of drugs for serious chronic or recurrent disorders likely to affect pregnant women.

In psychiatry, treatment of pregnant and lactating women is largely uncharted territory. Historically, women of childbearing age were excluded from early phases of clinical trials of psychotropic agents due to concern over possible adverse effects on their reproductive function or on their fetuses, should they become pregnant. Even with policies explicitly encouraging inclusion and analysis, there is little information about the impact of treatments on women versus men, and almost no information about treated or untreated mental disorders during pregnancy and lactation. In principle, effective treatments for women of this age group are likely to have a significant public health impact. A decision made ostensibly to protect women of childbearing age from untoward medication effects has led to a dearth of information about treatments for such women.

Record numbers of women are taking antidepressants and may conceive during a course of antidepressant therapy. Many women with bipolar disorder and schizophrenia are on maintenance medications. These women are in danger of relapse if they discontinue medication after becoming pregnant. On the other hand, there is little systematic data with which women or their clinicians can weigh the potential risks not only to themselves, but also to their unborn or breastfeeding children.

A substantial literature indicates that children of depressed mothers arc at higher risk themselves for childhood behavioral disorders (Goodman & Gotlib, 1999). The consequences of a relapse or recurrence of serious mental illness during pregnancy or postpartum may be to incapacitate the mother, and thereby put to the child at high risk for adverse developmental outcomes. Nonetheless, there is little data to indicate how or whether pregnancy alters the course of major mental disorders, except that it is increasingly clear that pregnancy does not protect against recurrence of such major disorders as depression and bipolar disorder. Little is known about the biological consequences to a child of having a mother with an untreated episode of bipolar disorder, major depression, or schizophrenia during pregnancy. Similarly, information is needed about the longer-term or subtler behavioral consequences to a child of having received psychotropic treatments as a fetus or during breastfeeding. For many of the newer serotonin selective reuptake inhibitors and the atypical antipsychotics, there is very little postmarketing data available on effectiveness, dosing or side effects during pregnancy. The newer atypical antipsychotics do not elevate prolactin levels as much as did the older neuroleptics and therefore may have less of an adverse impact on fertility in women. As a consequence, increasing numbers of chronically treated women with psychoses may become pregnant in the coming years. Women with psychotic disorders are in need of answers to questions of safety and effectiveness of treatments in relation to childbearing.

The ethical issues in providing versus discontinuing treatment are largely unexplored for psychotropic drug treatment in childbearing women. In the clinical situation, the clinician evaluates risks versus benefits and acts in the best interests of the patient. In the research situation, there has traditionally been a requirement for random assignment to treatment versus placebo or to different treatments. The current climate in which clinical research is conducted has highlighted a number of complex issues such as whether patients who are maintained on a drug may be withdrawn from the drug for purposes of testing new compounds, or whether placebos are ever advisable when effective treatments exist. In this climate, ethical issues in the treatment of pregnant and lactating women are yet more complicated by issues of safety for their children.

The clinical research community has responded to this need and the challenges of research in this area by designing naturalistic prospective studies. In such studies, some factors other than treatment versus nontreatment are identified and controlled for, but yet other factors may nonetheless confound findings. Methodologically, a naturalistic design is less desirable than a randomized controlled trial for efficacy and effectiveness. In naturalistic studies, the patients themselves, in consultation with treating clinicians, ultimately make an informed decision to maintain or discontinue medications. As more evidence accrues indicating safety and effectiveness of different treatments during pregnancy and breastfeeding, randomized trials may be contemplated by more and more researchers, or more innovative statistical models may be used to analyze observational data. No study to date has randomly assigned women to different treatments during pregnancy. A further complication for treatment of pregnant women is a fear that women, or even years later their children, may initiate litigation because of behavioral or developmental problems.

For childbearing women, psychotherapies may be a desirable alternative to pharmacological treatments. Research to address the effectiveness of psychotherapies in primary care settings is sparse. A recent review of psychotherapies in primary care (AHCPR, 1999) noted that only two studies addressed the issue of the portability and effectiveness of psychotherapies in primary care settings.

Although there is evidence that psychotherapies are effective both as prevention and as treatment for childbearing depression (Stuart & O'Hara, 1995), these therapies require specialized training A variety of less intensive psychosocial interventions, including support groups and counseling, have been reported to be effective in reducing postpartum mood disorders (Stuart et al., 1998; Ray & Hodnett, 1999). From a public policy perspective, consideration needs to be given to the cost-effectiveness of different types of psychosocial interventions in treating postpartum mental disorders.

CONCLUSIONS

In this chapter we have only partly covered the range of issues that could be considered from a public policy perspective for women with mental illness. Our focus has been primarily on women of childbearing age. From a public health perspective, mental disorders in this age group are associated with the highest proportion of mental-health-related disability among females. Women of this age have special roles due both to their reproductive and their social roles. We have raised several research questions that are in need of answers to improve their clinical care and outcomes of these women. This focus may also optimize around a strategy of having a major impact on the public health status of women with mental disorders. However, our chapter has not covered issues in adolescent women and in older women.

We note a pressing need to develop more information about the effectiveness of different preventive interventions, as well as psychotherapeutic and pharmacological interventions, for adolescent women. Currently little information is available to address general questions of efficacy in adolescents, so that there is insufficient data to analyze outcomes by gender of study participants. It is possible that different issues have personal salience for young women as compared to adult women. For example, eating disorders primarily affect young women during adolescence. The context of effective care for adolescent females may also be different than for adult women. Adolescent females may benefit from the delivery of integrated mental health care in their general care settings. However, neither pediatric settings nor internal medicine or obstetrics/gynecology settings may be appropriately designed and staffed to address the special issues of adolescent females.

We have not had time to discuss policy issues in relation to mental health treatment and services for older women. Older women face special psychosocial issues such as loss of social networks through death of close friends, bereavement following death of spouse, and depression related to health problems, and related disabilities. There are preliminary reports of differences in response to pharmacological agents in pre- and postmenopausal women (Kornstein et al., 2000). There is some support for beneficial effects of hormone replacement therapy on cognitive function in postmenopausal women (LeBlanc et al., 2001). The relationship between enhanced cognitive function and mental health outcomes is a high-priority area for research ranging from neuroscience research to clinical trials. With the aging of the "baby boomers," disability related to cerebrovascular disease and Alzheimer's Disease is anticipated to increase. Both conditions are associated with affective disturbances as well as cognitive disabilities and both may have common etiological factors.

In summary, a focus on gender-related issues in treatment and services research needs to take into account hormonal, social role, developmental and cognitive and affective variables. This focus can be seen as a potential benefit in terms of the public health goal of reducing disability burden associated with mental disorders in women.

REFERENCES

Agency for Health Care Policy and Research (AHCPR). (1993). *Depression in primary care: Vol 1. Detection and diagnosis: Clinical practice guideline* (AHCPR Publication No. 93–0550). Rockville, MD: Author.

Agency for Health Care Policy and Research (AHCPR). (1999). *Treatment of depression—Newer pharmacotherapies* (AHCPR Publication No. 99-EO14). Rockville MD: Author.

American Psychiatric Association. (1994). *Diagnostic and statistical manual of mental disorders* (4th ed.). Washington, DC: Author.

Bird, C. (1999). Gender, household labor and psychological distress: The impact of the amount and division of housework. *Journal of Health and Social Behavior, 40*(1), 32–45.

Blehar, M. C., DePaulo, J. R., Jr., Gershon, E. S., et al. (1998). Women with bipolar disorder: Findings from the NIMH Genetics Initiative sample. *Psychopharmacology Bulletin, 34*(3), 239–243.

Breslau, N., Kessler, R. C., Chilcoat, H. D., et al. (1998). Trauma and posttraumatic stress disorder in the community: The 1996 Detroit area survey of trauma. *Archives of General Psychiatry, 55*(7), 626–632.

Brown, G. W., & Harris, T. O. (1978). *Social origins of depressions: A study of psychiatric disorder in women.* New York: Free Press.

Burke, K. C., Burke, J. D., Rae, D. S., et al. (1991). Comparing age at onset of major depression and other psychiatric disorders by birth cohorts in five U.S. community populations. *Archives of General Psychiatry, 48*, 789–795.

Campbell, V. (1999, August). *Prevalence of depression among women with disability.* Paper presented at the Conference on Promoting the Health and Wellbeing of Women with Disabilities, San Antonio, TX.

Cox, J. L., Holden, J. M., & Sagovsky, R. (1987). Detection of postnatal depression: Development of the Edinburgh Postnatal Depression Scale. *British Journal of Psychiatry, 150*, 782–786.

Eisenberg, L. (1992). Treating depression and anxiety in primary care: Closing the gap between knowledge and practice. *New England Journal of Medicine, 326*, 1080–1084.

FDA/NIH Conference. (2000, December 4–5). *Clinical pharmacology during pregnancy: Addressing clinical needs through science,* Bethesda, MD.

Feingold, A. (1994). Gender differences in personality: A meta-analysis. *Psychological Bulletin, 116,* 429–456.

Gazmararian, J. A., Lazorick, S., Spitz, A. M., et al. (1996). Prevalence of violence against pregnant women. *Journal of the American Medical Association, 275*(24), 1915–1920.

Goodman, S. H., & Gotlib, I. H. (1999). Risk for psychopathology in the children of depressed mothers: A developmental model for understanding mechanisms of transmission. *Psychological Review, 106*(3), 458–490.

Hoff, A. L., Wieneke, M., Horon, R., et al. (1997). Estrogen levels relate to neuropsychological function in female schizophrenics. *Schizophrenia Research, 24,* 107–108.

Holt, W. J. (1995). The detection of postnatal depression in general-practice using the Edinburgh Postnatal Depression Scale. *New Zealand Medical Journal, 108,* 57–59.

Horan, D. L., Chapin, J., Klein, L., et al. (1998). Domestic violence screening practices of obstetrician–gynecologists. *Obstetrics and Gynecology, 92*(5), 785–789.

Kessler, R. C., Brown, R. L., & Broman, C. L. (1981). Sex differences in psychiatric help seeking: Evidence from four large-scale surveys. *Journal of Health and Social Behavior, 22,* 49–64.

Jensvold, M. F., Halbreich, U., & Hamilton, J. A. (1996) Gender-sensitive psychopharmacology: An overview. In M. F. Jensvold, U. Halbreich, & J. A. Hamilton (Eds.), *Psychopharmacology and women: Sex, gender, and hormones* (pp. 3–6). Washington, DC: American Psychiatric Press.

Katon, W., Robinson P., Von Korff, M., et al. (1996). A multifaceted intervention to improve treatment of depression in primary care. *Archives of General Psychiatry, 23,* 924–932.

Kessler, R. C., McGonagle, K. L., Swartz, M., et al. (1993). Sex and depression in the National Comorbidity Survey: I. Lifetime prevalence, chronicity and recurrence. *Journal of Affective Disorders, 29*(2–3), 85–96.

Kessler, R. C., McGonagle, K. L., Zhao, S., et al. (1994). Lifetime and 12-month prevalence of DSM-III-R psychiatric disorders in the United States: Results from the National Comorbidity Survey. *Archives of General Psychiatry, 51,* 8–19.

Kornstein, S. G., Schatzberg A. F., Thase, M. E, et al. (2000). Gender differences in treatment response to sertraline versus imipramine in chronic depression. *American Journal of Psychiatry, 157*(9), 1445–1452.

Kornstein, S. G., & Wojcik, B. A. (2000). Gender effects in the treatment of depression. *Psychiatric Clinics of North America, 7,* 23–57.

LeBlanc, E. S., Janowsky, J., Chan, B. K., et al. (2001). Hormone replacement therapy and cognition: Systematic review and meta-analysis. *Journal of the American Medical Association, 285*(11), 1489–1499.

Maciejewski, P. R., Prigerson, H. G., & Mazure, C. M. (2001). Sex differences in event-related risk for major depression. *Psychological Medicine, 31,* 593–604.

Mazza, D., & Dennerstein, L. (1996). Psychotropic drug use by women: Could violence account for the gender difference? *Journal of Psychosomatic Obstetrics and Gynecology, 17*(4), 229–234.

Miranda, J., Azocar, F., Komarony, M., et al. (1998). Unmet mental health needs of women in public sector gynecologic clinics. *American Journal of Obstetrics and Gynecology, 178*(2), 212–217.

Moldin, S. O., Scheftner, W. A., Rice, J. P., et al. (1993). Association between major depressive disorder and physical illness. *Psychological Medicine, 23,* 755–761.

Murray, C. J., & Lopez, A. D. (1996). *The global burden of disease.* Cambridge, MA: Harvard University Press.

Nazroo, J. Y., Edwards, A. C., & Brown, G. W. (1997). Gender differences in the onset of depression following a shared life event: A study of couples. *Psychological Medicine, 27*(1), 9–19.

Nolen-Hoeksema, S., Larson J., & Grayson, C. (1999). Explaining the gender difference in depressive symptoms. *Journal of Personality and Social Psychology, 77,* 1061–1072.

O'Hara, M. W. (1986). Social support, life events, and depression during pregnancy and the puerperium. *Archives of General Psychiatry, 43,* 69–73.

Ray, K. L., & Hodnett, E. D. (1999). *Caregiver support for postpartum depression: Cochrane Review* (The Cochrane Library, Issue No. 3) [Computer software]. Oxford: Update Software.

Robins, L. N., & Regier, D. A. (Eds.). (1990). *Psychiatric disorders in America: The Epidemiologic Catchment Area study.* New York: Free Press.

Shear, M. K., & Mammen, O. (1995). Anxiety disorders in pregnant and postpartum women *Psychopharmacology Bulletin, 31*(4), 693–703.

Stuart, S., & O'Hara, M. W. (1995). Interpersonal psychotherapy for postpartum depression: A treatment program. *Journal of Psychotherapy Practice Research, 4,* 18–29.

Stuart, S., O'Hara, M. W., & Blehar, M. C. (1998). Mental disorders associated with childbearing: Report of the biennial meeting of the Marce Society. *Psychopharmacology, 34*(3), 333–338.

Substance Abuse and Mental Health Services Administration. (1993). *Pregnant, substance-using women* (DHHS Publication No. SMA 93–1998). Rockville, MD: U.S. Department of Health and Human Services.

Warner, L. A., Kessler, R. C., Hughes, M., et al. (1995). Prevalence and correlates of drug use and dependence in the United States. *Archives of General Psychiatry, 52,* 219–229.

Way, K., Young, C. H., Opland, E., et al. (1999). Antidepressant utilization patterns in a national managed care organization. *Behavioral Health Trends, 11*(9), 6–11.

Weiss, E. L., Longhurst, J. G., & Mazure, C. M. (1999). Childhood sexual abuse as a risk factor for depression in women: Psychosocial and neurobiological correlates. *American Journal of Psychiatry, 156*(6), 816–828

Willis, A. G., Willis, G., Male, A., et al. (1998). Mental illness and disability in the US adult household population. In R. Manderscheid & M. J. Henderson (Eds.), *Mental health, United States, 1998* (pp. 113–123). Rockville, MD: U.S. Department of Health and Human Services.

Wolk, S. I., & Weissman, M. M. (1995). Women and depression: An update. In J. Oldham & M. Riba (Eds.), *American Psychiatric Press review of psychiatry* (Vol. 14, pp. 227–259). Washington, DC: American Psychiatric Press.

Yonkers, K. A. (1998). Assessing unipolar mood disorders in women. *Psychopharmacology Bulletin, 34*(3), 261–266.

Index